The Safe and Effective Use of Pesticides
Third Edition

The Pesticide Application Compendium

Volume 1. The Safe and Effective Use of Pesticides
ANR Publication 3324

Volume 2. Residential, Industrial and Institutional Pest Control
ANR Publication 3334

Volume 3. Wood Preservation
ANR Publication 3335

Volume 4. Forest and Right-of-Way Pest Control
ANR Publication 3336

Volume 5. Aquatic Pest Control
ANR Publication 3337

Volume 6. Demonstration and Research Uses of Pesticides
ANR Publication 9001

Volume 7. Landscape Maintenance Pest Control
ANR Publication 3493

Volume 8. Lawn and Residential Pest Control
ANR Publication 3510

PESTICIDE APPLICATION COMPENDIUM

1

THE SAFE AND EFFECTIVE USE OF PESTICIDES

THIRD EDITION

University of California
Statewide Integrated Pest Management Program
Agriculture and Natural Resources
Oakland, California

Publication 3324

To order or obtain ANR publications and other products, visit the ANR Communication Services online catalog at http://anrcatalog.ucanr.edu/ or phone 1-800-994-8849. Direct inquiries to

University of California
Agriculture and Natural Resources
Communication Services
2801 Second Street
Davis, CA 95618
Telephone 1-800-994-8849
E-mail: anrcatalog@ucanr.edu

© 1988, 1999, 2016, 2022
The Regents of the University of California
Agriculture and Natural Resources
Fourth reprint August 2024

All rights reserved. No part of this book may be reproduced or transmitted in any form or by any means, electronic or mechanical, including photocopying, recording, or by any information storage and retrieval system, without written permission of the Publisher. For permission requests, please contact Permissions@ucanr.edu.

Third Edition, 2016
Volume 1 in the Pesticide Application Compendium series

Publication 3324
ISBN-13: 978-1-60107-895-7

Library of Congress Cataloging-in-Publication Data

Names: University of California Integrated Pest Management Program, author.

Title: The safe and effective use of pesticides / University of California, Statewide Integrated Pest Management Program, Agriculture and Natural Resources.

Other titles: Pesticide application compendium ; 1. | Publication (University of California (System). Division of Agriculture and Natural Resources) ; 3324.

Description: Third edition. | Oakland, California : University of California Agriculture and Natural Resources, 2016. | Series: The pesticide application compendium ; v. 1 | Series: Publication ; 3324 | Includes bibliographical references and index.

Identifiers: LCCN 2016009659 | ISBN 9781601078957

Subjects: LCSH: Pesticides--California--Safety measures. | Pesticides--Application--California. | Pesticides--Toxicology--California.

Classification: LCC SB952.5 .S24 2016 | DDC 628.5/2909794--dc23 LC record available at http://lccn.loc.gov/2016009659

Editing and project management: Stephen Barnett. Design: Celeste Rusconi. Proofreading and indexing: Hazel White. Archivist: Evett Kilmartin. Print coordination: Ann Senuta. Illustrations by UC ANR staff, except as noted in the captions. Cover photos: Cheryl A. Reynolds (top); Shannah Markow Whithaus (bottom). Photo p. 161, Fernando "Marty" Martino; photo p. 279, Steve H. Dreistadt; photo p. 319, Michael L. Poe. All other photos by Jack Kelly Clark, except for the following figures: Joseph M. DiTomaso: 2-22; Draeger: 6-31; GoatThroat Pumps: 6-30, 7-9; Kenzo Estate Winery (Napa, CA): 10-19; Ferdinando "Marty" Martino: 6-4, 6-8 (A and B), 6-18, 6-19, 6-20A, 6-22, 6-23A, 6-23B, and Sidebar 6-1; Ross O'Connell: 3-10; Suzanne Paisley: 8-32, 8-34, 8-51, 8-52, 8-53, 8-59; Michael L. Poe: 6-15; Cheryl A. Reynolds: 3-6, 6-20B, 7-6, 7-10, 8-30, 8-31, 8-33, 8-44, 9-1, 10-18; Larry L. Strand: 3-14, 10-12; Shannah Markow Whithaus: 1-12, 6-9; unidentified photographer: 2-53.

The University of California, Division of Agriculture and Natural Resources (UC ANR) prohibits discrimination against or harassment of any person in any of its programs or activities on the basis of race, color, national origin, religion, sex, gender, gender expression, gender identity, pregnancy (which includes pregnancy, childbirth, and medical conditions related to pregnancy or childbirth), physical or mental disability, medical condition (cancer-related or genetic characteristics), genetic information (including family medical history), ancestry, marital status, age, sexual orientation, citizenship, status as a protected veteran or service in the uniformed services (as defined by the Uniformed Services Employment and Reemployment Rights Act of 1994 [USERRA]), as well as state military and naval service.

UC ANR policy prohibits retaliation against any employee or person in any of its programs or activities for bringing a complaint of discrimination or harassment. UC ANR policy also prohibits retaliation against a person who assists someone with a complaint of discrimination or harassment, or participates in any manner in an investigation or resolution of a complaint of discrimination or harassment. Retaliation includes threats, intimidation, reprisals, and/or adverse actions related to any of its programs or activities.

UC ANR is an Equal Opportunity/Affirmative Action Employer. All qualified applicants will receive consideration for employment and/or participation in any of its programs or activities without regard to race, color, religion, sex, national origin, disability, age or protected veteran status.

University policy is intended to be consistent with the provisions of applicable State and Federal laws.

Inquiries regarding the University's equal employment opportunity policies may be directed to: Affirmative Action Contact and Title IX Officer, University of California, Agriculture and Natural Resources, 2801 Second Street, Davis, CA 95618, (530) 750-1397. Email: titleixdiscrimination@ucanr.edu. Website: http://ucanr.edu/sites/anrstaff/Diversity/Affirmative_Action/.

To simplify information, trade names of products have been used. No endorsement of named or illustrated products is intended, nor is criticism implied of similar products that are not mentioned or illustrated.

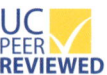 This publication has been anonymously peer reviewed for technical accuracy by University of California scientists and other qualified professionals. This review process was managed by ANR Associate Editor for Urban Pest Management Mary Louise Flint.

 Printed in Canada on recycled, acid-free, paper

Contents

Contributors and Acknowledgments vi
Introduction viii
1. Pest Management 1
    Historical Development of Pest Management Programs 2
    Creating a Pest Management Plan 3
    Integrated Pest Management 4
    Monitoring: The Key to Successful Pest Management 16
2. Pest Identification 19
    How Plants and Animals Are Named 20
    Identifying Pests 22
    Weeds 24
    Invertebrates 35
    Vertebrates 52
    Pathogens and Abiotic Disorders 65
3. Pesticides 67
    Pesticide Toxicity 69
    How Pesticides are Organized 73
    Pesticide Mixtures 94
4. Environmental Hazards Associated with Pesticide Use 99
    The Environment 100
    Pesticide Characteristics 100
    How Pesticides Move in the Environment 102
    Sources of Pesticide Contamination 105
    Environmental Impacts of Pesticide Application 110
5. Human Hazards Associated with Pesticide Use 119
    Potential for Human Injury 120
    Other Effects on People 127
    Pesticide Toxicity and Health Concerns 128
    Delayed Effects 129
6. Personal Protective Equipment and Personal Safety 131
    Worker Training and Personal Safety 132
    Personal Protective Equipment 134
    Engineering Controls 156
7. Using Pesticides Safely 161
    Pesticide Applicator Safety 162
    Fieldworker Safety 166
    Public Safety 168
    Handling Pesticides Safely 168
    Mixing Pesticides Safely 177
    Applying Pesticides Safely 180
    Cleanup and Disposal 187
    Recordkeeping 188
    Liability 190

8. Pesticide Application Equipment 193
    Application Methods 194
    Liquid Application Equipment 195
    Dust and Granule Application Equipment 231
    Livestock and Poultry Application Equipment 233
    Bait Application Equipment 234
    Application Equipment Maintenance 235

9. Calibrating Pesticide Application Equipment 245
    Why Calibration Is Essential 246
    Equipment Calibration Methods 248
    Calculation for Active Ingredient, Percentage Solution,
        and Parts per Million Dilutions 269
    Using System Monitors and Controllers 276

10. Using Pesticides Effectively 279
    Pest Detection and Monitoring 280
    Making Pesticide Use Decisions 287
    Choosing the Right Pesticide 289
    Making Pesticides More Selective 294
    Mixing Pesticides 299
    Pesticide Resistance 303
    Preventing Offsite Movement of Pesticides 306
    Follow-Up Monitoring 316

11. Reading the Label 319
    Pesticide Registration and Labeling 321

12. Pesticide Emergencies and Emergency Response 333
    First Aid 335
    Pesticide Leaks and Spills 341
    Pesticide Fires 344
    Stolen Pesticides 344
    Misapplication of Pesticides 345
    Reviewing Emergency Response to Accidents 346

Answers to Review Questions 349

Glossary 351

References 368

Index 370

Contributors and Acknowledgments

This manual was prepared by the University of California Agricultural and Natural Resources Statewide Integrated Pest Management (IPM) Program under a memorandum of understanding with the California Department of Pesticide Regulation (DPR).

Prepared by the University of California

Statewide IPM Program at Davis
Shannah M. Whithaus, Writer/Editor
Lisa A. Blecker, Technical Editor
Joyce F. Strand, Associate Director for Communications
Kassim Al-Khatib, Director, Statewide IPM Program at Davis
Mary Louise Flint, UC Agriculture and Natural Resources Associate Editor

Previous Edition
Patrick J. O'Connor-Marer, Pesticide Training Coordinator

Technical Advisory Committee and Principal Contributors (Third Edition)

The following people provided ideas, information, and suggestions and reviewed manuscript drafts:

Steve Fennimore, University of California Cooperative Extension Weed Specialist
Glen Foth, Grounds Services Manager, State Center Community College District
Adolfo Gallo, Pest Management and Licensing Branch, DPR
Ken Giles, Professor, Biological and Agricultural Engineering, University of California, Davis
Kurt Hembree, University of California Cooperative Extension Farm Advisor, Fresno County
Barbara Huecksteadt, County Agricultural Commissioner, San Joaquin County
Judy Letterman, CEO, Pesticide Applicators Professional Association (PAPA)
Franz Neiderholzer, University of California Cooperative Extension Farm Advisor, Sutter-Yuba Counties
Michael O'Malley, M.D., Associate Clinical Professor, Center for Health and the Environment, University of California, Davis
Renee Rianda, PCA, The Morning Star Company
Cathy Roache, Deputy Agricultural Commissioner, Alameda County
John Roncoroni, University of California Cooperative Extension Weed Science Farm Advisor, Napa County
Lucia Varela, University of California Cooperative Extension IPM Advisor, North Coast
Cheryl Wilen, University of California Cooperative Extension IPM Advisor, South Coast

The following people generously provided information, offered suggestions, reviewed draft manuscripts, or assisted in setting up photographs for the third edition:

Vic Acosta, Enforcement Branch, DPR
Maria Alfaro, Statewide IPM Program
Jodi Azulai, Statewide IPM Program
Tom Babb, Pest Management and Licensing Branch, DPR
Roger A. Baldwin, University of California Cooperative Extension Wildlife Specialist
Romy Basler, Statewide IPM Program
Rick Bergin, Environmental Monitoring Branch, DPR
Scott Birchfield, Syngenta Crop Protection
Carol Black, National Association of State Departments of Agriculture Research Foundation
Laurie Brajkovich, Pest Management and Licensing Branch, DPR
Robert Budd, Environmental Monitoring Branch, DPR
Randy Dahlgren, Professor, Soils and Biogeochemistry, University of California, Davis
Surendra Dara, University of California Cooperative Extension Strawberry and Vegetable Farm
    Advisor, San Luis Obispo County
Steve Dreistadt, Statewide IPM Program
Jim Farrar, Statewide IPM Program
Harvard Fong, Worker Health & Safety Branch, DPR
Adolfo Gallo, Pest Management and Licensing Branch, DPR
Doug Gubler, Professor, Plant Pathology, University of California, Davis
Linda Hall, Worker Health & Safety Branch, DPR
Leilani Hansen, Pesticide Registration Branch, DPR
April Holland, Worker Health & Safety Branch, DPR
Rick Melnicoe, Office of Pesticide Information and Coordination, Retired
Steve Peaslee, GIS Specialist, National Soil Survey Center
Margaret Reiff, Pesticide Registration Branch, DPR
Cheryl Reynolds, Statewide IPM Program
Frank Schneider, Worker Health & Safety Branch, DPR
Larry Schwankl, University of California Cooperative Extension Irrigation Specialist
Kevin Solari, Worker Health & Safety Branch, DPR
James Stapleton, University of California Cooperative Extension IPM Advisor, Central Valley
Joyce F. Strand, Statewide IPM Program
Parissa Tehrani, Worker Health & Safety Branch, DPR
Nancy Westcott, GoatThroat Pumps
Miglena Wilbur, Worker Health & Safety Branch, DPR
Karey Windbiel-Rojas, Statewide IPM Program
Nino Yanga, Worker Health & Safety Branch, DPR
Michael Zeiss, Enforcement Branch, DPR

Thank you to the following institutions for providing materials for reproduction: the National Association of State Departments of Agriculture Research Foundation (NASDARF), the U.S. Environmental Protection Agency, and the U.S. Occupational Safety and Health Administration.

INTRODUCTION

Handling pesticides requires many special skills and responsibilities. It is an important occupation on its own and a necessary part of many other jobs. If you handle pesticides, you need to recognize their hazards and how to avoid them. You must also be familiar with all local, state, and federal laws regulating the sale, use, storage, transportation, application, and disposal of pesticides. If you supervise pesticide handlers, you are responsible for seeing that these employees handle and use pesticides properly and safely.

You may need to become a certified pesticide applicator by taking one or more of the California Department of Pesticide Regulation's (DPR) Qualified Applicator Certificate (QAC), Qualified Applicator License (QAL), or apprentice or journeyman Pest Control Aircraft Pilot's Certificate examinations. If you apply restricted-use pesticides only on property under your control, you will need to take the Certified Private Applicator examination administered by local agricultural commissioner offices. While regulations may not require an applicator to possess one of these credentials, employers frequently require this certification as a condition of continued employment for employees handling pesticides.

This book is Volume 1 in the Pesticide Application Compendium series. This updated version reflects changes in laws, the scientific understanding of our environment and its ecosystems, and application technology. Its purpose is to help you learn safe and effective ways of using pesticides. It describes how to prevent accidents and how to avoid injury and environmental problems.

How to Use This Book

Use this book as a study guide if you are preparing for any of the QAC, QAL, or Pest Control Aircraft Pilot's Certificate examinations. DPR uses these tests to certify individuals, pest control businesses, commercial applicators, landscape maintenance personnel, researchers, designated agents, and others who apply pesticides as part of their work.

Use the knowledge expectations (descriptions of what you should know about pesticides, pesticide use and safety, and pest management) at the beginning of each chapter to guide you as you study. Individual knowledge expectations appear alongside the relevant content throughout each chapter, which will help you focus on the information in this book that you will be tested on during the examination.

What DPR Is Testing

DPR exams assess your competence in handling and/or supervising handling of restricted-use pesticides. Questions on these tests are similar to the review questions at the end of each of this book's chapters. You will be tested on the knowledge expectations provided at the beginning and throughout each chapter to ensure that you know how to safely and effectively handle or supervise the handling of restricted-use pesticides according to California law. The following paragraphs describe each chapter, and the important information the chapter contains.

1. **Pest Management.** Knowledge expectations in this chapter cover integrated pest management (IPM) concepts, as well as the various goals of pest management. You will learn about economic injury or treatment thresholds, pest monitoring techniques used before and after pesticide applications, various pest control methods and how they fit into IPM plans, and the ways that pest biology and the environment impact pest management planning.

2. **Pest Identification.** Knowledge expectations in this chapter cover pest biology and the tools you can use to identify pests and the damage they cause. You will also need to recognize common pests in California, as well as the symptoms and signs of infestation. This chapter also explains how pests are organized and named.

3. **Pesticides.** This chapter's knowledge expectations cover all aspects of pesticides, starting with the definition of a pesticide according to California law. You will learn about the relationship among the hazards of, exposure to, and toxicity of pesticides; pesticide toxicity categories and signal words; and the various ways pesticides are organized. After reading this chapter you will be able to define terms such as active ingredient, mode of action, contact, and systemic. You will also understand why pesticides are sold as formulated products and be able to list various formulations and the advantages and disadvantages of each. Adjuvants are also covered in this chapter.

4. **Environmental Hazards Associated with Pesticide Use.** Knowledge expectations in this chapter cover the ways in which pesticides move away from the application site and the chemical characteristics that create hazards in the environment. You will learn about the factors that influence the offsite movement of pesticides; point and nonpoint sources of pesticide contamination; the problems associated with pesticide residues and the conditions that favor its buildup; and the impacts pesticides have on nontarget organisms, especially pollinators. You will also learn how to identify various features of an application site that influence the ability of pesticides to reach surface water and groundwater.

5. **Human Hazards Associated with Pesticide Use.** This chapter's knowledge expectations cover the hazards to people who are exposed to pesticides as handlers or fieldworkers or when they live, work, or play near application sites. You will be able to describe how people get exposed to, the routes of entry for, and the tasks most associated with pesticide exposure. In addition, you will find out about application errors that can create exposure hazards and learn about how changing conditions at the application site can increase the probability of exposure. You will also become familiar with chronic and acute symptoms of pesticide poisoning and learn how to differentiate between symptoms of heat stress and an overexposure to pesticides.

6. **Personal Protective Equipment and Personal Safety.** Knowledge expectations in this chapter cover personal protective equipment (PPE) and the safety training required for pesticide handlers and fieldworkers, as well as an employer's responsibility to provide all label-mandated PPE for employees who handle pesticides. You will learn about the many different kinds of PPE available, be able to select the most effective PPE for any situation, and avoid heat stress that can result from wearing required PPE while mixing, loading, and applying pesticides. In addition, you will find out how to properly clean, maintain, and store your PPE, including information on fit-testing and fit-checking respiratory devices. You will also learn the limits of protection provided by PPE and the additional engineering controls that can protect you.

7. **Using Pesticides Safely.** Knowledge expectations in this chapter cover best practices for ensuring everyone's safety before, during, and after pesticide applications. You will learn about communicating with neighbors and others before an application, ways to restrict access to sites during and after an application, and how to clean equipment and contain rinse water after an application. You will also find out about how to protect yourself and others during the transportation, storage, mix-

ing, and loading of pesticides. In addition, you will be able to recognize and avoid hazardous weather conditions and environmentally sensitive areas that could be adversely affected by pesticide handling activities.

8. **Pesticide Application Equipment.** This chapter's knowledge expectations deal with the many types of application equipment available. The chapter describes the advantages and disadvantages of this equipment in a variety of scenarios. You will find out how to recognize components of different application equipment, including liquid, dry, and chemigation systems, and how to select the right nozzles and other parts so the machines work optimally at the site. You will also learn about proper equipment maintenance, cleaning, and storage techniques, and how to recognize wear in various components.

9. **Calibrating Pesticide Application Equipment.** Knowledge expectations in this chapter cover the calibration of various types of application equipment, including liquid, dry, and chemigation systems. After reading this chapter you will be able to define calibration and explain why it is important; list the tools needed and the variables that must be measured for proper calibration of equipment; and use formulas to calculate equipment output, amount of active ingredient needed in a given situation and in areas of various shapes. You will also find out about various ways to change the output of your application equipment and the consequences of the changes, as well as how rate controllers impact calibration activities. In addition, you will be able to describe how to calibrate liquid and dry application equipment, including chemigation systems.

10. **Using Pesticides Effectively.** Knowledge expectations in this chapter cover the goals of pesticide applications and how to achieve them using a variety of tools that increase effectiveness, such as monitoring before and after applications, evaluating spray coverage, preventing offsite movement, and using GPS units and other technology in the field. In addition, you will learn which factors should be considered during pesticide selection to maximize effectiveness, increase selectivity, and ensure that it is compatible with adjuvants or other pesticides used at the site. You will also learn mixing procedures for single and multiple pesticides, and methods for keeping pesticides on target. After reading this chapter you will understand pesticide resistance, why it is a problem, and the factors that contribute to it.

11. **Reading the Label.** In this chapter, knowledge expectations cover reading and understanding pesticide labels and associated labeling information. You will be able to recognize the various parts of a pesticide label and the associated Safety Data Sheet. In addition, you will be able to explain the legal requirement to read, understand, and follow directions on a pesticide label. You will also be able to describe the type of safety information provided by pesticide labeling and Safety Data Sheets.

12. **Pesticide Emergencies and Emergency Response.** Knowledge expectations in this chapter cover first aid, the procedures to follow when seeking medical treatment for exposure episodes, and setting up and executing an emergency response plan. You will learn how to recognize symptoms of heat stress, pesticide poisoning, and common illnesses so you can distinguish among them and deliver appropriate first aid as needed. You will also be able to find first aid information to use to help yourself or others when accidents occur, as well as react to spills, fires, misapplications, or thefts safely and appropriately. This chapter helps you understand why you should review every accident and response, and how to do this effectively.

Using the Review Questions

At the end of each chapter are several review questions to test your grasp of the knowledge expectations in that chapter. Some of these questions are similar to the questions on DPR's tests.

Begin your study of each chapter by reading through the knowledge expectations and the review questions. Make notes of the material you do not fully understand. Then, review the chapter to locate the sections that deal with that information. Read those sections carefully before you review the rest of the chapter.

When you finish studying the chapter, answer each of the review questions. Check your answers with the correct answers in the "Answers to Review Questions" at the end of the book. If you missed any of the questions, go back and reread the appropriate sections of the chapter that cover that information.

Useful Pesticide Resources

This and the other volumes in the Pesticide Application Compendium series are useful references for growers, structural pest control operators, pest control advisers, pest management students, homeowners, and anyone involved in pesticide use decisions. Books in this series are also helpful instructional guides for training people to use pesticides properly and safely.

Other volumes of the Pesticide Application Compendium cover the many different occupational areas in which people use pesticides (table 1). Applicants for a Qualified Applicator Certificate or Qualified Applicator License must take a test in one or more of these specialized areas.

Besides this text, there are two important sources you should rely on for information regarding pesticides and pest management.

- County agricultural commissioners (CACs) are DPR regulatory officials. Their offices throughout the state have the responsibility, among other functions, for issuing permits for restricted-use pesticides; monitoring pesticide use, storage, and disposal; and enforcing pesticide laws and regulations. Agricultural commissioners' offices provide local information on pesticide use, storage, transportation, disposal, and hazards. Contact your local CAC office if there is any pesticide emergency.
- The University of California, through its Cooperative Extension program, maintains offices in most counties of the state. Experts who staff these offices are able to help you locate pest identification, pest management, and pesticide use information you need, or they can access a network of University of California scientists when additional assistance is needed.

TABLE I-1.

Pesticide categories and subcategories in California

Category of Pest Control	Description of Pesticide Applicator's Work	Type of Pests
Residential, industrial, and institutional pest control	Performs pest control in apartments, restaurants, hospitals, offices, warehouses, grocery stores, and other buildings as part of employment by the building's owner or operator. Selects pest control methods and pesticides to use. Performs postharvest fumigation and insecticide and fungicide applications to agricultural products. Applies pesticides to stored agricultural products. Controls weeds around commercial and industrial structures. Work is often closely associated with people and pets. Special subsections of this category requiring separate examinations, relate to applying: (1) pesticides for preservation of wood products such as lumber, posts, and other structural wood; (2) antifouling paints to boat hulls; (3) pesticides to control roots in sewer lines; and (4) microbial pesticides.	*Invertebrates:* cockroaches, bugs, stored product pests, flies, fleas, mosquitoes, termites, ants, other insects; spiders and mites; marine organisms *Vertebrates:* rats, mice, bats, birds *Weeds:* weeds and unwanted vegetation; tree roots in sewer lines *Microorganisms:* wood-decaying fungi
Landscape maintenance pest control	Controls pests on or around ornamental and fruit trees, shrubs, small fruits and berries, turf, and flowers; works around homes, businesses, cemeteries, theme parks, public parks, indoor malls, and house plants. Pesticide application is often part of a landscape maintenance business. Applicator makes decisions regarding pest control methods, irrigation, and plant nutrition. Work is closely associated with human activities. A separate exam for maintenance gardeners is available as a subcategory in this area.	*Invertebrates:* aphids, scales, flies, bees, wasps, earwigs, moths, beetles, bugs; spiders, mites, centipedes; snails, slugs *Vertebrates:* rats, mice, gophers, moles, squirrels, rabbits, birds, snakes, lizards *Microorganisms:* fungi, bacteria, viruses *Weeds:* various types of terrestrial weeds
Right-of-way pest control	Performs pesticide applications along roads, rail lines, utility accesses, and drainage ditches to keep these areas free of weeds and to prevent fire hazards and obstruction of access or view. Applies pesticides to control vertebrates and insects that interfere with desirable foliage or water drainage. A special subsection of this category requiring a separate examination relates to applying pesticides for the preservation of wood products and utility poles.	*Invertebrates:* pests of foliage and wood products *Vertebrates:* squirrels, mice, gophers, moles, rabbits, birds *Weeds:* various types of terrestrial weeds
Forest pest control	Applies pesticides in forest locations and commercial Christmas tree plantations. Is responsible for protecting wildlife, watersheds, and lakes and streams.	*Invertebrates:* boring and defoliating insects of forest trees; mites *Vertebrates:* squirrels, voles, gophers, rabbits, deer, others *Weeds:* mostly undesirable plant species competing with forest trees; parasitic plants *Microorganisms:* plant disease agents affecting forest trees
Aquatic pest control	Applies pesticides for control of aquatic weeds, pest fish, arthropods, and mollusks. Requires special skills to protect aquatic environments and nontarget organisms. Familiarity with aquatic ecosystems and the ultimate use of water is very important to protect people, crops, and the environment.	*Invertebrates:* snails, clams, mussels, crabs *Vertebrates:* pest fish, rodents, beavers, others *Weeds:* aquatic weeds; algae

Category of Pest Control	Description of Pesticide Applicator's Work	Type of Pests
Plant agriculture pest control	Applies pesticides in and around agricultural crops. Often employed by a commercial applicator. Usually supervises pest control applicator. Responsible for protecting fieldworkers, groundwater, and environment. May work with highly toxic materials. A special subsection of this category, which requires a separate examination, relates to the application of fumigants in fields.	*Invertebrates:* many different agricultural pest insects; mites, snails, nematodes *Vertebrates:* squirrels, gophers, rabbits, birds. *Weeds:* many types of agricultural weeds and poisonous plants *Microorganisms:* fungi, bacteria, viruses, other microorganisms that cause crop diseases
Animal agriculture pest control	Applies pesticides for control of livestock and poultry pests. Requires familiarity with livestock and poultry and unique pest control techniques. Pesticide use is closely associated with animals.	*Invertebrates:* mosquitoes, lice, flies, bugs; ticks, mites *Vertebrates:* livestock and poultry predators *Weeds:* poisonous plants and undesirable range weeds
Seed treatment	Performs or supervises the application of insecticides and fungicides to seeds used to produce agricultural crops. Requires familiarity with different methods of protecting seeds. Usually employed by a seed treatment company.	*Invertebrates:* seed-feeding or damaging insects *Microorganisms:* fungi, bacteria
Regulatory pest control	Involved in detecting and eradicating imported pests that pose threats of economic harm to agriculture, livestock and poultry, or other segments of society. Must be familiar with suppression and eradication methods. Requires understanding of how pests enter and disperse through an area. Usually works for a public agency.	*Invertebrates:* exotic insects and mites that threaten to cause economic or health damage; nematodes, snails, clams, mussels, and crabs-damaging species that might be introduced from other areas *Weeds:* aquatic, terrestrial, exotic weeds *Vertebrates:* reptiles, birds, rodents, other mammals *Microorganisms:* exotic plant disease organisms
Demonstration and research pest control	Evaluates pesticides for efficacy. Studies interactions between pests, nonpests, and environmental factors when pesticides are applied. Demonstrates proper and effective methods of using pesticides. May be pesticide chemical company field representative, farm advisor, university researcher, independent consultant, or contract researcher.	All types of agricultural and nonagricultural pests may be involved
Public health pest control	Involved in applying pesticides to control pests that transmit disease organisms to people. Usually employed by public agencies. Pesticide use is often closely associated with homes and workplaces or public areas.	*Invertebrates:* flies, fleas, cockroaches, mosquitoes, lice, bugs; ticks, mites, spiders *Vertebrates:* rats, mice, bats, birds

Chapter 1
Pest Management

Historical Development of Pest Management Programs 2
Creating a Pest Management Plan 3
Integrated Pest Management 4
Monitoring: The Key to Successful Pest Management 16
Chapter 1 Review Questions 17

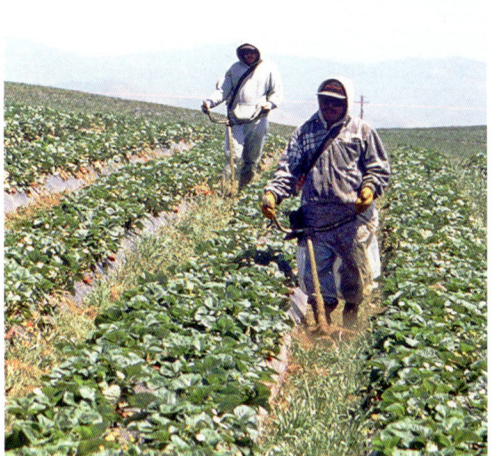

Knowledge Expectations

- Define integrated pest management.
- Differentiate among key pests, occasional pests, and secondary pests.
- Define prevention, suppression, and eradication of pests.
- Describe the methods used to achieve prevention, suppression, and eradication of pests.
- Explain the importance of site-specific variables; pest, host, and natural enemy populations; and pest life stage in pest management planning.
- Describe integrated pest management control options.
- Identify the five major components common to all integrated pest management programs.
- Describe monitoring and explain why it is important.
- Define economic injury (treatment) thresholds and describe what happens when these are reached.
- Explain the importance of evaluating pest management results.

Pest management is the science of safely preventing, suppressing, or eliminating unwanted organisms. Carrying out a successful pest management program involves choosing the right prevention or control techniques and timing their application correctly. Integrated pest management (IPM) incorporates a variety of these pest control techniques in a way that minimizes effects on human health and the environment while maximizing reductions in pest populations. Due to its effectiveness, IPM has become the system preferred by pest management professionals around the world.

Historical Development of Pest Management Programs

Since the earliest days of agriculture, people have found ways to produce a better, more abundant, and more reliable harvest. Chemical control of agricultural pests has helped humans increase yields and quality for over 4,000 years, beginning with the use of substances such as sulfur, copper, and arsenic to kill or drive away pests. Over time, new chemicals have been developed to control particular problem insects, plant diseases, or weeds and are now used widely in homes, landscapes, and agriculture. Experience shows us, however, that though chemical controls may start out working well, eventually they fail to produce desired results and have occasionally caused substantial harm to people and the environment.

Define integrated pest management.

DDT is the classic example of a chemical solution that began as promising but ended up causing serious problems for people and the environment. During the late 1940s, farmers embraced DDT and other chlorinated hydrocarbon-based pesticides to solve agricultural pest problems and boost production. It didn't take long, however, before people discovered that these new pesticides weren't performing as anticipated. In the 1950s, many researchers began to document increased pest insect populations when heavy applications of DDT (and related compounds) destroyed their natural enemies. In the 1960s and 70s, additional peer-reviewed studies reported that DDT harmed not only beneficial insects but also other animals in the ecosystem. Eventually, the evidence against DDT resulted in its ban by the U.S. Environmental Protection Agency (U.S. EPA). Since that time, many other highly toxic pesticides have been banned due to their ill effects on nontarget organisms, groundwater, and people.

> **SIDEBAR 1-1**
>
> ### WHAT IS IPM?
>
> Integrated pest management (IPM) is an ecosystem-based strategy that focuses on long-term prevention of pests or their damage through a combination of techniques such as biological control, habitat manipulation, modification of cultural practices, and use of resistant varieties. Pesticides are used only after monitoring indicates that they are needed according to established guidelines, and treatments are made with the goal of removing only the target organisms. Pest control tools are selected and applied in a manner that minimizes risks to human health, to beneficial and nontarget organisms, and to the environment.

Since the 1950s, many scientists have validated the conclusion that ecosystems benefit when pesticide treatments are carefully chosen, timed, and integrated with other pest management methods. Scientific findings report that, in areas where people repeatedly apply a single insecticide, natural enemies and wildlife populations are negatively affected, and strains of pesticide-resistant pests develop. These resistant species can no longer be managed using the pesticides that formerly controlled them. Developing new chemicals to control these pests is expensive, and new materials may be more harmful to the environment, more toxic to people, or less effective overall than the original pesticide. To combat these problems, researchers have developed integrated pest management programs that rely on a variety of pest control methods, including naturally occurring biological control and changes in cultural practices, to provide more reliable long-term relief from pests.

Integrated pest management, or IPM, programs can result in good control of pest organisms while reducing negative impacts on the environment and human health (see Sidebar 1-1 for the official definition of IPM). Farmers, scientists, and consumers have become aware that our environment is a complex system, requiring us to approach problems within it from many directions. We now see that when we take action to eliminate just one pest in an ecosystem, or boost production of just one agricultural commodity, it affects more than just that pest or commodity. Often it creates a cascade of unanticipated, interrelated effects on people and the environment.

Armed with growing evidence in support of IPM practices, government agencies, such as the U.S. EPA, USDA, and FDA started working together with university and other agency scientists to help farmers and others develop IPM programs. In 1994, these three agencies worked together to form the Pesticide Environmental Stewardship Program (PESP), which had two major goals: to develop specific use/risk reduction strategies that include reliance on biological pesticides and other approaches considered to be safer than traditional chemical methods; and to have 75% of U.S. agricultural acreage adopt integrated pest management programs (the practice of using a variety of methods—cultural, pesticidal, biological, etc.—to control pests) by the year 2000.

In addition, the federal government has enacted fifteen different regulations since 1918 that eventually led to the creation by university scientists of a formal definition of IPM in the 1960s. This definition led to the implementation of a national IPM policy in 1972 aimed at agricultural and urban pest management professionals.

As the years go by, research continues to show the effectiveness of IPM programs. For instance, we now know that the most effective, least disruptive pest management systems are based on a combination of chemical, biological, cultural, and mechanical/physical controls applied according to local needs and conditions. These combined approaches help preserve and maintain vital ecosystems, save money, and protect human health.

Creating a Pest Management Plan

The first step in creating a pest management plan is to determine the identity of the pest to be managed. Monitoring, sampling, knowing common pests at the site, and using identification keys can help identify a pest and the damage it is causing (see "Identifying Pests" in Chapter 2 and "Pest Detection and Monitoring" in Chapter 10). Another early step that helps ensure the effectiveness of any plan involves finding out whether the identified organism is a key, occasional, or secondary pest.

- **Key pests** are those that cause major damage on a regular basis unless you successfully manage them. Many weeds are key pests because they compete with desired plants for resources. These weeds require regular control efforts to prevent damage.
- **Occasional pests** are those that become pests once in a while due to their life cycles, environmental conditions at the site, or as a result of human activity. For instance, ants become pests when sanitation practices change, providing them with food where none previously existed. Ants will also move into buildings after a rainfall destroys their outdoor food source.
- **Secondary pests** are not normally problems but become problems after a key pest is controlled. Some weed species become pests after more competitive weeds have been controlled. Particular species of fleas, ticks, and blood-feeding bugs attack people only after their natural hosts are eliminated. Certain secondary plant-feeding pests begin to cause damage when the plant's key pest is under control. Secondary insect and mite pests often become problems because insecticides applied to control a key pest killed their natural enemies.

Differentiate among key pests, occasional pests, and secondary pests.

APPROACHES TO PEST MANAGEMENT

A pest management program is created with a particular goal in mind. Goals of a pest management program can include one or more of the following: prevention, suppression, or eradication. The most effective pest management programs are IPM programs, combining prevention and suppression of pest populations.

Define prevention, suppression, and eradication of pests.

Describe the methods used to achieve prevention, suppression, and eradication of pests.

Prevention

When you prevent pest populations from invading and populating an area, you stop them before they damage plants or reach treatment thresholds. Usually there are economical and environmentally sound ways to prevent pest infestation or buildup. Such techniques include planting weed- and disease-free seeds and growing varieties of plants that resist diseases or insects. Fencing can be used to prevent damage from vertebrate pests such as rabbits. Other control options include using cultural methods to prevent weedy plants from seeding or choosing planting and harvesting times that minimize pest problems. Often, sanitation practices reduce pest buildup. Additional preventive methods involve excluding pests from the target area, structure, or host. An important preventive measure uses pest management practices that conserve natural enemies. Keeping plants, poultry, and livestock healthy by making sure they receive adequate water and nutrients may also make them less susceptible to diseases or other pests.

There are also preventive practices that use pesticides. These include
- using preplant or preemergence herbicides on areas where weed seeds are present
- using fungicides to protect plants from disease when environmental conditions favor infection
- applying preservatives to structural lumber before construction to protect it from insects, fungi, or marine borers

Suppression

Common pest control methods suppress pest populations but usually do not eliminate them. These methods reduce pest numbers below an economic injury threshold or to a tolerable level. Suppression sometimes lowers pest populations so that natural enemies are able to maintain control. Suppression is the goal of most pesticide applications used to manage weeds, insects and mites, and microorganisms. Examples of suppression techniques include cultivating or mowing weeds and releasing biological control agents.

Eradication

Eradication is the total elimination of a pest from a designated area. This goal is common for pest control efforts in buildings or other small, confined spaces. Over larger areas, however, eradication is a radical approach to pest control. Eradication can be very expensive and often has limited success. Government agencies are the main organizations conducting large-scale eradication programs to eliminate exotic or introduced pests that pose area-wide public health or economic threats. These eradication programs are conducted using quarantine orders that refer to particular foreign or introduced pests proven to severely damage the local environment (see "Special Pest Management Methods," later in this chapter for more on regulatory pest control methods). Certain pests of commodities shipped from one state to another or shipped outside the United States may have to be eradicated before these commodities are allowed into the state or country. An example of pests that require eradication before shipping is snails or slugs that infest nursery plants. Other pests that are often targeted for eradication include the Mediterranean fruit fly and hydrilla in California and Florida.

Integrated Pest Management

Integrated pest management (IPM) is a process that helps to solve pest problems while minimizing risks to people and the environment. IPM can be used to manage any pest anywhere—in urban, agricultural, and wildland or natural areas.

IPM focuses on long-term prevention of pests or their damage by managing the ecosystem. IPM programs use techniques that keep pests from becoming a problem, such as growing healthy plants that can withstand pest attacks, using disease-resistant plants, or caulking cracks to keep insects or rodents from entering a building.

Rather than simply eliminating the pests that are problems right now, IPM requires a more careful look at environmental factors that affect the pest and its ability to thrive. Armed with this information, pest management professionals can create conditions that are unfavorable for the pest.

Determining when to take action. Accurate predictions of when you should act to control a pest are made by

- identifying the pest correctly
- monitoring pest populations or signs of a pest's presence
- assessing the extent of pest damage
- monitoring and recording weather conditions conducive to pest development
- monitoring plant growth stages for vulnerability to pests

Monitoring means checking a field, landscape, forest, building, or other site to identify which pests are present, how many there are, and what damage they've caused (see "Monitoring: The Key to Successful Pest Management" later in this chapter and "Pest Detection and Monitoring" in Chapter 10). Identifying the pest is key to knowing whether it is likely to become a problem as well as in determining the best management strategy. For many pests, including plant pathogens, it is also important to monitor plant growth and weather to determine when damage is likely to occur.

Defining pest management methods. IPM programs are effective because they use information gathered through monitoring to help determine the best management tools for the situation. Often, two or more management methods are combined for the most effective control. Relying on multiple approaches to managing pests can increase long-term effectiveness. Methods for managing pests are often grouped into the following categories, which are defined in greater detail in "Pest Management Methods" later in this chapter.

- **Biological control** is the use of living biological control agents or natural enemies—predators, parasites, pathogens, and competitors—to control pests and their damage. Invertebrates, plant pathogens, nematodes, weeds, and vertebrates have many natural enemies.
- **Chemical control** is the use of naturally occurring or synthetic pesticides. In IPM, pesticides are used only when needed and in combination with other approaches for more effective, long-term control. Also, pesticides are selected and applied in a way that minimizes their possible harm to people and the environment. With IPM you'll use the most selective pesticide that will do the job and is the safest for other organisms and for air, soil, and water quality, for example, using a pesticide in a bait station rather than a spray or spot-spraying a few weeds instead of an entire area.
- **Mechanical and physical controls** kill a pest directly or make the environment unsuitable for it. Traps for rodents are examples of mechanical controls. Physical controls include mowing for weed management, steam sterilization of the soil for disease management, and using barriers such as screens to keep birds or insects out.
- **Cultural controls** are practices that reduce pest establishment, reproduction, dispersal, and survival. For example, changing irrigation practices can reduce pest problems, since too much water can increase root disease and weeds, and crop rotation can be used to reduce nematode populations (see Flint 2012).

Key Components of IPM Programs

The following IPM principles and practices are combined to create IPM programs. While each situation is different, five major components are common to all IPM programs:

1. Identifying pests (see Chapter 2)
2. Monitoring and assessing pest numbers, damage, and favorable field conditions (see Chapter 10)
3. Using economic injury or treatment thresholds to determine when management action is needed
4. Preventing pest problems
5. Combining biological, cultural, physical/mechanical, and chemical management tools as needed (see the UC IPM website, ucipm.ucanr.edu)

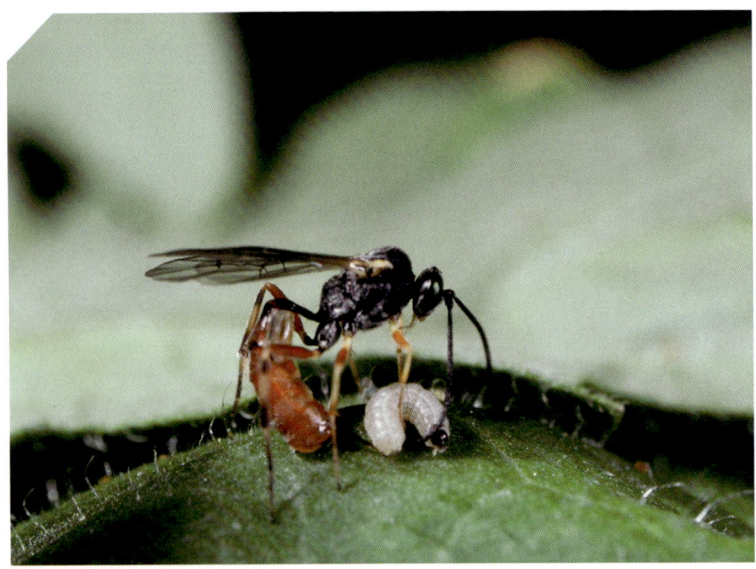

FIGURE 1-1

Classical biological control involves locating the native home of a pest (usually outside of the United States), finding and rearing one or more of its natural enemies, and releasing these natural enemies into the pest-infested area. In this photo, the parasitic wasp *Hyposoter exiguae* is laying an egg inside a beet armyworm larva.

Pest Management Methods

You can often manage a pest or pest complex using a single method (such as application of a pesticide), but it is always most effective to combine several compatible methods into an IPM program. In order to put together an effective IPM program, you need to know which management techniques are available and how they can be combined. Consider methods that are both effective and least harmful to people and the environment before resorting to other, more hazardous possibilities.

Biological Control

You can implement any of the following types of biological control as part of a pest management program:

- classical biological control
- augmentation
- naturally occurring control

Classical Biological Control. Researchers and pest managers use classical biological control to manage pests that are not native to a geographical area. These introduced pests are often problems in their new location because there are no natural enemies to help control them. Classical biological control involves locating the native home of the new pest and finding suitable natural enemies there. After extensive testing and evaluation, researchers select certain natural enemies to import, rear, and release (Fig. 1-1). If successful, the introduced natural enemies become established within large areas and effectively lower target pest populations. The control lasts for long periods of time without further intervention. Establishing new natural enemy populations is a difficult process because the native homes of some pests are hard to locate. Also, researchers must prove that imported natural enemies will not cause problems in the new location. Laws strictly control importation of all organisms, including biological control agents, into the United States. Other countries have similar restrictions.

Augmentation. Augmentation involves rearing and releasing large numbers of certain natural enemies that probably already occur in an area. However, their natural populations are too low to be effective in controlling the target pest. Augmentation usually does not have a long-term effect because environmental or other conditions do not favor large populations of these natural enemies. Therefore, pest managers must make periodic releases to maintain sufficient population levels. Commercial insectaries raise many natural enemies. These include predatory mites to control plant-infesting spider mites and parasitic wasps and lacewings to control various insect pests. Certain species of nematodes are used as biological control agents for some soil-dwelling insects. Some companies sell general predators such as praying mantids and lacewings and make claims for their use in biological control. In many cases, however, researchers have not established the effectiveness of these predators.

Naturally Occurring Control. Many factors influence pests, including natural enemies, environmental and geographical features, and climatic conditions. Maintaining naturally occurring populations of natural enemies can be one of the most economical means of control. Do this by avoiding damaging cultural practices or indiscriminate pesticide use. If pesticides will be part of your control program, select types that are less toxic to natural enemies. Spot-treating with insecticides or timing applications to avoid natural enemy mortality can also protect natural enemies. It may be

PEST MANAGEMENT

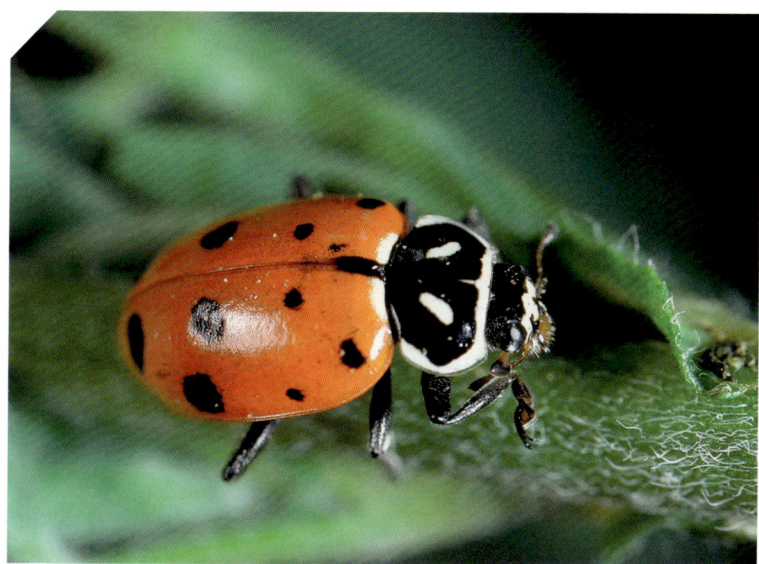

FIGURE 1-2

The convergent lady beetle, *Hippodamia convergens*, is a common predator and is often found in gardens, landscapes, trees, and field crops whenever aphids are abundant.

possible to modify certain parts of the environment to maintain or enhance natural enemies. Examples include strip-cropping or alternate mowing, planting flowering plants that produce nectar for parasitic wasps, or planting ground covers that compete with weeds.

Biological Control Agents

You can use several types of biological control agents to suppress pest populations, including predators, parasites, herbivores, competitors, and organisms that release substances that are toxic or repellent to pests (known as antibiosis).

Predators. A predator is an animal that attacks, feeds on, and kills more than one prey organism during its lifetime. Predators are usually larger and stronger than their prey. Some predators feed only on one or a few closely related species. Many predators, however, feed on a variety of similar types of organisms, such as soft-bodied insects or free-living nematodes in the soil. Predators range from large carnivores, such as coyotes and raptors, to microscopic amoebae and other soil-dwelling microorganisms. The most recognized predators in biological control, however, are the predatory arthropods, such as lady beetles (Fig. 1-2), carabid beetles, lacewings, syrphid flies, predatory true bugs, spiders, and predatory mites. In some insect species, both the adult and immature (larval or nymphal) stages are predaceous. Other species of insects are predaceous only during their immature stages. Adults of many of these predators feed on honeydew and plant nectar or pollen.

Parasites. A parasite feeds in or on a larger host organism. Parasitic organisms have a prolonged and specialized relationship with their host, usually parasitizing only one or a few individuals in their lifetime. True parasites often weaken the host but do not kill it outright; in some cases, they may have little negative impact. Only those that significantly weaken or kill their host are important in biological control.

Insects that parasitize and kill other insects are often called parasitoids. Parasitoids are parasitic during their immature stages and kill their host as they reach maturity. Most parasitoids are wasps or flies with adults that feed on insect honeydew and plant nectar and pollen. In certain species, the adult female parasitoid also feeds on hosts.

Because they kill their hosts, insect parasitoids are not considered true parasites. However, in this book and most of the other pest management literature, parasitoids are simply referred to as insect parasites.

Pathogens are microorganisms that cause disease or malfunctioning of host cells and tissues and are a kind of parasite. Pathogens may or may not kill their host. Beneficial pathogenic organisms include certain bacteria, fungi, protozoa, viruses, and nematodes (Fig. 1-3) that cause disease in pest insects, weeds, nematodes, and mites.

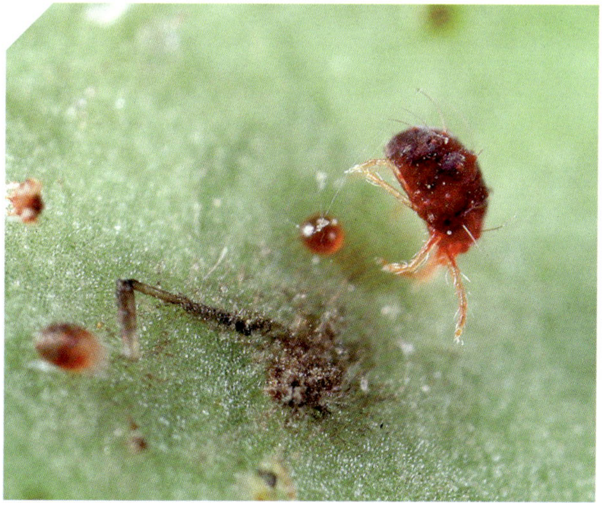

FIGURE 1-3

Its swollen, darkened body suggests that this citrus red mite, *Panonychus citri*, is infected by a virus. As the disease progresses, shriveled bodies on plants provide further evidence of infection.

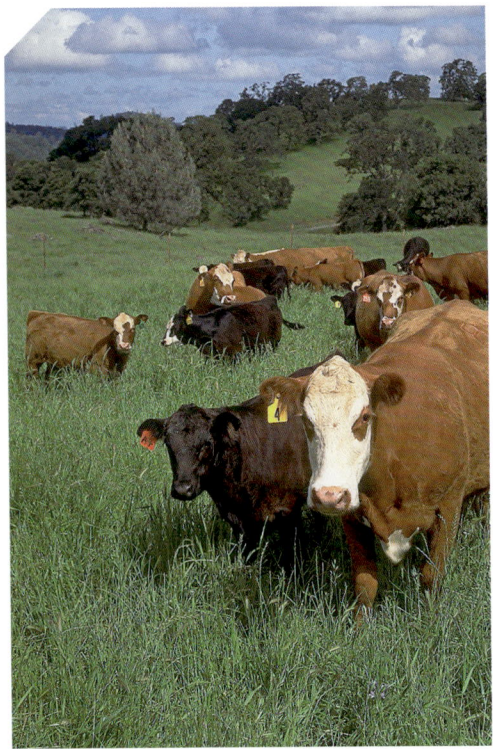

FIGURE 1-4

The grazing of herbivores such as cattle, when well managed, can contribute to the control of yellow starthistle.

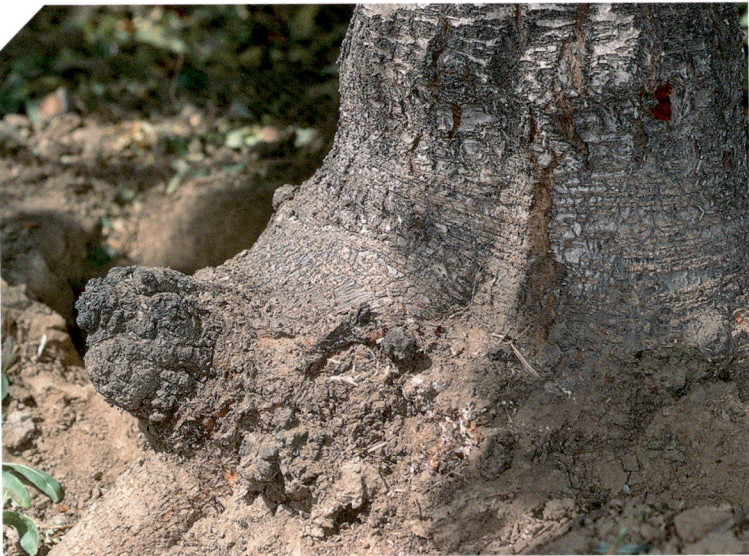

FIGURE 1-5

The crown gall, *Agrobacterium tumefaciens*, shown here, might have been prevented by treating the roots before planting with *Agrobacterium radiobacter* strain K84.

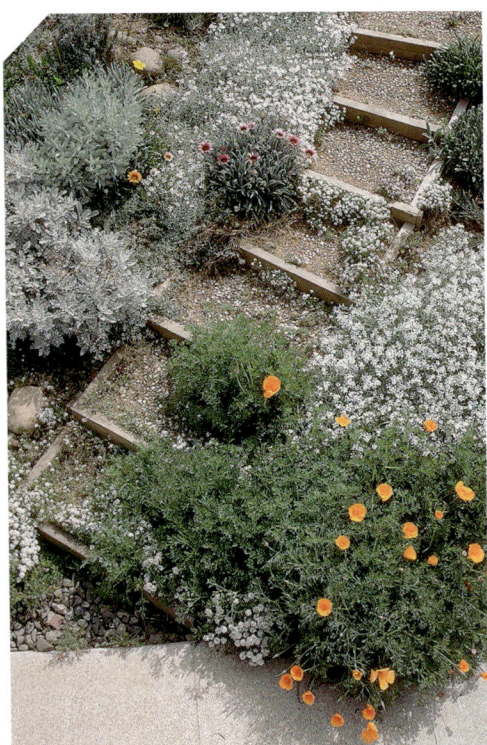

FIGURE 1-6

Planting ground covers and other plants close together in the landscape uses plant competition to suppress weeds.

Herbivores. Herbivores are animals that feed on plants. Herbivores are important natural enemies of weeds, especially when they specialize and feed on only one or several closely related weed species. The most effective natural enemies of weeds limit weed reproduction by feeding on flowers or seeds. Birds feeding on weed seeds after harvest, for example, can help keep the weed seed bank in check. Geese have also been used to control weeds in organically grown cotton, tomato, pepper, and lettuce crops. Livestock such as cattle, sheep, and goats can also play a role in weed suppression, especially on rangelands (Fig. 1-4).

Antibiosis. Some organisms release toxins or otherwise change conditions so that pest activity or growth is reduced. Many bacteria and molds secrete antimicrobial substances that inhibit the growth of other microorganisms. Injecting fruit tree rootstocks with strain K84 of the bacterium *Agrobacterium radiobacter* can prevent infection by damaging strains of *Agrobacterium tumefaciens*, the pathogen that causes crown gall (Fig. 1-5). The K84 strain also produces an antibiotic against other *Agrobacterium* bacteria.

Another form of antibiosis is allelopathy, in which one plant releases substances that are toxic to another plant species. Allelochemicals are released into the environment as volatile gases, secreted from living roots, leached from shoots, or released through the decomposition of dead plant material.

Competitors. Competition occurs when two organisms compete for limited supplies of essential resources, such as food in the case of animals and water, nutrients, and light in the case of plants. Due to their superior ability to secure resources, competitors limit populations of pest organisms, sometimes with little negative impact on the crop or other managed resource. Competition can be used in weed control: for instance, highly competitive ground covers in landscape plantings can rapidly outgrow and shade out weedy species (Fig. 1-6). Competitors

PEST MANAGEMENT

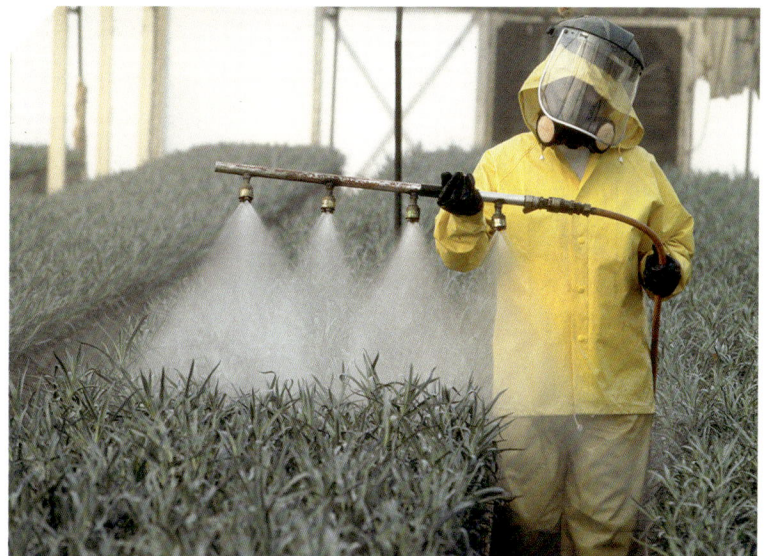

FIGURE 1-7

Pesticides provide an effective way to control pests. Usually, pest damage stops within a few hours to a few days after a pesticide application. This photo shows a fungicide being applied to carnation plants in a greenhouse.

may also be important in the biological control of pathogens, as in the use of strains of bacteria or fungi as protective seed coatings. A soil with a diverse array of harmless nematodes or pathogens may help limit numbers of damaging species (Flint 2012).

Chemical Control: Pesticides

Pesticides often play a key role in pest management and occasionally may be the only management method available. Major benefits associated with the use of pesticides include

- their effectiveness
- the speed and ease of controlling pests
- their reasonable cost compared with other control options (in many instances)

For example, after applying a pesticide, pest damage usually stops within a few hours (for arthropods) to a few days (for weeds); also, fungicides provide plants with immediate, short-term protection against microorganisms (Fig. 1-7).

According to the Federal Insecticide, Fungicide, and Rodenticide Act (FIFRA), a pesticide is "any material applied to plants, the soil, water, harvested crops, structures, clothing and furnishings, or animals to kill, attract, repel, or regulate or interrupt growth and mating of pests." Some pesticides also regulate plant growth. Herbicides, insecticides, fungicides, rodenticides, nematicides, and miticides are common types of pesticides. Chapter 3 describes pesticide types and classifications.

Mechanical and Physical Controls

An important way to control pests or protect crops, livestock and poultry, people, and manufactured products is by using mechanical and physical control methods, which include

- excluding or trapping pests
- physically removing and destroying pests
- modifying the environment so that it is not suitable for pest survival
- using cultivation to disrupt pest life cycles

Exclusion. Exclusion consists of using barriers to prevent pests from getting into an area. Window screens, for example, exclude flies, mosquitoes, and other flying insects (Fig. 1-8).

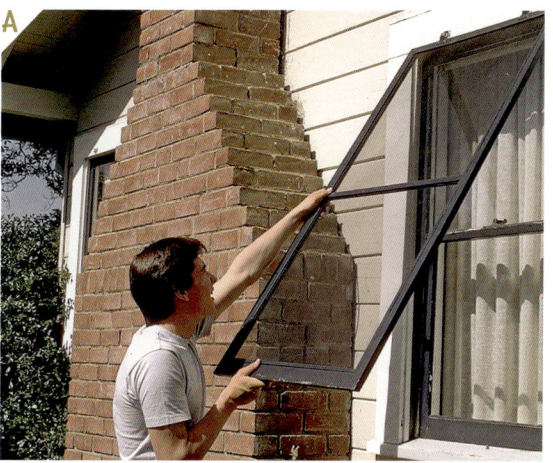

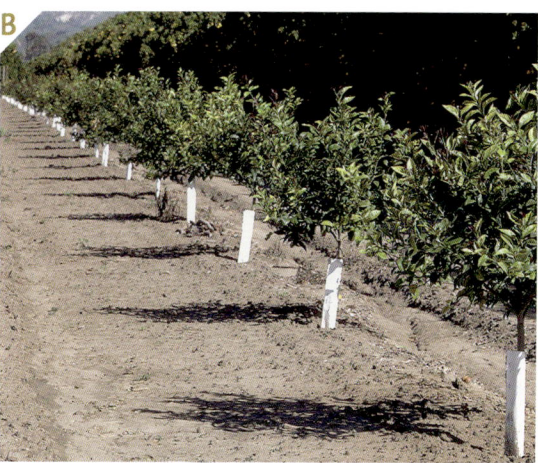

FIGURE 1-8

Window screens and paper tree protectors are mechanical devices that exclude certain pests.

TABLE 1-1

Various traps used for pest control and some of the pests they control

Trap	Pest controlled
automatic multicatch house sparrow trap; double funnel trap	house sparrows
box-type squirrel trap; multicatch box-type squirrel trap	ground squirrels, tree squirrels
conibear trap	ground squirrels
snap trap	mice, rats, meadow voles
Macabee trap	pocket gophers, moles
box trap	pocket gophers
electronic trap	rats, house mice
glue boards	mice
live traps	rats, mice, birds, skunks, opossums, other small animals
bait traps	Indian meal moths, fruit flies
sticky traps	flies, some cockroaches, whiteflies, thrips
walk-through traps	horn fly
cone-shaped bait traps	yellowjackets, flies

Source: Flint 2012.

Patching or sealing cracks, crevices, and small openings in buildings excludes insects, rodents, bats, birds, and other pests. Fences and ditches make effective barriers against many vertebrate pests. Wire or cloth mesh excludes birds from fruit trees. Sticky material painted onto tree trunks, posts, wires, and other objects prevents crawling insects from crossing.

Trapping. Traps are practical devices for controlling many vertebrate and invertebrate pests. Traps are especially important in the management of vertebrate species such as ground squirrels, moles, meadow voles, pocket gophers, rats, mice, and some species of large animals. Insect traps used for control include fly traps, roach traps, and other types of sticky traps. Some of these traps are regularly used for monitoring but can also be used to assist in management efforts.

Traps are of various designs and are specific to a pest species. Some traps are designed to kill, while others catch the offending individuals. An alternative trap type for mice is the glue board. Glue boards work much in the same way as flypaper; as mice travel across the glue board, they get stuck. Mice trapped on glue boards do not die immediately and you must dispose of them. Table 1-1 lists various types of traps used in pest control.

When using traps, placement is very important (Fig. 1-9). For vertebrates, the most effective locations are usually in natural travel ways and near or in runways, depending on the species. Be aware of legal requirements when trapping vertebrate pests. Some species are classified as nongame mammals by the California Fish and Game Code and can be controlled whenever they injure crops, while other species are classified as game animals and fall under special provisions of the Fish and Game Code. If you use a live trap, be aware that the trapped animal must be killed: you cannot legally release it in another location. Check with the county agricultural commissioner's office for specific information on trapping.

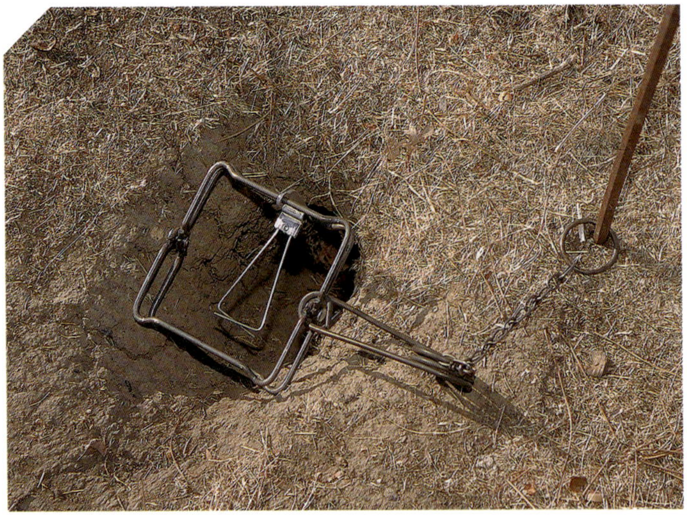

Soil Tillage. Tillage, or cultivation, contributes to pest management by killing weeds, disrupting the life cycle of some insect pests, and burying disease inoculum. Tillage has many purposes and is often combined with other management practices to turn under crop debris, incorporate fertilizer, improve

FIGURE 1-9

Conibear traps are placed over the entrance to ground squirrel burrows and secured with a stake.

water penetration, or enhance growing conditions for the crop. Cultivation is the most important and widely used weed management tool in many crops and, with proper timing, kills annual weeds, biennial weeds without a taproot, and seedlings of annual and perennial weeds. Mature perennial weeds can be sufficiently controlled by repeated cultivations under dry soil conditions. Improper timing, however, can increase perennial weeds. Tillage can also bring additional weed seeds to the surface, resulting in germination flushes after each cultivation, while some perennial weeds, such as johnsongrass, bermudagrass, and field bindweed, can increase due to regrowth from chopped-up underground stems.

All cultivation techniques have advantages, but the disadvantages should be considered before starting a program of soil tillage. Tillage can
- destroy soil structure and contribute to soil erosion
- cause a loss of fertilizer
- increase compaction
- disrupt the life cycle of beneficial organisms
- produce air pollution

Mowing. Correct mowing height and frequency of mowing are critical for preventing weed invasion in turf. Different turf species have different mowing height requirements. Mowing Kentucky bluegrass too short (below 1.5 inches) weakens the turf and encourages weed growth. Conversely, mowing bermudagrass too long (above 1 to 2 inches) results in a buildup of thatch, which reduces the competitive ability of the grass (Flint 2012).

Cultural Controls

Many different cultural practices influence the survival of pests. In turf, mowing, irrigation, aeration, and fertilization are important ways to prevent pest buildup and damage. In agricultural crops, you can reduce populations of weeds, microorganisms, insects, mites, and other pests by
- timing planting and harvesting to avoid pests
- managing the amount and timing of irrigation water
- using crop rotations

Sanitation practices, habitat modification, and the selection of resistant plant varieties (also known as host resistance) can also significantly reduce pest problems.

Site Selection. Sometimes you can prevent pest problems by selecting a site that is pest-free or by choosing a crop, plant species, or variety that is particularly well suited to the site. Before planting, evaluate the site with the resource being planted in mind. Ask yourself whether planting in this location will create or aggravate pest problems. For example, planting trees or shrubs in landscapes where conditions do not support them can result in more damage by insects and diseases. Plants in the wrong environment generally do not perform well (Fig. 1-10). Likewise, it is good management to avoid fields with weeds that are potentially troublesome and hard to control in a crop. Instead, plant an alternative crop where available herbicides, cultural practices, or crop competitiveness will help reduce these weeds. Sampling for nematodes, pathogens, and weed seeds and looking at the field history prior to planting can help determine whether the site will work for a given crop. For sampling methods, see "Establishing a Monitoring Program" in Chapter 10.

Sanitation. Sanitation practices control pests in many locations. Sanitation, or source reduction, involves eliminating food, water, shelter,

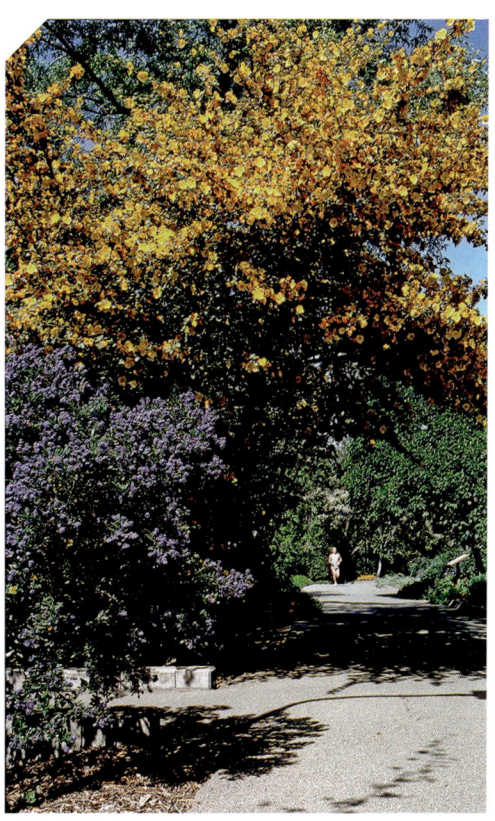

FIGURE 1-10

In landscape situations, choosing plants that are adapted to local conditions and grouping plants that have similar requirements can avoid many pest problems. The ceanothus and flannel bush shown are well adapted to dry areas in Central and Southern California.

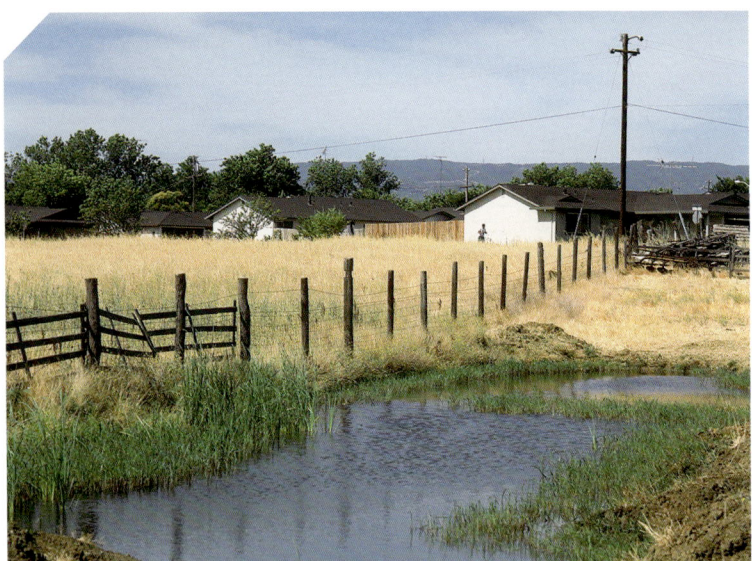

FIGURE 1-11

Draining standing water is an important cultural practice that reduces mosquito populations.

or other necessities important to the pest's survival. In agriculture, sanitation includes removing weeds that harbor pest insects or rodents and removing weed plants before they produce seeds. Sanitation also involves destroying diseased plant material and removing and destroying unharvested produce and crop residues. It includes keeping field borders or surrounding areas free of pests and pest breeding sites. Properly storing feeds and preventing feed waste reduce rodent problems in these locations. In nonagricultural areas, draining standing water (Fig. 1-11) and managing wastes control certain pests. Waste management is very important—closed garbage containers and frequent garbage pickup eliminate food sources for flies, cockroaches, and rodents (Fig. 1-12). Removing soil, trash, and other debris from around and under buildings reduces pest habitat.

Habitat Modification. Pest problems occur when conditions essential for survival (food, shelter, alternate hosts, and proper environmental conditions) are favorable. Habitat modification changes the environment, limiting availability of one or more of these requirements so pest populations cannot find what they need to survive. Habitat modification is very important in vertebrate control. For example, weeds, ground cover, and litter provide food and cover for meadow mice. Mowing can reduce both food and hiding places for these pests, causing them to leave the area or be more exposed to prey animals. Habitat modification can help limit numerous insect pests as well. For example, draining areas of standing water reduces breeding sites for mosquitoes and is an important management technique.

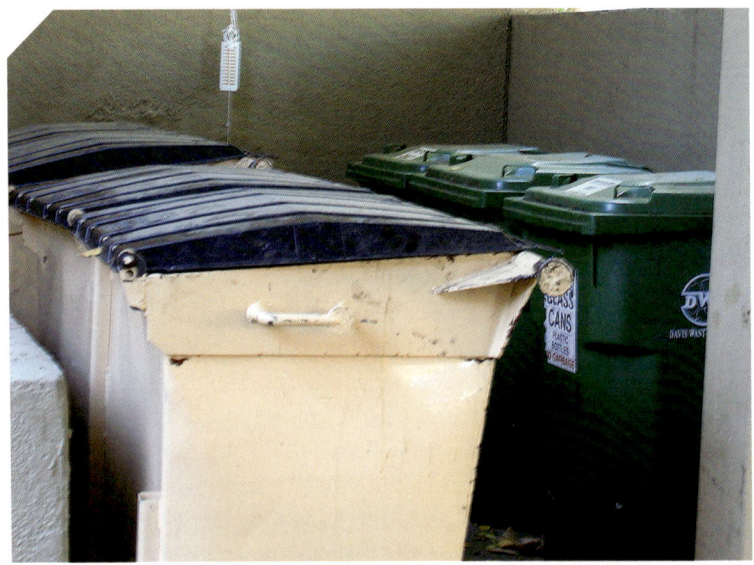

FIGURE 1-12

Sanitation around homes, restaurants, and businesses reduces populations of cockroaches, ants, and rodents. Garbage and trash containers must have tight lids to keep out pests.

Habitat modification is also a critical element in the management of pest flies in poultry houses and dairies. Flies have three basic developmental requirements: food, warmth, and moisture. Eliminating any of these in the poultry house, barn, or barnyard can break the life cycle of the fly and reduce the problem. Warm weather combined with moist organic matter encourages the production of large numbers of flies. Manure, silage stored on a cement base, waste feed, and contaminated animal bedding provide ideal sources for feeding, egg laying, and development of pest flies. However, even if eggs hatch, larvae cannot develop into flies without food, warmth, and moisture. Barns and poultry houses designed for easy removal of manure and barn floors surfaced and sloped to facilitate drainage help eliminate the conditions that larvae rely on for survival (Fig. 1-13). Moist bedding, old feed, and other decomposing organic matter should be

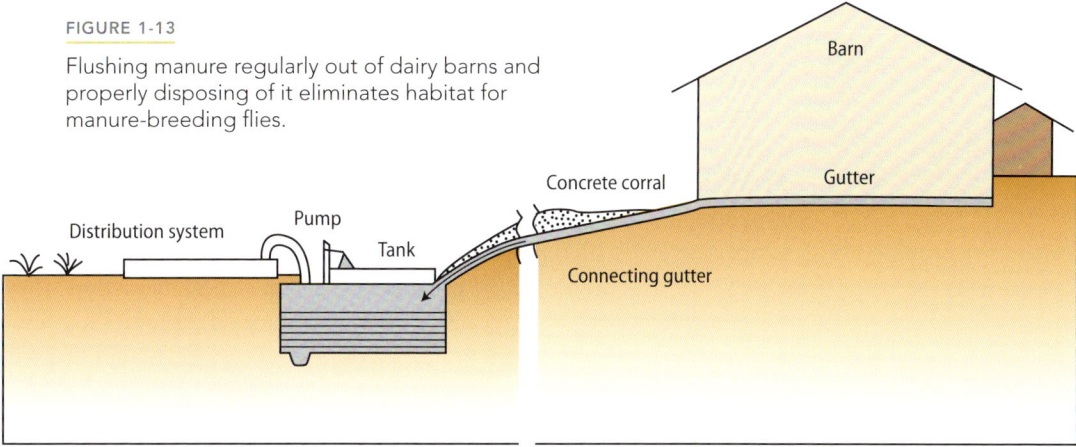

FIGURE 1-13

Flushing manure regularly out of dairy barns and properly disposing of it eliminates habitat for manure-breeding flies.

regularly removed. Manure-breeding flies have many natural enemies, and certain practices can enhance their activities. For instance, in poultry houses, when fresh manure is being removed, a single pad of manure 6 to 8 inches thick can be left on the house floor to provide habitat for natural enemies such as ants, mites, beetles, and parasitic wasps. This manure pad allows predators to quickly invade adjacent fresh droppings that the flies use for breeding.

Host Resistance. Breeding or selecting plants and animals to resist specific pest problems is another method of pest control. For example, animal breeders select livestock for physical characteristics that prevent attack by some pests. They also select for physiological resistance to disease or parasitic organisms. Plants are bred to be resistant to pests such as nematodes and certain plant pathogens. The host's health and nutritional needs also influence resistance. Certain plant varieties are naturally resistant to insects, pathogens, or nematodes. Other plants are genetically modified to produce pest-specific toxins.

Inoculating growing plants with certain microorganisms sometimes induces resistance. Genetic engineering research demonstrates that it is possible to build pest resistance into the genetic makeup of some plants so that future generations then have this resistance. These plants are commonly referred to as transgenic plants or genetically modified organisms (GMOs) (see Flint 2012).

Special Pest Management Methods

Quarantine. Quarantine is a pest control process designed to prevent entry of pests into areas free of that pest. The state of California maintains inspection stations at all major entry points into the state. The goal of the inspection stations is to intercept pests or materials that might harbor pests. There are sixteen border stations for inspecting vehicles entering the state from Oregon, Nevada, Arizona, and Mexico (Fig. 1-14). The California Department of Food and Agriculture, in cooperation with the U.S. Department of Agriculture and local offices of county agricultural commissioners, monitors airports and ocean ports as well.

Quarantine is also used to prevent movement of designated pests within the state. Quarantine orders require that you

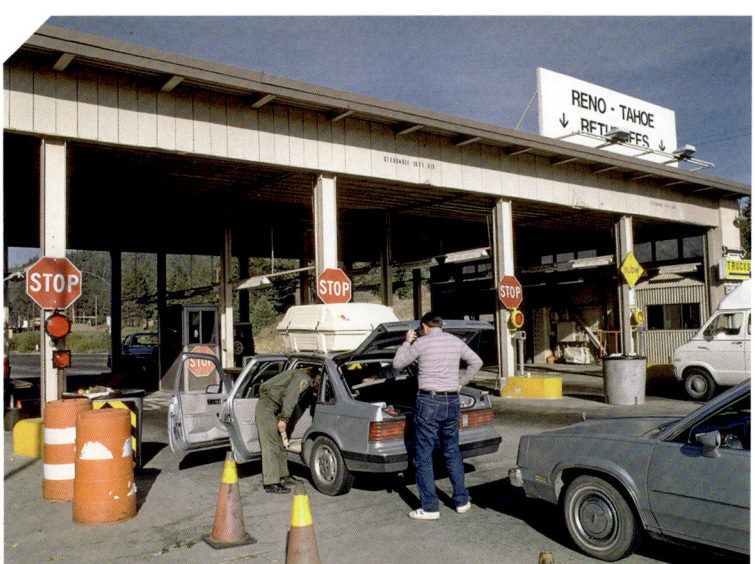

FIGURE 1-14

This border inspection station, located in Truckee, is part of the effort to control the movement of pests into California. Inspection stations are in operation on all major highways into the state from Oregon, Nevada, Arizona, and Mexico.

apply pesticides to destroy pests on produce, nursery plants, and other identified items before these items leave a quarantine area.

Nursery stock, plant cuttings, and budding and grafting material are regulated to prevent the spreading of pests. As part of this program the state of California maintains a registry of certified pest-free plant material that can be shipped throughout the state.

Eradication. For pests that are unacceptable at any level, eradication is generally the only control option. These pests are usually also under quarantine restrictions. State or federal agencies supervise eradication programs. Once monitoring information confirms the presence of the pest, state agencies determine the geographical extent of pest infestation. They then begin eradication efforts to eliminate this pest from the defined area. Procedures may include

- an area-wide spray program
- releasing sterile insects
- using mechanical and cultural practices
- intensively monitoring for pests within and around the borders of the infested area

Regulations prohibiting the planting or growing of certain host plants (host-free areas) or prohibiting the planting and growing of these plants during certain periods (host-free periods) may also be part of eradication programs.

Abatement. Weedy areas and neglected or abandoned crops create fire hazards and may harbor vertebrate, invertebrate, or microorganism pests. They also provide a reservoir of weed seeds that threaten adjoining areas or crops. Specific host plants attract or promote the buildup of certain pest invertebrates or disease-causing organisms. Some weedy plants are noxious to people or livestock. Government agencies tell owners to destroy weeds and plants that cause fire hazards, harbor harmful pathogens or animals, or are noxious to people or livestock in and around agricultural areas. Similar authority applies to diseased or infected livestock or poultry and also extends to weeds and nuisance plants in residential, commercial, and industrial areas.

Mosquito abatement is an important pest control function undertaken to protect public health. Under the authority of mosquito abatement laws, state agencies drain or treat standing water that serves as breeding sites for mosquitoes.

Organic Agriculture. In 1979, the Organic Foods Act became part of the California Health and Safety Code, and in 1990 the Organic Foods Production Act (OFPA) was enacted on the federal level. These laws specify the types of pesticides people can use in organic agriculture. It covers crops, livestock, poultry, and dairy products sold as organic. The California law applies to any labeling using the terms *organically grown*, *naturally grown*, *wild*, *ecologically grown*, or *biologically grown*. Food certified as organic is produced according to federal standards set by the USDA National Organic Program.

Pesticides allowed for use on organically produced food include microorganisms, microbiological products, and materials derived or extracted from plant, animal, or mineral-bearing rock substances. Permitted pesticides include Bordeaux mixes, trace elements, soluble aquatic plant products, botanical lime sulfur, naturally mined gypsum, dormant oils, summer oils, fish emulsion, and insecticidal soaps. All materials used as pesticides must have current labels for such use. Table 1-2 lists many of the materials that currently are allowable or have been used as organic pesticides. A complete, updated list of approved and banned substances is available in the Electronic Code of Federal Regulations (search for Title 7 at the website ecfr.gov).

In general, pesticides approved for use on organically grown produce break down rapidly. These materials are often less disruptive to natural enemies and other organisms in the environment. However, the modes of action of many chemicals acceptable under the Organic Foods Act are similar to some synthetically manufactured pesticides. For example, copper materials interfere with cell respiration, and pyrethrins interfere with nerve transmission, similar to DDT. These pesticides can have *Caution*, *Warning*, or *Danger* signal words.

TABLE 1-2
Pesticides accepted for use on or around selected types of organically grown produce

Compound*	Type	Use and comments
Insecticides		
Bacillus thuringiensis (Bt)	microbial	Controls many species of lepidopteran larvae and mosquito larvae, depending on the variety of the Bt used.
boric acid powder	inorganic	A sorptive dust with a desiccant action. Controls cockroaches, ants, and other household pests. Ineffective if dust gets wet.
diatomaceous earth	inorganic	A sorptive dust derived from the skeletons of microscopic marine organisms. As a desiccant, controls household pests such as cockroaches and ants. Also controls some plant pests.
granulosis virus	microbial	Controls codling moth.
lime	inorganic	Controls mites and certain plant-sucking insects.
lime sulfur	inorganic	Controls mites and psylla.
petroleum oils	hydrocarbon	Controls aphids, psylla, scale insects, mites, and aphid and mite eggs. May provide some control of other overwintering insects.
pheromones	attractant	Used mainly for monitoring to time other control measures. Sometimes used to confuse insects in localized area to disrupt mating. Occasionally used to catch large numbers of specific insects to reduce future generations.
pyrethrum	plant derivative	Broad spectrum of pests controlled, including mosquitoes, flies, aphids, beetles, moth larvae, thrips, and mealybugs. Provides rapid knockdown of flying pests.
sabadilla	plant derivative	Has contact and stomach poison action against cockroaches, several species of bugs, potato leafhopper, imported cabbageworm, house fly, citrus thrips, and the cattle louse. Is toxic to honey bees. Not highly toxic to mammals.
soap	soap	Controls mites, aphids, and other plant-sucking arthropods. Can be phytotoxic under certain conditions. Soap must be specifically labeled for use as an insecticide.
sulfur	inorganic	Controls mites.
vegetable oils	plant derivative	As a contact spray, controls scale insects, aphids, and mites.
Fungicides		
basic copper sulfate	inorganic	Controls early and late blight, scab, blotch, bitter rot, fire blight, downy mildew, black rot, leaf spot, melanose, greasy spot, brown rot, anthracnose, angular leaf spot, and others.
Bordeaux mixture	inorganic	A slurry made of hydrated lime and copper sulfate. Controls brown rot and shot hole diseases in tree fruits. Controls some grape diseases. Also controls apple scab, blotch, apple black rot, melanose, anthracnose, early and late blight of potatoes and tomatoes, downy mildew, fire blight, leaf spot, peach leaf curl, and many other fungal diseases.
copper hydroxide	inorganic	Controls cercospora leaf spot, bacterial blight, septoria, leaf blotch, anthracnose, halo blight, helminthosporum, downy mildew, leaf curl, early and late blight, angular leaf spot, melanose, scab, walnut blight, and others.
copper oxychloride sulfate	inorganic	Controls peach blight, peach leaf curl, damp-off, anthracnose, fire blight, shot hole fungus, pear blight, bacterial spot, walnut blight, brown rot, celery blight, downy mildew, early and late blight of vegetables, cherry leaf spot, septoria leaf spot, powdery mildew, melanose, scab, and others.
copper sulfate	inorganic	Suppresses development of fungal and bacterial organisms such as fire blight, cercospora leaf spot, early and late blight, bacterial blight, and others.
lime sulfur	inorganic	Controls powdery mildew, anthracnose, apple scab, brown rot, peach leaf curl, and others.
sulfur	inorganic	Controls brown rot, peach scab, apple scab, powdery mildew, downy mildew, rose black spot, and others.

Note: *Some pesticides on this list may not be currently approved for use on organically grown produce. Many materials listed in this table may no longer be registered as pesticides or their labels may restrict their use to specific pests, crops, or sites. Use all pesticides only in accordance with current federal and state labels.

Monitoring: The Key to Successful Pest Management

Describe monitoring and explain why it is important.

Monitoring to detect and track the development of pests is your key to building an effective pest management program. Detection verifies the presence of pests and helps you anticipate pest outbreaks. Continued monitoring provides important information about a pest's life stages and habits as well as site-specific variables that can affect the outcome of pest control measures. Also, you need the information provided by monitoring to choose a pesticide and to know when, where, and how to apply it. Establishing a monitoring program not only allows you to detect pests, it also lets you

- observe seasonal changes in pest populations
- track natural enemy populations
- properly time control applications
- assess the effectiveness of control measures

WHY MONITORING MATTERS

Define economic injury (treatment) thresholds and describe what happens when these are reached.

A major objective of monitoring is to obtain information to help make pest management decisions. Monitoring can provide immediate data for decision making, comprehensive data on the far-reaching effects of a pest organism over time or over an area, and a site-specific historical record that can measure the effectiveness of management actions at that site. Monitoring can also be useful in predicting the location and abundance of a pest population. Monitoring is key to determining when economic injury (or treatment) thresholds have been, or might be, reached. Predicting when a site might experience expensive pest damage helps you perform pesticide applications that make economic sense.

Monitoring is fundamental to IPM and is a prerequisite for effective decision making. Monitoring includes a variety of procedures used to observe, measure, and record over time the activities, growth, development, and abundance of organisms. It may also include observations of the factors that affect them, including site-specific variables. Pest monitoring provides information on populations, life stages, and infestation levels of pests. Additionally, it provides information on weather, crop development, the effectiveness of management practices, and populations of beneficial organisms, including natural enemies. The records generated by monitoring establish a pest history for the field, orchard, or managed site (see Flint 2012).

Your local pest control adviser (PCA) will make recommendations for pesticide applications based on treatment thresholds that vary according to pest type, crop type, and environmental conditions. It is up to you to monitor and record pest activity to improve the effectiveness of any recommended applications.

For more information about pest monitoring and guidelines for creating a comprehensive monitoring program, see "Pest Detection and Monitoring" in Chapter 10.

FOLLOW-UP MONITORING

Explain the importance of evaluating pest management results.

Monitor after every treatment to learn whether the control activity was successful. Follow-up monitoring includes checking a site even if no treatment has been recommended; nontreatment decisions should include follow-up monitoring until the pest is no longer a threat to the crop. After treatment, monitor to look for signs indicating that the level of control achieved is adequate. For instance, after a fungicide application, perform follow-up monitoring to verify that coverage was thorough and the pathogen has been suppressed. Also, if the conditions for disease development continue, continue monitoring to determine whether further management actions are required as unprotected foliage becomes susceptible (see Flint 2012).

If a pesticide application is determined to be unsuccessful, regular follow-up monitoring and recordkeeping allow you to assess the problem(s), and institute corrective measures or change faulty procedures for the next application.

Chapter 1 Review Questions

1. Match the pest control technique with its IPM method.

1. augmentation	a. cultural control
2. exclusion	b. chemical control
3. habitat modification	c. biological control
4. pesticide application	d. mechanical and physical control

2. Match the situation to the pest control approach you should use.

1. An invasive species is threatening crops in a new area.	a. prevention
2. Environmental conditions are beginning to favor the development of disease.	b. suppression
3. Pest populations need to be lowered so natural enemies can take over and maintain control.	c. eradication

3. Match the pest type with its definition.

1. key pests	a. A pest that becomes a problem as the result of the control of another pest.
2. secondary pests	b. A pest that causes major damage on a regular basis.
3. occasional pests	c. A pest that causes problems only under specific circumstances or at certain times.

4. Which would be considered a preventive pest management strategy?
    - ☐ a. planting weed-free seeds
    - ☐ b. releasing natural enemies
    - ☐ c. eliminating rodents from a building

5. Which statement is *true* about treatment thresholds?
    - ☐ a. Treatment thresholds are usually easy to establish by searching the Internet.
    - ☐ b. In an urban landscape, treatment thresholds are usually more related to economics than aesthetics.
    - ☐ c. Treatment thresholds vary considerably depending on pest, host, and environmental conditions.

6. Which of the following is *true* about monitoring?
    - ☐ a. You may not always need it to make good pest management decisions.
    - ☐ b. It helps you predict the location and abundance of key pest populations.
    - ☐ c. Use it primarily in spring and summer, when pest populations are high.

7. Which of the following principles are combined to create an IPM program? Select all that apply.
    - ☐ a. eliminating all insects present in an area
    - ☐ b. identifying pests accurately
    - ☐ c. preventing pest problems
    - ☐ d. using guidelines to determine the best control techniques
    - ☐ e. removing vegetation completely at a location
    - ☐ f. monitoring for pests and pest damage
    - ☐ g. combining pest management tools

8. Which statement is *true* about biological control methods?
   - ☐ a. If pesticides are part of a biological control program to control an exotic pest, it is better to apply them at the highest label rate.
   - ☐ b. Modifying the environment to enhance natural enemies is a recommended practice in biological control.
   - ☐ c. Biological control involves the importation of exotic pests to control natural enemies.

9. Which of the following is an example of cultural control?
   - ☐ a. discing weeds in a field
   - ☐ b. making spot treatments using an herbicide
   - ☐ c. releasing imported natural enemies

10. The use of barriers such as screens, fences, and cloth mesh is known as _____.
    - ☐ a. eradication
    - ☐ b. elimination
    - ☐ c. exclusion

11. Sanitation is important in order to control _____.
    - ☐ a. insects and rodents only
    - ☐ b. many pest and disease organisms
    - ☐ c. all natural enemy populations

12. Which statement is *true* about pest management strategies in IPM?
    - ☐ a. The goal is often to tolerate pests at economically acceptable levels.
    - ☐ b. Eradication is never the goal of an IPM program.
    - ☐ c. Pesticides are not included in an IPM strategy.
    - ☐ d. Nonchemical methods usually provide only short-term control of a pest.

13. When pesticide treatments are carefully chosen, timed, and integrated with plant biology, wind conditions, and certain agronomic practices, pest control efforts _____.
    - ☐ a. will always be successful when guidelines are strictly followed
    - ☐ b. will often be expensive and time consuming over the long term
    - ☐ c. can control pests while preserving natural enemy populations

14. Why is it important to track the life stage of pests you are trying to control?
    - ☐ a. You might look foolish at work if you can't identify a pest by its life stages.
    - ☐ b. Certain pests at certain life stages are best to avoid, even when trying to control them.
    - ☐ c. Successful pest control efforts must coincide with a pest's most vulnerable life stage.

15. Monitor after every treatment to learn _____.
    - ☐ a. whether the control activity was successful
    - ☐ b. how much residue remains on leaves
    - ☐ c. whether the landowner is satisfied with the results

Chapter 2
Pest Identification

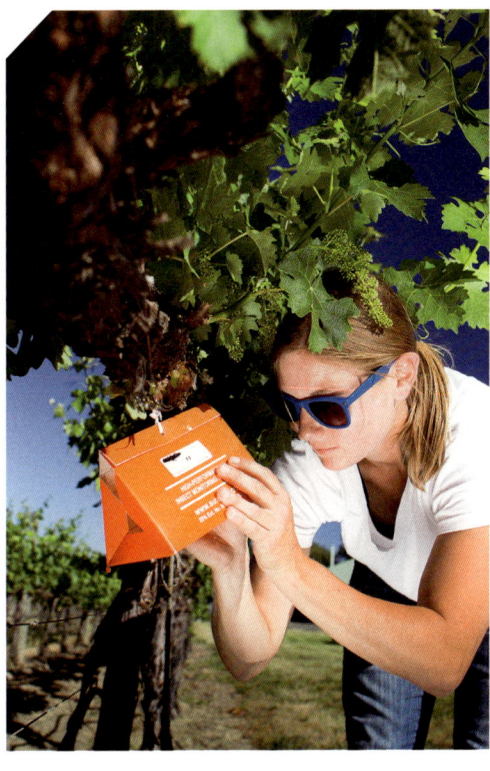

How Plants and Animals Are Named 20
Identifying Pests 22
Weeds 24
Invertebrates 35
Vertebrates 52
Pathogens and Abiotic Disorders 56
Chapter 2 Review Questions 65

Knowledge Expectations

- Explain why understanding pest biology is important when managing pests.
- Explain why identifying pests correctly is important.
- List the main groups of common pests.
- Explain how pests are organized and identified using scientific names.
- List and describe the types of resources and references available for identifying pests, symptoms of infestation, and damage caused by pests.
- List examples of common pests in California from each main group and describe the damage they cause.
- Distinguish between damage caused by pathogens and abiotic factors.

Explain why understanding pest biology is important when managing pests.

Explain why identifying pests correctly is important.

List the main groups of common pests.

Explain how pests are organized and identified using scientific names.

Pests are organisms that cause problems in various ways. Some compete with people for food or fiber. Others interfere with raising crops, livestock, or poultry. Certain types of pests damage property and personal belongings or disfigure ornamental plantings. A few transmit or cause plant, animal, or human diseases.

Before trying to control a pest, you must identify it and understand its biology. Be certain any injury or observed damage is actually due to the identified pest and cannot be attributed to some other cause. Once you have identified the pest and its damage, become familiar with its life cycle, growth, and reproductive habits, as well as the life cycle and growth of the host plant or crop. Then, use this information to form your pest control plans. Misidentification, lack of information about a pest, and poor understanding of a plant or crop's most vulnerable growth stages could cause you to choose the wrong control method or apply the control at the wrong time. Making poor choices based on poor information is the most frequent cause of pest control failure.

This chapter reviews some of the ways to identify pests. The four main groups of pests include
- weeds (undesired plants)
- invertebrates (insects, mites, and their relatives; nematodes and worms; and snails and slugs)
- vertebrates (birds, reptiles, amphibians, fish, and mammals)
- disease agents (bacteria, viruses and viroids, fungi, phytoplasmas and other microorganisms, and abiotic factors)

How Plants and Animals Are Named

Names of plants and animals are your doorways to information about them. Once you know the name of a pest, you can more easily select control methods. Control methods include specific pesticides that prevent a particular pest from causing injury.

SCIENTIFIC NAMES

Classification systems are sets of rules used for organizing and naming living things. An elegant, standardized classification system used throughout the world is the basis for the scientific names given to plants and animals. This system reveals relationships among different species of plants or animals. Scientific names are very useful when trying to locate information about organisms.

Most living organisms belong to one of two major groups: the plant kingdom or the animal kingdom. Usually it is easy to distinguish between living organisms and nonliving objects and between plants and animals. However, microorganisms and algae are more difficult to classify because of characteristics that make them intermediate between plants and animals.

There are six subcategories within a kingdom in the standardized classification system—phylum, class, order, family, genus, and species. Unique physical characteristics set some organisms apart from others. For example, in the phylum Arthropoda all organisms have jointed appendages and external skeletons; animals in the phylum Chordata have backbones, spinal nerve cords, and internal skeletons. Within a phylum there are several orders, each containing one or more families. A family is a group of related genera (the plural of genus), and a genus is a collection of species. A species is unique from all other organisms. The genus and species names make up an organism's scientific name. There may be variations among individuals of the same species. These include color and size differences and ability to attack a specific type of crop or plant. There may even be differences in the ability to resist certain pesticides.

COMMON NAMES

Besides a scientific name, most plants and animals have one or more common names. Pesticide labels refer to most pests by their common names. These names are usually descriptive, such as house fly, American cockroach, roof rat, field bindweed, yellow foxtail, apple scab, and fire blight. The disadvantage of using common names is that they do not provide any information about the relationship of one organism to another. For example, johnsongrass (*Sorghum halepense*) is a weed, while Sudan grass, grain sorghum, and milo (all *Sorghum bicolor*) are grains. All three belong to the genus *Sorghum*, but their common names do not indicate any relationship. Their scientific names, however, show that they all belong to the genus *Sorghum*, indicating a close relationship.

Because common names vary with locality or host, an organism will often have more than one common name. The insect *Helicoverpa zea*, for example, is called the corn earworm, bollworm, and tomato fruitworm, depending on which crop it is attacking (Fig. 2-1). Organizations such as

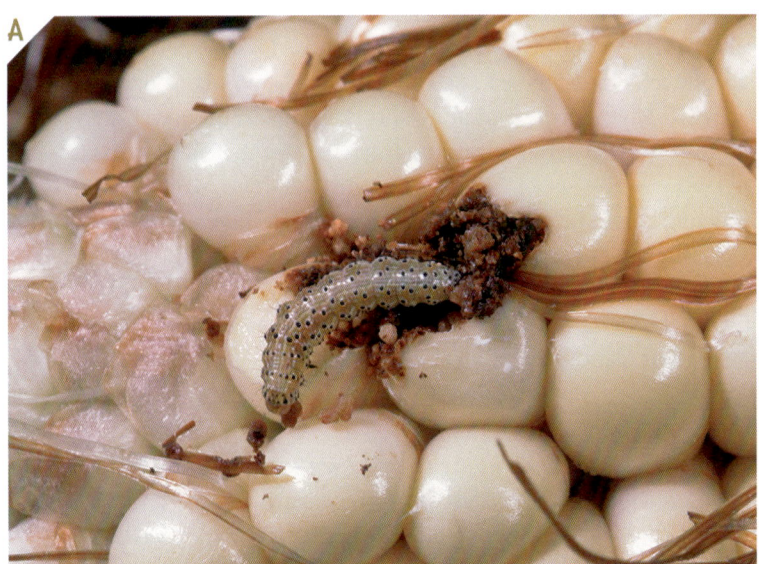
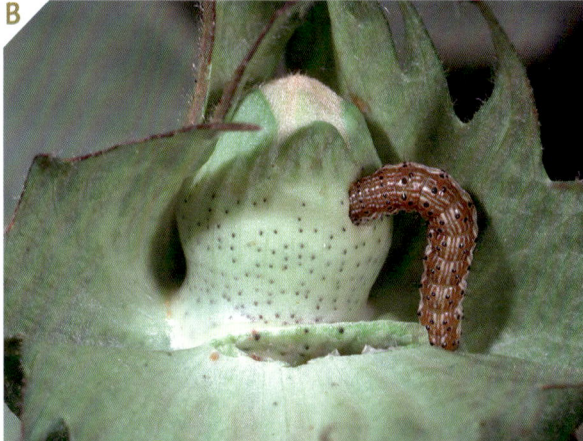
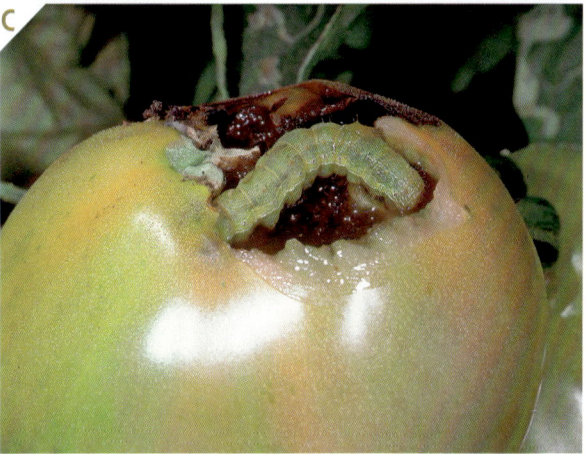

FIGURE 2-1

Common names are not always a dependable way to identify pests because some pests may have more than one common name. The *Helicoverpa zea* shown here, for example, becomes the corn earworm (A), bollworm (B), or tomato fruitworm (C), depending on which crop it is infesting.

the Weed Science Society of America and the Entomological Society of America have developed lists of accepted common names.

Identifying Pests

You can identify pests by using the guidelines included in this chapter and consulting identification books or the University of California's online resources. Or, have the pest examined and identified by specialists. When having pests identified, always collect several specimens.

The difficulty in identifying certain insects and most mites, nematodes, and plant pathogens in the field is their small size. Accurate identification requires the use of a hand lens or microscope, special tests, or careful analysis of damage. Often, the pest's host association and location are important to making positive identifications. Information on the environmental conditions where you collect pests and the time of year of collection provides clues to the pest's identity. Resources on the UC IPM website, ipm.ucdavis.edu, can help you associate pests with their common hosts and the time of year they will be most prevalent.

Pest species may have different physical forms depending on their life cycles or the time of year. Weed seeds, for example, do not resemble seedlings or mature weeds. Many insect species undergo extreme changes in appearance as they develop from eggs through larval, pupal, and adult stages.

IDENTIFICATION EXPERTS

Only trained experts using special techniques and equipment can positively identify pests such as nematodes and most pathogens. Private laboratories exist that can identify nematodes, mites, insects, plant pathogens, and other pests. Farm advisors in each county have expertise in pest identification and are in close contact with other University of California experts. County agricultural commissioners and their staff are helpful resources. In addition, the California Department of Food and Agriculture (CDFA) maintains a pest identification laboratory. Many pest control companies have licensed pest control advisers on their staffs. These experts can identify some types of pests. To contact a farm advisor at a University of California Cooperative Extension office near you, see the UC Division of Agriculture and Natural Resources website, ucanr.edu/County_Offices; to find your local agricultural commissioner, see the CDFA website, cdfa.ca.gov/exec/county/countymap.

When sending samples for identification, be sure to keep the material fresh and undamaged. Provide complete information on where you found the pest and, if appropriate, include examples of pest damage. Weeds, pathogens, and arthropods require different types of sampling and handling. Sidebars in the following sections provide suggestions on how to collect and prepare specimens for shipment to an expert or identification laboratory.

IDENTIFICATION KEYS

Identification keys provide descriptive clues to the identity of living organisms. Unless you are familiar with the terms used to describe the pest's physical structures, many keys are difficult to use. This is because experts develop these keys for use by other experts. However, simple keys are usually available for common pests. A dichotomous key consists of a series of sequentially paired statements. To use a key, begin by selecting the descriptive statement from the first pair that best fits the pest you are trying to identify. The statement you select will lead you to another pair of statements. Continue working through the paired statements in this manner until the key leads you to the pest's identity. Dichotomous keys mainly use structural features, but sometimes they rely on the organism's color or size, especially with weeds. Many keys include photographs or drawings to help illustrate features referred to in the key. Table 2-1 is an example of a dichotomous key.

List and describe the types of resources and references available for identifying pests, symptoms of infestation, and damage caused by pests.

TABLE 2-1

Example of a dichotomous key: Key to common adult cockroaches

Characteristics	Species
1a. Small, about ⅜ in or shorter 1b. Medium to large, longer than ⅜ in	go to line 2 go to line 4
2a. Pronotum without longitudinal black bars 2b. Pronotum with two longitudinal black bars	go to line 3 German cockroach (*Blattella germanica*)
3a. Wings covering about half of abdomen; pronotum narrower 3b. Wings covering nearly all of abdomen or extending beyond; pronotum narrower	western wood roach (*Parcoblatta americana*) brownbanded cockroach (*Supella longipalpa*)
4a. Wings covering abdomen, often extending beyond 4b. Wings absent or shorter than abdomen	go to line 5 Oriental cockroach (*Blatta orientalis*)
5a. Pronotum more than ¼ in wide 5b. Pronotum about ¼ in wide with pale border	go to line 6 wood cockroach (*Parcoblatta* spp.)
6a. Front wing without pale streak; pronotum solid color or with pale design only moderately conspicuous 6b. Front wing with outer pale streak at base; pronotum strikingly marked	go to line 7 Australian cockroach (*Periplaneta australasiae*)
7a. Pronotum usually with some pale area; general color seldom darker than reddish chestnut 7b. Pronotum solid dark color; general color very dark brown to black	go to line 8 smokybrown cockroach (*Periplaneta fuliginosa*)
8a. Last segment of cercus not twice as long as wide 8b. Last segment of cercus twice as long as wide	brown cockroach (*Periplaneta brunnea*) American cockroach (*Periplaneta americana*)

Source: Adapted from Platt 1953.

PHOTOGRAPHS AND DRAWINGS

Whenever possible, use photographs and drawings to help with identification because they provide good visual information about the pest (Fig. 2-2) and its damage and can help you locate the pest's unique or distinguishing features. Use publications such as the California Department of Food and Agriculture *Vertebrate Pest Control Handbook* (available online at the CDFA website, www.vpcrac.org/about/vertebrate-pest-handbook) and the University of California publications *Weeds of California and Other Western States* (DiTomaso and Healy 2007), *Pests of Landscape Trees and Shrubs: An Integrated Pest Management Guide* (Dreistadt 2016), *Pests of the Garden and Small Farm* (Flint 1998), *Wildlife Pest Control Around Gardens and Homes* (Salmon et al. 2006), and the various UC IPM manuals. Also see the UC IPM website, ipm.ucanr.edu, for additional resources, such as weed gallery pages, *Pest Management Guidelines*, IPM manuals for various crops, and *Pest Notes* that can help you identify pests.

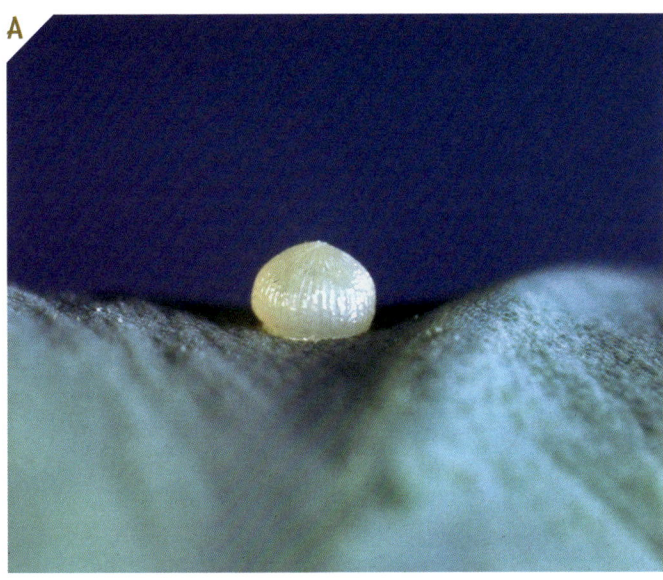

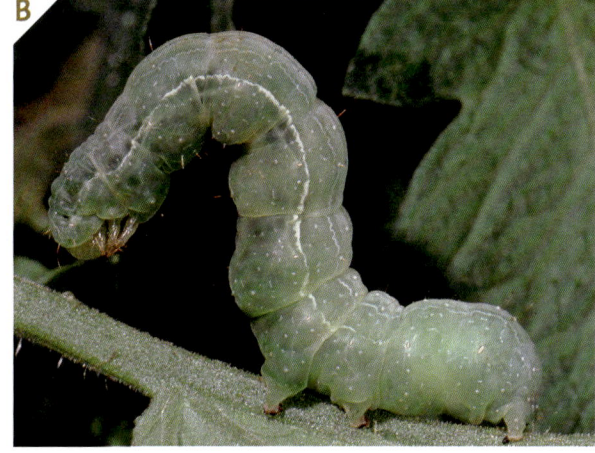

FIGURE 2-2

Photographs such as these of a cabbage looper egg (A) and larva (B) show the unique physical characteristics or coloration patterns that are useful identification aids.

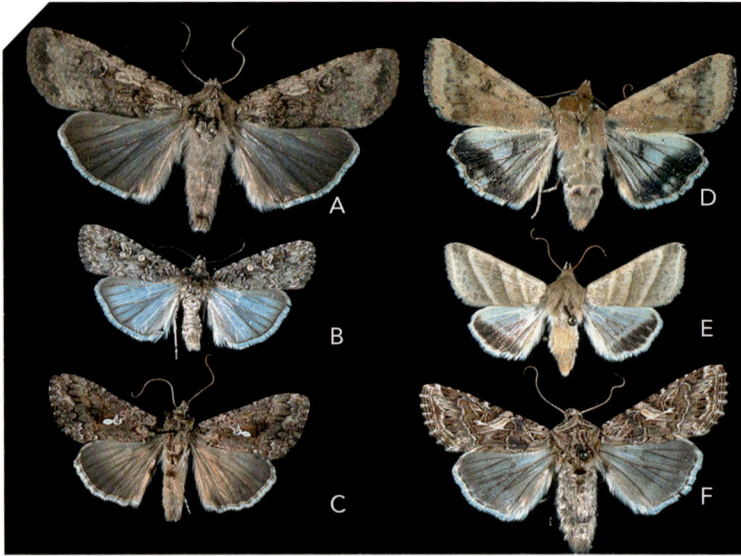

FIGURE 2-3

Preserved specimens, such as these mounted insects, aid in pest identification. These are the adults of (A) the variegated cutworm, (B) the beet armyworm, (C) the cabbage looper, (D) the tomato fruitworm, (E) the tobacco budworm, and (F) the western yellowstriped armyworm.

Preserved Specimens

Experts preserve identified plants, insects and other arthropods, reptiles, and mammals for study and comparison (Fig. 2-3). Museums and herbaria at universities or other institutions are the most common locations for large collections of preserved specimens. You can also buy individual specimens and small collections of more common household and structural pests. Collections of weed seeds are available as helpful identification aids. Most preserved material is fragile, so handle it carefully. Store specimens in a cool, dry place to prevent damage and deterioration.

Characteristic Signs

Pests may leave signs of their presence that help you determine what they are. Birds and rodents build nests that are often characteristic to each species. The type of feeding damage helps you identify many insects. Rodents and other mammals dig unique burrows in the ground and often leave identifying gnaw marks on tree trunks or other objects. Sometimes trails in grass or tracks in dirt are helpful clues to rodent identification. Rodent fecal pellets and insect frass are also distinctive and important identification aids. Weeds may have unique flowers, seeds, fruits, or unusual growth habits. Also look for remains of weed plants from the previous season. Fungi and other pathogens sometimes cause specific types of damage, deformation, or color changes to host tissues.

Weeds

Weeds are plants that interfere with the growing of crops or ornamental plants or cause other types of damage. Some weeds are noxious and endanger livestock. Others affect the health of people or interfere with the safety or use of roads, utilities, and waterways. Invasive weeds can cause ecological damage by displacing native plants and the organisms that feed on them. Weeds compete with agricultural crops for water and nutrients, causing them to become more susceptible to disease or other pests. Many weeds are visual or physical nuisances due to their growth habits and size. Grasses, broadleaved herbaceous plants, shrubs, and even trees are "weeds" if they interfere with the activities of people (Fig. 2-4).

Important weeds, however, possess special characteristics that distinguish them from the occasional out-of-place plant. True weeds

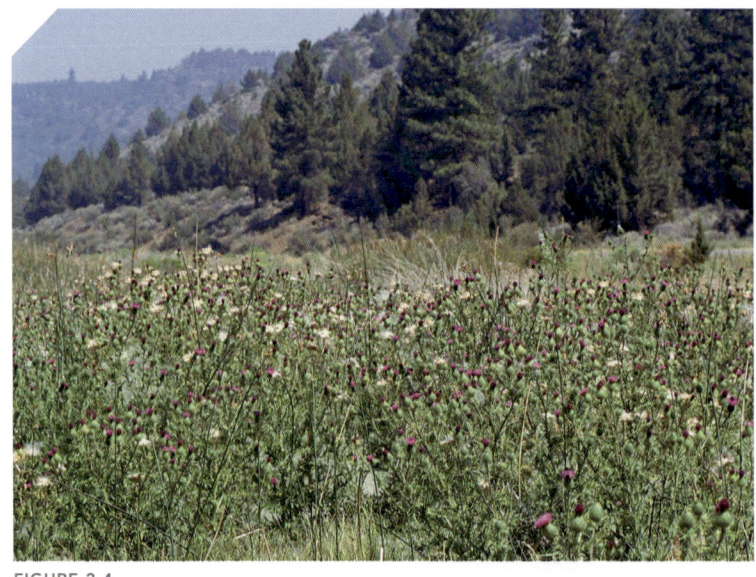

FIGURE 2-4

Weeds are plants that interfere with the growing of desirable plants or endanger the health or safety of people or animals. This photo shows an infestation of bull thistle in rangeland.

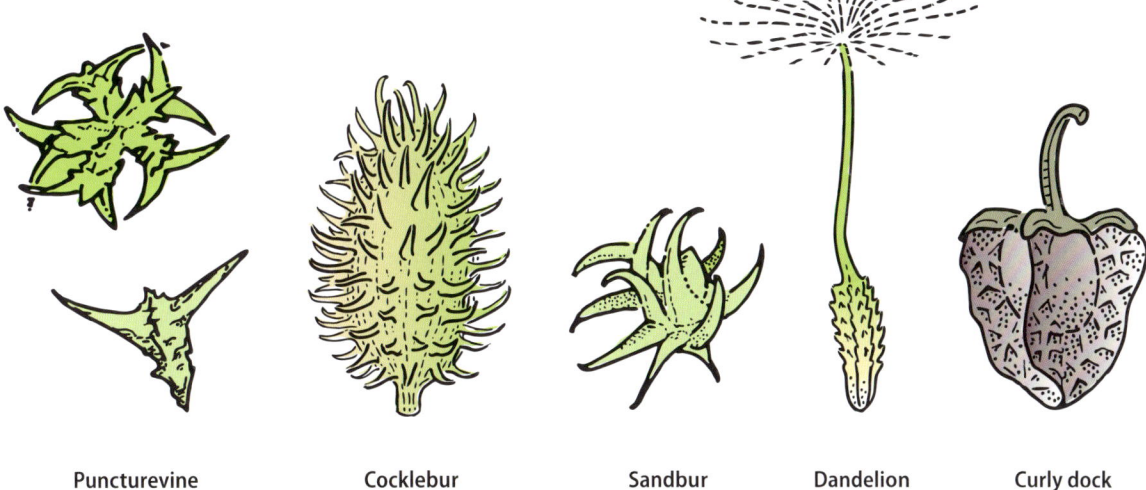

| Puncturevine | Cocklebur | Sandbur | Dandelion | Curly dock |

FIGURE 2-5

Weed seeds such as those shown here have many adaptations enabling them to disperse. These special characteristics are one of the ways weeds compete with other plants.

adapt well to local climates, soils, and other external conditions. They compete successfully with cultivated plants for available resources. Most weeds produce lots of seeds, even under adverse conditions. Seeds of some weeds remain dormant in the soil for extended periods, sometimes 20 years or more, before germinating. Some weed seeds or fruits have special adaptations to promote dispersal (Fig. 2-5). Perennial weeds are capable of reproducing through vegetative structures such as stolons, rhizomes, and tubers (see "Physical Features of Weeds" later in this chapter). Cultural activities that break up these structures, such as hoeing, mowing, or discing, can produce new plants (Fig. 2-6). Consequently, many perennial weeds are persistent and difficult to eliminate.

Some weeds are native plants, while most are exotic species imported inadvertently or intentionally from other parts of the world. In their new location, many imported weeds become serious pests because they lack natural enemies or diseases to suppress them. The weeds thrive if local environments are ideal for their growth.

Weed experts consider only about 3% of the identified plant species found in the world to be weeds. Usually, there are no more than 25 to 35 weed species at any one crop or landscape site. It is common for specific sites to have certain groups of weed species associated with them. Sometimes weeds found in crops or other cultivated areas are difficult to control with herbicides because they are similar to the cultivated plants. You can find discussions and illustrations of some of the major weed families at the end of this section.

How Weeds Are Pests

Weeds compete with agricultural crops for water, nutrients, light, and space, and they may also interfere with farming operations. Some weed species are toxic to livestock. Others release compounds into the soil that inhibit the growth of other plants. Weeds clog irrigation canals and drainage ditches. Uncontrolled weeds contaminate products at harvest (such as forage crops harvested to feed livestock) and can harbor insects and pathogens.

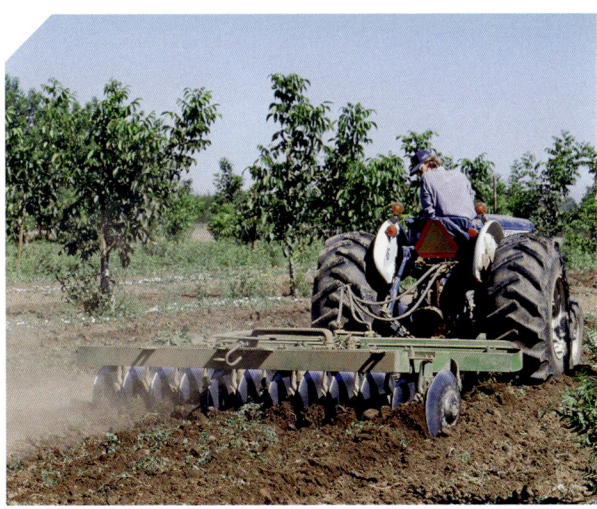

FIGURE 2-6

Cultural activities such as discing can disperse some weeds. Cultivation breaks plants up into smaller segments that can reroot and form new plants.

> **SIDEBAR 2-1**
>
> ### SAMPLING AND SENDING WEEDS FOR IDENTIFICATION
>
> **SAMPLING**
> 1. Choose several plants that represent the species.
> 2. Include stems, leaves, flowers (if present), and roots.
> 3. Dig up weeds to prevent damage to roots.
> 4. Shake plants lightly after digging to remove excess soil.
>
> **PREPARATION**
> 1. Keep plants in an ice chest while you are in the field. If they cannot be shipped immediately, store them in a refrigerator.
> 2. Place plants in plastic bags without moisture, or press them between sheets of absorbent paper, and encase them in heavy cardboard for protection.
>
> **LABELING**
>
> Attach a label to the outside of each sample. Include the following information on labels:
> 1. Location where samples were taken, including names of nearby crossroads.
> 2. Description of specific characteristics of the site where the weeds were growing.
> 3. Whether plants are annuals or perennials.
> 4. Your name, address, telephone number, and email address (if you have one).
> 5. Date samples were taken.
> 6. Any other information that would help in the identification of the weeds.
>
> **SHIPPING**
> 1. Contact the person or laboratory that will receive samples to determine the best method of shipping and to inform them that samples will be arriving.
> 2. Pack samples in a sturdy, well-insulated container to prevent crushing or heat damage.
> 3. Mark package clearly and request shipper to keep it in a cool location.
> 4. Ship packages early in the week so they will arrive before a weekend.

Around homes, businesses, and industry, heavy populations of weeds often infest lawns, ground covers, and ornamental plantings. Weeds sometimes harbor insect or vertebrate pests and detract from the appearance of landscaping. Dry weeds are fire hazards. Various weed pollens cause allergies in some people, and certain weeds produce skin irritation.

Along roadsides and rights-of-way, large weeds interfere with travel and maintenance operations. Tall roadside weeds obscure signs, while creeping species clog road drains or erode pavement edges. In commercially operated forests, weeds compete with tree seedlings and become fire hazards; they also interfere with normal cultural activities. Some weeds, such as mistletoe and dodder, parasitize trees. Overgrown aquatic weeds clog irrigation canals, ditches, streams, rivers, and lakes. These cause harm to native aquatic life and make the use of waterways difficult for people and animals. Large infestations of aquatic weeds also hinder fish growth and reproduction. Aquatic weeds promote mosquito problems by decreasing normal water flow and wave action.

Invasive plants can cause significant economic and ecological damage in natural areas. Invasive species can
- reduce livestock forage quality and quantity
- jeopardize animal and human health
- increase the threat of fire or flooding
- interfere with recreational activities
- lower land value

Invasive plants are sometimes the cause of dramatic ecological changes that impact plant and animal communities. They can also transform environments in many ways, including changing the soil fertility of the ecosystem, promoting soil erosion by increasing water runoff down slopes, building up of leaf litter that acts as a suppressive mulch, and preventing the establishment of more desirable species.

Overall, uncontrolled growth of invasive plants creates a more suitable environment for additional species to invade, resulting in a decrease in plant diversity as non-native plants crowd out native species.

IDENTIFYING WEEDS

Specialists identify plants, including weeds, by recognizing differences and similarities among flowers, leaves, stems, and roots. Fruits, seeds, and special structures such as tubers or rhizomes are also useful identification characteristics, as are the plant's growth habits. If you can't identify a weed right away, you may need to send it to an expert for identification (see Sidebar 2-1).

Weed Classification. Most weeds fall within two major plant groups, the dicots and the monocots. Dicots, also called broadleaves, are plants that produce two seedling leaves (cotyledons); leaves of dicots usually have netlike veins. Dicots generally grow as herbaceous plants (leafy and herblike) or as woody plants (shrub- or treelike).

Monocots produce only a single grasslike leaf in the seedling. Leaves of these plants typically have veins that run parallel to their length. Grasses, sedges, and rushes are monocots.

Mosses and liverworts belong to a unique group of plants known as bryophytes. Bryophytes are different from land plants because they lack a vascular system. They are occasional pests in aquatic settings and sometimes cause problems in greenhouses or on buildings or ornamental plants.

Algae are primitive, nonflowering aquatic plants that often clog streams, lakes, drainage ditches, and rice fields. Pest managers usually include algae among weed pests. Like more highly developed plants, algae carry out photosynthesis to convert light into energy. However, algae lack true stems, leaves, and flowers that are characteristic of higher plants. They reproduce through cell division or production of spores.

It is usually easy to determine whether the weed is a land plant, bryophyte, or alga. However, when identifying land weeds, you must distinguish between a woody or herbaceous dicot (broadleaf) or a monocot (grass, rush, or sedge), because herbicides are often developed to control particular weed types.

Weed Development. Annual and some perennial weeds pass through several stages of development, beginning with the seed. Sprouted seeds, known as seedlings, are usually tender and vulnerable to environmental extremes and are often quite susceptible to herbicides. Seedlings differ in appearance from mature plants, which can make identifying weeds difficult. Because they are the stage most readily controlled, learn to identify weed seedlings.

From seedlings, weeds progress through a vegetative growth stage marked by rapid foliage development as they attain their maximum size. They then enter a reproductive period in which they divert most of their energy to flowering and seed production. Once they form seeds, weeds reach maturity, which is often referred to as their post-reproductive period. Perennial plants continue to repeat vegetative growth and reproductive cycles each year.

For identification, learn to recognize the different growth stages of weeds (Figs. 2-7, 2-8).

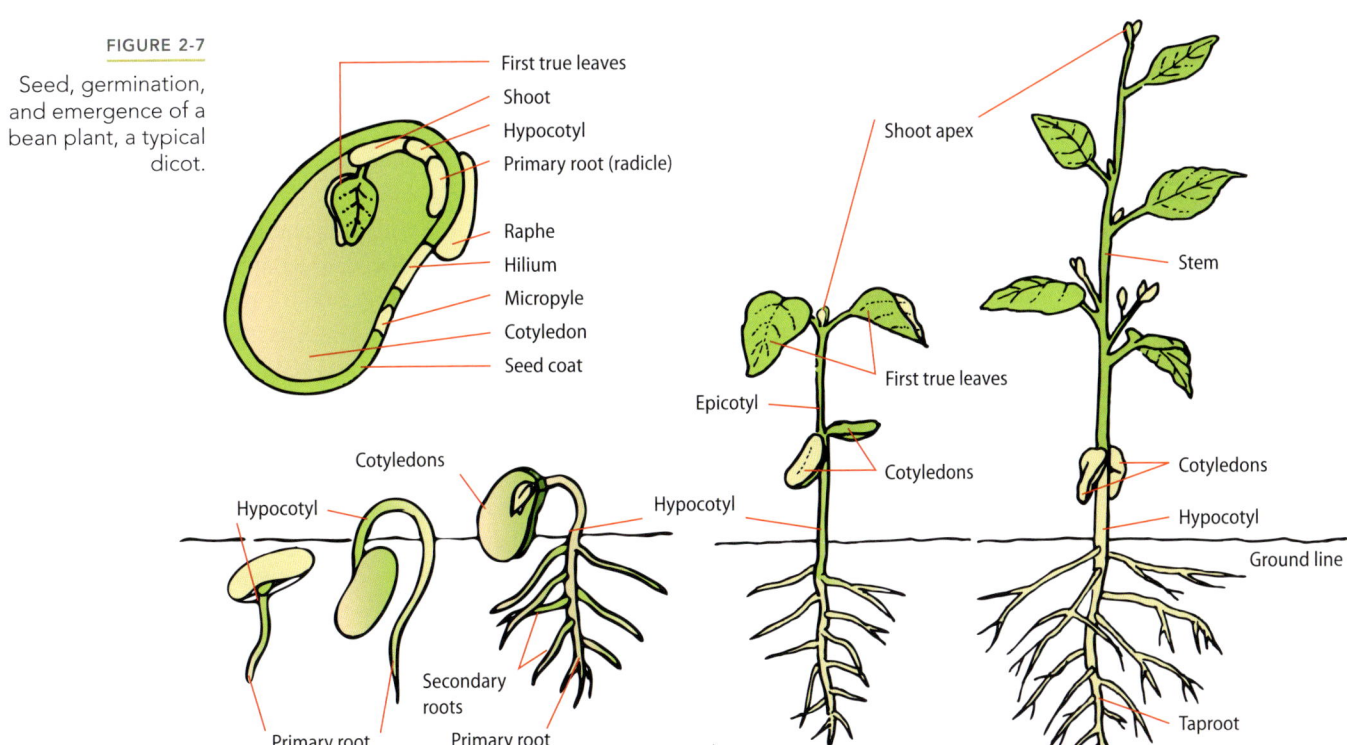

FIGURE 2-7

Seed, germination, and emergence of a bean plant, a typical dicot.

FIGURE 2-8

This illustration shows the difference in the growth periods of winter and summer annual weeds and the growth stages of perennial weeds.

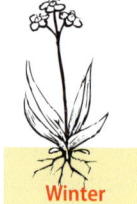 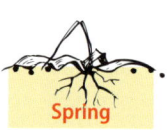 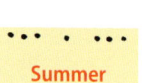 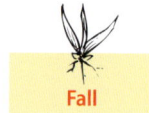

Winter annual
Winter annuals germinate in the fall, mature in the winter, and die in early summer. The seeds remain dormant until the fall.

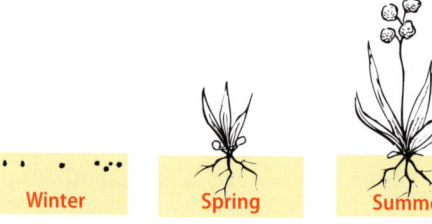 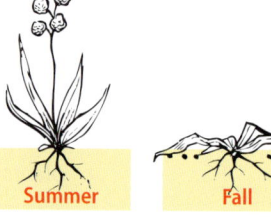

Summer annual
Summer annuals germinate in the spring, mature in the summer, and die in the fall. The seeds remain dormant until the spring.

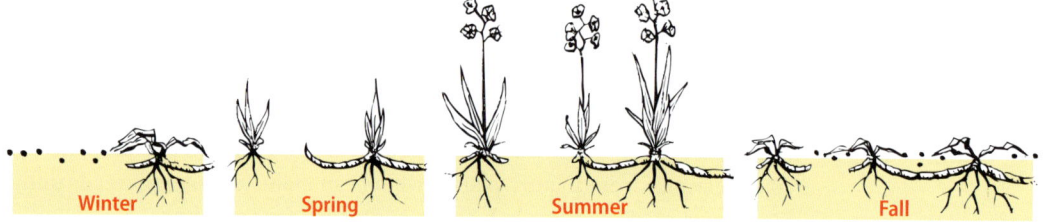

Perennial
Herbaceous perennials grow new plants from seeds or vegetative parts, such as rhizomes, bulbs, tubers, or rootstocks, in the spring. They mature in the summer and die in the fall; seeds and underground parts overwinter.

Understanding growth stages is also important when selecting and using herbicides or other methods of weed control.

Weed Life Cycles. Weed life cycles may be annual, biennial, or perennial. Occasionally, some weed species with one type of life cycle may behave as if they have a different life cycle due to favorable weather or abnormal or unusual changes in environmental influences. Milder temperatures, for example, promote longer life cycles. Once you are familiar with the life cycle of a weed, you can properly time herbicide applications so they are maximally effective. For instance, most perennial weeds are not very susceptible to herbicides during early bloom stages, so you should avoid making applications at that time.

Annual weeds live 1 year or less. They sprout from seeds, mature, and produce seeds for the next generation during this period. Annual weeds are either summer annuals or winter annuals (Fig. 2-8). Seeds of summer annuals sprout in the spring, and the plants produce seeds and die during the summer or fall. Some common summer annual weeds include pigweed, puncturevine, barnyardgrass, Russian thistle, common purslane, and yellow foxtail. Seeds of winter annuals sprout in the fall, then grow over the winter. These plants produce seeds in the spring and usually die before summer. Mustard, wild oat, annual bluegrass, burclover, and filaree are examples of winter annual weeds. When environmental conditions in an area are suitable for growth, however, both winter and summer annuals may be found year-round.

Biennial plants live for two growing seasons. They sprout and undergo vegetative growth during the first season, then flower, produce seeds, and die the following season. Bristly oxtongue, poison hemlock, wild carrot, mullein, and Scotch thistle are biennials.

Perennial weeds live 2 or more years; some species live indefinitely. Many perennials lose their leaves or die back entirely during the winter (herbaceous perennials). These plants regrow each spring from roots or underground storage organs such as tubers, bulbs, or rhizomes. These storage organs provide the chief means of dispersal for a number of major perennial weeds as

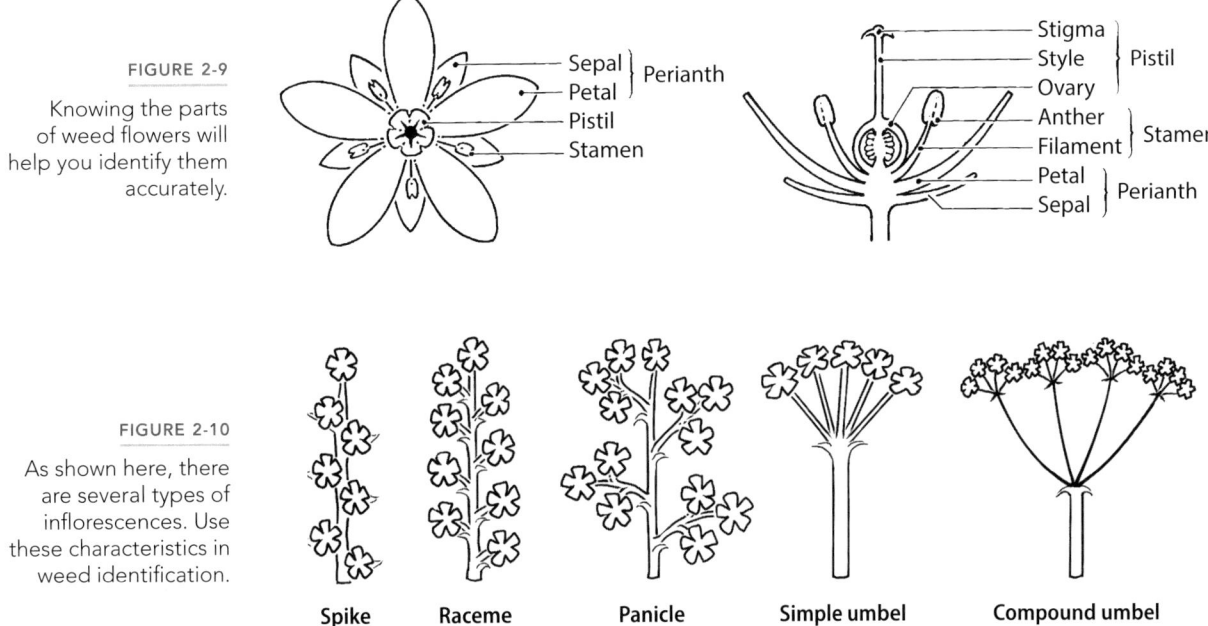

FIGURE 2-9
Knowing the parts of weed flowers will help you identify them accurately.

FIGURE 2-10
As shown here, there are several types of inflorescences. Use these characteristics in weed identification.

well. Examples of perennial weeds include curly dock, silverleaf nightshade, field bindweed, alkali sida, dandelion, yellow nutsedge, Pacific poison oak, johnsongrass, and bermudagrass. Woody plants such as trees and shrubs are perennials and can be weeds under certain circumstances. Perennial weeds are the most difficult type of weed to control.

Physical Features of Weeds. Flowers, leaves, stems and special rooting structures, roots, and fruits and seeds are used to identify weeds.

Flowers. Flowers contain sexual reproductive organs and differ widely among species. To use flowers as an identification aid, become familiar with the different flower parts (Fig. 2-9). Flowers occur singly or as compound inflorescences, groups of flowers arising from a common main stem. Various names, such as panicle, raceme, spike, head, umbel, and catkin, describe the arrangement of flowers in an inflorescence (Fig. 2-10).

Leaves. The arrangement and shape of leaves, vein patterns, and presence of spines or hairs are helpful identifying characteristics. When identifying seedlings, leaves are the only easily visible structures. Cotyledons and occasionally the first true leaves of broadleaved plants differ from the plant's mature foliage. For grasses, experts rely on the collar region of the plant, where leaves separate from the main stem.

Stems. Stems form the weed's basic framework or skeleton. They connect roots to other structures, providing support for leaves and flowers as well as channels for transport of nutrients

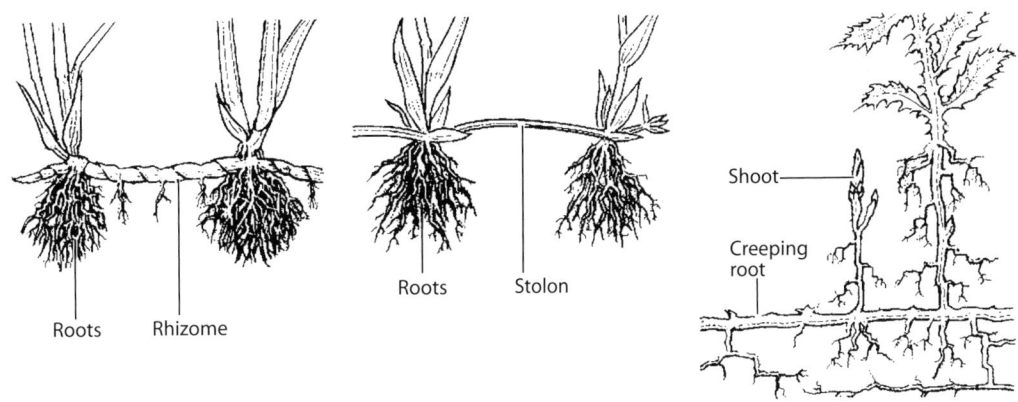

FIGURE 2-11
Many weeds reproduce by underground and aboveground rooting structures such as those illustrated here.

and water. Specialized stem modifications enable some weeds to reproduce vegetatively (Fig. 2-11). Rhizomes are elongated underground stems that grow horizontally from the plant. Tubers also grow underground and are enlarged fleshy growths arising from stems, rhizomes, or roots. A stolon is a stem that grows horizontally above the ground surface and roots at nodes.

Roots. Roots absorb water and nutrients from the soil and store food. The creeping roots of some plants give rise to stems. Some weeds have thick, elongated taproots from which short lateral rootlets grow (e.g., dandelions). Other weeds have networks of fine, branching fibrous roots, as seen in grasses.

Fruits and seeds. A fruit is the ripened ovary of a plant's flower. Seeds are the primary way weeds reproduce. Fruits and seeds help you identify weeds because they are unique in their shape, size, markings, and color.

> List examples of common pests in California from each main group, and describe the damage they cause.

Algae

Important Characteristics. Algae are primitive plants closely related to some fungi and protozoans. They reproduce by means of spores, cell division, or fragmentation. There are more than 17,000 identified species of algae. Pest algae fall within three general groups: planktonic or microscopic, filamentous, and attached-erect (Fig. 2-12A). Microscopic algae impart greenish or reddish colors to water. They often float on the water surface as scums. Filamentous algae form dense, free-floating mats or mats attached to aquatic plants or rocks. Attached-erect algae, known as *Cham* and *Nitella*, resemble flowering plants with leaflike and stemlike structures.

Algae clog irrigation channels, irrigation equipment, waterways, and ponds and render swimming pools unsightly (Fig. 2-12B). Large algal buildup may deplete oxygen within a body of water and kill fish. Some forms release toxins into water as they decompose, which may poison people or livestock.

Where Found. Algae occur in swimming pools, ponds, lakes, streams, rivers, and other bodies of water. They also become pests in irrigation canals. Some forms of algae are problems in flooded rice fields and greenhouses.

Sedge Family

Important Characteristics. Many sedges and rushes (Fig. 2-13) are perennial plants. They are grasslike and have fibrous root systems, and their perennial species produce rhizomes or tubers. Sedges have elongated, V-shaped leaves arising from triangular stems. Rushes have round leaves and a solid, round

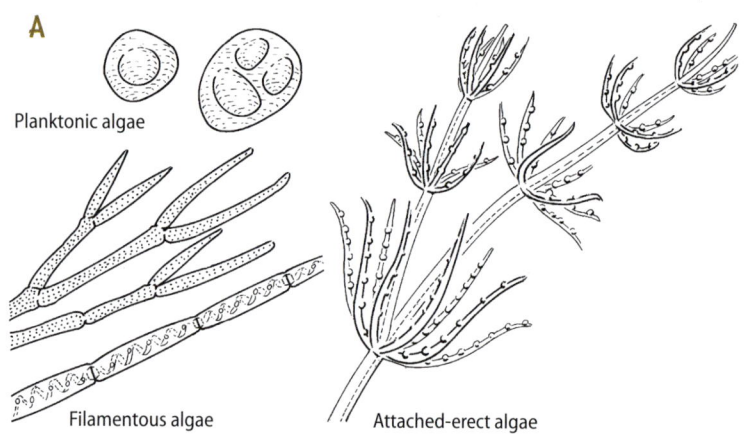
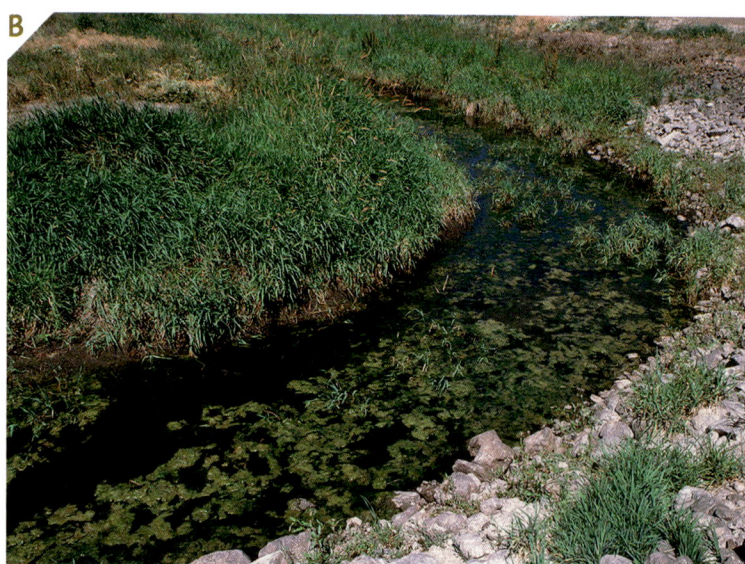

FIGURE 2-12

There are three types of algae: planktonic, filamentous, and attached-erect. (Drawings are greatly enlarged.) Algae often clog waterways, as seen in the photograph.

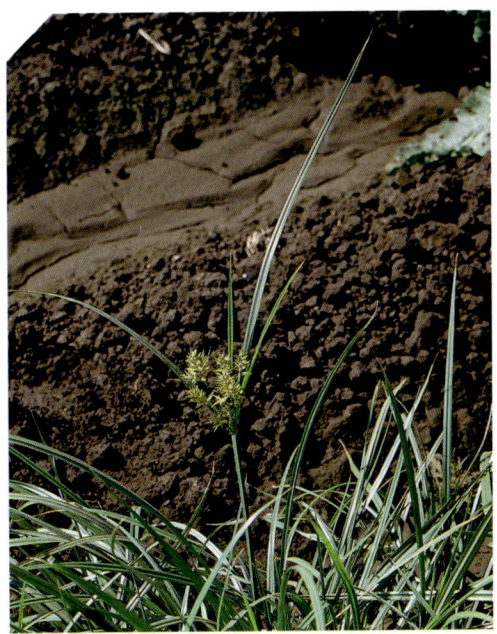

FIGURE 2-13

Sedges are grasslike plants with fibrous root systems. They are usually found in marshy or poorly drained areas.

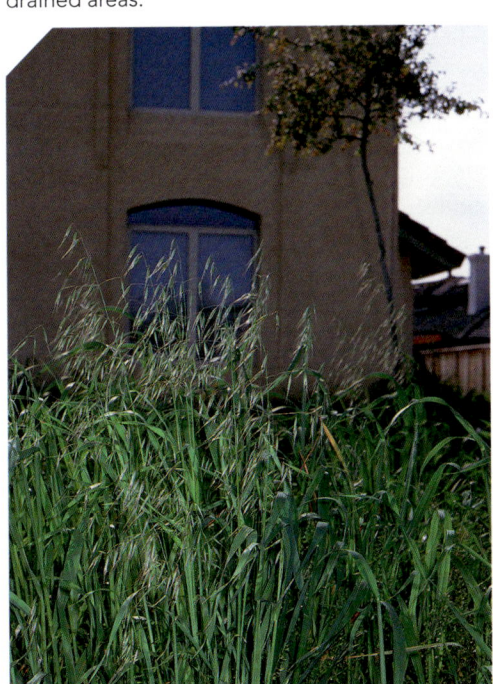

stem. These stem characteristics distinguish sedges and rushes from grasses, which have a hollow, round stem.

Where Found. Sedges are pests in orchards, vineyards, irrigated crops, and home gardens. They cause severe problems in rice fields. Sedges usually occur in marshy or poorly drained areas and along edges of ditches and ponds. Rushes are generally problems in aquatic systems and inhabit ecosystems similar to those of sedges.

Examples. Yellow nutsedge (*Cyperus esculentus*), purple nutsedge (*C. rotundus*). Rushes include blunt spikerush (*Eleocharis obtusa*), hardstem bulrush (*Scirpus acutus*), and river bulrush (*S. fluviatilis*).

Grass Family

Important Characteristics. Grasses (Fig. 2-14) are a large family of annual or perennial plants. They include many notable weeds as well as important cultivated crops such as grains. Some species provide substantial food sources for grazing livestock. Roots of grasses are dense and fibrous; several species reproduce by rhizomes. A major feature used in grass identification is the collar region (Fig. 2-15). A thin outgrowth or fringe of hairs known as the ligule occurs at the collar region in many species of grasses.

Several important grassy weeds are winter annuals. Wild oat, for example, is one of the most widely distributed, troublesome winter annual weeds in California.

Where Found. Most cultivated and natural areas contain grassy weeds. They are often pests in fields, pastures, rangelands, orchards, vineyards, landscaped areas, turf, along roadsides and ditch banks, and in other locations.

Examples. Wild oat (*Avena fatua*), foxtail brome (*Bromus rubens*), bermudagrass (*Cynodon dactylon*), smooth crabgrass (*Digitaria ischaemum*), barnyardgrass (*Echinochloa crus-galli*), deergrass (*Muhlenbergia rigens*), dallisgrass (*Paspalum dilatatum*), annual bluegrass (*Poa annua*), yellow foxtail (*Setaria glauca*), and johnsongrass (*Sorghum halepense*).

FIGURE 2-14

Grasses, like the wild oat shown here, are one of the largest families of important weeds.

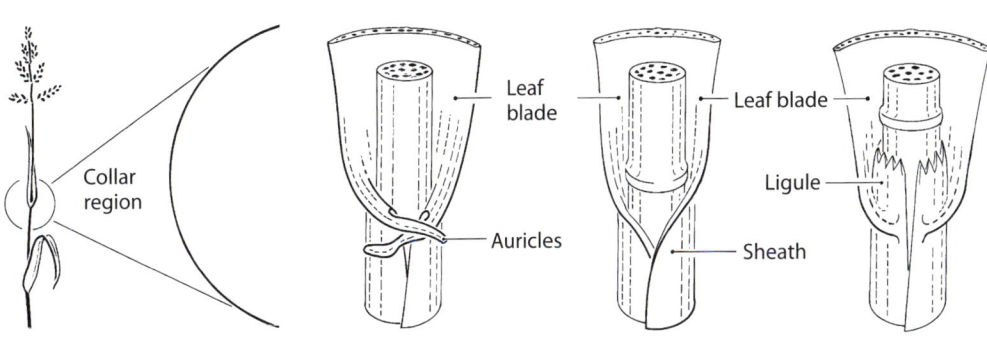

FIGURE 2-15

The collar region of a grass leaf contains unique structures that are very important in identifying grass species.

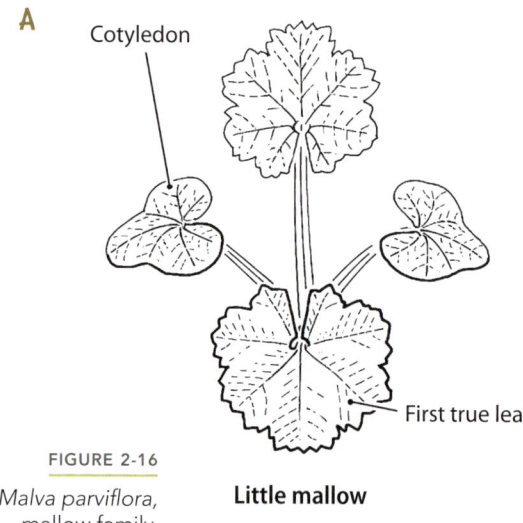

FIGURE 2-16
Malva parviflora, mallow family.

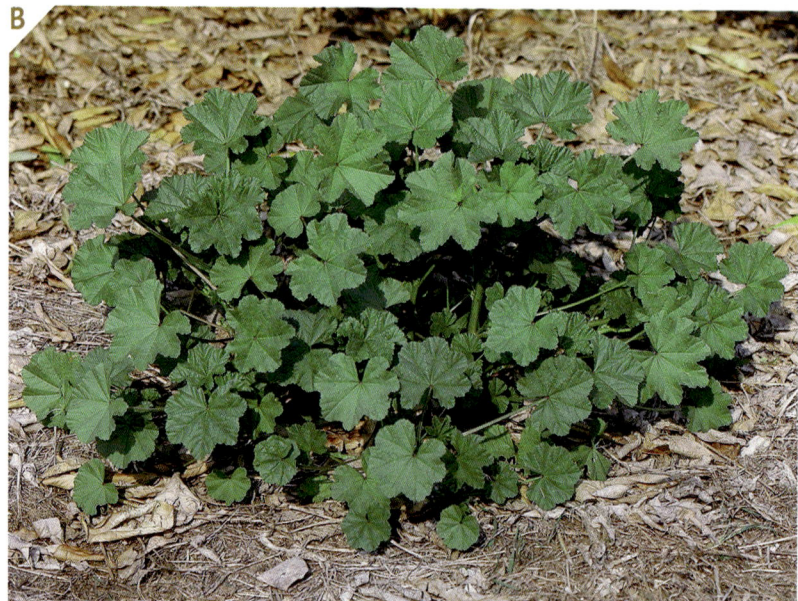

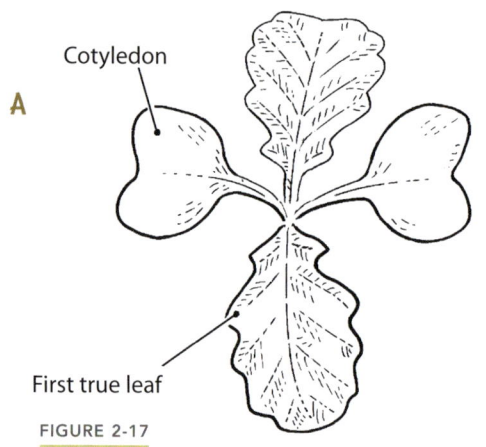

FIGURE 2-17
Brassica rapa, mustard family.

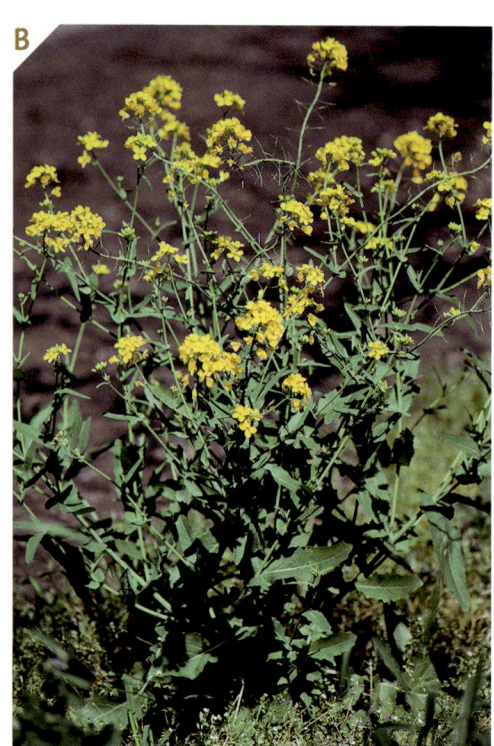

Mallow Family

Important Characteristics. Mallows are annual or perennial broad-leaved weeds, depending on the species (Fig. 2-16). Most are tolerant to many of the widely used herbicides, making them persistent pests. Most species are herbaceous plants that grow from ½ to 7 feet tall. They produce capsule- or disclike fruits that enclose several seeds. Their leaves are usually round with serrated edges and have a characteristic palmate vein structure (the veins radiate from a common center). The cotyledons are roundish to heart shaped or pear shaped.

Where Found. Weeds in the mallow family are pests in annual crops, orchards, vineyards, and along roadsides, ditch banks, and in waste areas.

Examples. Venice mallow (*Hibiscus trionum*), velvetleaf (*Abutilon theophrasti*), little mallow (*Malva parviflora*), and alkali sida (*Malva leprosa*).

Mustard Family

Important Characteristics. Mustards are usually upright broad-leaved weeds that grow from 1 to 5 feet tall, depending on the species (Fig. 2-17). Many have yellow flowers. Seedlings usually have broad cotyledons, which in some species are kidney shaped or indented at the tip. They have annual or biennial life cycles.

Where Found. Mustards occur in fields, orchards, vineyards, pastures, along roadsides and ditch banks, and in vacant lots and waste areas.

Examples. Black mustard (*Brassica nigra*), birdsrape mustard (*B. rapa*), shepherdspurse (*Capsella bursa-pastoris*), hoary cress (*Cardaria draba*), wild radish (*Raphanus raphanistrum*), and London rocket (*Sisymbrium irio*).

PEST IDENTIFICATION   33

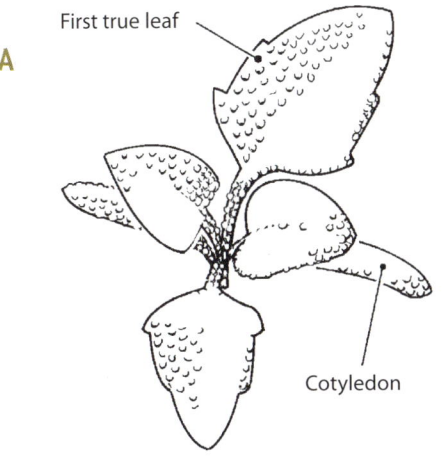

Goosefoot Family

Important Characteristics. Weeds of the goosefoot family include annuals, biennials, and perennials (Fig. 2-18). These broadleaved plants are variable in size, depending on the species and where they are growing. Some reach heights of 6 feet; other species range in height from 8 to 24 inches. Mature leaves often have notches and are usually tinged with purple. Many species have elongated cotyledon leaves that are four to six times longer than their width.

Where Found. Weeds in the goosefoot family are widespread and are found in agronomic, horticultural, and vegetable crops. They grow abundantly in waste places, along roadsides, and along irrigation and drainage ditches.

Examples. Australian saltbush (*Atriplex semibaccata*), common lambsquarters (*Chenopodium album*), nettleleaf goosefoot (*C. murale*), and Russian thistle (*Salsola iberica*).

Amaranth Family

Important Characteristics. Amaranths are mostly upright, broadleaved, herbaceous plants that can be annual, biennial, or short-lived perennials. Some species reach 8 feet in height (Fig. 2-19), but there is also a low-growing, prostrate species. Amaranths have small, inconspicuous greenish flowers. The cotyledons are narrow and elongate and are four to five times as long as they are wide. Seedling leaves are dull green to reddish on upper surfaces and magenta to bright red underneath. Some amaranths can cause nitrate poisoning in livestock under certain environmental conditions.

Where Found. Amaranths are pests in most cultivated crops, orchards, and vineyards. They often grow along ditch banks and roadsides and in waste areas.

Examples. Tumble pigweed (*Amaranthus albus*), prostrate pigweed (*A. blitoides*), and redroot pigweed (*A. retroflexus*).

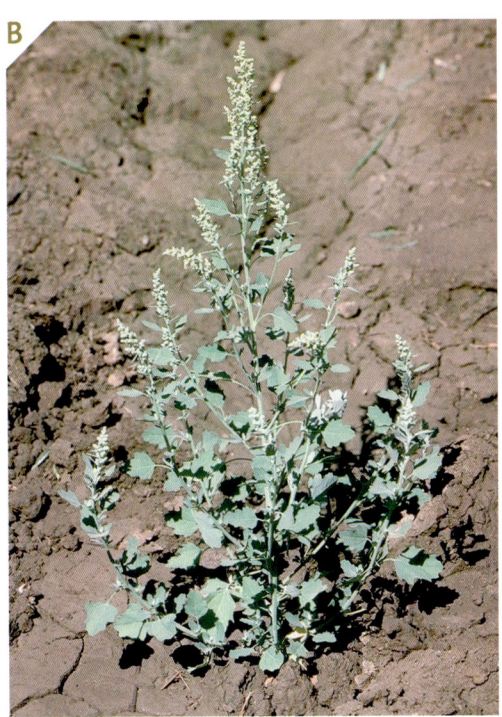

FIGURE 2-18

Chenopodium album, goosefoot family.

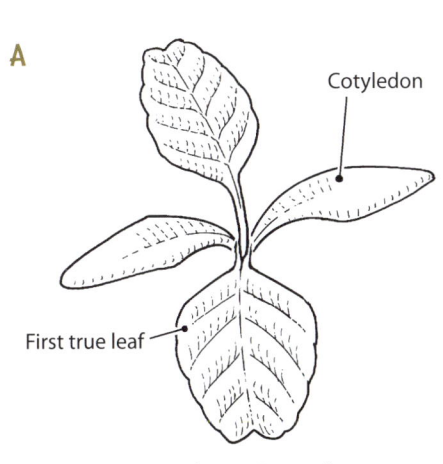

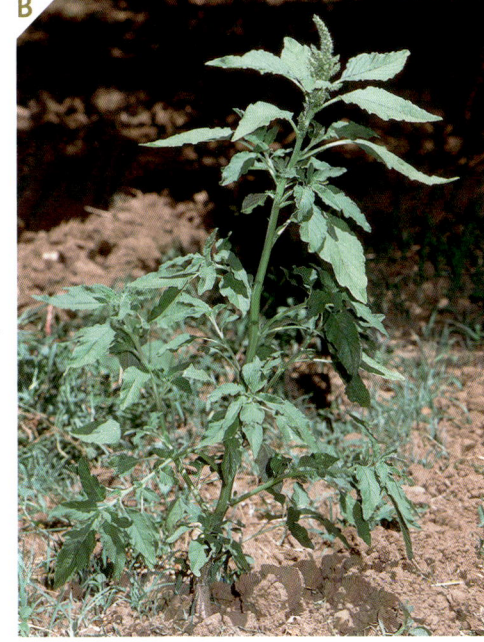

FIGURE 2-19

Amaranthus retroflexus, amaranth family.

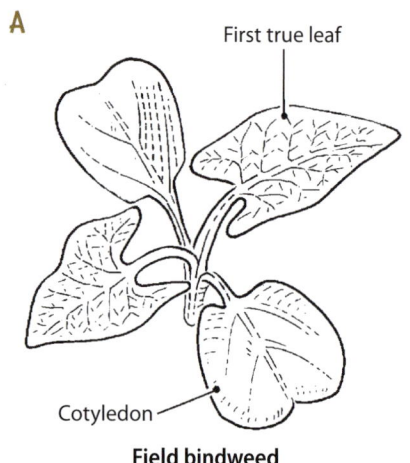
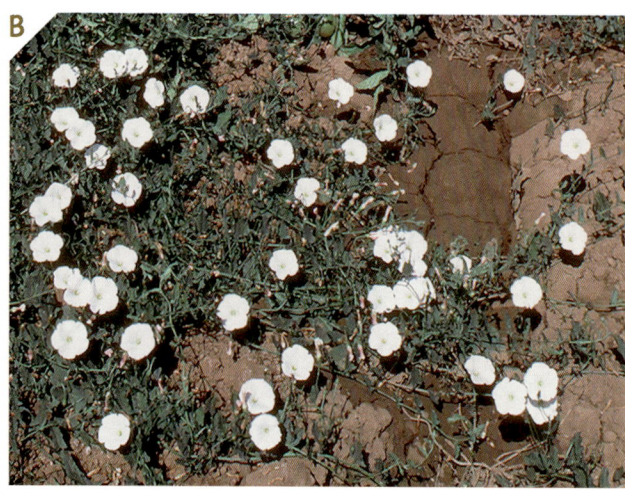

FIGURE 2-20
Convolvulus arvensis, morningglory family.

Field bindweed

Morningglory Family

Important Characteristics. Weeds in the morningglory family include annuals and perennials. These are low-growing vines (Fig. 2-20). One species, field bindweed, is one of the most difficult perennial broadleaved weeds to control in California. Cotyledons of plants in this family are large and roundish and notched on the end. The first true leaves are triangular.

Where Found. Weeds of the morningglory family occur in all agronomic and vegetable crops as well as along roadsides and ditch banks.

Examples. Field bindweed (*Convolvulus arvensis*), ivyleaf morningglory (*Ipomoea hederacea*), and tall morningglory (*I. purpurea*).

Potato Family

Important Characteristics. The potato family contains a large number of pest weeds that can be annuals or perennials. Most are low-growing, bushy, broadleaved plants reaching heights of about 3 feet (Fig. 2-21). Tree tobacco grows to 12 feet. Cotyledons are longer than they are wide, sometimes by as much as eight to ten times. This leaf gently tapers to a point at the end. Some species produce thorny seedpods, while others produce rounded berries with many seeds. Several species are poisonous to people and livestock because seeds and young leaves contain high levels of alkaloids.

Where Found. Weeds in the potato family occur in agronomic crops and along roadsides, ditch banks, and fencerows. They are also pests in vineyards and orchards.

Examples. Chinese thornapple (*Datura ferox*), jimsonweed (*D. stramonium*), Indian tobacco (*Nicotiana quadrivalvis*), tree tobacco (*N. glauca*), Wright groundcherry, lanceleaf groundcherry, and tomatillo groundcherry (*Physalis* spp.). Also silverleaf nightshade, black nightshade, and hairy nightshade (*Solanum* spp.).

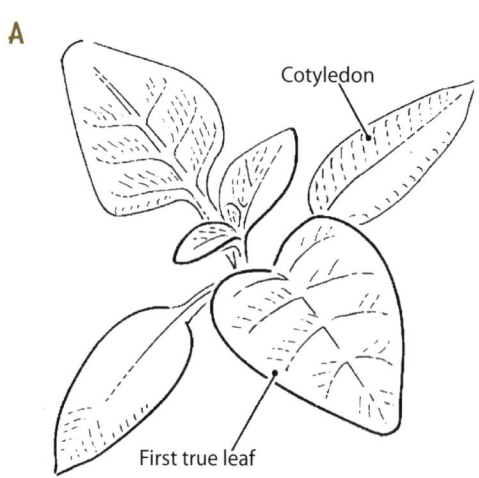
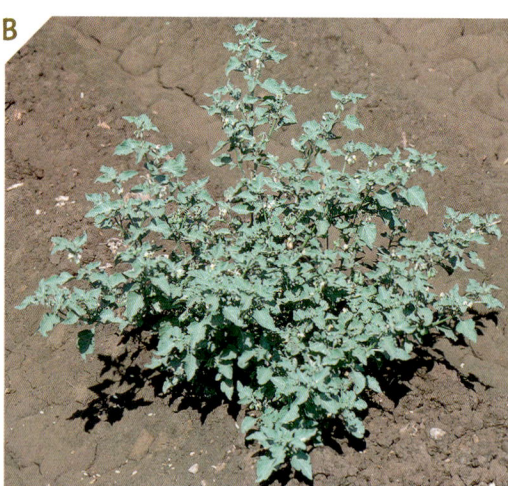

FIGURE 2-21
Centaurea solstitialis, aster family.

Black nightshade

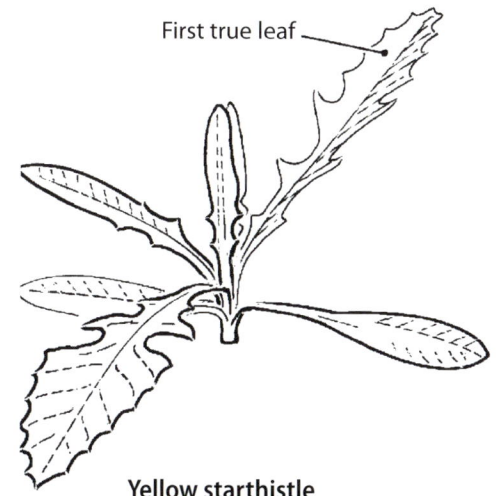

Yellow starthistle

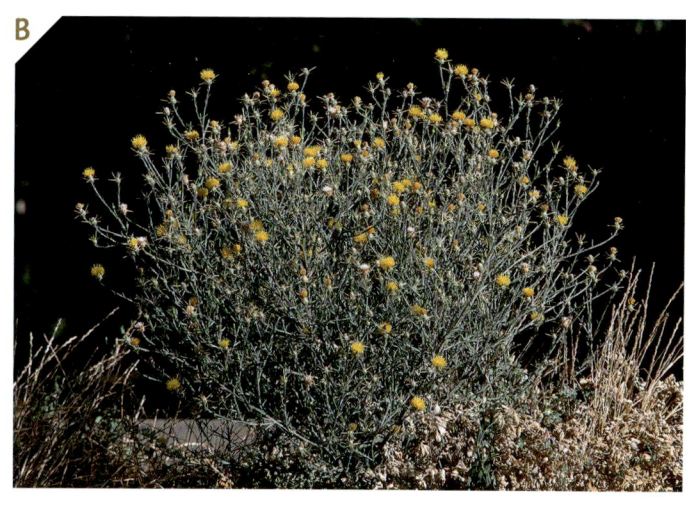

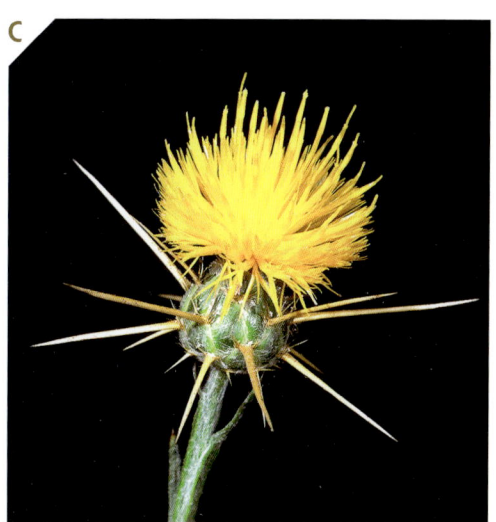

FIGURE 2-22

Centaurea solstitialis, aster family.

Aster Family

Important Characteristics. The very large aster family contains many important annual and perennial broadleaved weeds. Many weeds in this family are "thistles" (Fig. 2-22), characterized by spines on their leaves, stems, or flowers. These weeds are usually erect plants; many grow to heights of 1 to 3 feet while others are much taller. Most have showy flowers.

Where Found. Weed species in this family grow in almost all open or cultivated areas. These include rangelands, along roadsides and ditch banks, along fencerows, and in vacant lots, cultivated crops, orchards, vineyards, and lawns.

Examples. Common yarrow (*Achillea millefolium*), California mugwort (*Artemisia douglasiana*), Russian knapweed (*Acroptilon repens*), yellow starthistle (*Centaurea solstitialis*), Canada thistle (*Cirsium arvense*), bull thistle (*C. vulgare*), common sunflower (*Helianthus annuus*), Jerusalem artichoke (*H. tuberosus*), telegraphplant (*Heterotheca grandiflora*), prickly lettuce (*Lactuca serriola*), pineapple weed (*Matricaria matricarioides*), Scotch thistle (*Onopordum acanthium*), bristly oxtongue (*Picris echioides*), common groundsel (*Senecio vulgaris*), California goldenrod (*Solidago californica*), annual sowthistle (*Sonchus oleraceus*), dandelion (*Taraxacum officinale*), and common cocklebur (*Xanthium strumarium*).

Invertebrates

Invertebrates are animals without backbones (vertebrae). These include nematodes and all other worms, snails and slugs, and arthropods (insects, spiders, mites, and their relatives). Pest invertebrates affect people in many ways. Some are parasites of livestock, poultry, or human beings; they feed on skin, hair, and blood or invade internal tissues. Many invertebrates transmit disease organisms to people, pets, livestock, poultry, or plants. A large number of invertebrate pests are herbivores and feed on growing plants. Invertebrates also consume or contaminate stored food products. Some invertebrates even damage buildings and other structures, as well as books, fabrics, furniture, equipment, and other items.

ARTHROPODS

Arthropods are one of the largest groups in the animal kingdom. The word *arthropod* means "jointed foot" and refers to organisms with an external skeleton and jointed body parts. Insects, spiders, ticks, and mites are part of this group, as are crabs, crayfish, shrimp, and lobsters. Centipedes, millipedes, scorpions, and sowbugs are also arthropods. Only about 3% of the arthropod species that occur in the United States are pests, however. Table 2-2 lists some of the ways that arthropods interfere with human activities. Most arthropod species are beneficial to people, plants, or livestock (Table 2-3).

Sometimes an arthropod may be a pest in one situation but beneficial in another. For example, venomous spiders are pests when they disturb or endanger people or animals. However, in gardens and agricultural situations they help control harmful insects and other arthropod pests.

In addition, arthropods that attack or parasitize pests or serve as pollinators are considered beneficial organisms and should be protected whenever possible.

How to Identify Arthropods. Identify pest arthropods by distinguishing between the various types of body structures that are unique to different groups. Some insects undergo changes in their body form during their life (e.g., caterpillars turn into moths or butterflies, a process known as metamorphosis). Also learn to recognize developmental stages, because immature forms are often the ones that damage plants or products. Adults of many pest insects possess

TABLE 2-2

Ways in which arthropods are pests

Type of pest	Type of damage	Example of arthropod pest
plant pests	chewing on leaves	caterpillars, beetles, grasshoppers
	boring or tunneling into leaves, stems, fruits	twig borers, leafminers, beetles
	sucking plant juices	aphids, mites, scales, thrips, plant bugs
	feeding on roots	beetles, aphids, flies
	feeding on fruits, nuts, berries	moth larvae, beetles, earwigs
	causing malformations such as galls	flies, wasps, mites
	transmitting diseases	aphids, mites, leafhoppers
pests of animals and people	have venomous bite or sting	bees, wasps, ants, spiders, scorpions
	feed on flesh or blood	flies, mosquitoes, bugs, ticks, fleas, lice, mites
	transmit diseases	mosquitoes, bugs, flies, fleas, ticks, cockroaches
	cause allergic reactions	bugs, bees, wasps, mites
	have offensive odors	beetles, lacewings, bugs
	cause fear or are nuisances	insects, spiders, scorpions, centipedes
	cause loss in livestock weight gain or reduction of milk or egg production	fleas, ticks, mites
	damage and devalue hides and pelts; cause loss of carcasses used for meat	sheep keds, lice, ticks, mites, cattle grubs
	cause reduction in livestock's worth and reproduction efficiency	flies, mites
stored product pests	eat or damage grains and other stored products	beetles, cockroaches, moths, crickets
structural pests	damage buildings and other wood structures	termites, beetles, ants, bees
pests of human belongings	feed on clothing, carpeting, paper products	moths, beetles, cockroaches, crickets
	feed on furniture and other wood products	termites, beetles

SIDEBAR 2-2

SAMPLING AND SENDING ARTHROPODS FOR IDENTIFICATION

SAMPLING

1. Collect plant-feeding insects and mites by snipping off portions of foliage or stems containing the pest and placing these into a plastic bag.
2. Use an insect net to collect flying insects.
3. For other insects, shake plant foliage onto a light-colored cloth sheet and funnel arthropods into a plastic bag or glass or plastic jar.
4. Keep all collected specimens cool by placing them into an ice chest or refrigerator.

PREPARATION

1. Place insects, mites, and other arthropods into a glass vial with 70% isopropyl alcohol (rubbing alcohol also may be used). Vials must be sealed so that alcohol cannot leak out.
2. Include more than one individual of each species whenever possible. If other life stages are present (eggs, larvae, pupae, adults), include representative samples of these.
3. If the pest is associated with plants, send samples that show pest damage. Do not put plant material in the alcohol. Keep plants as fresh as possible by keeping them cool.

LABELING

Attach a label to the outside of each vial and plant sample bag. Include the following information on labels:

1. Your name, address, telephone number, and email address (if you have one).
2. Name and variety of host plant, if applicable.
3. Date specimens were collected.
4. Whether pest is in commercial, agricultural, residential, nursery, or other setting. If the pest is not associated with plants, describe the site where it was collected.
5. Location where samples were taken, including names of nearby crossroads.

SHIPPING

1. Contact the person or laboratory that will receive samples to determine the best method of shipping and to inform them that samples will be arriving.
2. Pack samples in a sturdy, well-insulated container to prevent crushing or heat damage.
3. Mark package clearly and request shipper to keep it in a cool location.
4. If plant material is included, ship packages early in the week so they will arrive before a weekend.

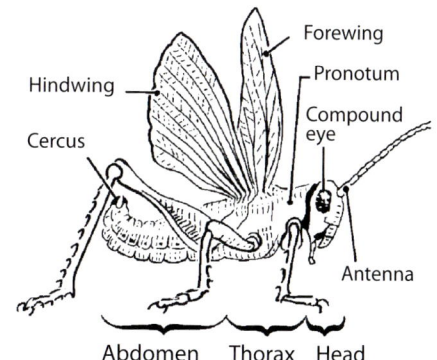

FIGURE 2-23

The body parts of this grasshopper represent the structures that you usually see on most adult insects. Some adult insects are wingless, however.

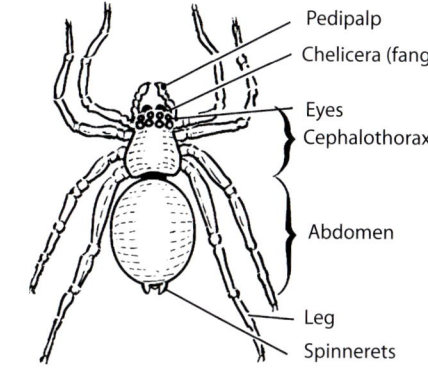

FIGURE 2-24

Spiders have two main body regions rather than the three found in insects. They have four pairs of legs, a pair of pedipalps, and a pair of chelicerae. The chelicerae terminate in fangs that spiders use to inject venom. At the end of the abdomen is a cluster of spinnerets, part of the spider's web-producing mechanism.

FIGURE 2-25

The body arrangement of mites and ticks is different from that of insects or spiders. Adults generally have four pairs of legs; immature forms usually have three pairs.

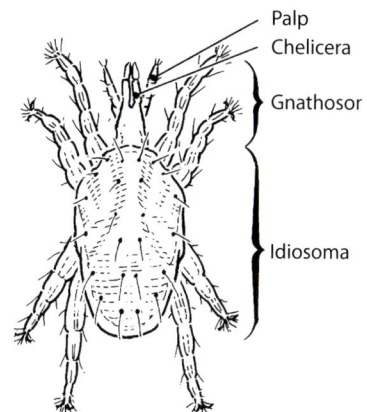

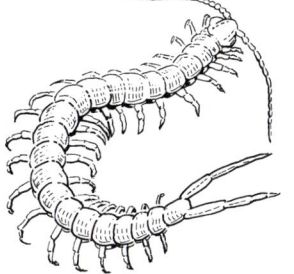

FIGURE 2-26

Centipedes have many body segments, most of which give rise to pairs of legs. Centipedes have a pair of poisonous fangs that arise from the head segment.

wings that can be used for identification. If you cannot identify an arthropod using available tools, send a specimen for evaluation by a trained specialist. Sidebar 2-2 explains how to prepare arthropods for shipment to identification specialists.

Arthropod Body Structure

Insects. The body of an adult insect has three distinct parts: the head, thorax, and abdomen (Fig. 2-23). Eyes and one pair of antennae arise from the head. Also, several pairs of appendages that make up the mouthparts are usually on the head. The thorax has three pairs of legs and often one or two pairs of wings. Insects have segmented abdomens. Sometimes the folded wings partially or entirely cover the abdomen. Some insects have appendages extending from the tip of the abdomen, such as pinchers, a sting, or other structures.

Spiders. Spiders have two major body parts (Fig. 2-24). The head and thorax combine into one section called a cephalothorax. The cephalothorax gives rise to four pairs of legs, eyes, and mouthparts, including a pair of fangs (chelicerae). The remaining body part is a nonsegmented abdomen that terminates with several pairs of spinnerets, the spider's web-spinning organs.

Ticks and Mites. Ticks and mites have only two body segments, but these are different from spiders' (Fig. 2-25). A small head (called a gnathosoma) with a few mouth appendages is attached to a large, combined thorax and abdomen called an idiosoma. Adult mites and ticks have four pairs of legs arising from the idiosoma; immature forms usually have only three pairs.

Other Arthropods. Other arthropod groups have varying arrangements of body parts and legs. For example, centipedes and millipedes have many body segments with large numbers of legs (Fig. 2-26). Scorpions have a long, segmented tail.

Arthropod Developmental Stages

Most arthropods hatch from eggs into immatures that increase in size by molting or shedding their outer body covering (exoskeleton) and growing a new, larger one. Often they modify their shape with each successive molt, a process known as metamorphosis. The period between one molt and the next is known as an instar. Immature arthropods pass through several instars before becoming adults.

Some species of insects undergo major morphological or structural changes between the immature stages and adulthood. This transformation occurs within a nonfeeding pupal stage; these insects are said to have complete metamorphosis (Fig. 2-27). Immatures in these groups are called larvae and, in many cases, have different feeding habits from adults, so that only either the larval or adult stage causes damage. Examples of insects with complete metamorphosis include flies, wasps, moths, butterflies, and beetles.

Other insects, such as grasshoppers, aphids,

TABLE 2-3

Beneficial arthropods

Type of benefit	Arthropod
Useful products	
beeswax, honey	honey bees
shellac	scale insects
silk	silkworm moths
pigments and dyes	scale and gall insects
Pollination	
of figs	wasps
of many fruits and vegetables	honey bees, wild bees, bumble bees, flies, other insects
Food	
for birds	butterflies, moths, beetles, many more
for fish	mosquitoes, flies, many others
Parasites and predators of harmful insects and mites	
parasites	wasps, flies
predators	beetles, lacewings, flies, bugs, spiders, wasps, mites
Natural control of weeds	
feeding damage	moths, beetles, others
introducing disease agents	beetles
Other benefits	
improved soil conditions	beetles, other soil-inhabiting insects
scavengers of dead plant and animal matter	beetles, flies, many others
use in scientific studies	fruit flies, cockroaches, others
medicinal uses	bees, wasps, flies

PEST IDENTIFICATION   39

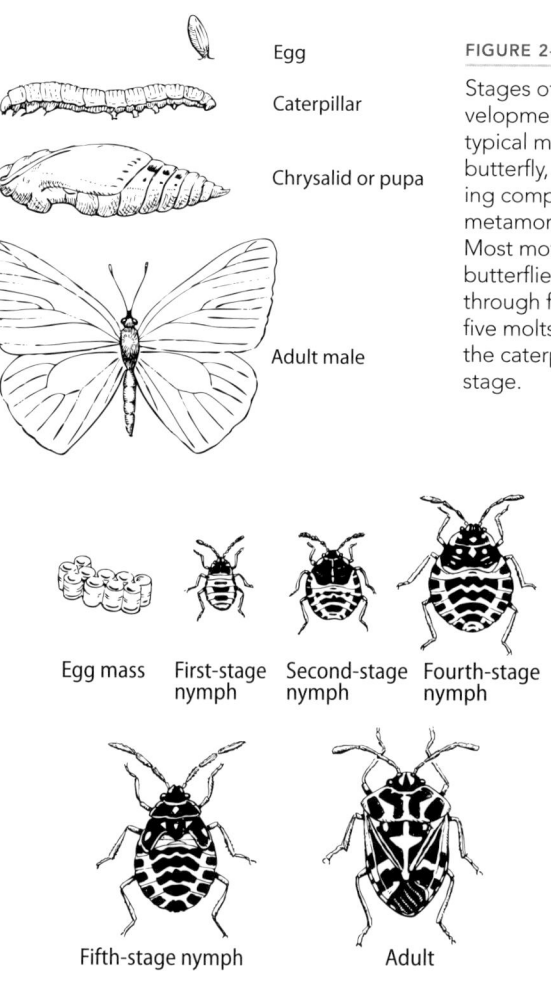

FIGURE 2-27
Stages of development of a typical moth or butterfly, showing complete metamorphosis. Most moths and butterflies go through four or five molts during the caterpillar stage.

FIGURE 2-28
Development of the harlequin bug, showing incomplete metamorphosis and wing development.

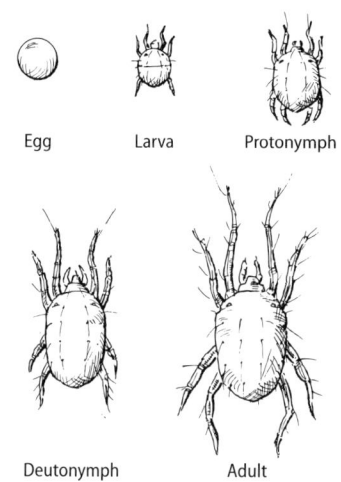

FIGURE 2-29
Development of a typical plant-feeding spider mite. The stage that hatches out of the egg is called a larva. Remaining immatures are called nymphs.

and true bugs, go through gradual, simple, or incomplete metamorphosis and do not have a pupal stage (Fig. 2-28). Their immatures are called nymphs; they differ from adults primarily in their size and absence of wings and reproductive organs. Adults and immatures of these insects have the same food habits.

The development of mites, spiders, and other arthropods is similar to the incomplete metamorphosis of some insects. For instance, mites hatch from eggs and pass through several immature stages before becoming adults; the stage that hatches out of the egg is normally called the larva (Fig. 2-29). Later-stage nymphs look similar to adult mites. Immature mites and spiders have feeding habits similar to adults of the same species.

Arthropods have one to many generations per year, depending on species, location, and environmental conditions. In hot weather, species such as spider mites or aphids reproduce rapidly, and in warmer areas such as some parts of California, they can reproduce all year. Other arthropods, such as some borers, take more than a year to mature. The number of generations and the length of time for each generation to develop are important in determining monitoring activities and control methods (Flint 2012).

Spiders

Important Characteristics. Spiders have four pairs of legs and an unsegmented abdomen. The abdomen attaches to the other main body part (the cephalothorax) by a narrow waist. At the tip of the abdomen are spinnerets, special organs used for producing different types of webbing.

Life Cycle. Immature spiders hatch from eggs and pass through several instars before becoming adults. Each instar begins with molting. During this process the spider sheds its outer body covering, allowing it to grow larger. Most spiders live for 2 or 3 years, although some species may live as long as 20 to 30 years. Females generally live longer than males. Spiders feed on insects and other small arthropods.

Where Found. In buildings, spiders congregate in corners of ceilings, behind and underneath furniture, and in basements, attics, and crawl spaces. Outdoors, spiders appear in most types of environments. They frequently live among agricultural crops and landscape plants.

Damage. In California, black widow, recluse, hobo, and a few other spider species can inflict painful bites. These bites may require prompt medical attention. Other large spiders may bite occasionally. Spiders leave webbing on inside and outside surfaces of buildings. Their presence in shipped produce has caused concern.

Beneficial Aspects. Spiders are general predators of arthropods, including insects, and contribute to the natural control of many pest species.

Ticks, Mites

Important Characteristics. Mites and ticks have their abdomen broadly joined to the head and thorax (Fig. 2-30). Adults usually have four pairs of legs, while immatures most often have three or fewer pairs. Some species of mites produce fine webbing from silk glands located near their mouth. Most mites are very small and difficult to see without the aid of a hand lens or microscope.

Life Cycle. Ticks and mites hatch from eggs and pass through several immature stages before becoming adults. Immature ticks and mites resemble adults. Mites usually develop quickly from eggs to adults; some overwinter as adults, while other species overwinter as eggs. Ticks generally live much longer. Some require 1 to 2 years to reach maturity and may live an additional 2 or 3 years as adults.

Where Found. Depending on the species, mites are parasites on plants or animals. Certain species are predatory on other mites. Ticks are blood-feeding parasites of vertebrates and require blood meals to develop and reproduce. They commonly occur on animal hosts or in or near their nests. Plant-feeding mites live on upper or lower leaf surfaces. Mites in homes can be found in ventilation systems, pillows, couches, and other places where dust collects.

Damage. Plant-feeding mites often produce serious economic or visual damage, including leaf discoloration and defoliation. Some plant-feeding mites transmit disease-causing microorganisms (such as citrus leprosis virus). Feeding injuries produced by mites that infest animals and people may itch severely. Toxins injected by ticks during feeding sometimes cause paralysis of hosts; some tick species transmit microorganisms that cause disease (such as Lyme disease).

Beneficial Aspects. Several species of mites are predators of pest mites or small insects. These serve as an important component of natural and biological control programs.

Springtails

Important Characteristics. Springtails are minute, wingless arthropods about $1/16$ inch long (Fig. 2-31). Springtails get their name from the ability to jump up to several inches high by means of a tail-like "spring" (furcula) tucked under the abdomen. When disturbed, they use this furcula to spring into the air away from danger.

Life Cycle. These arthropods lay their round eggs in small groups in moist soil, especially where organic matter is abundant, and go through incomplete metamorphosis. The immature stage is usually whitish, and adults tend to be whitish, bluish, or dark gray to black. The immature stage differs from the adult stage only in size and color, so the young resemble adults but are smaller. Individuals of some species live for 2 to 3 years.

Where Found. Springtails live in soil, especially soil amended with compost, in leaf litter and organic mulches, and under bark or decaying wood. They feed on decaying plant material, fungi, molds, and algae. They are also found on the surface of stagnant water or on sidewalks that border flowerbeds or swimming pools. Mushroom houses and greenhouses also provide the damp environment required for their development.

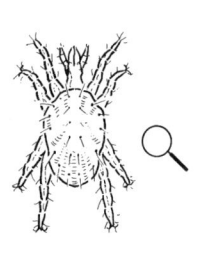
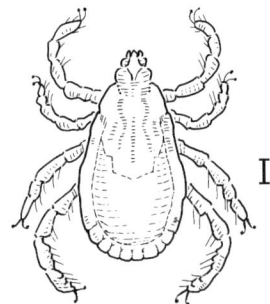

FIGURE 2-30

Ticks and mites are closely related, although ticks are much larger. Ticks are parasites of vertebrates and feed on blood. Some mites are parasites of vertebrates, although many are serious plant pests.

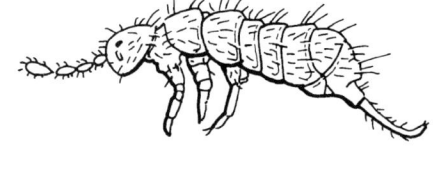

FIGURE 2-31

Springtail.

Springtails may invade homes or other areas such as swimming pools in search of moisture. After entering a house, they crawl in search of moisture and are often trapped in sinks, washbasins, and bathtubs. They may also occur around floor drains, in damp basements, crawl spaces, and wall voids. They soon die after entering a home unless they find moisture.

Damage. Some springtail species may damage plants by chewing on the roots and leaves of seedlings, especially when the soil is moist and rich in organic matter. They can become a nuisance around swimming pools when they fall in and drown in large numbers, often coating the pool surface. Their large populations can also make them a nuisance in homes, greenhouses, and other locations where there is a source of moisture. They do not bite or otherwise harm people or pets.

Bristletails (Silverfish and Firebrats)

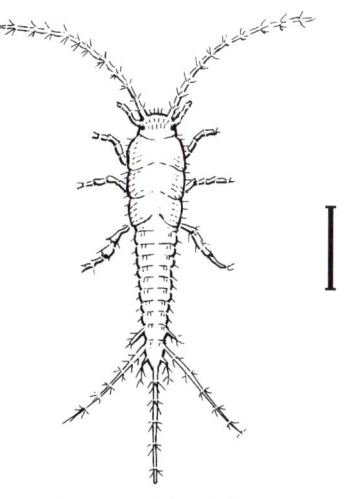

FIGURE 2-32

Silverfish, order Thysanura.

Important Characteristics. Silverfish and firebrats have no wings. They usually have two or three long, tail-like structures (Fig. 2-32). Mouthparts are of the chewing type. Most are brownish or silver in color. They are often nocturnal.

Life Cycle. Bristletails undergo incomplete metamorphosis, so the young resemble adults but are smaller. Individuals of some species live for 2 to 3 years.

Where Found. Silverfish and firebrats occur in homes, businesses, and libraries. They hide in cracks and crevices and other dark places. Silverfish prefer areas of high humidity and often may become trapped in sinks and tubs. Firebrats prefer drier habitats.

Damage. These insects infest paper, cereals, and fabrics (including synthetics). They also feed on resins and glue used in books and picture mountings.

Crickets, Grasshoppers, Locusts, Katydids

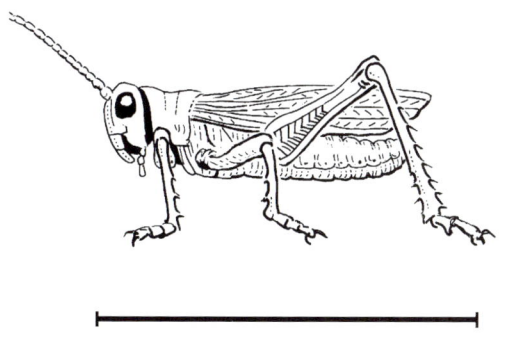

FIGURE 2-33

Grasshopper, order Orthoptera.

Important Characteristics. Immature insects in this group resemble adults. They have chewing mouthparts, and many species have wings, although most are not good fliers (Fig. 2-33). Wingless species also exist. They have powerful hind legs that they use for jumping. Crickets, locusts, and katydids make distinguishing chirping or buzzing sounds. Many grasshopper species make clicking or buzzing sounds when they fly.

Life Cycle. Orthopterans hatch from eggs that adult females glue to plant surfaces, insert into plant tissues, lay in soil, or lay freely on the ground. Immature forms do not have wings; they undergo incomplete metamorphosis. Most orthopterans live 1 or more years.

Where Found. Orthopterans occur in most agricultural crops, landscaped areas, and gardens. Many live in the soil, while others live in trees or shrubs.

Damage. Grasshoppers, locusts, and katydids feed on plants and can cause serious injury or defoliation. Crickets sometimes infest residences and stain or damage fabrics and paper products.

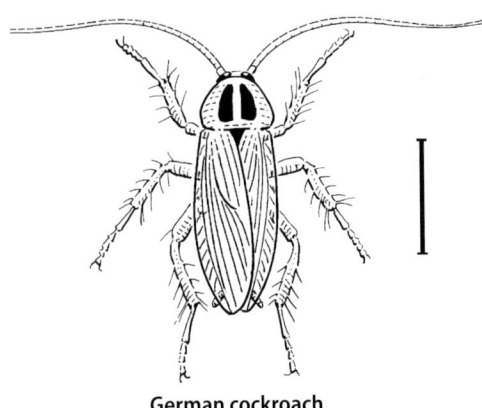

FIGURE 2-34
Cockroach, order Blattodea.

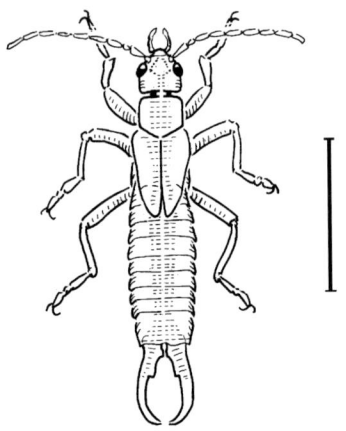

FIGURE 2-35
Earwig, order Dermaptera.

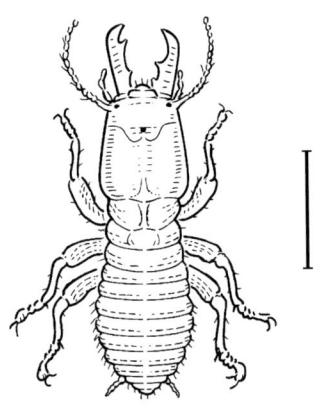

FIGURE 2-36
Termite, order Isoptera.

Cockroaches

Important Characteristics. Most cockroaches are poor fliers. Immature cockroaches resemble adults. They have chewing mouthparts. A great range of size differences exists among species. Although more than fifty species of cockroaches have been identified in the United States and more than thirty-five hundred worldwide, only five species are major pests in California (Fig. 2-34). Cockroaches are nocturnal. They hide in dark, warm areas, especially narrow spaces where surfaces touch them on both sides. Cockroaches tend to congregate in corners and generally travel along the edges of walls or other surfaces.

Life Cycle. Cockroaches hatch from eggs that are usually laid in capsules made by the adult female. Females of some species carry their egg capsules about with them. They undergo incomplete metamorphosis. Adults usually live from 1 to 2 years.

Damage. Several species of cockroaches inhabit buildings and may become persistent and troublesome pests. Cockroaches that have come into contact with human and animal waste carry bacteria responsible for food poisoning, such as *Salmonella* and *Shigella*. They can also pass along viral hepatitis organisms through their frass. Cockroaches are also believed capable of transmitting staphylococcus, streptococcus, and coliform bacteria through their frass, which is also responsible for allergy and asthma problems.

Earwigs

Important Characteristics. Earwigs are elongated, sometimes wingless insects having characteristic forceplike pinchers (cerci) extending from the end of the abdomen (Fig. 2-35). They use these pinchers for defense and for catching prey. The pinchers of female European earwigs are straight, while those of the male are curved. Earwigs have chewing mouthparts.

Life Cycle. Earwigs hatch from eggs deposited in a nest in the soil. Adult females protect their eggs and newly hatched young. Earwigs pass through incomplete metamorphosis. They develop from egg to adult in 2 to 3 months. They hibernate as adults.

Where Found. Earwigs usually nest in the ground and hide under boards, stones, and ground litter. Earwigs are very common insects in some parts of California.

Damage. Earwigs feed on vegetables, ripe fruits, garden flowers, and garbage; some prey on other arthropods (predaceous). They are occasional nuisances in buildings when they wander in from outdoors.

Termites

Important Characteristics. Termites superficially resemble ants but have an abdomen broadly joined to the thorax. Compared with ants, there also are differences in body coloration and the shape and size of wings and antennae (Fig. 2-36). Some termites have wings but lose them after dispersing from the colonies where they hatched. Termites' wings are much longer than the body, and both pairs of wings are of equal length. The wings of ants are shorter—no longer than the body, with the front pair of wings being longest. Termites live in colonies having different subgroups of individuals, called castes. Each caste performs specific func-

PEST IDENTIFICATION

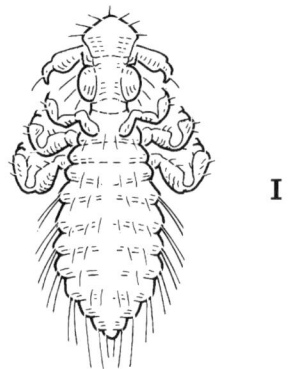

Chicken head louse

FIGURE 2-37

Chewing lice, order Mallophaga.

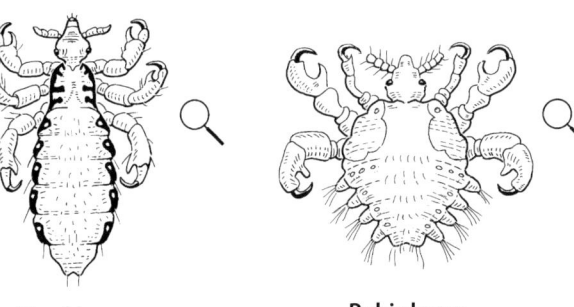

Head louse   **Pubic louse**

FIGURE 2-38

Sucking lice, order Anoplura.

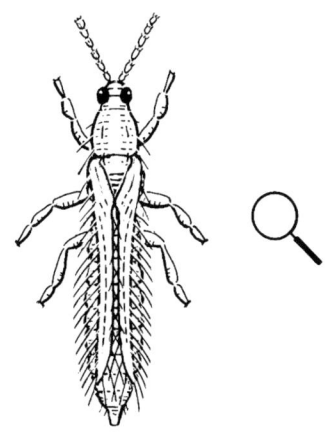

Western flower thrips

FIGURE 2-39

Thrips, order Thysanoptera.

tions in the colony. Many soldiers have enlarged heads with powerful, pincerlike jaws. Queens have greatly enlarged abdomens. Termites have chewing-type mouthparts.

Life Cycle. Adult termites feed and tend to newly hatched termites. The nymphal stage lasts 3 to 4 months or longer. Adult workers may live 3 to 5 years, while queens live much longer. Termite colonies survive for many years as younger individuals replace older ones.

Where Found. Some species of termites live in the soil, but others construct nests in trees and wooden structures. Soil-nesting species usually construct tunnels or tubes to the wood sources they use as food.

Damage. Termites cause serious damage to wood structures by feeding and constructing tunnels or galleries.

Chewing Lice

Important Characteristics. Chewing lice (Fig. 2-37) are very small, oval or elongated wingless insects with chewing mouthparts. They have flattened bodies, sometimes with dark brown or black spots or bands. Chewing lice have a head that is wider than their thorax. You need a hand lens or microscope to examine these tiny insects.

Life Cycle. Chewing lice lay their eggs on hosts, usually attached to hair or feathers. They may pass through three or more nymphal stages before developing into adults. Most chewing lice develop into adults within 2 or 3 weeks after hatching.

Where Found. Chewing lice are parasites of birds, fowl, and a few mammals. Species are host-specific—each species occurs only on one type of animal.

Damage. These parasites feed on feathers and the outer skin and skin debris of birds, and on hair, blood, and skin of mammals. Poultry infested with chewing lice usually become restless and uncomfortable, have decreased weight gain, and have lowered egg production.

Sucking Lice

Important Characteristics. Sucking lice (Fig. 2-38) are flat-bodied, wingless insects with piercing-sucking mouthparts. The head is narrower than the thorax. A hand lens or microscope is necessary to examine these insects.

Life Cycle. Females cement their eggs to hairs of the host. After hatching, sucking lice pass through several instars and become adults within 1 to 2 weeks. Sucking lice pierce the skin of their hosts to feed on blood.

Where Found. Sucking lice are host-specific parasites of mammals, including people. The human body louse remains on clothing when removed and can survive off its host for short periods of time. Other species must always remain on their hosts.

Damage. Feeding by sucking lice causes irritation and itching. Some lice are capable of transmitting disease-causing organisms.

Thrips

Important Characteristics. Thrips are tiny, elongated insects with two pairs of wings (Fig. 2-39). Their wings have a fringelike appearance. Thrips have modified sucking-rasping mouthparts.

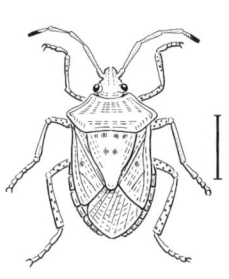 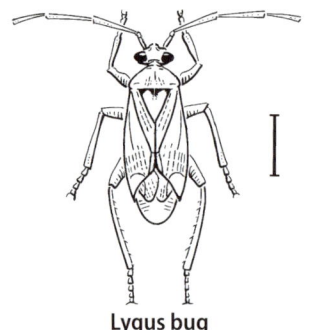 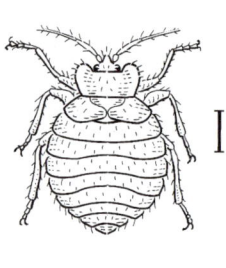

FIGURE 2-40

True bug, order Hemiptera.

Consperse stink bug   Lygus bug   Bed bug

Life Cycle. Thrips hatch from eggs, and most species pass through four instars. Thrips actively feed during their first two instars. The final instars are more of a resting stage, which often takes place in the soil. Wings are present after the thrips' final molt.

Where Found. Thrips commonly infest plants and are often found in flowers and on tender, developing parts of leaves and fruits.

Damage. Thrips puncture plant cells and suck the fluid that escapes. This type of feeding damages cells, resulting in deformed fruits and other plant structures. Some thrips are serious pests in greenhouses, gardens, and agricultural areas.

Beneficial Aspects. A few species of thrips are predatory. Predatory thrips play an important role in the natural control of several plant pests, including aphids and mites.

True Bugs (True Bugs, Plant Bugs, Damsel Bugs, Assassin Bugs, Bed Bugs)

Important Characteristics. You can recognize most true bugs (Fig. 2-40) by the triangular-shaped plate or scale on the thorax (scutellum) seen from above. They also have a long, needle-like beak (piercing-sucking mouthparts) that folds under their bodies. Their forewings are hard at the base and thinner (membranous) and more flexible at the tip. True bugs are various sizes depending on the species; some are nearly 2 inches long. They have two pairs of wings and most fly well. The second pair of wings is not visible while the insect is at rest. They sometimes have brightly colored wings.

Life Cycle. True bugs undergo incomplete metamorphosis after hatching from eggs. Young resemble adults but lack wings. Life cycles vary among the many species of true bugs.

Where Found. True bugs feed on plants and animals, depending on the species. Most are free living, searching out appropriate hosts for food. There are several aquatic species.

Damage. Some species feed on blood of livestock, birds, rodents, and people. Feeding sites may become inflamed or infected and usually are very tender. A few species of true bugs transmit disease-causing organisms. Plant-feeding true bugs damage plant cells. This causes deformities of fruits and other plant parts. Some true bugs also inject chemicals into the plant that prevent or alter the plant's normal growth. True bugs are often serious plant pests in agricultural, home garden, and landscaped settings.

Beneficial Aspects. Some species of true bugs are predators of other insects, including many insect pests. Examples of these are assassin bugs, bigeyed bugs, and minute pirate bugs.

Aphids, Whiteflies, Mealybugs, Scales

Important Characteristics. These insects are diverse, somewhat soft-bodied, and most have wings or have some winged forms. They all have piercing-sucking mouthparts. Figure 2-41 shows two of the many types of insects in this group.

Life Cycle. All insects in this group undergo incomplete metamorphosis, though the time it takes to go from egg to adult varies widely among species.

Where Found. These insects are plant feeders, so they are usually found on or near plants. Some occur in greenhouses and indoors on houseplants.

FIGURE 2-41

Whitefly, scale, and aphid, order Hemiptera.

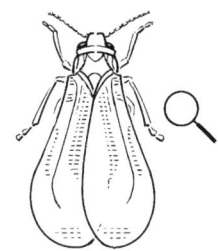
Greenhouse whitefly

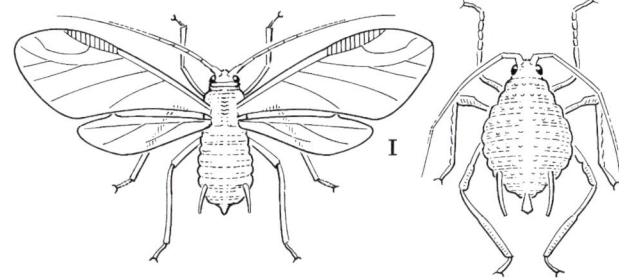
Rosy apple aphid

Damage. Insects in this group pierce plant tissues and suck out liquids. Feeding usually causes deformed leaves and fruits, loss of plant vigor, stunted growth, and dieback of plant parts. Most of these insects excrete a sticky substance called honeydew that supports the growth of black sooty mold fungi. Many species transmit disease-causing pathogens to host plants.

Leafhoppers, Cicadas, Psyllids, Phylloxerans, Spittlebugs, Treehoppers

Important Characteristics. Almost all insects in this group have piercing-sucking mouthparts. Most of them feed on plant sap (phloem or xylem), but a few planthoppers feed on fungi or mosses. They have short, bristlelike antennae, and some mature insects develop wings (Fig. 2-42).

Life Cycle. All insects in this group undergo incomplete metamorphosis, though the time it takes to go from egg to adult varies widely among species.

Where Found. These insects can be found in many different habitats, including landscapes, gardens, agricultural areas, recreational areas, and nurseries, to name a few.

Damage. Insects in this group feed on plants using piercing-sucking mouthparts, and many are vectors of viral and fungal diseases of plants. Their feeding causes scarring on fruits and can discolor or blacken leaves. The honeydew they leave behind is sticky, unsightly, and can result in the development of black sooty mold on infested plants.

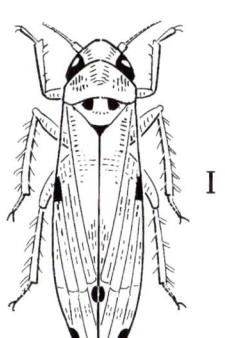
Grape leafhopper

FIGURE 2-42

Leafhopper, order Hemiptera.

Beetles, Weevils

Important Characteristics. Adult beetles and weevils range from the size of a pinhead to several inches in length, depending on the species (Fig. 2-43). Most adults have a pair of hardened and often black forewings. They completely cover the abdomen and hide the insect's second pair of wings when it is not flying. Larvae are very diverse in appearance. Both larvae and adults have chewing mouthparts.

FIGURE 2-43

Beetle and weevil, order Coleoptera.

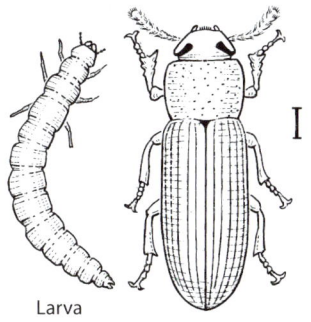
Larva
Confused flour beetle

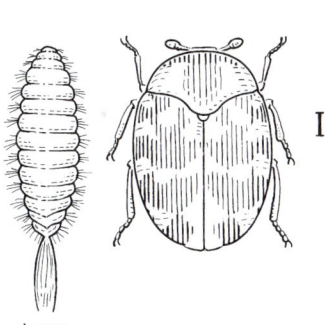
Larva
Carpet beetle

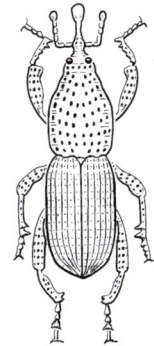
Granary weevil

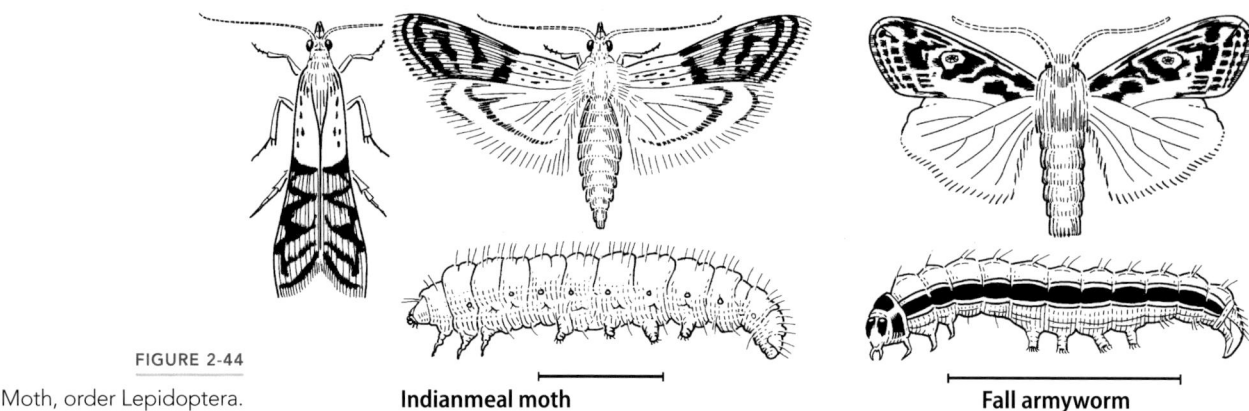

FIGURE 2-44

Moth, order Lepidoptera.   **Indianmeal moth**   **Fall armyworm**

Life Cycle. Beetles and weevils undergo complete metamorphosis. Larvae pass through several instars before pupating; pupation usually takes place in the soil. Some adults survive adverse weather by going into a dormant period—hibernating during cold winter periods or aestivating during hot or dry periods.

Where Found. Beetle and weevil pests infest plants, stored food products, wood, furniture, fabrics, and animal products; some even bore into metal. Many species actively bore into items they use for food.

Damage. Beetles and weevils damage or destroy agricultural products, forest trees, stored food, fabrics, furs, carpets, wood items, and landscape plants.

Beneficial Aspects. Several species of beetles are predatory on other insects and contribute to the control of plant-feeding pests such as aphids and mites.

Butterflies, Moths, Skippers

Important Characteristics. Adult butterflies, moths, and skippers (Fig. 2-44) are distinguishable from other insects by their large, scale-covered, and often brightly colored wings. Larvae are wormlike, with chewing mouthparts. Adults have modified mouthparts in the form of a coiled tube that they extend to suck up liquids. Butterflies and skippers differ from moths by their antennae. Moths have tapering hairlike or feathery antennae, while those of butterflies and skippers are clubbed (although certain rare moths and butterflies have antennae that resemble one another). Skippers have shorter, thicker bodies and smaller wings, setting them apart from butterflies. Moths are primarily nocturnal, while butterflies and skippers fly mostly during the day.

Life Cycle. These insects undergo complete metamorphosis. After hatching from eggs, larvae pass through several instars, then enter the pupal stage and change into winged adults. Pupation sometimes takes place in the soil. Many of these pests overwinter as pupae. Life cycles from egg through adult vary according to the species. Many species in this group produce three or four generations per year.

Where Found. These pests occur on or in plant parts (including fruits), in stored food products, and in fabrics. Adult moths are commonly attracted to lights.

Damage. Moth larvae are one of the most serious agricultural pests. They cause considerable damage to fruits and vegetables, nuts, grains, cotton, and forage crops. Moths are also prominent pests in stored food and cause extensive damage to fabrics.

PEST IDENTIFICATION   47

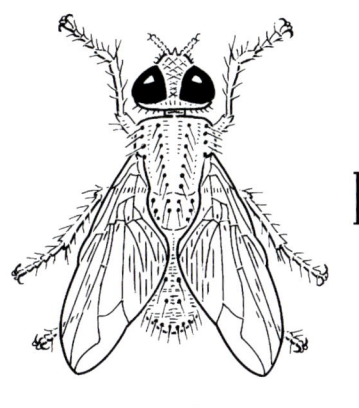
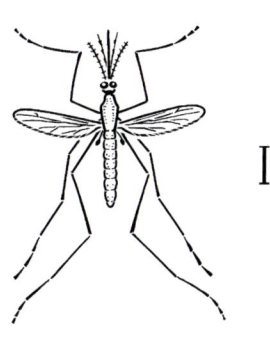

House fly   **Western malarial mosquito**

FIGURE 2-45
Fly and mosquito, order Diptera.

Flies, Mosquitoes, Gnats, Midges

Important Characteristics. Adults in this group (Fig. 2-45) have only one pair of wings. In place of the second pair of wings are small clublike organs believed to assist in balance. Their larvae, known as maggots, are usually wormlike. Most adults have modified mouth structures for sucking, lapping, or piercing. Some adults have biting mouthparts.

Life Cycle. These pests undergo complete metamorphosis. Most species deposit eggs onto surfaces or into tissues of hosts. In a few species, the eggs hatch inside the female's body, and these females deposit larvae rather than eggs. Many species undergo rapid development from eggs through the adult stages. This development may take as little as 3 or 4 days. Others have extended life cycles, taking 2 or more years to complete. Many species survive periods of adverse environmental conditions as resting pupae in the soil.

Where Found. Flies, mosquitoes, gnats, and midges occur in most outdoor areas and inside buildings. Some larvae are internal parasites of animals; others invade plant tissues. Larvae of mosquitoes live in aquatic habitats. House fly larvae congregate in garbage and on animal feces.

Damage. Many species in this group are serious pests. Larvae of some invade living animal tissues. Adult mosquitoes and the adults of some species of flies, midges, and gnats feed on blood. Many of these insects transmit serious disease-causing pathogens. Some species of flies are pests in agricultural crops and landscape settings. Others are nuisances in and around buildings and livestock or poultry areas.

Beneficial Aspects. A few fly species are parasitic on pest insects, and others are predators. These species are often important natural and biological control agents.

Fleas

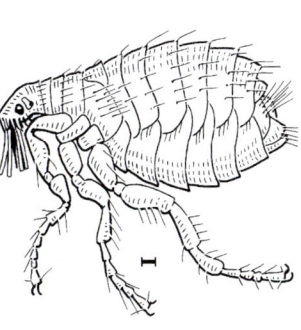

FIGURE 2-46
Cat flea, order Siphonaptera.

Important Characteristics. Adult fleas are tiny, dark brown or black, wingless insects with laterally compressed bodies (Fig. 2-46). Fleas are capable of hopping great distances for their small size: cat fleas have been observed to jump 8 inches vertically and 15 inches horizontally. Larvae are wormlike. Fleas have piercing-sucking mouthparts.

Life Cycle. Fleas undergo complete metamorphosis. They usually pass through one complete cycle, from eggs to adults, in 30 to 40 days.

Where Found. Females lay their eggs on the host, although the eggs usually drop off before hatching. Larvae are free living, usually on the ground. They feed on skin debris and hair of their host. Adults must feed on the blood of warm-blooded animals. Therefore, they live on their hosts or in their host's nest. They are usually host specific.

Damage. Flea bites are uncomfortable and may cause an allergic reaction in some people and animals. Some species of fleas can transmit pathogens of diseases such as bubonic plague and murine typhus. Certain fleas serve as the intermediate hosts of tapeworms.

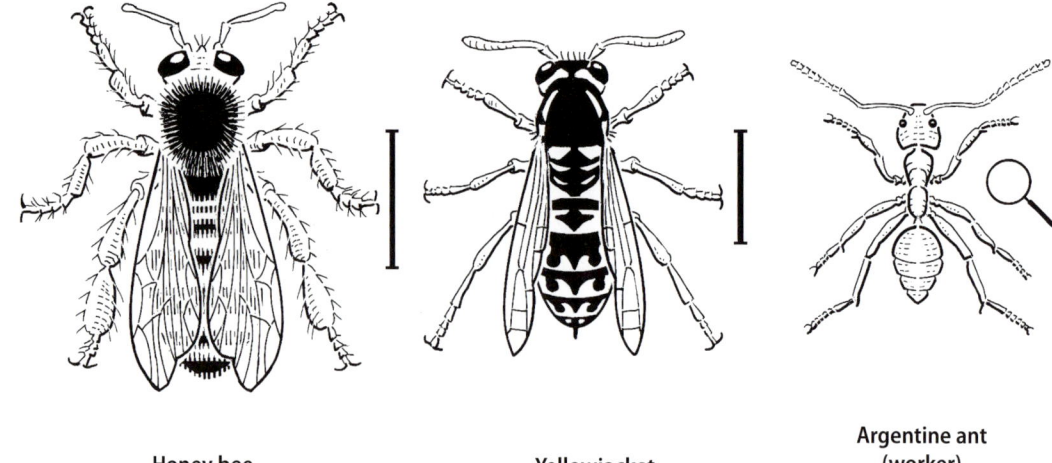

FIGURE 2-47

Honey bee, yellowjacket, and ant, order Hymenoptera

Honey bee   **Yellowjacket**   **Argentine ant (worker)**

Bees, Wasps, Ants, Sawflies, Horntails

Important Characteristics. Adults in this group differ from other insects by usually having their abdomen joined to the thorax by a very narrow "waist" (Fig. 2-47). Winged forms have two pairs of transparent, sometimes colored wings. Larvae are grublike. Certain species of bees, wasps, and ants are venomous and have a sting at the tip of their abdomen. Several species are social rather than solitary. Large numbers of individuals live together in a colony, and members of the colony perform different tasks, depending on their caste. Larvae and some adults have chewing mouthparts.

Life Cycle. These insects undergo complete metamorphosis. Their larvae may be internal or external parasites of insects, spiders, and other arthropods; some species feed on plants. Species that live in colonies forage for food for their larvae. Colonies of social species live for many years, although individuals survive for only a few months to 1 or 2 years. Some species produce several generations per year.

Where Found. Adults in this group forage for food on flowers and other plant parts. Many congregate on sweets and meat. Social species live in nests in the ground or in buildings, trees, and other structures.

Damage. Many species in this group are venomous and inflict painful stings that, in some people, may be fatal. They can also cause galls to form on plants. Certain species of sawflies are serious agricultural and forest pests. Many bees and wasps are nuisances around homes and outdoor areas. Ants are persistent pests in food preparation areas and in agricultural crops. Some bees and ants damage wood structures.

Beneficial Aspects. Bees and other species in this group are important pollinators of agricultural and horticultural plants. Parasitic wasps play an extremely important role in the control of pest insects. Some are egg parasites and others attack the larval or adult stages of their hosts. Some species, such as yellowjackets, are predators.

NEMATODES

Nematodes belong to the phylum Nemata (or Nematoda), the third-largest phylum in the animal kingdom. Nematodes are unsegmented

TABLE 2-4

Important genera and species of nematodes

Common name	Scientific name
Plant pests	
citrus nematode	*Tylenchulus semipenetrans*
cyst nematode	*Heterodera* spp.
dagger nematode	*Xiphinema* spp.
foliar nematode	*Aphelenchoides* spp.
lesion nematode	*Pratylenchus* spp.
needle nematode	*Logidorus africanus*
pin nematode	*Pratylenchus* spp.
potato rot nematode	*Ditylenchus destructor*
rice root nematode	*Hirschmanniella* spp.
ring nematode	*Criconemoides* spp.
root-knot nematode	*Meloidogyne* spp.
seed gall nematode	*Anguiana* spp.
stem nematode	*Rotylenchus* spp., *Heliocotylenchus* spp.
stubby root nematode	*Trichodorus* spp., *Paratrichodorus* spp.
stunt nematode	*Tylenchorhynchus* spp.
Animal pests	
canine heartworm	*Dirofilaria immitis*
filariasis nematode	*Wucheria bancrofti*
hookworm	*Ancylostoma duodenale*
pig lungworm	*Metastrongylus apri*
pinworm	*Enterobius vermicularis*

PEST IDENTIFICATION

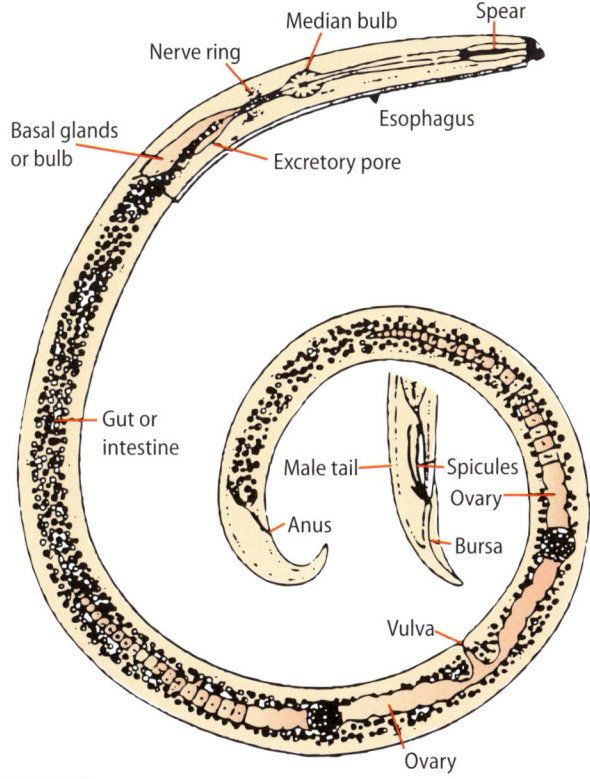

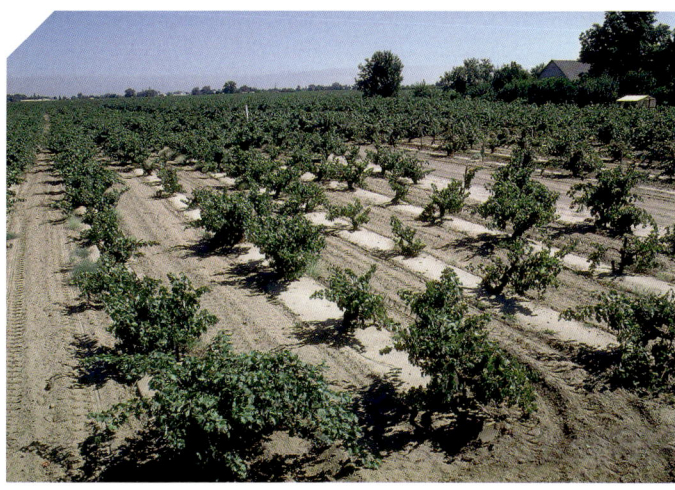

FIGURE 2-49

Root-feeding nematodes impair plants' ability to take up water and nutrients, resulting in a decrease in aboveground growth. The small grapevines shown here are suffering from a root-knot nematode infestation.

FIGURE 2-48

Anatomy of a typical plant-parasitic nematode. *Source:* McKenry and Roberts 1985.

roundworms that can be found in soil, water, plant tissues, and animals; they feed on a diversity of organisms, including plants, insects, and animals. The nematodes of most concern in pest management are plant-parasitic species that attack crops and species that cause disease in domestic animals (Table 2-4). Most nematodes, however, are not pests; some are beneficial, breaking down organic matter or attacking insects, weeds, plant-pathogenic organisms, or other nematodes.

Plant-parasitic nematodes live on or in a particular plant host. Close association with the host influences nematode behavior, reproduction, and dispersal. Nematodes occur in practically all soils, are common in high mountain soils, and can occur to depths of at least 17 feet in some agricultural soils.

Important Characteristics. Nematodes are microscopic roundworms that are unsegmented, generally transparent, and colorless. Most are slender, range in size from about $1/10$ to $1/2$ inch) in length, and most cannot be seen without a microscope. A typical plant-parasitic nematode is pictured in Figure 2-48. Nematodes are difficult to identify because of their small size. Identification of plant-parasitic nematodes requires samples of surrounding soil, roots, and other affected plant parts. Send samples to a laboratory for identification (see Sidebar 2-3).

Nematodes may be spindle shaped, pear shaped, lemon shaped, or sac shaped. The mouth opening is located on the nematode's blunt, rounded front end. All plant-parasitic nematodes have a stylet that they use to penetrate and feed on plant cells. Nematodes are covered with a multilayered cuticle that has various surface markings.

Because of their size, field identification of nematodes requires knowledge of specific pest and crop associations. Nematodes attack specific crops, and their presence can be determined by symptoms visible above the ground, such as stunting, chlorosis (yellowing or blanching), or leaf drop, and symptoms existing below the ground on the roots, such as galls, lesions, or stunting. Nematode infestations should be suspected whenever a general decline of a particular plant species is observed (Fig. 2-49). Delayed plant maturity might also indicate nematode damage. If no other causes for the decline of the plant are obvious, examine the roots for signs of nematodes. Signs include root galls or stubby, stunted, or overgrowing roots. Darkened roots

FIGURE 2-51

Root-knot nematodes may have infested this sugar beet. To be sure, send this and other random samples from the same field to a laboratory for analysis.

SIDEBAR 2-3

SAMPLING AND SENDING PLANTS FOR IDENTIFICATION OF PLANT-INFESTING NEMATODES

SAMPLING

1. Take random samples, but sample in a consistent manner. Mark off area to be sampled into grids. Randomly select areas to be sampled.
2. Keep samples from suspected diseased areas separated from samples taken in healthy areas.
3. Dig up and include roots and soil of diseased and healthy plants. Take root samples from below the level of surface feeder roots, because temperature and moisture fluctuations at the surface will affect the nematode species living there.
4. Include partially rotted or decayed roots.
5. Include aboveground plant parts if it is suspected that the nematodes are infesting these areas. Keep aboveground parts separate from root and soil samples.

PREPARATION

1. Place samples in clean plastic bags and keep them out of the sunlight. Keep samples in an insulated ice chest or refrigerator until they can be shipped. Do not freeze.
2. Pack samples in a well-insulated carton or disposable foam ice chest. Be sure container is sturdy enough to prevent damage to its contents.

LABELING

Attach a label to the outside of each sample bag. Include the following information on labels:

1. Name and address of grower or property owner.
2. Crop or plant types, including variety.
3. Location of field or property (names of nearby crossroads).
4. Portion of planted area that sample represents. Include a map if necessary.
5. Brief description of the field's crop history (previous crops).
6. Observations by you and the owner or operator of previous problems and of when present problem was first detected.
7. Date samples were taken.

SHIPPING

1. Contact the person or laboratory that will receive samples to determine the best method of shipping and to inform them that samples will be arriving.
2. Mark package clearly and request shipper to keep it in a cool location.
3. If plant material is included, ship packages early in the week so they will arrive before a weekend.

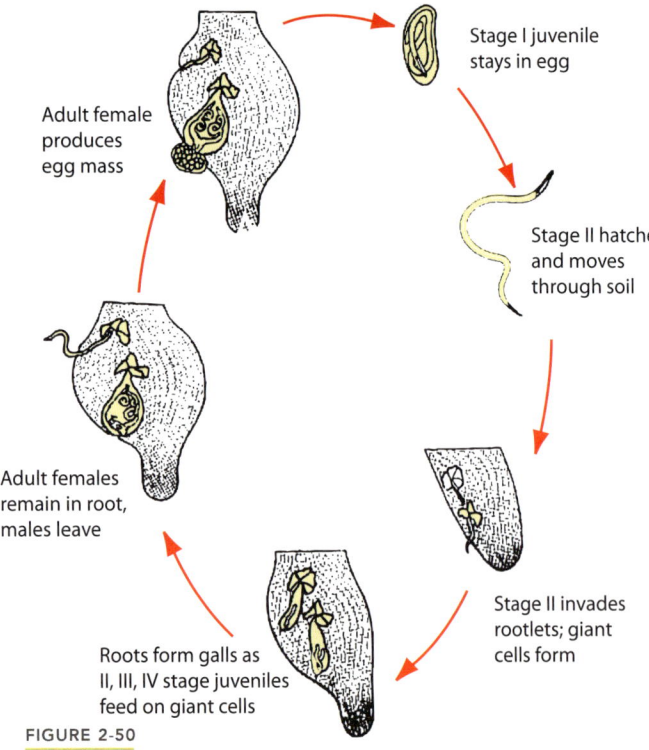

FIGURE 2-50

Root-knot nematodes spend most of their life cycle in galls on roots. Second-stage juveniles invade new sites near root tips, and the host produces a gall in response to the nematodes' feeding.

with lesions or plants with fewer roots than normal can also indicate a nematode infestation. Again, accurate identification is important. Collect samples and send them to a laboratory for analysis (see Sidebar 2-3). Contact the county University of California Cooperative Extension office to locate a testing laboratory.

Life Cycle. The nematode life cycle consists of six distinct stages: an egg stage, four juvenile stages, and an adult stage (Fig. 2-50). The nematode molts between each juvenile and adult stage. There is no metamorphosis in nematodes; the young resemble the adults but are smaller. Differences between males and females can be seen at the third juvenile stage.

Some nematodes lay their eggs singly in the soil; others lay them in the root tissue. Some species encase their eggs in a jellylike material. Female cyst nematodes, *Heterodera* spp., produce a brown protective case that keeps the eggs viable for several years. The number of eggs laid varies among species. Some lay from 2 to 10 per day over an extended period; the total laid can vary from 100 to 500 for each female.

In some nematode species, the first molt occurs in the egg, and a second-stage juvenile emerges. The juvenile molts twice more while passing through the third and fourth juvenile stages to become a fully developed adult. The length of the life cycle varies by species and is influenced by environmental conditions.

Where Found. Generally, wherever plants are cultivated, some species of plant-parasitic nematode will be present in the soil. Nematodes have evolved successful survival mechanisms that enable them to withstand unfavorable environmental conditions such as desiccation, brief periods without food, and various soil reactions. Most nematodes are encouraged by agricultural activities.

Plant-parasitic nematodes are active only when in moist habitats. They can be classified into three groups based on their life habits:

- Migratory ectoparasitic species feed on root surfaces without becoming attached and are free living throughout their life.
- Migratory endoparasitic species move about freely but enter the plant during certain life stages and feed from within.
- Sedentary endoparasitic species do not move about once they are within host tissue or other organs.

Dispersal and Movement. Nematodes are spread easily when infested plants, farm equipment, soil, irrigation water, and animals move from place to place. Movement over long distances primarily occurs when farm produce, nursery plants, seeds, tubers, or bulbs are transported. Nematodes move very slowly through soil by themselves; their movement is aided when soil pores are lined with a thin film of water.

Damage. Plants infected with root nematodes can show damage symptoms on upper portions as well as on the root. Symptoms such as stunting, chlorosis, wilting, curling and twisting of leaves and stems, delayed or uneven maturation of crops, and fruit drop can be associated with nematodes and with many other pests as well. Nematodes may inject saliva into the plant, which brings about much of the plant distortion. Root symptoms produced by various nematodes include galls (Fig. 2-51), swelling, stubby roots, lesions, and stunting. These symptoms can warn you of the presence of nematodes but do not tell you for sure whether they are present. An expert should confirm that nematodes are the cause of the symptoms you observe. Some nematodes develop an association with pathogens to create a nematode-disease complex. For instance, Fusarium wilt is more severe in cotton when nematodes are present. Nematode vectors transmit several plant viruses, including tomato ring spot and grapevine fanleaf.

Beneficial Aspects. Some nematode species (*Steinernema carpocapsae*, *S. glaseri*, and *Heterorhabditis bacteriophora*) are used to control caterpillars or grubs, usually in turf. They attack armyworms and cutworms, craneflies, white grubs, and other soil-dwelling pests (Flint 2012).

Snails and Slugs

Snails and slugs belong to the phylum Mollusca. They are related to clams, scallops, abalone, octopi, and squid (Fig. 2-52). Other pests that belong to this group are the shipworms and the pholads. Shipworms bore into wood that is in contact with salt or brackish water. Pholads are clamlike marine organisms that attack and destroy submerged wood. Snails have visible shells into which they can retreat. Slugs have shells that are internal; semi-slugs have a small visible shell. In Southern California, a predatory snail controls pest snails in citrus.

Important Characteristics. Snails prefer cool, moist surroundings. However, their shells afford them protection from heat and dryness. This enables them to exploit many different environments. They seal themselves into their shells and become dormant for up to 4 years during dry periods. Slugs do not have protective shells and so are vulnerable to high temperatures and dry weather; they prefer cool, damp locations.

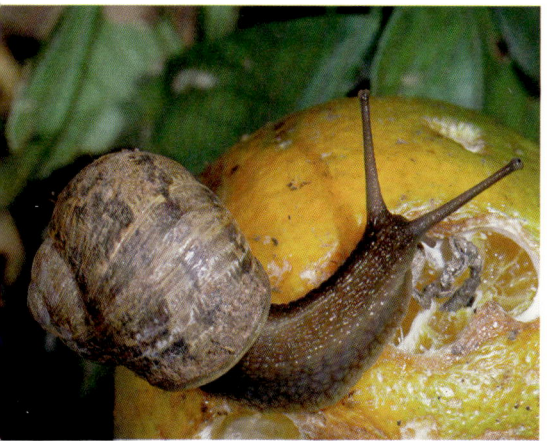

FIGURE 2-52
Snail, phylum Mollusca.

Life Cycle. Snails and slugs lay between 10 and 200 eggs beneath the surface of the soil. They lay egg masses several times each year from spring through fall. In cooler areas, egg-laying activity stops during the winter. It takes from 1 to 3 years for newly hatched snails or slugs to reach maturity.

Where Found. Snails and slugs inhabit damp areas, soil litter, and foliage of plants. They are usually nocturnal and hide during the day under boards or stones, or among ivy, dense shrubbery, or damp refuse. At night and early in the morning, or during cool, damp periods, they forage for food. They often return to the same resting area each day unless the area becomes too dry or disturbed.

Damage. Snails and slugs feed on foliage, fruits, berries, and vegetables. Snails can be serious pests in citrus, where they feed on developing fruits. They are also pests in greenhouses. Besides feeding damage, both snails and slugs leave slime trails that detract from the appearance of produce and foliage. Some aquatic snails carry disease-causing organisms that can be transmitted to people.

Beneficial Aspects. Some species of snails are predaceous, making them useful in biological control programs aimed at pest snails.

Vertebrates

Vertebrates belong to the phylum Chordata and have internal skeletons and backbones. They include fish, amphibians (frogs, toads, and salamanders), reptiles (turtles, lizards, and snakes), birds, and mammals. They become pests if they

- are reservoirs of pathogens that cause disease (such as plague and rabies)
- damage crops or stored products
- prey on livestock
- interfere with the activities or needs of people

Identification of vertebrates is often easier than microorganisms, invertebrates, and weeds because fewer species are involved. Endangered species, migrant species, or other wildlife laws protect many vertebrates. Therefore, you must know the species' identity before beginning any control program. Identify vertebrates by comparing them to photographs and drawings, such as those in the *Vertebrate Pest Control Handbook Online* (vpcrac.org/about/vertebrate-pest-handbook) and in *Wildlife Pest Control around Gardens and Homes* (Salmon et al. 2006). For help in identifying vertebrates, contact the U.S. Fish and Wildlife Service or the California Department of Fish and Wildlife. These agencies require permits for control of some vertebrate species.

Besides observing the animals, another useful way to identify vertebrates is by recognizing certain indirect damage, such as burrows, nests, tracks, and fecal droppings. You can also recognize some pests by the direct damage they do to crops, structures, or lawns; teeth marks or feeding habits can be checked against identification keys to help narrow down the pest.

FISH

Some fish are pests because they eat other fish that are more important to people. Some also compete with important fish for limited food and space. Others occur in places where they are unwanted. Certain fish species may be undesirable because they serve as intermediate hosts for parasites, such as nematodes, that infect animals and people.

Life Cycle. The life cycles of fish vary, depending on the species. The following cycle represents the general life stages of fish.

Fish begin as eggs, then hatch into larvae that feed off the yolk sac, which remains attached to their bodies. Once the larvae have consumed the entire yolk sac, they are known as fry for the next several months (and for up to 1 year in some species). Fry feed on their own and eventually develop into juveniles, the final stage before they become mature (adults) and can reproduce (spawn).

Damage. Pest fish populations compete with desirable species and may crowd them out, especially where ponds are stocked for recreational fishing. They can also strip a pond of its plants, reducing oxygen levels and destroying habitat for smaller fish and other aquatic species.

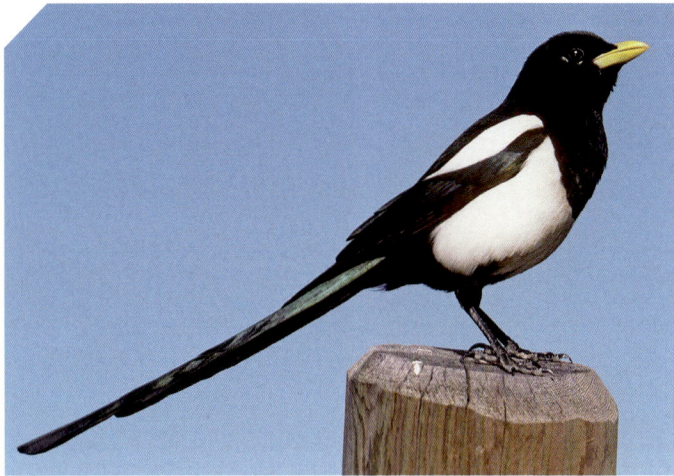

FIGURE 2-53
Birds can be pests when they damage agricultural crops, nest on buildings, or interfere with aircraft operation.

Beneficial Aspects. Sterilized grass carp are sometimes used in ponds with overgrown vegetation to control plant populations. In California, grass carp can be purchased only if they have been sterilized. If unsterilized, they will reproduce quickly and eat all vegetation in a pond. Check with the agricultural commissioner in your county to be sure you can use grass carp to control pond vegetation.

Many ponds are stocked with fish that eat mosquito larvae—the fish keep mosquito populations under control naturally and reduce the need for pesticide applications to standing water.

AMPHIBIANS AND REPTILES

A few species of toads, frogs, snakes, lizards, and their relatives are poisonous to people and livestock. These species are pests if they occur in areas where people or livestock live. Amphibians occasionally clog water outlets, filters, pipes, hoses, and other equipment associated with irrigation systems and drains. Be aware that the taking and possession of lizards is regulated by the California Department of Fish and Wildlife, with specific regulations depending on the species.

BIRDS

People appreciate birds because of their song, beauty, or predaceous habits. Many birds catch insects, and some kill snakes, rats, mice, and other pests. However, some pest birds harbor pathogens that insects or other organisms transmit to commercial poultry. Also, they eat or damage crops (Fig. 2-53) and roost in massive numbers in trees or on window ledges. Some birds interfere with aircraft, cause damage to buildings, or make too much noise. Bird lice and mites associated with nesting areas can infest homes, hospitals, and offices. Some bird species can be removed only with a depredation permit from the California Department of Fish and Wildlife or while under the supervision of the local county agricultural commissioner. Check with your local Fish and Wildlife warden or agricultural commissioner before removing birds, even on your own property (Stetson and Baldwin 2010).

MAMMALS

Pest mammals interfere with the activities of people or cause harm to their crops, livestock, or possessions. Some of the most important mammalian vertebrate pests are rodents such as rats and mice. These animals inhabit buildings and damage or soil furnishings and other items. They also consume and destroy stored food. They sometimes harbor disease organisms and compete with people and livestock for food. These animals often carry fleas and mites that harbor and transmit disease-causing organisms. Infected skunks and bats transmit rabies. Larger mammals, like foxes, coyotes, mountain lions, and bears, are occasional pests when they endanger

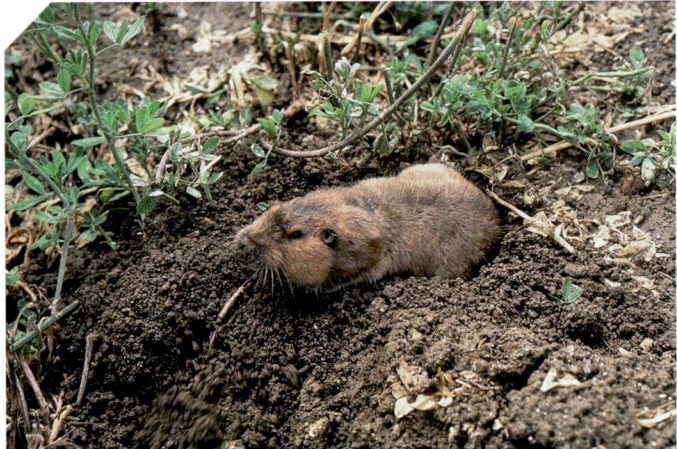

FIGURE 2-54

Adult pocket gophers are rarely seen above ground except when pushing soil from their burrow, as shown here, and sometimes when clipping small plants near a burrow opening.

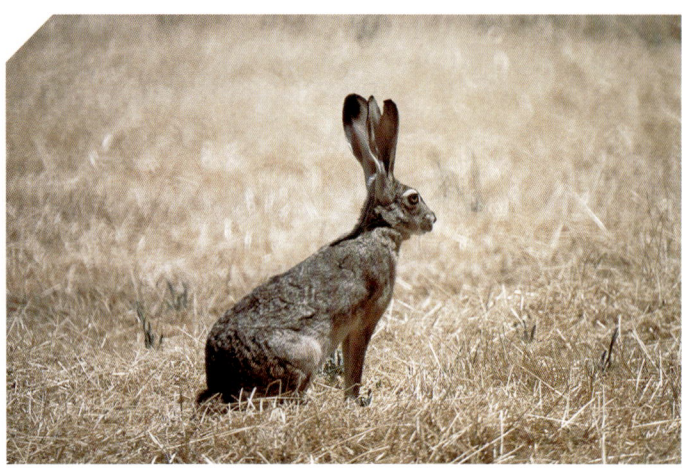

FIGURE 2-55

Jackrabbits are the most common pest rabbits. In contrast to brush rabbits, jackrabbits live in areas that are more open. They have much longer ears and longer hind legs.

people and their possessions or prey on pets or livestock. Foraging deer can be serious pests of agricultural crops and residential landscaping.

The life stage of mammals matters when you are planning pesticide applications. For instance, in the case of ground squirrels, the best time to apply fumigants is when the young are still in the burrows, before they are ready to emerge. More important is knowledge of rodent biology, such as the food they eat during particular times, and whether they aestivate or hibernate. Again, ground squirrels provide a good example. In late winter and spring, they feed on green vegetation but switch to seeds and fruits in late spring and early summer, so baiting with grain or seeds in winter will yield poor results. Below you will find information about some of the more troublesome pests of gardens, landscapes, and agricultural and recreational areas.

Pocket Gophers. Pocket gophers (*Thomomys* spp., Fig. 2-54) are burrowing rodents that get their name from the fur-lined external cheek pouches, or pockets, they use for carrying food and nesting materials. They are well equipped for digging and tunneling with their powerfully built forequarters; large-clawed front paws; fine, short fur that doesn't cake in wet soils; small eyes and ears; and highly sensitive facial whiskers that assist with moving about in the dark. A gopher's lips also are unusually adapted for their lifestyle: they can close them behind their four large incisor teeth to keep dirt out of their mouths when using their teeth for digging. Gophers don't hibernate and are active year-round, although you might not see any fresh mounding. They also can be active at all hours of the day.

Gophers live alone within their burrow system, except when females are caring for their young or during breeding season. Gopher densities can be as high as sixty or more per acre in irrigated alfalfa fields or in vineyards. Gophers reach sexual maturity about 1 year of age and can live up to 3 years. In nonirrigated areas, breeding usually occurs in late winter and early spring, resulting in one litter per year; in irrigated sites, gophers can produce up to three litters per year. Litters usually average five or six young.

Pocket gophers often invade yards, gardens, and fields, feeding on the roots and trunks of many food and forage crops, ornamental plants, vines, shrubs, and trees. A single gopher moving down a planted row can inflict considerable damage in a very short time. Gophers also gnaw and damage buried irrigation systems. Their tunnels can divert and carry off irrigation water, which wastes water and leads to soil erosion. Mounds on lawns interfere with mowing equipment and ruin the aesthetics of well-kept turfgrass or the safety and playability of golf and other sports turf (Salmon and Baldwin 2009).

Rabbits. Rabbits are enjoyed by many people, but they can also be very destructive to gardens, cultivated areas, and landscapes. Eight species of rabbits are found in California. Three of these species—the black-tailed hare or jackrabbit (*Lepus californicus*), the desert cottontail (*Sylvilagus audubonii*), and the brush rabbit (*S. bachmani*)—are widespread and cause the majority of problems. Because of its greater size and abundance, the jackrabbit (Fig. 2-55) is the most destructive.

The breeding season for jackrabbits runs from late January through August, although breeding is possible during any month of the year where winters are mild. Litters average between two and three young, and jackrabbits can have as many as five or six litters per year. Young jackrabbits are born fully furred and with their eyes open. Within a day they can move about quite rapidly. For both cottontails and brush rabbits, breeding begins in December and ends in June. The average litter size is usually three or four, and there can be up to six litters per year. These rabbits give birth in a shallow depression on the ground. The newborn rabbits, which are nearly furless and have closed eyes, remain in the nest for several weeks.

Rabbits can be very destructive in gardens, agricultural fields, and landscaped places. They are particularly prevalent where wild or uncultivated lands border residential zones, parks, greenbelts, or croplands. Open lands such as uncultivated wild areas provide resting and hiding cover during the day within easy travel distances to prime irrigated food sources. Rabbits feed on leaves, stems, and other plant parts. They also gnaw and cut plastic irrigation lines, especially small-diameter tubes (Salmon and Gorenzel 2010b).

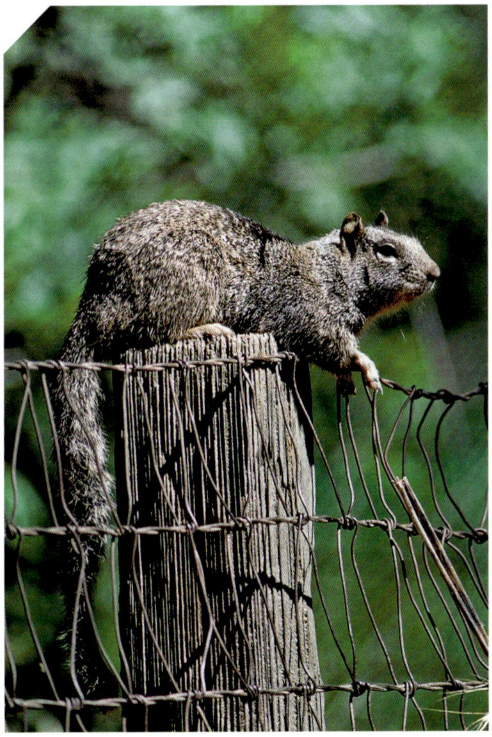

Ground Squirrels. Ground squirrels are troublesome pests for homeowners, farmers, and gardeners. The California ground squirrel (*Spermophilus beecheyi*) is the species most commonly reported as problematic (Fig. 2-56). This squirrel's habitat includes nearly all regions of California except for the Owens Valley. Ground squirrels are active during the day, mainly from midmorning through late afternoon, especially on warm, sunny days. They have two periods of dormancy during the year. During winter months, most ground squirrels hibernate, but some young can be active at this time, particularly in areas where winters are not severe. During the hottest times of the year, most adults go into a period of inactivity (aestivation) that can last a few days to a week or more.

Ground squirrels breed once a year, averaging seven or eight per litter. Aboveground activity by adults is at a maximum at the height of the breeding season. The young are born in the burrow and grow rapidly. When they are about 6 weeks old, they usually emerge from the burrow. At 6 months they resemble adults.

Ground squirrels damage many plants. Particularly vulnerable are grains as well as nut and fruit trees such as almond, apple, apricot, orange, peach, pistachio, prune, and walnut. They can damage young shrubs, vines, and trees by gnawing bark, completely removing a strip of bark from a tree's outer circumference (girdling), and eating twigs and leaves. Their burrowing around tree roots and buildings, and in yards or fields can be quite destructive. Ground squirrels will burrow in hillsides, berms, and the sides of dirt-lined canals. This activity can result in loss of these structures' integrity and their ultimate collapse (Salmon and Gorenzel 2010a).

FIGURE 2-56

Ground squirrels are often pests because they compete with people for agricultural products. Squirrels also damage levees and bridge foundations through their burrowing activities. Some vector diseases that fleas or other insects transmit to people and livestock.

Distinguish between damage caused by pathogens and abiotic factors.

Pathogens and Abiotic Disorders

Plant diseases cause many problems on farms, in landscapes, and in recreational and natural areas, so accurate diagnosis, treatment, and preventive action are very important. Plant and animal diseases can be caused by nonliving (abiotic) factors and living (biotic) pathogenic microorganisms. Biotic and abiotic factors alter or interfere with the chemical processes that take place within an organism's cells. This interference produces disease symptoms or disorders. To avoid unnecessary pest management treatments, you must accurately identify the cause of the symptoms you observe in plants and animals. For a more detailed discussion of pathogens and abiotic disorders, see Flint 2012.

Biotic Factors Causing Disease (Pathogens). Biotic disease-causing agents, or pathogens, are capable of spreading from one host to another and producing disease symptoms. The ability of the organism to spread and infect may depend on climatic factors, the host's genetic makeup or nutritional state, and other factors. Although several types of pathogens produce disease in plants and animals, the most important are fungi, bacteria (Table 2-5), viruses, viroids, and phytoplasmas.

Many pathogens are submicroscopic, making identification difficult. Often, only the use of electron microscopes or complex biochemical or genetic tests confirms the identity of a pathogen. It may even be necessary to grow the organism in the laboratory or inject plants or laboratory animals with the pathogen to make a positive identification. These types of tests require trained technicians and specialized laboratory equipment. Sidebar 2-4 contains information on using laboratory identification services and how to send material for analysis.

Another way to identify disease-causing microorganisms in plants and animals is by studying the observed symptoms. Each host plant or animal usually has specific diseases to which it is susceptible and produces specific symptoms or groups of symptoms for a given disease. Learning to recognize disease symptoms helps you sort through and reject some pathogens as causes of the observed symptoms. In some cases, specific disease-causing pathogens are more

---

SIDEBAR 2-4

SAMPLING AND SENDING PLANTS FOR IDENTIFICATION OF DISEASE-CAUSING PATHOGENS

SAMPLING

1. Select plants that are most representative of the observed disease symptoms. Collect several plants.
2. Include roots by digging up plant and shaking off soil.
3. Place plants in plastic or paper bags. Keep plant materials cool. Put them in an ice chest while you are in the field. Store samples in a refrigerator until they can be shipped.

LABELING

Attach a label to the outside of each sample bag. Include the following information on labels:

1. Your name, address, and telephone number.
2. Crop or plant type, including variety.
3. Location of field or property (names of nearby crossroads).
4. Portion of planted area that sample represents. Include a map if necessary.
5. Brief description of the field's crop history (previous crops) or any information on what was planted in the area before diseased plants were grown there.
6. Observations made by you and the owner/operator of the property of previous problems and of when present problem was first detected.
7. Date samples were taken.

SHIPPING

1. Contact the person or laboratory that will receive samples to determine the best method of shipping and to inform them that samples will be arriving.
2. Pack samples in a sturdy, well-insulated container to prevent crushing or heat damage.
3. Mark package clearly and request that the shipper keep it in a cool location.
4. Ship packages early in the week so they will arrive before a weekend.

TABLE 2-5

Examples of bacterial diseases in plants

Symptom	Disease	Pathogen
galls	crown gall	*Agrobacterium* spp.
leaf spots	bacterial blight of walnuts	*Pseudomonas* spp.
	leaf spot of cucurbits	*Pseudomonas* spp.
	halo blight of beans	*Xanthomonas* spp.
	bacterial spot of tomato	*Xanthomonas* spp.
systemic infections	fire blight of apple, pear, and quince	*Erwinia* spp.
	bacterial wilt of cucurbits	*Erwinia* spp.
soft rot	blackleg of potato	*Erwinia* spp.
	vegetable soft rots	*Pseudomonas* spp.
scab	common potato scab	*Streptomyces* spp.
	gladiolus scab	*Pseudomonas* spp.

prevalent in particular locations or under certain conditions. Knowing these limitations helps you to narrow the choices. Also, lesions or rotted areas of infected plants may provide clues to the type of organism causing the damage. Inspect the plant's vascular system for damage. Be sure to dig up some infected plants and examine their root systems.

If possible, check the disease symptom distribution throughout a population of plants or animals. Do many individuals show signs of infection or only a few? Are the diseased plants distributed evenly, or are they confined to specific locations? Try to associate the distribution of infection with conditions that would favor specific diseases. This association may provide valuable clues to the identity of the pathogen.

Signs of infection can also be observed for some pathogens. For instance, fungi produce distinctive structures such as molds or spore-producing bodies that aid in identification. Remember that fungal or bacterial infections may not be the primary cause of observed signs; they may be secondary infections breaking down already-dead tissue.

Abiotic Factors Causing Disease. Abiotic disorders are noninfectious diseases induced by adverse environmental conditions, often as a result of human activity. These include nutrient deficiencies or excesses; low or high temperatures; toxic levels of salt, herbicides, or other pesticides; air pollution; and too little or too much water (Table 2-6). Activities that compact soil, change the soil grade, or injure trunks or roots can also predispose plants to abiotic disorders. In addition to direct damage, abiotic disorders can predispose plants to attack by insects and pathogens.

Although some abiotic disorders can be recognized by characteristic symptoms such as distortion or discoloring of foliage, roots, stems, fruits, or flowers, abiotic disorders are difficult to identify with certainty. A field history, records of pesticide and fertilizer use, and testing soil or leaf tissue samples may help in diagnosis. Patterns of injured plants in the field can also help you identify abiotic disorders. In general, symptoms of abiotic disorders arise suddenly and do not spread through a plant or to other plants over time as pest damage can.

TABLE 2-6

Common abiotic disorder symptoms and their causes

Symptoms*	Possible cause
Foliage wilts, droops, discolors, and drops prematurely. Twigs and limbs may die back. Bark cracks and develops cankers. Plant may be attacked by wood-boring insects.	water deficiency
Foliage yellows and drops. Twigs and branches die back. Root crown diseases develop.	water excess or poor drainage
Foliage is discolored, undersized, sparse, or distorted and may drop prematurely. Plant growth is slow. Limbs may die back.	mineral deficiency
Foliage turns brown, dry, and crispy. Limbs may die back. Odor of natural gas may be detectable.	natural gas line leak underground
Foliage or shoots turn yellowish, are undersized or distorted. Leaves may appear burned, with dead margins and drop.	pesticide toxicity
Yellow, brown, then white areas develop on upper side of leaves, beginning between veins. Foliage may die.	sunburn
Leaves or needles turn yellowish, brownish, or have discolored flecks. Foliage may be sparse, stunted, and drop prematurely.	air pollution
Leaves turn yellowish or brownish, especially along margins. Foliage may drop prematurely. Bark becomes corky.	mineral deficiency
Foliage is abnormally dark.	excess light
Excess growth of succulent foliage. Foliage may appear burned and die. Plant is infested with many mites, aphids, psyllids, or other insects that suck plant juices.	nitrogen excess
Shoots, buds, or flowers curl, darken, and die. Limbs and entire plant may die.	frost
Foliage, twigs, or limbs injured. Cankers may develop.	hail or ice
Bark or wood dead, often in a streak or band.	lightning
Bark is cracked or sunken, often on south and west sides. Wood may be attacked by boring insects or decay fungus.	sunscald

Note: *Many of these symptoms can have other causes, including pathogens and insects.
Source: Flint 2012.

Poor irrigation practices can cause diseaselike symptoms in plants. Plants that do not get enough water wilt, discolor, and drop leaves, fruits, or flowers prematurely. If plants do not get water for long periods of time, you may see stunted growth, dieback, and a greater susceptibility to insects and other pests. Too much water drowns and kills roots and weakens the plant's resistance to attack from pathogens such as *Phytophthora* spp. As roots die, discolored and dying foliage appear on the aboveground portions of the plant.

Nutrient deficiencies cause foliage to discolor, fade, distort, or become spotted, causing symptoms that are sometimes confused with those caused by pathogens. Fewer leaves, flowers, and fruits may be produced; they can also develop late and be undersized. More severely deficient plants become stunted and exhibit dieback. Excess nutrients and salts can also be toxic to plants. Toxicity symptoms include chlorosis on leaf edges, necrosis, branch dieback, and increased pests.

Weather conditions can contribute to disorders in plants that can be mistaken for pathogen-caused diseases. Too much or too little sunlight can damage plants. Sunburn, sunscald, and deficient pigmentation are associated with improper light levels. Frost damage can cause shoots, buds, and flowers to curl, turn brown or black, and die. Frost damage to foliage often looks like leaf anthracnose diseases. Plant damage from hail can provide entry sites for pathogens such as fire blight on susceptible species. Wind injury may cause scarring similar to insect feeding. If several species of plants in an area show similar damage, the cause is likely to be abiotic because most plant pathogens and many pest arthropods attack only one or a few species of related plants.

THE DISEASE TRIANGLE

For a pathogen to attack a plant, the plant and pathogen must come in contact with one another and interact. Plant and pathogen are often present and in contact but disease does not develop, either because the host is resistant to attack or the environment does not support disease development. These three components—susceptible host plant, causal agent (pathogen), and the right environment—are known as the disease triangle (Fig. 2-57). One side of the triangle represents each component. If any of the sides is absent, the disease will not develop.

It is essential to understand that a pathogen and the disease it causes are not the same: a pathogen may be present, but unless the other two conditions of the triangle (the right environment and a susceptible host) are also present, the disease will not develop. In practice, pest managers must take preventive measures when conditions in the environment favor the development of disease because unseen pathogens may already be present on the host.

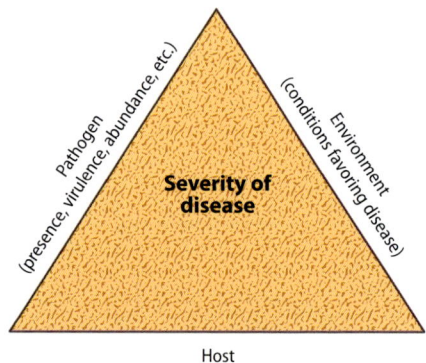

FIGURE 2-57

The disease triangle. All sides of the triangle must be present for disease to occur. The disease becomes more severe as conditions on each side become more favorable.

THE DISEASE CYCLE

Specific events unfold that lead to the development and spread of a disease; together these events are called the disease cycle (Fig. 2-58). The disease cycle consists of the appearance, development, and spread of the disease on a host plant (i.e., inoculation, penetration, infection, and growth), as well as the pathogen's life cycle. The disease cycle also includes changes that occur in the host plant, the plant's symptoms during the growing season, and the survival of the pathogen into the next season.

Inoculation occurs when inoculum, the form of the pathogen that initiates infection, comes into contact with a susceptible plant. In fungi, inoculum can be spores, sclerotia, or mycelia. Bacteria, phytoplasmas, viruses, and viroids do not produce specialized structures for survival or spread. Primary inoculum survives the winter and causes the primary infection, or first infection,

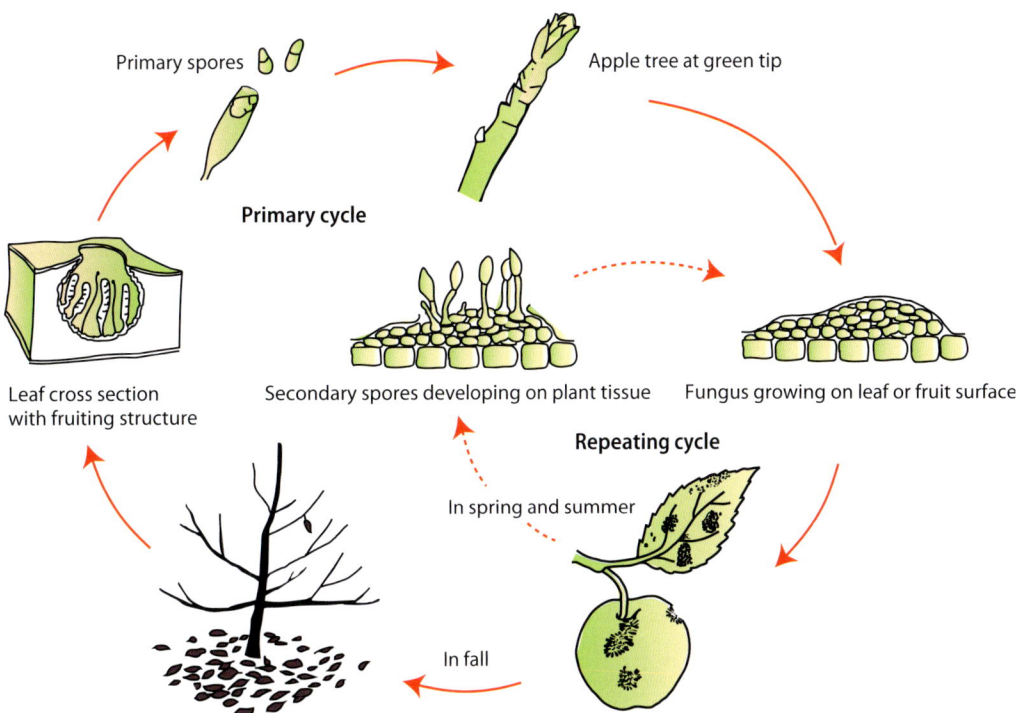

FIGURE 2-58

The disease cycle of apple scab. The disease cycle includes the life cycle of the pathogen and how it interacts with the host to cause disease and perpetuate within the ecosystem.

of the season. In multicycle pathogens, primary infections produce secondary inoculum, which in turn causes secondary infections that can rapidly spread disease within a crop. Sources of inoculum may be nearby plants, seeds, transplants, or other disease-spreading structures. Inoculum may already be present on the host or in the field or may be spread by wind, water, or insects. Some types of inoculum survive in the soil for less than a season; other types survive for many years.

Pathogens enter the host by direct penetration through natural openings or through wounds. Most bacteria enter plants through natural openings such as stomata, lenticels, nectaries, or through wounds. Viruses, viroids, and phytoplasmas enter through wounds, through feeding by vectors or, in perennial plants, through grafts. Fungi commonly penetrate directly through intact plant surfaces, although some enter through wounds to the plant.

A pathogen has successfully infected a host once the pathogen begins to withdraw nutrients, grow, and multiply in the plant tissues. Successful infections usually result in symptoms such as necrosis that are associated with specific pathogens. When symptoms do not appear right away, the infection is said to be latent. In most diseases, however, symptoms appear a few days after infection.

Understanding the cycle of a disease can help identify possibilities for control. Opportunities to break the disease cycle exist through the selection of disease-resistant stock, seed treatment, well-timed fungicide application, and many cultural control practices such as rotation, removal of overwintering inoculum or alternate hosts, solarization, and crop-free periods to reduce inoculum or avoid the presence of a vector.

FUNGI

Fungi are a diverse group of organisms that get their nutrients from living or dead plant or animal material. Although once classified in the plant kingdom, fungi are not plants; most are in the kingdom Fungi. Most fungi feed on decaying material (saprophytes), helping to break down dead organic matter and build up soil fertility. Certain fungi live on dead and living plants; some of these cause plant disease. Still other fungi require living host plants to grow and reproduce; these fungi are called obligate parasites and include many of the major plant pathogen species, such as rusts, downy mildews, and powdery mildews.

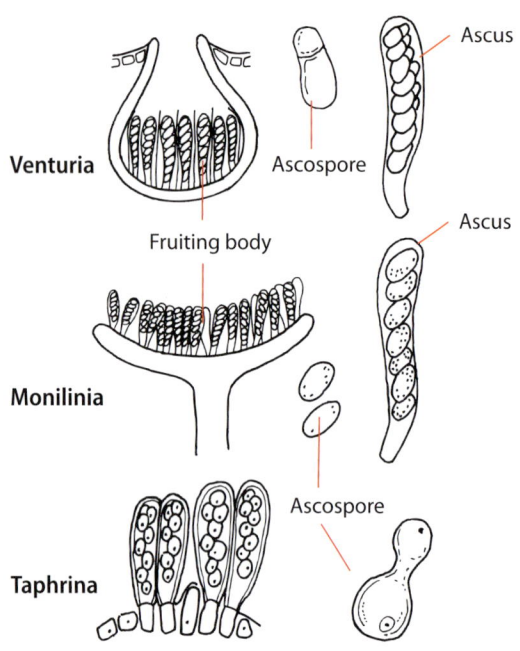

FIGURE 2-59

These footprint-shaped spores were produced by *Venturia inaequalis*, the causal agent of apple scab. These drawings show fruiting bodies, ascospores, and asci for the apple scab pathogen in the genus *Venturia* along with two other types: the genus *Monilinia*, which includes the agent causing brown rot of stone fruits, and the genus *Taphrina*, which includes the agent causing peach leaf curl.

Identification. Fungi are mostly microscopic organisms, but some have forms, such as mushrooms, that are large and identifiable without magnification. The body of the fungus is made up of tiny tubular filaments called hyphae. Growth of the fungus occurs at the tips of the hyphae. Hyphae may be colorless or variously pigmented. The mass of hyphae growing together is referred to as the mycelium. Reproductive structures called spores may be produced on specialized hyphae or fruiting bodies.

Spores and spore-bearing structures are what people use to identify fungi. Size, shape, color, arrangement of spores, and the shape and color of the fruiting body can be used to help determine the genus and species of the fungus. (Fig. 2-59).

Field identification of disease symptoms caused by fungi can often help determine the species causing the damage. However, when in doubt, enlist the assistance of an expert.

Types of damage that may be associated with fungus infection include leaf spots; blight on leaves, branches, twigs, and flowers; cankers; dieback of twigs; root rot; seedling damping off; stem rots; soft and dry rots; scab on fruits, leaves, or tubers; and the overall decline of the host. All of these symptoms also contribute to the stunting of infected plants.

Fungal infections can also result in distortion of plant parts. Examples of symptoms you can see include enlarged roots (clubroot); enlarged growths filled with mycelia (galls); warts on tubers and stems; profuse upward branching of twigs (witches' broom); and distorted, curled leaves (leaf curl). Other symptoms of fungus infections include wilting or powdery accumulations such as rust and mildew.

In diagnosing disease, plant pathologists distinguish between symptoms and signs (Fig. 2-60). The symptoms of a disease refer to changes in the appearance of the infected plant, such as the necrotic, sunken, ulcerlike lesions of an anthracnose infection. The signs of a

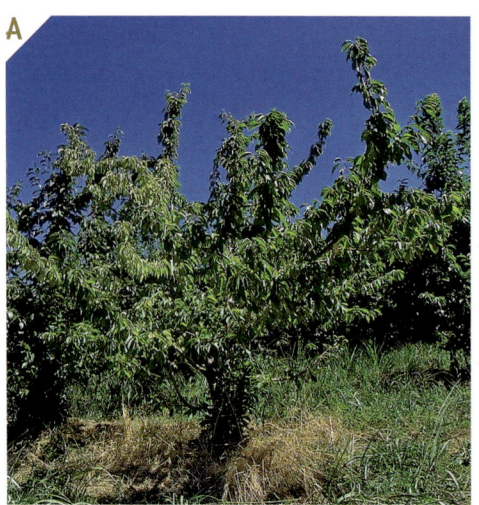
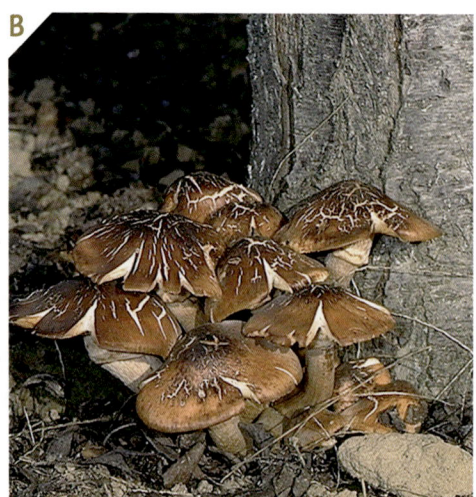
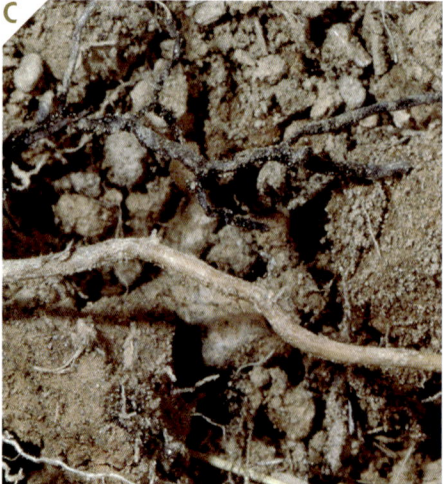

FIGURE 2-60

One of the symptoms of Armillaria root rot in tree crops is the yellowing and wilting of foliage, often on one side of the tree (A). Signs of the disease include *Armillaria mellea* mushrooms that may appear around the trunk of infected trees following rain in fall or winter (B), and the dark strings of fungal mycelia called rhizomorphs, which can extend from diseased wood to infect the roots of healthy trees. In the photo (C), a rhizomorph is shown above a light brown healthy root.

PEST IDENTIFICATION   61

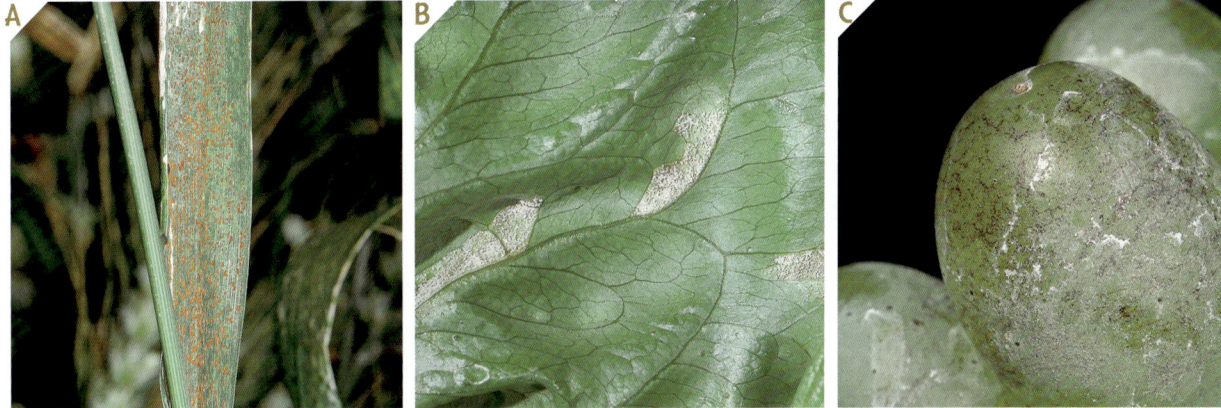

FIGURE 2-61

Some major fungal diseases and their causal organisms that can be identified by the signs (or fungal growth) that appear on the host include leaf rust (*Puccinia recondita*) spores on wheat (A); downy mildew (*Bremia lactucae*) spores on lettuce (B); and powdery mildew (*Uncinula necator*) spores on grapes (C).

disease, on the other hand, are structures that the pathogen may produce on the surface of the host, such as mycelia, sclerotia, sporophores, fruiting bodies, and spores (Fig. 2-61). For example, the white, cottony mycelia and hard black clusters of dormant sclerotia found on the lower stem of lettuce plants are signs of the *Sclerotinia* fungus; symptoms of *Sclerotinia*-caused diseases include wilting of the lower leaves and limpness of the entire plant.

Life Cycle. The life cycles of fungi vary. Generally, fungi reproduce through spore production. Spores are specialized reproductive bodies that may be formed sexually or asexually. Almost all fungi have an asexual cycle, and asexual reproduction can occur several times within a growing season. In most of the fungi that have a sexual reproductive cycle, reproduction occurs only once a year. Fungi that are not known to have a sexual cycle are called imperfect fungi.

Fungi have evolved a number of mechanisms to survive when conditions are unfavorable (Fig. 2-62). Fungi overwinter as mycelia or spores in or on infected tissue. Resting spores of some species are resistant to extremes in temperature and moisture. Infected plant debris, bud scales, or bark cankers in trees, shrubs, or soil can provide overwintering habitat for the mycelia, sclerotia, or spores of many fungi. Seeds and other vegetative organs or alternative hosts such as weeds provide other survival sites for overwintering fungi. Some soil-inhabiting fungi survive as saprophytes or by producing resistant oospores.

Dispersal and Movement. Most fungi cannot move long distances without the assistance of people, insects, animals, or environmental factors such

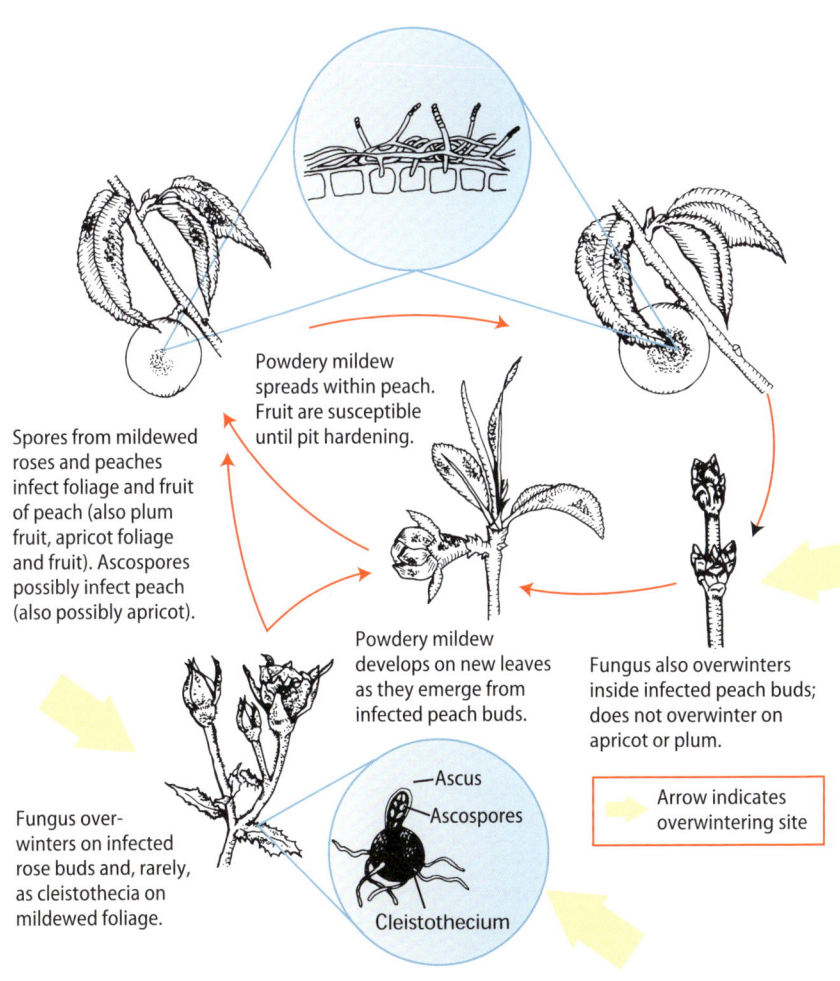

FIGURE 2-62

Seasonal cycle of powdery mildew caused by the *Sphaerotheca pannosa* fungus in apricots, peaches, and plums. The pathogen can overwinter as mycelia on rose buds or peach buds or as cleistothecia on rose foliage, but it cannot survive on plum or apricot.

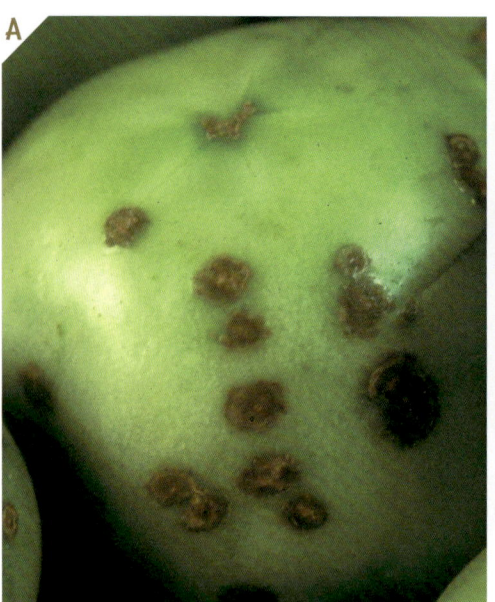 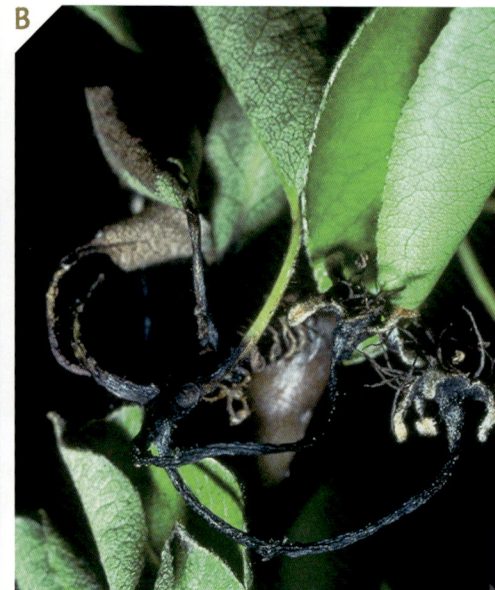 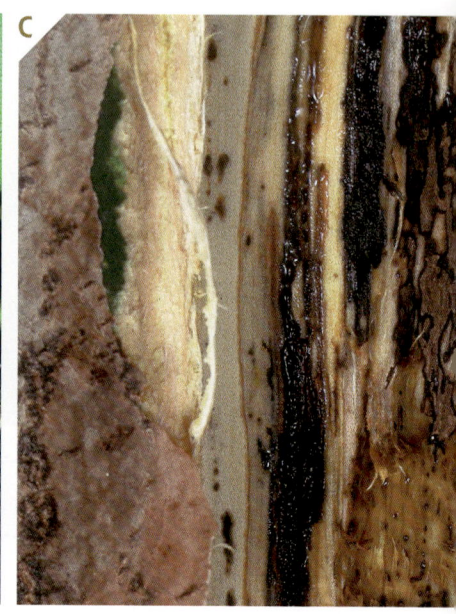

FIGURE 2-63

Disease symptoms of some bacterial diseases. Bacterial spot lesions caused by *Xanthomonas vesicatoria* on tomato fruits have a rough, scabby texture (A). When they first develop, the lesions are surrounded by a white halo, similar to bacterial speck. As with all bacterial diseases, laboratory analysis is required for identification. Pear fruits, flowers, and leaves infected with fire blight turn black (B). Tan droplets of ooze are also typically present. A walnut trunk damaged by deep bark canker bacteria, *Erwinia rubrifaciens*, typically shows dark spots underneath the bark (C).

as wind or rain. A few fungi are able to move from one host to another by extending rhizomorphs through the soil. Most fungal spores spread in air currents and can be carried over long distances. Spores, sclerotia, and mycelial fragments can be picked up and dispersed by water; some fungi depend on rain to spread. Insects can spread fungal pathogens. For example, the elm bark beetle (*Scolytus multistriatus*) brings Dutch elm disease (DED) to new areas. Once the tree is infected, DED can continue its spread from one tree to another through root grafts between adjoining trees. Animals, people, and contaminated equipment can carry fungal spores. People also spread pathogens through the transport of infected seeds, transplants, nursery stock, and contaminated containers.

BACTERIA

Bacteria are microscopic one-celled organisms that are classified as prokaryotes and belong to the kingdom Procaryotae. Bacterial diseases affect almost every kind of plant and can occur wherever moist, warm conditions are present.

Identification. Bacteria are very small, typically under 0.002 mm, or about one twelve-thousandths of an inch, long. They can be rod shaped, spherical, ellipsoidal, spiral, comma shaped, or filamentous. Most bacteria have flagella that allow for some limited movement. The cell wall of bacteria is hard and enveloped by a slime layer. In some species, the slime layer forms a large mass and is referred to as a capsule.

Field diagnosis of bacterial disease relies on recognition of disease symptoms (Fig. 2-63). Plants generally have specific reactions to bacterial infections; however, laboratory analysis is required for positive identification. Common symptoms include cankers, galls, wilts, slow growth, distorted fruits, rots, discoloration of plant parts, slow ripening, distorted leaves, brooming, and leaf spots. Some bacterial diseases produce a slimy ooze on the plant surface.

Certain bacteria cause the formation of galls on specific plant parts; examples include olive knot and crown gall. Galls are typified by large, swollen, rapidly dividing cells and disorganized vascular tissues. Galls may interfere with the movement of food and water in the plant. Bacterial wilts generally affect the entire plant; slime is produced that plugs the water-conducting tissue of the infected plant. Destructive wilts include those found in tomato, cotton, cucumber, and corn. Cankers are the result of widespread tissue destruction caused by certain bacteria such as those that cause tomato cankers and

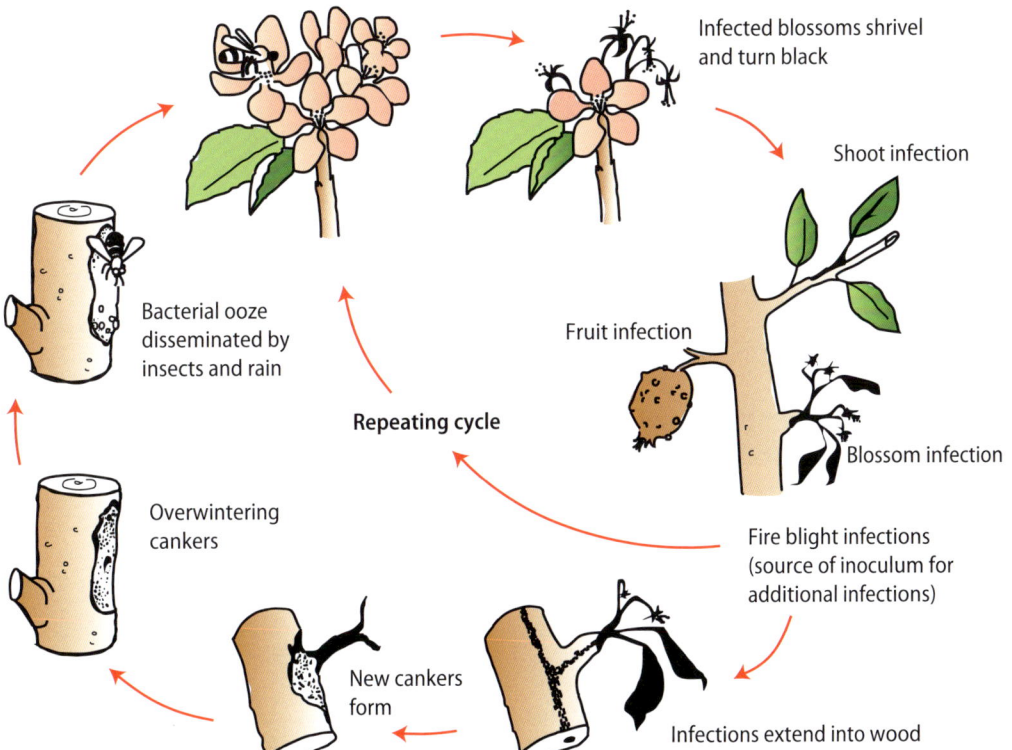

FIGURE 2-64

The disease cycle of fire blight of pear and apple caused by the bacterium *Erwinia amylovora*. The bacteria overwinter at the margins of cankers on branches and twigs and are disseminated in spring when trees start growing and sap flows out of the cankers. Splashing rain and insects attracted to the ooze move the bacteria to blossoms. Bacteria multiply rapidly in the blossoms and enter other tree tissues through stomata, lenticels, and wounds.

fire blight. Localized spotting occurs most commonly on leaves and fruits; potato scab, for instance, appears as local spots on tubers. Rots invade fleshy tissue and often result in a slimy, foul-smelling ooze. Soft rots often enter secondarily, after another pathogen has invaded.

Life Cycle and Growth Requirements. Each bacterial cell is an individual organism. Reproduction occurs by an asexual process known as binary fission: the cytoplasmic membrane grows toward the center of the cell, dividing it, and the bacterium's DNA separates into two equal pieces. When conditions are favorable, a bacterium can reproduce every 20 minutes. Over time, the offspring of a single bacterial cell produces a visible mass called a colony.

Bacteria enter plants through natural openings and wounds. Once inside the plant, some bacteria move along the sap stream; others move about with the flow of fluids between the cells. In early stages of disease, bacteria often develop between the cells of a plant. As cell walls become injured, the bacteria penetrate the cell and continue growing. The disease cycle of fire blight, caused by the bacterium *Erwinia amylovora*, is shown in Figure 2-64.

Disease symptoms appear at varying times after bacteria enter and develop in plant tissue. Soft rots and leaf spots are usually visible within a day; crown gall infections can take up to 2 years to become evident. The time between the establishment of the bacteria and the appearance of symptoms is referred to as the incubation period.

Survival Characteristics. Bacteria survive mostly within plant hosts as parasites, on seeds, or in plant debris in soil. They do not produce overwintering spores as fungi do; however, many are able to overwinter, using plant debris as an energy source, until host plants return.

Dispersal and Movement. Bacteria can be carried from one place to another in splashing or flowing water and rainwater, by moisture, and by various management practices. Bacteria that survive in organic debris in the soil can be spread by any practice that involves moving soil from one place to another, such as cultivation. Bacterial pathogens are frequently carried on infected seeds, cuttings, or transplants. Insects and animals often aid in spreading bacteria. Cucumber beetles, for example, transmit the cucumber wilt organism, and sharpshooters transmit *Xylella fastidiosa*, the bacterium that causes Pierce's disease of grape and oleander leaf scorch.

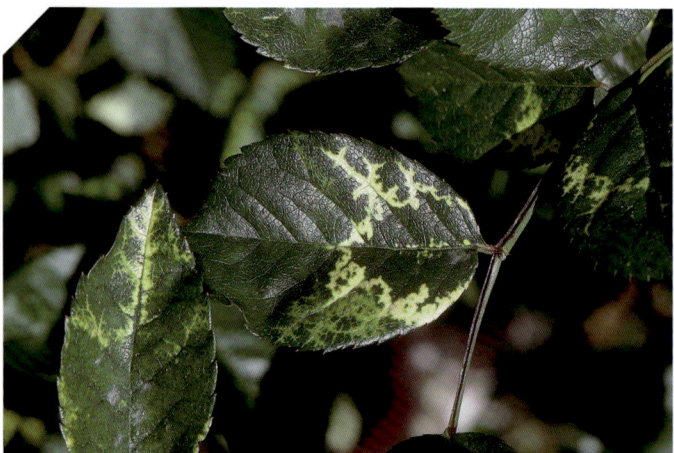

FIGURE 2-65

Discolored bands, lines, and ring patterns, such as on these rose leaves infected with rose mosaic virus, are typical symptoms of certain viruses.

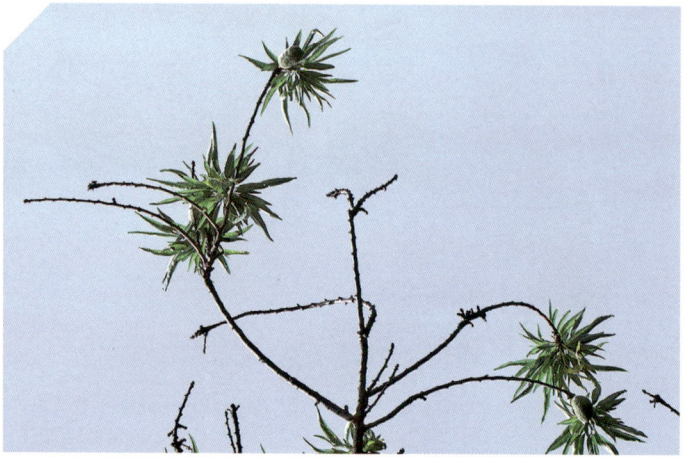

FIGURE 2-66

Some viruses can cause severe stunting and tight, bunchy growth (rosetting). This almond tree has been infected with yellow bud mosaic for several years and shows severe stunting and concentration of leaves on terminals.

VIRUSES

A virus is a parasite of submicroscopic size that is composed of genetic material and is surrounded by a layer of protein. Viruses multiply only in living cells and are unable to complete their life cycle without a host (obligate). They are among the smallest and simplest of plant pathogens. Viruses cause disease by disrupting normal processes in plant cells.

Identification. Because of their small size and transparency in the host cells they inhabit, viruses cannot be viewed or detected in the same way as other pathogens. Virus particles in infected plant cells can sometimes be seen with light microscopes in a plant pathology lab, but this method is not practical for the field. The main detection clues for the pest manager are plant symptoms.

Viral diseases produce a variety of injury symptoms on plants. Common field symptoms associated with plant viruses include growth reductions, color changes, malformations, and necrosis of tissue; severe stunting and a reduction in yield may be evident. Mosaic patterns (Fig. 2-65), a mottling of healthy and discolored tissue on leaves, are a common virus symptom. Some viruses roll or crinkle leaves; the affected leaves may be a deeper green. Vein clearing or leaf yellowing is typical of some viral infections. Some viral diseases cause the plant to become dwarfed, while others stimulate short, sporadic shoots or stunting and rosetting (Fig. 2-66). Positive identification of a virus in a plant can be determined only through the use of an electron microscope, serology, or a nucleic acid probe.

Life Cycle and Growth Requirements. All viruses are parasitic on cells and require a host cell for survival and reproduction. They are not cellular organisms themselves. Nucleic acid is released from the virus particle when the virus infects the host; the host cell is then directed to form more viruses. Viruses do not divide, nor do they produce any reproductive structures. Plant viruses have different sizes and shapes, but they are usually elongate, bacilluslike, or spherical.

Viruses enter plants through wounds made by insect or nematode vectors, mechanical injury, or from an infected pollen grain or grafting. The first virus particles may appear about 10 hours after inoculation. For infection to occur, the virus must move from cell to cell and multiply in the cells to which it moves. The movement of viruses in the plant varies with the virus and the host.

Survival Characteristics. Viruses cannot survive in dead plant debris or outside living plant tissue. Alternate hosts such as perennial plants, weeds, or volunteer crop plants provide overwintering sites for many viruses and are often suitable hosts for virus vectors as well. Insect vectors also provide an important overwintering mechanism for viruses.

Dispersal and Movement. Viruses can enter plants only through wounds. They are dispersed mechanically from plant to plant through vegetative propagation, sap, seeds, and pollen; by vectors; and by the use of contaminated pruning tools. Vectors of one or more plant viruses include aphids, leafhoppers, whiteflies, beetles, thrips, mites, nematodes, fungi, and dodders. Vectors are specific to certain viruses and hosts.

VIROIDS

Viroids are nucleic acids with a low molecular weight that can infect plant cells, replicate themselves, and cause disease. Viroids lack a protein coat and contain only RNA. Viroids consist of 250 to 400 nucleotides and exist as free RNA. Symptoms of disease from viroids are similar to viruses. Viroids cannot survive in dead plant matter or outside the host for long periods of time. They overwinter and oversummer in perennial hosts. Viroids are spread by equipment, propagation tools, pruning tools, vegetative propagation, and sometimes with seeds. Only a few viroid-caused diseases have been identified. Potato spindle tuber, citrus exocortis, chrysanthemum stunt, chrysanthemum chlorotic mottle, and cucumber pale fruit are caused by viroids.

PHYTOPLASMAS

Phytoplasmas are the smallest cells known to multiply independently of other living cells, and they can survive for extended periods outside plant cells. Phytoplasmas have a cellularlike structure without a true cell wall and may assume a wide variety of shapes and sizes. They reproduce by budding and binary fission and are transmitted primarily by leafhoppers or psyllids; mites may also transmit phytoplasmas. Phytoplasmas are also readily transmitted among woody crop plants by grafting. Phytoplasmas are responsible for several insect-transmitted diseases, including pear decline, aster yellows, western-X disease of peach, and citrus stubborn disease.

Chapter 2 Review Questions

1. **Which of the following is *most* likely to happen if you fail to understand a pest's biology?**
   - ☐ a. The pest may attack you while you are performing monitoring activities, so you will not be able to complete the job.
   - ☐ b. The pesticide you select will not take full advantage of the pest's vulnerabilities, so your application will not be very successful.
   - ☐ c. You may use the wrong application equipment, accidentally killing nontarget organisms in the treatment area.

2. **Which of the following is *most* likely to happen if you identify pests incorrectly?**
   - ☐ a. Pests may escape before they can be killed by pesticide applications.
   - ☐ b. You may confuse beneficial insects with pest insects in the field.
   - ☐ c. Your pest control efforts will often fail regardless of site conditions.

3. **Match the characteristic to the weed type.**

1. leaves have parallel veins	a. monocots
2. plants are woody	
3. leaves have netlike veins	b. dicots
4. seedlings have a single leaf	

4. **Invertebrate pests can include which of the following organisms?**
   - ☐ a. crayfish, shrimp, and eels
   - ☐ b. slugs, snails, and salamanders
   - ☐ c. spiders, insects, and nematodes

5. Match the pest with its group.

1. vertebrates	a. tick
	b. little mallow
2. invertebrates	c. ground squirrel
	d. fungi
3. weeds	e. yellow nutsedge
	f. termite
4. disease-causing agents	g. high temperatures
	h. pocket gopher

6. Which of the following is *true* about the system of scientific names used to identify living things?
   - a. It reveals relationships among various organisms so people can identify them more easily.
   - b. It reduces confusion because it relates closely to the common name of most organisms.
   - c. It is the only way of correctly identifying organisms in a written pest management plan.

7. Definitive identification for nematodes and pathogens can only be made by consulting _____.
   - a. identification keys
   - b. trained experts
   - c. farm advisors
   - d. photographs

8. When monitoring an area, you should look for which of the following to help you correctly identify pests?
   - a. characteristic signs
   - b. a pest control adviser
   - c. preserved specimens
   - d. distinguishing features

9. Match the symptom or sign with its causal agent.

	a. lesions
1. abiotic cause	b. rotted areas
	c. discolored foliage
	d. mold
2. pathogen	e. distorted fruits
	f. premature flowering

10. Match the pest with its characteristic signs or symptoms.

1. ground squirrels	a. galls filled with mycelia
	b. tree girdling
2. root nematodes	c. stubby roots
	d. fruit drop
3. aquatic weeds	e. stem rots
	f. clogged irrigation canals
4. fungal infections	g. burrows seen around tree trunks
	h. decreased fish reproduction

Chapter 3
Pesticides

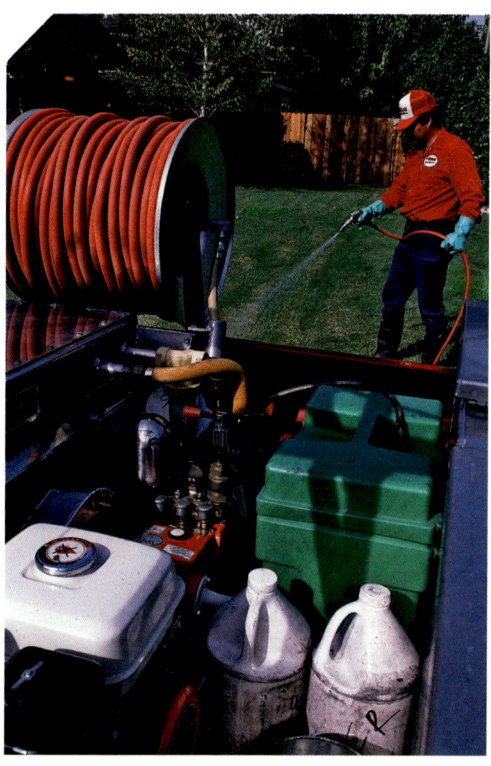

Pesticide Toxicity 69
How Pesticides are Organized 73
Pesticide Mixtures 94
Chapter 3 Review Questions 96

Knowledge Expectations

- Define a pesticide.
- Explain the concepts of hazard, exposure, and toxicity and how they relate to one another.
- List pesticide toxicity categories and signal words and explain what each category means in terms of a pesticide's effects on humans and animals.
- Identify factors that should be considered when selecting pesticides.
- List groups of pesticides according to pest target and describe the functions of each group.
- List major chemical families and describe the particular hazards associated with each one.
- Define *mode of action* and provide examples of the different modes.
- Explain how various modes of action influence pesticide selection.
- Explain how contact and systemic pesticides control pests differently.
- Define a pesticide formulation.
- List the various formulations available and the advantages and disadvantages of each.
- Explain the role of adjuvants in pesticide applications.

Define a pesticide.

The Federal Insecticide, Fungicide, and Rodenticide Act (FIFRA) defines a pesticide as "any substance or mixture of substances intended for preventing, destroying, repelling, or mitigating any insects, rodents, nematodes, fungi, or weeds, or any other forms of life declared to be pests; and any substance or mixture of substances intended for use as a plant regulator, defoliant, or desiccant."

Pesticides represent a broad range of hazardous and unique substances. Many are toxic and present risks to users as well as the environment. As a result, selecting, using, and handling pesticides requires that you have special skills and training. You must understand the different ways in which pesticides control pests. Also, you need to recognize how different pesticide formulations react within target pests, nontarget organisms, and the environment. Understanding the hazards and actions of pesticides helps you to choose the most effective and safe product for the job.

In order to find the right pesticide for your application, you should understand how pesticides are organized for reference and selection purposes. Pesticides can be grouped based on the organism they target, their mode of action, their chemical makeup, or their specific formulation. Pesticides are categorized according to their toxicity (or level of human hazard) from Category I, DANGER, to Category IV, which does not require a signal word.

Pesticides can be produced in nature, or may be manufactured synthetically, and may be chemical compounds or microbial agents. Microbial agents include naturally occurring organisms and those made through genetic manipulation. A few pesticides are chemicals not commonly thought of as pest control agents. For instance, chlorine added to swimming pools for algae control is a pesticide. So are household disinfectants, insect repellents, and plant growth regulators.

Do not confuse organic chemicals with the pesticides approved for use in organic agriculture. For more information about pest control in organic agriculture, see "Special Pest Management Methods" in Chapter 1.

This chapter focuses on the following key concepts:
- pesticide toxicity categories and how toxicity levels are determined
- pesticide groupings that help you find the right product for your specific situation
- adjuvants and their uses

Pesticide Toxicity

Toxicity, just like color or boiling point, is one of the characteristics used to describe chemicals. Toxicity is the capacity of a chemical to cause injury, sometimes referred to as potency. Most pesticides, by their nature, are toxic in order to destroy pests. Like other toxic chemicals, pesticides are hazardous because they have a potential for causing injury. Not all pesticides present the same hazard—some are more toxic or potent than others. Because highly toxic pesticides cause injury at smaller doses, they are recognized as more hazardous.

Explain the concepts of hazard, exposure, and toxicity and how they relate to one another.

PLANT AND ANIMAL TESTING

One way to measure the toxicity of pesticides is to give known doses to laboratory animals and observe the results. Animal testing is the way researchers find out the lethal dose or lethal concentration of each pesticide. Through animal testing, researchers also decide the maximum dose to which organisms can be exposed without causing injury. They use the results from these types of tests to predict hazards to people and nontarget organisms.

Animal testing establishes exposure risks and provides information on mode of action. Researchers conduct different types of tests depending on what kind of information they need. In some cases, they feed the laboratory animals small, sublethal doses of a pesticide on a daily basis. Such studies establish no observable effect levels (NOEL) and give information on the long-term, or chronic, effects of pesticides. An array of special studies assesses the potential for causing sterility, birth defects, cancer, or other problems in people.

Short-term toxicity testing predicts the acute (or immediate) health effects of pesticides. During a study, researchers give groups of laboratory animals single, high doses of a certain pesticide. They measure immediate responses and study the pesticide's mode of action. Exposing animals for short periods to large doses of a pesticide predicts possible human hazards from similar short-term exposures.

Research workers test pesticides on mice, rats, rabbits, and dogs. They also perform toxicity tests on nontarget plants and animals if these organisms are at risk from pesticide exposure. Nontarget animals may include insects (such as bees), fish, amphibians (frogs, toads, salamanders), deer, birds, and other wildlife. Researchers also test pesticides on target pests to set the dosage rates listed on pesticide labels. These tests also tell how well the pesticide works under different conditions. The effectiveness of a pesticide on its target pest is known as its efficacy.

Lethal Dose and Lethal Concentration. Researchers divide laboratory animals into several groups and test different routes of exposure (skin, mouth, eyes, lungs). They rate a pesticide's toxicity by determining the amount, or lethal dose (LD_{50}), that kills 50% of a test population (Fig. 3-1). LD_{50} is expressed as the milligrams of pesticide per kilogram of body weight of the test animal (mg/kg). Research workers also determine how much pesticide vapor or dust in the air or what amount of pesticide diluted in rivers, streams, or lake water causes

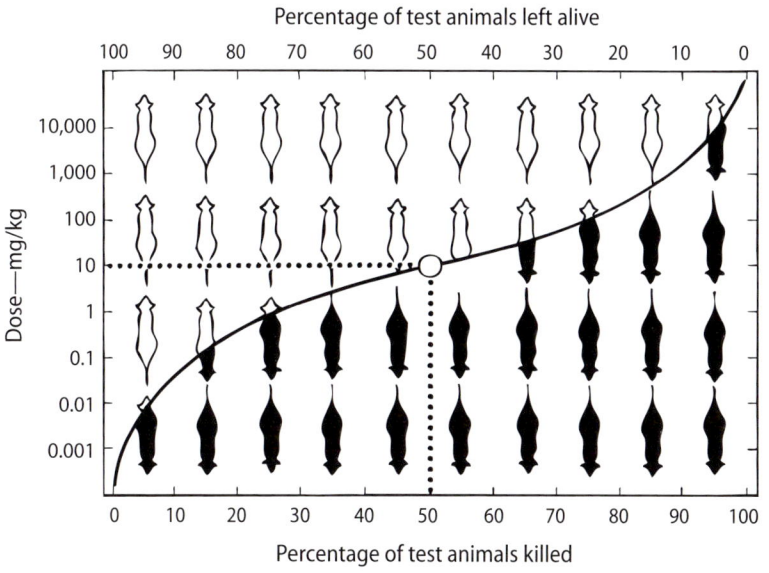

FIGURE 3-1

The amount of pesticide that will kill half of the group is the LD_{50}. The smaller the LD_{50}, the more toxic or hazardous a pesticide. LD_{50} values are established for both oral and dermal (skin) exposure. In this illustration, the LD_{50} is 10 mg of pesticide per kg of body weight of test animal.

death in 50% of test animal populations. This level is the lethal concentration, or LC_{50}, which is expressed as micrograms (1 one-millionth g) per liter of air or water (µg/l).

The more toxic pesticides present higher hazards, or risks of injury, to people and the environment (Table 3-1). Besides toxicity, pesticide hazards also vary according to the way they enter the body. Normal routes of entry include the mouth, skin, eyes, and lungs.

Lethal dose or lethal concentration classifications do not provide information about chronic, long-term toxic effects. A pesticide that has a high LD_{50} (relatively nontoxic) may not necessarily be harmless. Low exposure to some pesticides may cause health problems that only appear months or even years later.

No Observable Effect Level. The no observable effect level (NOEL) is the maximum dose or exposure level of a pesticide that produces no noticeable toxic effect on test animals. NOEL is a guide for establishing maximum exposure levels for people and residue tolerance levels on pesticide-treated produce. Usually, the U.S. Environmental Protection Agency (U.S. EPA) sets exposure levels and residue tolerances at 100 to 1,000 times less than the NOEL. U.S. EPA takes this precaution to provide a wide margin of safety.

Threshold Limit Value. The threshold limit value (TLV) for a chemical is its airborne concentration in parts per million that produces no adverse effects over time. The TLV applies to pesticides used as fumigants. The most common TLV protects workers who are exposed to low-level concentrations of a toxic chemical 8 hours per day for 5 consecutive days. Sometimes regulations set a TLV for short-term exposure to protect workers who must briefly enter recently treated areas. Although this concentration of airborne chemical is higher than the long-term TLV, injury will not result because of the limited exposure period. Researchers establish safe TLVs by exposing laboratory animals to different airborne concentrations and analyzing the results.

Factors that Influence Pesticide Toxicity

A number of factors affect the toxicity of a pesticide. These include the passage of time, characteristics of the water used for mixing, features of the application site, formulation and dosing, and chemical reactions that occur during mixing.

Once applied, pesticides usually break down into different chemicals or chemical compounds over time. These new chemicals may be less toxic or more toxic than the original pesticide. The time it takes for half of what you apply to break down into its component parts is called the pesticide's half-life. Soil microbes, ultraviolet light, temperature, quality of the water used in mixing, or impurities combined with the pesticide increase or decrease the half-life and can influence toxicity. Sometimes impurities contaminate pesticides during manufacture, formulation, storage, or while you are mixing them. In addition to the environment, the chemical nature of the pesticide, its formulation, and the dose applied affect its toxicity. Combining a pesticide with other pesticides can also change its toxicity or alter its half-life.

Pesticide Toxicity Categories

> List pesticide toxicity categories and signal words, and explain what each category means in terms of a pesticide's effects on humans and animals.

Federal regulations place pesticides into one of four categories according to their toxicity and potential to injure people or the environment (Table 3-2). Pesticide labels indicate these categories by the following signal words:
- Category I, DANGER
- Category II, WARNING
- Category III, CAUTION
- Category IV, no signal word or optional signal word CAUTION

DANGER pesticides are the most toxic or hazardous, and regulations normally restrict their use. Category IV pesticides are the least toxic to people and are generally less hazardous. Different label and regulatory requirements apply to each category. For example, you must use a closed mixing system and other safety equipment when mixing liquid DANGER pesticides. In California you need permits to buy, possess, and use most DANGER pesticides. To get a permit you must be a certified applicator.

TABLE 3-1

Oral LD_{50} values for selected formulated pesticide products. Pesticide products are grouped by toxicity according to Table 3-2.

Brand name*	Active ingredient*	LD_{50}**	Type of pesticide	Signal word
Diphacin	diphacinone	7	vertebrate	DANGER/Cat I
Telone	dichloropropene	224	fumigant	WARNING/ Cat II
Agri-Mek	abamectin	300	acaricide	
Gramoxone	paraquat	310	herbicide	
Sevin	carbaryl	406	insecticide	CAUTION/ Cat III
Ziram	ziram	478	fungicide	
Comite	propargite	600	acaricide	
Diazinon	diazinon	787	insecticide	
Weedone	2,4-D	863	herbicide	
Omite	propargite	960	acaricide	
C-O-C-S	copper hydroxide	1,131	fungicide	
Rovral	iprodione	1,170	fungicide	
Malathion	malathion	>2,000	insecticide	
Treflan	trifluralin	3,738	herbicide	
Roundup	glyphosate	3,794	herbicide	
Prowl	pendimethalin	5,000	herbicide	
Deadline	metaldehyde	>5,000	molluscicide	Cat IV
Bravo	chlorothalonil	>5,000	fungicide	
Entrust	spinosad	>5,000	insecticide	
Princep	simazine	>5,000	herbicide	
Talon	brodifacoum	>5,000	vertebrate	
Surflan	oryzalin	>5,000	herbicide	
Dipel	B. thuringiensis	>5,050	insecticide	
Precor	methoprene	>34,000	insect growth regulator	

Notes: *Some a.i.'s or products listed may not be currently registered as pesticides or may have had their registration cancelled.

**LD_{50} values are from product Safety Data Sheets and may be different from LD_{50} values for unformulated active ingredients. LD_{50} values may also vary by formulation type. These values are shown for comparative purposes only. Some chemicals listed may no longer be in use as pesticides.

TABLE 3-2

Signal words and pesticide toxicity categories that appear on U.S. EPA–approved labels

	Toxicity category (signal word)			
	High toxicity (DANGER/ DANGER-POISON) Category I	Moderate toxicity (WARNING) Category II	Low toxicity (CAUTION) Category III	Very low toxicity (Optional signal word = CAUTION) Category IV
acute oral LD_{50}*	up to and including 50 mg/kg	>50 through 500 mg/kg	>500 through 5,000 mg/kg	>5,000 mg/kg
acute inhalation LC_{50}*	up to and including 0.05 µg/liter	>0.05 through 0.5 µg/liter	>0.5 through 2 µg/liter	>2 µg/liter
acute dermal LD_{50}*	up to and including 200 mg/kg	>200 through 2,000 mg/kg	>2,000 through 5,000 mg/kg	>5,000 mg/kg
primary eye irritation	corrosive (irreversible destruction of ocular tissue) or corneal involvement or irritation persisting more than 21 days	corneal involvement or other eye irritation clearing in 8-21 days	corneal involvement or other eye irritation clearing in 7 days or less	minimal effects clearing in less than 24 hours
primary skin irritation	corrosive (tissue destruction into the dermis and/or scarring)	severe irritation at 72 hours (severe erythema or edema)	moderate irritation at 72 hours (moderate erythema)	mild or slight irritation at 72 hours (no irritation or slight erythema)

Note: *LD_{50} values represent milligrams (mg) of the pesticide per kilogram (kg) of body weight of the test animals. LC_{50} values represent the milligrams of pesticide per liter of air inhaled by the test animals.

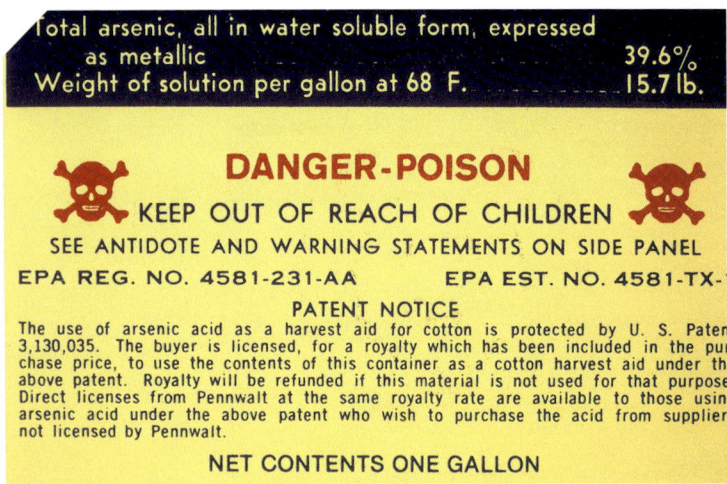

FIGURE 3-2

The most hazardous pesticides are recognized by the signal word DANGER and a skull and crossbones with the word POISON on the label. A few drops to a teaspoon of these pesticides, taken internally, would probably cause death. These pesticides have an oral LD_{50} of 50 mg/kg or less and a dermal LD_{50} of 200 mg/kg or less.

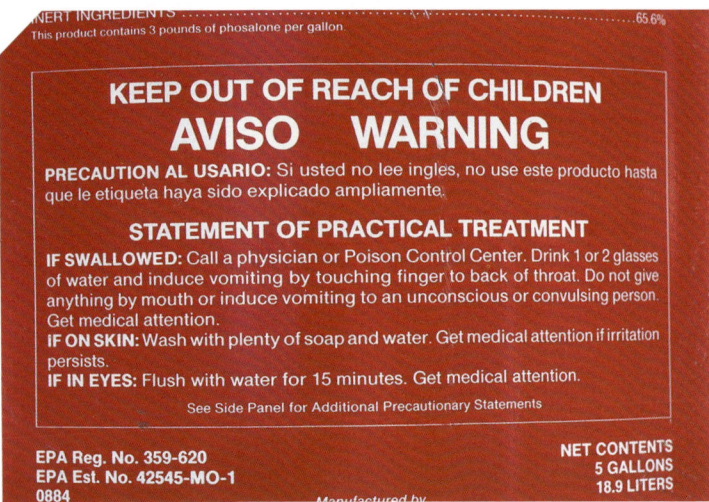

FIGURE 3-3

Moderately hazardous pesticides have the signal word WARNING on their labels. One teaspoonful to 1 ounce of pesticide in this category would probably kill a person if taken internally. These pesticides have an oral LD_{50} in the range of 50 to 500 mg/kg and a dermal LD_{50} in the range of 200 to 2,000 mg/kg

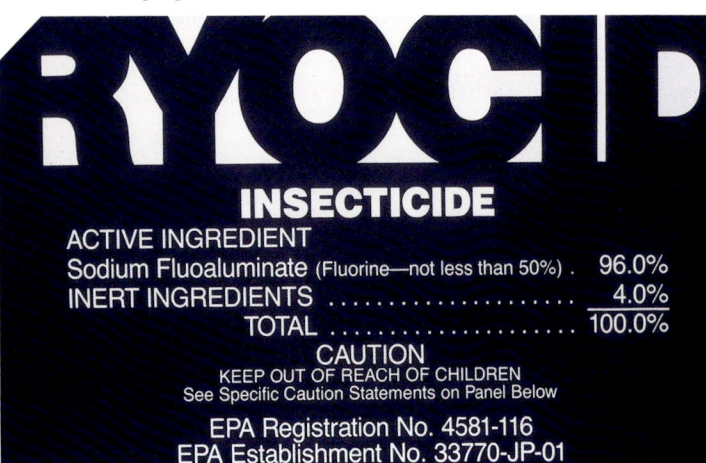

DANGER Pesticides

DANGER pesticides have an oral LD_{50} up to 50 mg/kg or a dermal LD_{50} up to 200 mg/kg. Some of these also have the word POISON and the skull and crossbones on their labels (Fig. 3-2). DANGER pesticides with the skull and crossbones are the most hazardous because they are the most toxic. A few drops to a teaspoonful of some of these pesticides could possibly cause death if swallowed, inhaled, or absorbed through the skin. Less-toxic pesticides may still have the signal word DANGER on their labels if they cause specific hazards. These hazards include severe skin or eye injury. For those, the signal word DANGER appears on the label, but not the word POISON or the skull and crossbones.

WARNING Pesticides

WARNING pesticides have an oral LD_{50} between 50 and 500 mg/kg or a dermal LD_{50} between 200 and 2,000 mg/kg. These are moderately hazardous (Fig. 3-3). If swallowed, from 1 teaspoon to 1 ounce (6 teaspoons) of many pesticides in this group would probably kill an adult.

CAUTION Pesticides

CAUTION pesticides have an oral LD_{50} between 500 and 5,000 mg/kg and a dermal LD_{50} between 2,000 and 5,000 mg/kg (Fig. 3-4). The signal word CAUTION indicates they may be slightly hazardous. An adult would probably need to swallow over 1 ounce of these types of pesticides for them to cause death or serious injury.

Category IV Pesticides

A signal word is not required for Category IV pesticides; however, they may carry an optional CAUTION on their labels. Pesticides in this category have an oral LD_{50} over 5,000 mg/kg and a dermal LD_{50} greater than 5,000 mg/kg and are generally deemed safer than pesticides in the other categories.

FIGURE 3-4

The least hazardous pesticides are recognized by the signal word CAUTION on their labels. It would probably take more than 1 ounce of material in this category, taken internally, to kill an adult. These pesticides have an oral LD_{50} between 500 and 5,000 mg/kg and a dermal LD_{50} between 2,000 and 5,000 mg/kg.

Identify factors that should be considered when selecting pesticides.

How Pesticides Are Organized

Pesticides are organized in a variety of ways to help people easily locate and select an appropriate product for controlling particular pests in particular circumstances. In this section, you will find pesticides sorted by pest targeted (Table 3-3), chemical family (Table 3-4), mode of action (Table 3-5), and formulation. Some pesticides do not fit well into any one group and will be treated in "Pesticides with Special Functions."

TABLE 3-3

Pesticides organized by pest targeted

Pesticide target	Pesticide type	Example of pesticide* Chemical	Example of pesticide* Brand name
algae[†]	algaecide	copper sulfate endothall sodium hypochlorite	 Hydrothol 191 Clorox
bacteria	bactericide	copper compounds oxytetracycline	Basic Copper Mycoshield
birds	avicide	aminopyridine	Avitrol
fish	piscicide	rotenone	Prentox
fungi[†]	fungicide	chlorothalonil copper sulfate metconazole	Bravo C-O-C-S Quash
insects	insecticide	diazinon imidacloprid permethrin petroleum oils	Diazinon Gaucho Ambush
mammal predators	predacide	sodium cyanide	M-44
microbes	antimicrobial	alkyl dimethylbenzyl ammonium caprylic acid chloride chlorine dioxide hydrogen peroxide sodium hypochlorite	3DT Vortexx Lysol Cryocide Clorox
mites	acaricide	abamectin propargite	Agri-Mek Comite
nematodes	nematicide	dicloropropene	Telone
rodents	rodenticide	brodifacoum chlorophacinone diphacinone strychnine bromadiolone	Talon Diphacin Gopher Getter Maki
snails and slugs	molluscicide	iron phosphate metaldehyde	Sluggo Deadline
trees and woody shrubs	silvicide	imazapyr petroleum oils tebuthiuron	Imazapyr, Arsenal Spike
viruses[†] (antimicrobial products for cleaning)	virucide	alkyl dimethylethylbenzyl ammonium chloride peroxyacetic acid sodium hypochlorite	 Minncare Cold Sterilant Clorox
weeds	herbicide	bromoxynil glyphosate paraquat petroleum oil simazine trifluralin	Buctril Roundup Gramoxone Princep Treflan

Notes: *Some a.i.'s or products listed may not be currently registered as pesticides or may have had their registration cancelled. Also, some chemicals may have more than one brand name or no brand name.
[†]Includes algae, bacteria, fungi, and viruses targeted by antimicrobial pesticides.

TABLE 3-4

Selected pesticides organized by chemical family

Chemical family	Pesticide type	Example of pesticide* Chemical	Example of pesticide* Brand name
carbamates	fungicide	mancozeb propamocarb hydrochloride	Manzate Pro-Stick Previcur Flex
	molluscicide	methiocarb	Mesurol
	nematicide, insecticide, herbicide	metam-sodium	Vapam
	insecticide, miticide	carbaryl methomyl	Sevin Lannate
neonicotinoids	insecticide, miticide	imidacloprid	Gaucho
organophosphates	insecticide, miticide	diazinon chlorpyrifos malathion	Diazinon Lorsban Malathion
pyrethroids	insecticide	bifenthrin cypermethrin permethrin	Brigade Demon Ambush, Pounce
strobilurins	fungicide	azoxystrobin pyraclostrobin/boscalid trifloxystrobin	Abound Pristine Gem
sulfonylureas	herbicide	chlorsulfuron rimsulfuron sulfometuron	Telar, Glean Matrix Oust
triazines	herbicide	atrazine prometryn simazine	Atrazine Caparol Princep

Note: *Some a.i.'s or products listed may not be currently registered as pesticides or may have had their registration cancelled.

TABLE 3-5

Selected pesticides organized by mode of action

Mode of action	Pesticide type	Example of pesticide* Chemical name	Brand name
Systemic			
acetylcholine receptor (nAChR) agonists	insecticide	imidacloprid	Admire
EPSP synthase inhibitor	herbicide	glyphosate	Roundup
mitosis inhibitor	herbicide	oryzalin	Surflan
signal transduction	fungicide	iprodione	Rovral
synthetic auxin	herbicide	2,4-dichlorophenoxyacetic acid	2,4-D
Contact			
attractant	insecticide	CPB pheromone	
chitin biosynthesis inhibitor	insecticide	buprofezin	Courier
enzyme inhibitor, multi-site inhibitor	herbicide, fungicide, nematicide, algaecide	metam-sodium	Vapam
mitochondrial ATP synthase inhibitor	miticide	propargite	Comite
multi-site contact inhibitor	fungicide	chlorothalonil	Bravo
photosystem I inhibitor	herbicide	paraquat	Gramoxone
photosystem II inhibitor	herbicide	propanil	Stam, SuperWham!
protectant, multi-site inhibitor	fungicide, miticide	sulfur	Microthiol Disperss
repellent, protectant	insecticide	kaolin	Surround

*Note: *Some a.i.'s or products listed may not be currently registered as pesticides or may have had their registration cancelled. Modes of action taken from IRAC, HRAC, and FRAC websites.*

> List groups of pesticides according to pest target and describe the functions of each group.

BY PEST TARGET

Pesticides are often organized by the pest they target. Some pesticides are effective on several pest types, such as petroleum oils, which can be used to manage weeds, insects, and woody plants like trees or shrubs. Others work only on one pest type, like atrazine, which targets weeds. See Table 3-3 for a list of pesticides (along with brand names) sorted by target pest. When you know which pest is damaging your site, having pesticides sorted by the target pest makes finding the most effective, safest pesticide easier.

BY CHEMICAL FAMILY

Experts group pesticides according to chemical family. This type of grouping often reveals common characteristics, such as mode of action, chemical structure, and types of formulations possible. There may also be similarities in environmental persistence (how long the pesticide lasts in the environment) and how related pesticides break down through biological processes. Table 3-4 lists the chemical groups for many commonly used pesticides. Organizing pesticides by chemical family can help you find the best pesticide for a given application. Below you can find descriptions of some of the most popular chemical families and the brand names of pesticides with active ingredients that belong to each family.

> List major chemical families and describe the particular hazards associated with each one.

Organochlorines. Organochlorines (also known as chlorinated hydrocarbons) were one of the original types of synthetic chemicals used as pesticides. They became the mainstay for controlling insects and mites in the early years of chemical pest management. Some of these materials are highly poisonous to mammals, including people, while others are reasonably harmless.

Many are fat-soluble, so traces of organochlorine pesticides frequently appear in animal tissues. Most organochlorines break down slowly in the environment. Their persistence made them attractive for structural pest control and public health applications.

The U.S. EPA has now banned most of the early organochlorines due to environmental persistence, impact on wildlife, or other concerns. DDT, chlordane, toxaphene, and dieldrin are some of these earlier organochlorine insecticides. Newer, less-persistent organochlorines are used today for controlling certain insects, mites, and rodents.

Organophosphates. Organophosphates are an important group of pesticides widely used to manage insect and mite pests. These pesticides are derivatives of phosphorous compounds, and some are among the most acutely toxic chemicals known. Many organophosphates are absorbed through the skin, lungs, or digestive tract. They interfere with animal and human nervous systems, effects that are shared by some of the carbamates. Organophosphate pesticides usually break down rapidly in the environment. Well-known organophosphate insecticides include malathion, diazinon, and chlorpyrifos.

Carbamates. Carbamates are a widely used group of synthetic organic pesticides. They are highly effective, moderately priced, and, under normal conditions, short-lived in the environment. Derivatives of carbamic acid, they include the sulfur-containing subgroups of dithiocarbamates and thiocarbamates. Besides being used as insecticides, some types of carbamates have uses as fungicides, herbicides, molluscicides, and nematicides.

In animals, some carbamate pesticides impair nerve function and are highly toxic to mammals, including human beings. Carbamate pesticides do not build up in animal tissue, so their toxic effects are often short-lived and reversible. Examples of carbamate pesticides include carbaryl (Sevin), methomyl (Lannate), metam-sodium, and metam-potassium.

Triazines. Triazines are a large, important chemical family and are used to control both broadleaved and grassy weeds either before they emerge (preemergent) or after (postemergent). Because herbicides in this family are so flexible, they are used in many situations, including residential, commercial, and agricultural. Triazines translocate through plants and inhibit photosynthesis.

Pesticides in the triazine family are frequently detected in streams, rivers, groundwater, and reservoirs because of their tendency to persist in soil and move with water. In California, applicators using pesticides that contain atrazine or simazine must check to see if the application site is in a Ground Water Protection Area (GWPA), because these two active ingredients are on the state's Groundwater Protection List. Exposure to triazines can negatively affect humans and other mammals, and fish. Herbicides in this family include atrazine, simazine, and prometryn.

Neonicotinoids. The neonicotinoid family of insecticides mimics the effects of nicotine, disrupting an insect's central nervous system, causing paralysis and death. Neonicotinoids were invented as an alternative to more dangerous chemical families such as organophosphates and carbamates and have become very popular worldwide. Although they are less toxic to humans than other chemical families, they can still cause health problems such as dizziness or vomiting in exposed people and animals.

One major drawback of systemic pesticides in this family is their potential effect on beneficial insects. Data suggest that the residues left by neonicotinioids can accumulate in pollen and nectar of treated plants on which honey bees and other pollinators might feed. Scientists are actively studying the effects of imidacloprid, a popular member of the neonicotinoid family, on bees and other invertebrates. As they finish their studies, new information will help define the risks to these animals.

Pyrethroids. Pyrethroids are a group of synthetic (laboratory-made) chemicals typically used as pesticides in commercial, agricultural, and domestic settings. Pyrethroids work by interfering with sodium transport in insect nerve cells and are often formulated as sprays, aerosols, dusts, and dilutable concentrates. While they have very low solubility in water and bind tightly to soil particles, surveys of urban and rural California waterways have revealed a widespread presence of toxic pyrethroid residues in the waterways' sediment.

Pyrethroids are often combined commercially with other chemicals called synergists that enhance their insecticidal activity. Synergists prevent some enzymes from breaking down the pyrethroids, which increases their toxicity. In humans and mammals, pyrethroids interfere with the function of the nerves and brain. If people are exposed to large doses of pyrethroid-based pesticides, they will become sick and may even lose consciousness. Some of the more popular pyrethroids are bifenthrin, permethrin, and cypermethrin.

Sulfonylureas. Sulfonylureas are a family of herbicides taken up by a plant's roots and foliage. They work on a broad range of grasses and broadleaved weeds but do not affect plants they are designed to protect. Crops like rice, wheat, barley, soybean, maize, and many others are able to metabolize sulfonylureas safely. They are safe for humans and animals because mammals do not have the enzyme that sulfonylurea molecules target. Because of the low application rates of sulfonylurea herbicides, overall herbicide use has gone down by about 200 million pounds per year. Sulfonylurea herbicides are generally only slightly toxic to freshwater fish and invertebrates.

Although application rates are low, resistance has developed to this family of pesticides, which disrupt protein synthesis (also known as acetolactate synthase, or ALS disruption). Worldwide, 131 weed species have shown resistance to herbicides with this mode of action. Rimsulfuron, sulfometuron methyl, and chlorsulfuron are some of the sulfonylurea herbicides used in California.

Strobilurins. Strobilurins are used frequently worldwide to fight pathogens and increase plant health in a variety of settings, from turfgrass to agriculture. Fungicides in the strobilurin (or Q_{oI}) family have a preventive mode of action, disrupting respiration and metabolism to suppress pathogen populations. Studies of strobilurins have shown them to be practically nontoxic to birds, mammals, and bees. However, they are highly toxic to freshwater fish, freshwater invertebrates, and estuarine and marine fish, and very highly toxic to estuarine and marine invertebrates. Pyraclostrobin, azoxystrobin, and trifloxystrobin are examples of fungicides in the strobilurin chemical family.

BY MODE OF ACTION

Define mode of action and provide examples of the different modes.

People sometimes organize pesticides by their modes of action. A pesticide's mode of action is the way it reacts with a pest organism to destroy it. For instance, an insecticide may act as a stomach poison, an herbicide may prevent root development in seedlings, and a biocide may disrupt cell membranes of microorganisms. Table 3-5 lists pesticides according to their modes of action.

Understanding mode of action makes it easier to select the right pesticide. It also helps you predict which pesticide works best in a particular situation. For instance, if pests show resistance to one pesticide, a material with a different mode of action can counteract the problem (see "Pesticide Resistance" in Chapter 10 for more information).

Explain how various modes of action influence pesticide selection.

Usually, pesticides within a chemical class have the same mode of action on specific types of pests. They may also have similar characteristics such as chemical structure, persistence in the environment, and types of formulations possible. Most modes of action fall under one of the following two umbrella terms.

- **Contact.** These pesticides work only on pests that they contact directly. For instance, weeds die when a contact herbicide covers a sufficient surface area of the plant. Only insects that are sprayed directly or have traveled across treated surfaces are affected by contact insecticides.

Explain how contact and systemic pesticides control pests differently.

- **Systemic.** These pesticides work when applied to a particular area of a plant or animal. The pesticide is then translocated, or moved, throughout the organism's system. For example, a systemic herbicide applied to a plant's roots moves throughout the whole plant and kills it. Some soil-applied insecticides are picked up by a plant's roots and translocated to the leaves, making the plant toxic to foliage-feeding insects.

TABLE 3-6
Suffixes of pesticide formulations

Suffix	Meaning
Type of formulation	
AF	aqueous flowable
AS	aqueous suspension
D	dust
DF	dry flowable
E	emulsifiable concentrate
EC	emulsifiable concentrate
ES	emulsifiable solution
F	flowable
FL	flowable
G	granulars
OL	oil-soluble liquid
P	pellets
PS	pellets
S	soluble powder, water-soluble concentrate/solution, low-concentration solution
SG	sand granules
SL	slurry
SP	soluble powder
ULV	ultra-low-volume concentrate
W	wettable powder
WDG	water-dispersible granules
WP	wettable powder
How a pesticide is used	
GS	for treatment of grass seed
LSR	for leaf spot and rust
PM	for powdery mildew
RP	for range and pasture
RTU	ready to use
SD	for use as a side dressing
TC	termiticide concentrate
TGF	turfgrass fungicide
WK	to be used with weed killers
Characteristics of the formulation	
BE	the butyl ester of 2,4-D
D	an ester of 2,4-D
K	a potassium salt of the active ingredient
LO	low odor
LV	low volatility
MF	modified formulation
T	a triazole
2X	double strength
Label for use in special locations	
PNW	for use in the Pacific Northwest (e.g., Benlate PNW)
TVA	for use in the waterways of the Tennessee Valley

Within these general terms, modes of action become quite specific and can help you effectively select and use a pesticide.

For instance, the mode of action of certain herbicides destroys weeds by damaging leaf cells and causing plants to dry out (desiccants). Others alter the uptake of nutrients or interfere with the plant's ability to grow normally (growth inhibitors) or convert light into food (photosynthetic inhibitors). A preemergent herbicide's mode of action inhibits seed germination or seedling growth, requiring the pesticide's incorporation into the soil to control weed seedlings before they emerge. A postemergence herbicide's mode of action destroys leaf and stem tissues on contact, so it is applied to foliage or soil after weeds emerge.

Insecticides can act as nerve poisons, muscle poisons, desiccants, growth regulators, or sterilants. Others have purely physical effects, such as clogging air passages. An insecticide may have more than one mode of action.

Some fungicides are called eradicants because they destroy fungi that have already invaded and begun to damage plant tissues. Their mode of action inhibits the metabolic processes of the growing fungal organisms. Others are protectants that prevent fungal infections. Their mode of action retards fungal growth or prevents the organisms from entering treated plants.

BY FORMULATION

Pesticide chemicals in their "raw," or unformulated, state are not usually suitable for pest control. These concentrated chemicals (active ingredients) may not mix well with water and may be chemically unstable. For these reasons, manufacturers add other ingredients to improve application effectiveness, safety, handling, and storage. "Other ingredients" are all the substances that manufacturers add to the pesticide active ingredient.

Define a pesticide formulation.

The final product is a pesticide formulation. This formulation consists of
- the pesticide active ingredient
- the carrier, such as an organic solvent or mineral clay
- surface-active ingredients, often including stickers and spreaders
- other ingredients, such as stabilizers, dyes, and chemicals that improve or enhance pesticidal activity, such as antifreeze to prevent them from freezing

Usually you need to mix a formulation with water or oil for final application. However, baits, granules, and dusts are ready for use without additional dilution. Manufacturers package specialized pesticides, such as products for households, in ready-to-use formulations.

The label lists the amount of actual pesticide in a dry formulation as percentage of active ingredient (a.i.). For instance, a 50-W wettable powder contains 50% by weight of actual pesticide. Ten pounds of Diazinon 50W contains 5 pounds of diazinon and 5 pounds of other (also sometimes called inert) ingredients. With liquid formulations, the label lists the pounds of active ingredient in 1 gallon of formulated pesticide. For example, in Lorsban 4E, the "4" indicates that the material contains 4 pounds per gallon of the active ingredient chlorpyrifos.

Labels usually indicate formulation type by letters that follow or are a part of the brand name of the pesticide (Table 3-6). In the examples above, the "W" represents a wettable powder and the "E" indicates that the pesticide is an emulsifiable concentrate. Sometimes these codes describe what the pesticide is used for or how it is used (e.g., "SD" indicates the pesticide is used as a side dressing). They may describe some special characteristics of the formulation, such as "LO" for low odor. In some cases, they indicate a use for a specific location, such as "PNW" for Pacific Northwest. Selecting the correct formulation among the many available can be difficult. The following paragraphs describe a wide variety of available formulations. See Chapter 10 for methods you can use to select the best formulation for your application.

> List the various formulations available and the advantages and disadvantages of each.

Wettable Powders (W or WP)

Wettable powder formulations do not dissolve in water. Instead, they form a milky suspension similar to mixing chocolate drink mix with water. Wettable powder formulations consist of the pesticide and a finely ground dry carrier, usually mineral clay. Manufacturers combine these with other ingredients that enhance the ability of the powder to remain suspended in water. Most wettable powder formulations contain from 15 to 75% active ingredient.

Choose formulations with the highest percentage of active ingredient if visible residues are a concern. Carriers and other (or inert) ingredients are the most common source of unsightly residues on sprayed surfaces. Also, the cost per unit of active ingredient is usually less in formulations with a high percentage of active ingredient. However, a higher percentage of active ingredient in the formulation makes the wettable powder more hazardous. These require more care in handling and mixing and often require special personal protective equipment (PPE).

Wettable powders are among the safest formulations to use if phytotoxicity (plant injury) is a concern. They are considered safer than other formulations because the carriers are inert minerals. These formulations are suitable to mix (compatible) with many other pesticides (especially other wettable powders) and fertilizers. A disadvantage is the abrasiveness of the inert carrier, which contributes to pump and nozzle wear. Wettable powders always require agitation during application to keep the mixture suspended. When you apply wettable powders to porous materials, water in the mixture penetrates, but the pesticide remains on the surface. On nonporous surfaces, water evaporates and leaves the pesticide as a residue.

A serious problem with wettable powders is the potential hazard of inhaling dust during handling and mixing. Dust particles usually contain high concentrations of pesticide active ingredient. These particles are very fine and can remain suspended in the atmosphere for several hours. To overcome this hazard, some manufacturers package wettable powders in water-soluble bags (WSB or WSP). If you choose a formulation packaged in water-soluble bags, do not open the bags during mixing. Calibrate your equipment so you can use one or more whole bags. Drop these premeasured, unopened bags into a filled spray tank. With agitation, the bags dissolve and release the wettable powder into the tank's water.

Dry Flowables, or Water-Dispersible Granules

Dry flowables (DF) also called water-dispersible granules, (WDG) are similar to wettable powders. Rather than being a powder, however, the formulated pesticide consists of small granules. These require mixing with water before use. The granules have a higher percentage of active ingredient per unit of weight because manufacturers use less carrier.

Dry flowables do not have the dust problems associated with wettable powders, so they are safer to handle. Measuring and mixing granules is simple because manufacturers package them in easy-to-pour plastic containers. Measure these out by volume, similar to liquids, rather than by weight. Like wettable powders, dry flowables require constant agitation during application and are abrasive to application equipment.

Soluble Powders (S or SP)

A soluble powder formulation is similar to a wettable powder. However, the pesticide, its carrier, and all other formulation ingredients completely dissolve in water to form a true solution. In this manner, they are similar to dissolving sugar or salt in water. Once dissolved, soluble powders require no additional mixing or agitation. They are not abrasive to spray nozzles or pumps. Only a few pesticides are available in this formulation because most pesticide active ingredients do not dissolve in water. While mixing, inhalation of soluble powders is a potential hazard. To overcome this hazard, manufacturers sometimes package these formulations in water-soluble bags, as they do for wettable powders.

Emulsifiable Concentrates (E or EC)

Many pesticides are not soluble in water but dissolve completely in petroleum solvents. Emulsifiable concentrates are petroleum-soluble pesticides formulated with emulsifying agents (soaplike materials) and other enhancers. When you add emulsifiable concentrates to water, they form an emulsion (a milky liquid), similar to mixing certain household disinfectants in water. After mixing, the emulsified pesticide disperses evenly in the water. Agitation during application is important to keep this emulsion uniform.

Emulsifiable concentrates are among the most versatile of all formulations and have many applications. They penetrate porous materials such as soil, fabrics, paper, and wood better than wettable powders. Since they are liquid, they pour easily for mixing. However, using emulsifiable concentrates introduces several handler hazards:

- If spilled, they spread easily and are difficult to clean up.
- Porous protective clothing and leather boots readily absorb them.
- They pass through the skin more readily than powders.
- They may cause serious injury if splashed into the eyes.

Emulsifiable concentrates are more risky to use (potentially phytotoxic) on sensitive plants than wettable powders because they contain petroleum solvents. These solvents also contribute to the deterioration of rubber and plastic hoses and gaskets. The solvents may damage some pump parts and corrode painted surfaces.

Flowables (F)

A flowable formulation combines many of the characteristics of emulsifiable concentrates and wettable powders. Manufacturers use this formulation when the active ingredient is an insoluble solid and will not dissolve in either water or oil. They combine finely ground pesticide particles with a liquid carrier and emulsifiers to form a concentrated emulsion (similar to liquid antacids). Flowables share the features of liquid emulsifiable concentrates and have similar disadvantages. They require agitation to keep them in suspension and leave visible residues, similar to wettable powders.

Flowables are easy to handle and apply. Because they are liquids, they are subject to spilling and splashing like emulsifiable concentrates. They contain solid particles, so they contribute to abrasive wear of nozzles and pumps. Flowable suspensions settle out in their containers, so always shake them thoroughly before mixing. Because flowables tend to settle, manufacturers package them in containers of 5 gallons or less to make remixing easier.

Water-Soluble Concentrates or Solutions (S)

Water-soluble concentrates or solutions are formulations that dissolve in water, similar to sugar-based syrups. Once dissolved, they require no further mixing or agitation. The same handler hazards are present with water-soluble concentrates as with other liquids, but they are nonabrasive to application equipment. Only a limited number of pesticide liquids dissolve in water.

Low-Concentrate Solutions (S)

Low-concentrate formulations are ready to use and require no dilution. They consist of a small amount of active ingredient dissolved in an organic solvent. They usually do not stain fabrics or have unpleasant odors. They are especially useful for structural and institutional pests as well as for household use. Major disadvantages to low-concentrate formulations include limited availability and high cost per unit of active ingredient. Many organic solvents are harmful to foliage, so they cannot be used as plant sprays.

Ultra-Low-Volume Concentrates (ULV)

Ultra-low-volume concentrates have high concentrations (from 80 to 100%) of active ingredient. These formulations require little or no dilution. However, they require application equipment suited to applying very small quantities of pesticide over a large area. This requirement results in less frequent refilling of spraying equipment, a major advantage when treating large areas. You usually dilute ULV formulations with vegetable oil rather than water when dilution is needed. Droplets of ULV formulations do not evaporate as rapidly as those from emulsions. Because of the high concentration of active ingredient, equipment calibration must be extremely accurate.

Slurry (SL)

A slurry is a thin, watery, paste-like mixture of finely ground dusts. Because they are dusts before mixing, slurries have similar respiratory hazards to the handler as other powdered formulations. Usually, mix a slurry first in a small container; combine water with the powder and stir to form a paste. Slowly add this mixture to water in a partially filled spray tank. Be sure to agitate the mixture constantly to prevent settling. After adding the paste, fill the tank with water. Allow it to mix thoroughly before applying. Pest managers apply slurries to seeds and plants to protect them against insects or fungi. After application, slurries dry and leave thick residues on treated surfaces, similar to paint. Usually these residues are highly visible. Slurries are abrasive and contribute to pump and nozzle wear.

A common slurry formulation is the Bordeaux mixture applied to plants as a fungicide. People who use a Bordeaux mixture combine hydrated lime and copper sulfate in various proportions with water to produce a slurry. They usually combine the dry materials just before application, although some premixed dry formulations are commercially available.

Fumigants

Fumigants have many uses because they penetrate hard-to-reach areas. They control insect pests of stored products as well as soil pests such as weeds, insects, nematodes, and microorganisms. Some fumigants control vertebrates such as ground squirrels and gophers. Fumigants are used in ships, boxcars, aircraft, trucks, dwellings, warehouses, greenhouses, and commercial buildings. Fumigants may be solid, liquid, or gas. Solids and liquids evaporate (volatilize) into a gas after or during application. Many fumigants are gases at room temperature. Manufacturers package these in steel cylinders for metering into treatment areas.

Fumigants introduce a serious inhalation hazard to applicators and other people in or near the treated area. Applicators often must wear supplied air breathing equipment and protective clothing. When applying, they use atmosphere-monitoring equipment to detect fumigant concentration. Atmosphere monitoring enables them to determine when people can safely enter the area without PPE. For more about respirators and atmosphere monitoring, see Chapter 6.

Pest managers apply many soil fumigants through irrigation systems or inject them directly into the soil. Usually, soil moisture needs to be high to prevent fumigants from volatilizing into the atmosphere. Tarping the soil with plastic sheeting also confines the fumigant and maintains its concentration. Soil texture and type, amount of organic material, and soil condition affect how well soil fumigants work. Soil temperature and weather during and after application also influence the effectiveness of soil fumigants.

People who fumigate structures seal the structures with tarps or make them airtight in some other way. They often use fans to circulate the air in the area and mix the fumigant uniformly. Treated areas must be thoroughly ventilated after fumigation and before they are reoccupied. Stored products are fumigated in airtight containers or specially designed rooms or buildings.

Invert Emulsions

Invert emulsions are liquid formulations of small water droplets suspended in oil. Pesticides dissolve in either oil or water (Fig. 3-5). Invert emulsion concentrates have the consistency of mayonnaise and usually require continuous agitation. Uses of invert emulsions are limited, and regulations prohibit some uses.

Invert emulsions aid in reducing drift. With other formulations, some drift results when water droplets begin to evaporate before reaching target surfaces. As a result, they become very small and light. Because oil evaporates more slowly than water, invert emulsion droplets shrink less, therefore more pesticide reaches the target. The oil helps to reduce runoff and improves rain resistance. It also serves as a sticker-spreader by improving surface coverage and absorption. Since droplets are larger and heavier, it is difficult to get thorough coverage on the undersides of foliage.

Dusts (D)

Dust formulations consist of finely ground pesticide combined with an inert dry carrier. Most dust formulations contain from 1 to 10% active ingredient. Some, such as sulfur dust, may be pure active ingredient. Dusts are appropriate in situations where moisture from liquid sprays would damage crops, foliage, or sprayed surfaces. You can apply dusts to many surfaces without harm, although they do leave visible residues (Fig. 3-6). Depending on the pesticide being used, dust formulations often provide long-term protection of treated surfaces.

Because of drift hazards, most pest managers prefer liquid sprays to dusts in agricultural applications. However, they work well in hard-to-reach indoor areas and for treating pests in home gardens. Pesticidal dusts control parasites on pets, livestock, and poultry. They also protect seeds. Fungicides, herbicides, insecticides, and rodenticides are available in dust formulations.

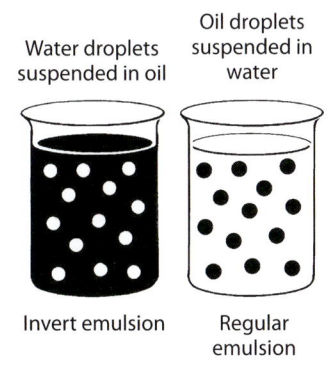

FIGURE 3-5

An invert emulsion consists of small water droplets suspended in oil. Compare this with the regular emulsion, in which oil droplets are suspended in water.

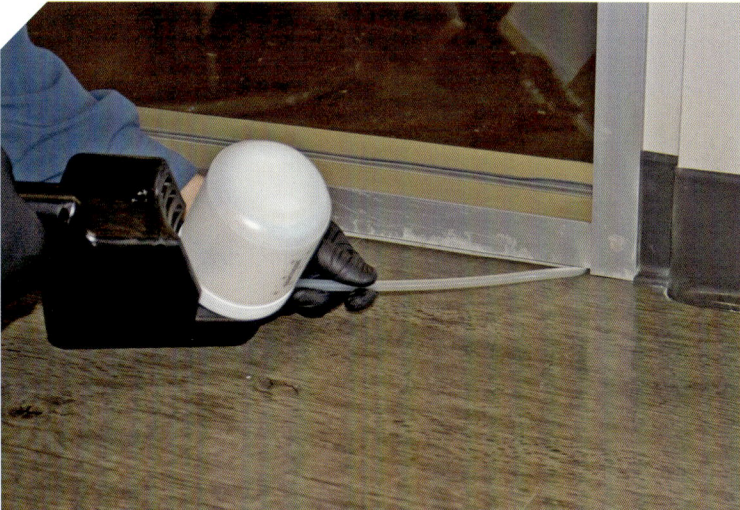

FIGURE 3-6

One type of pesticide formulation consists of a finely ground powder containing active and other ingredients applied dry as a dust. Here, insecticidal dust is blown into cracks and voids using a small electric dust blower.

Other problems associated with dust applications include the following:
- Dusts present serious inhalation hazards to applicators; to prevent poisoning, wear respirators whenever using dust formulations.
- Regulations restrict outdoor applications of dusts to periods when the air is still.
- Application equipment is difficult to calibrate, and dusts require agitation during application to prevent settling and caking in the hopper.

Tracking Powders. Special dusts known as tracking powders are used for rodent and insect monitoring and control. For rodent control, the tracking powder consists of finely ground dust combined with a stomach poison rodenticide. Rodents walk through the dust, pick it up on their feet and fur, and ingest it when they clean themselves. Tracking powders are useful when bait acceptance is poor due to an abundant, readily available food supply. Use nonpoisonous powders, such as talc or flour, to monitor and track the activity of rodents in buildings.

Granules (G)

Granules consist of a pesticide and carrier combined with a binding agent. They range in size from 4 to 80 mesh; the most common formulations are in the range of 15 to 30 mesh. *Mesh* is the term used to categorize the size of powder particles based on the number of wires in an inch of screen (Fig. 3-7); the higher the mesh size, the smaller the particles. The larger size and weight granules (lower mesh size) helps eliminate drift. You can minimize dust and spray mist hazards to the applicator and environment by using granular formulations. Granular formulations are more persistent in the environment than other formulations because the pesticide active ingredient releases slowly.

Some granular pesticide formulations that dissolve in water control aquatic pests such as algae, aquatic weeds, and fish. These have advantages over liquids in aquatic situations because liquids are hard to disperse. When sprayed, liquids may dry on plants or floating debris. Also, liquids may not pass through the surface film of the water. Granules bounce off vegetation and easily penetrate the surface film. Some aquatic granular formulations offer sustained, controlled release of pesticide because they dissolve slowly. However, slow-dissolving granules may be hazardous to waterfowl because birds can mistake the pesticide for food.

Pest managers apply granules to soil to control weeds, nematodes, and soil-dwelling insects. Manufacturers formulate some systemic insecticides as granules. The granules dissolve in the soil, and plants absorb the active ingredients through their roots. These materials control leaf- and stem-feeding insects. Some granular formulations require mechanical incorporation into the soil and often need moisture for activation. Granules are not suitable for conventional foliar application since they do not stick to leaves. However, when applied to plants like corn, the granules lodge in the leaf whorls, providing effective control for some corn insect pests. For this type of application, manufacturers weight granules with sand.

Pellets (P or PS)

Pellets are identical to granules, except manufacturers mold them into specific uniform weights and shapes. Pest managers apply pellets with equipment such as precision planters to achieve uniformity that is normally difficult to accomplish with granules.

FIGURE 3-7

The size of dust and granule particles is measured by passing the material through screens with different sizes of mesh. Mesh is the number of wires per inch of screen. As seen here, the larger the mesh number, the finer the screen, and the smaller the granules that pass through. Granules range in size from 4 to 80 mesh, while dusts are 80 mesh and finer.

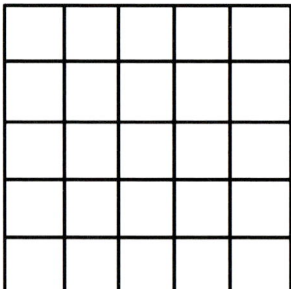
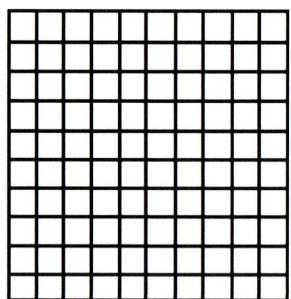

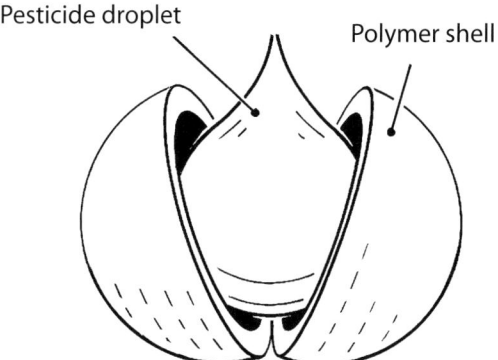

FIGURE 3-8

Microencapsulated formulations consist of pesticides enclosed in tiny plastic capsules. This often makes them safer to use and increases their effectiveness.

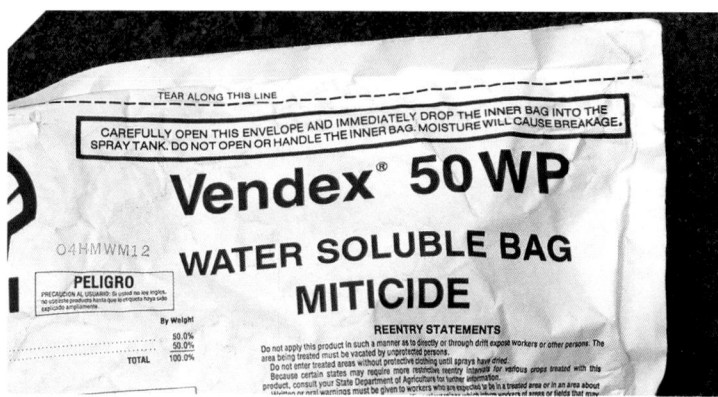

FIGURE 3-9

Water-soluble bags protect handlers during the mixing of some types of highly toxic or hazardous pesticides. A preweighed amount of formulated pesticide powder is in a plastic bag inside this paper envelope. Remove the bag from the envelope and drop it into your water-filled spray tank. The plastic bag dissolves in the water and releases the powder.

Microencapsulated Materials

Manufacturers cover liquid or dry pesticide particles in a plastic coating, producing a microencapsulated formulation (Fig. 3-8). You mix microencapsulated pesticides with water and spray them in the same manner as other sprayable formulations. After spraying, the plastic coating breaks down and slowly releases the active ingredient. Microencapsulated formulations have several advantages.

- They make it safer for applicators to mix and apply highly toxic materials.
- They prolong the active ingredient's effectiveness because release is delayed or slowed, allowing for fewer applications that are less precisely timed.
- They volatilize more slowly, so there is less drift from the application site.
- They reduce phytotoxicity.

In residential, industrial, and institutional applications, microencapsulated formulations offer several advantages. These include reduced odor, release of small quantities of pesticide over a long time, and greater safety. Microcapsules offer less hazard to the skin than do ordinary formulations. Microcapsules pose a special hazard to bees, however. Because microcapsules are about the same size as pollen grains, bees may carry them back to their hives. As the capsules break down, they release the pesticide, poisoning the adults and brood.

Breakdown of the microcapsules to release the pesticide sometimes depends on weather conditions. Under certain conditions, the microcapsules may break down more slowly than expected. This could leave higher residues of pesticide active ingredient in treated areas beyond normal restricted-entry or harvest intervals with the potential to injure fieldworkers. For this reason, regulations require long restricted-entry intervals for some microencapsulated formulations.

Water-Soluble Bags or Packets (WSB or WSP)

Water-soluble bags reduce the mixing and handling hazards of some highly toxic pesticides (Fig. 3-9). Manufacturers package preweighed amounts of wettable powder or soluble powder formulations in a special type of plastic bag. As you drop these bags into a filled spray tank, they dissolve and release their contents to mix with the water. There are no risks of inhaling or contacting the undiluted pesticide as long as you do not open the bags. Once mixed with water, pesticides packaged in water-soluble bags are no safer than other mixtures. They are also abrasive to application equipment.

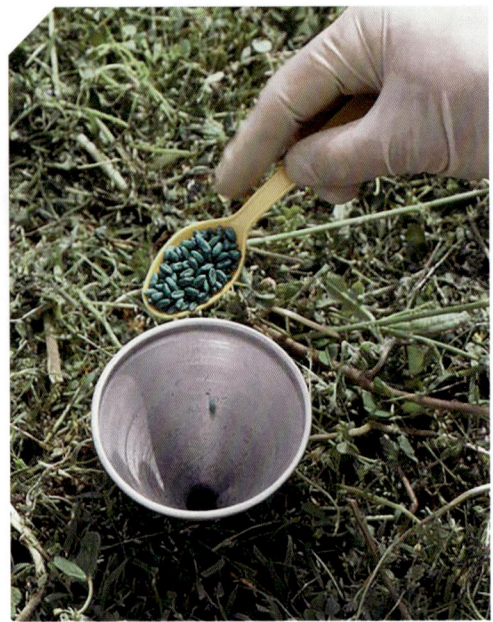

FIGURE 3-10

Manufacturers color some baits, such as these seeds, to distinguish them as being poisonous.

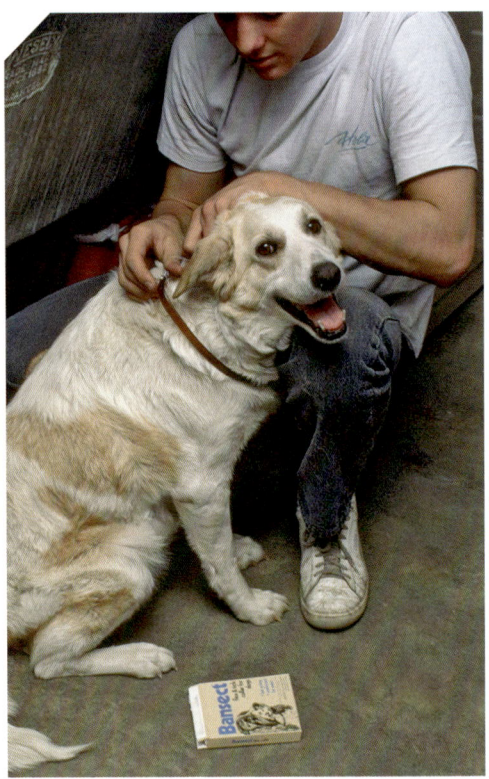

FIGURE 3-11

Manufacturers impregnate flea collars with an insecticide that kills fleas. A low level of this insecticide is slowly released by the collar.

Baits

Baits are pesticides combined with food, attractants, or feeding stimulants. Because baits attract target pests to a pesticide, they eliminate the need for widespread pesticide application. For example, target pests such as ants carry baits back to their nestbound young. Use baits indoors to control rodents, ants, roaches, and flies. Use them outdoors to control slugs, snails, insects, and vertebrates such as birds, rodents, and larger mammals. Dangers associated with baits include their attractiveness to nontarget animals and to children. When children, pets, or other nontarget species are present, place baits in specially designed bait stations that prevent other animals and children from accessing the bait. Manufacturers color some baits, such as grains, to distinguish them as being poisonous and to make them less attractive to birds (Fig. 3-10).

Attractants

Attractants include pheromones, sugar and protein hydrolysate syrups, yeasts, and rotting meat. Pest managers use these attractants in various traps. You can also combine them with pesticides and spray them onto foliage or other items in the treatment area.

Aerosols

Manufacturers package some insecticides and other pesticides in small aerosol cans. The pesticide combines under pressure with a chemical propellant in the can. Some aerosol containers emit pesticides as a fine airborne mist or fog (aerosol foggers). Usually, you use the aerosol foggers as one-time, total release units. Other aerosol containers produce a coarse spray of liquid or powder (pressure spray applicators). With pressure spray applicators, you apply a pesticide film directly onto surfaces.

Residential, industrial, and institutional pest control operators frequently use refillable aerosol applicators. In structural pest control, aerosol containers are convenient because they require no mixing or special application equipment. They are handy for situations when you apply only small amounts of pesticide at any one time. The remaining pesticide in the container does not lose its potency during storage.

Hazards from aerosol containers include risks of inhalation injury from breathing the spray or dust. Also, it is difficult to confine the spray, fog, or dust emitted from aerosol containers. Because of the flammable petroleum oil carriers, do not use pressure spray applicators around open flames or other sources of ignition.

Impregnates

Manufacturers impregnate pet collars, livestock ear tags, adhesive tapes, plastic pest strips, and other products with pesticides (Fig. 3-11). These pesticides evaporate over time, and the vapors provide control of nearby pests. Some paints and wood finishes have pesticides incorporated into them to kill insects or retard fungus growth. In residences and commercial buildings, cockroaches are controlled by insecticides incorporated into clear plastic or lacquer paint. Surfaces painted with this material provide 6 to 12 months of residual control. Sometimes manufacturers impregnate carpeting, furniture, bedding, fabrics, and clothing with pesticides to prevent damage from insects and fungi. Adhesive-backed impregnated strips provide long-term protection against insect damage when placed inside electrical boxes, electronic equipment, and appliances.

Repellents

Various types of insect repellents are available in aerosol and lotion formulations. People apply these to their skin, clothing, or to plant foliage to repel biting and nuisance insects. You can mix other types of repellents with water and spray these onto ornamental plants and agricultural crops. Use these to prevent damage from deer, dogs, and other animals.

Animal Systemics

Systemic pesticides protect animals against fleas and other external blood-feeding insects as well as against worms and other internal parasites. These pesticides enter the animals' tissues after being applied orally or externally. Oral applications include food additives and premeasured capsules and liquids. External applications involve pour-on liquids, liquid sprays, and dusts. Most animal systemics are used under the supervision of veterinarians.

Fertilizer Combinations

Pest managers frequently combine insecticides, fungicides, and herbicides with fertilizers. This provides a convenient way of controlling pests while fertilizing crops or ornamental plants. Homeowners commonly use these combinations, although the unit cost of pesticide in these preparations is usually high. In commercial applications, dealers or growers custom-mix pesticides with fertilizers to meet specific crop requirements.

PESTICIDES WITH SPECIAL FUNCTIONS

A few pesticides do not belong to specific chemical groups. Some occur naturally, some are produced by living organisms, and others are manufactured. These special types of pesticides include antibiotics, anticoagulants, botanicals, insect growth regulators, inert dusts, microbials, petroleum oils, pheromones, plant hormones, and soaps. The following sections describe these unique materials.

Antibiotics

An antibiotic is a substance produced by one organism that kills or inhibits another organism. The antibiotic penicillin, used to control bacterial infections in people and animals, comes from a fungus. Streptomycin, used to treat bacterial diseases in people, animals, and plants, occurs naturally and is also a synthetically produced antibiotic. Terramycin and other similar synthetic antibiotics resemble naturally occurring antibiotics. These control several plant diseases caused by fungi, viruses, and bacteria.

Anticoagulants

Anticoagulants interfere with the blood-clotting mechanism of mammals, causing them to die of blood loss after an injury. Pest managers use anticoagulants to control rodents such as rats and mice. First- and second-generation anticoagulant active ingredients are used to control rodents. Second-generation anticoagulants like brodifacoum and bromadiolone are designed to be toxic

TABLE 3-7

Examples of botanically derived insecticides

Insecticide	Source	Uses/comments
azadirachtin	extract from the neem tree (*Azadirachta indica*)	Acts as a natural insect growth regulator (IGR) and as an antifeedant. Azadirachtin also has nematicidal and fungicidal properties.
pyrethrum/pyrethrins	extract from dried flowers of certain chrysanthemum species	Derived from the extract of the chrysanthemum flower and comprised of two different types of pyrethrins. Has contact, stomach, and fumigant poisoning action on insects. Is also toxic to cold-blooded animals. Kills aphids, mosquitoes, flies, fleas, mealybugs, cabbageworms, thrips, beetles, leafhoppers, lice, loopers, and many others. Insecticidal action is degraded rapidly by sunlight. Action is often enhanced by addition of piperonyl butoxide, a synergist.
rotenone	derived by grinding roots of certain legume plants (68 different species); U.S. supplies come primarily from roots of the cube plant	Contact and stomach poison. Used to control unwanted fish. Rotenone is slow acting and has a short residual activity.
sabadilla	obtained from the dried ripe seed of a South American lily plant	Has contact and stomach poison action against cockroaches, brown soft scale, potato leafhopper, imported cabbageworm, house fly, thrips, and the cattle louse. Is toxic to honey bees but not highly toxic to mammals. Used on avocado and citrus, and in greenhouses.

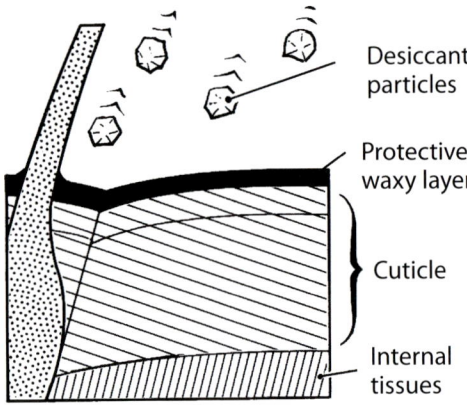

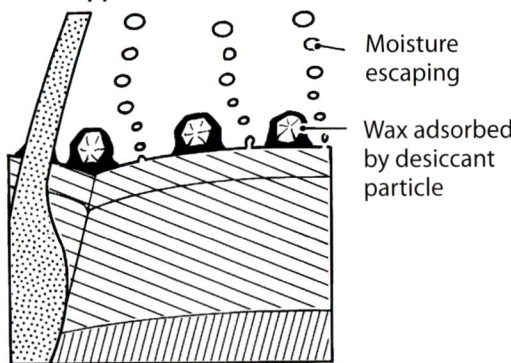

FIGURE 3-12

Desiccants (inert dusts and sorptive powders) destroy insects and mites by removing or disrupting their protective outer body covering. This causes the organism to lose body fluids.

in a single feeding but may take several days to kill the target pest. Since rodents do not die immediately and may feed multiple times before death, their bodies present a secondary poisoning hazard to predators or scavengers, including house pets. Rodents must feed on first-generation anticoagulants like warfarin or chlorophacinone several times before accumulating enough toxic material to cause death.

Botanicals

Certain plants contain substances that are naturally poisonous to insects and other animals. These include species of chrysanthemum flowers from which manufacturers extract pyrethrum. The roots of the cube plant supply rotenone. Species of lily plants provide sabadilla and hellebore. Strychnine comes from the dried seeds of a small tree found in India, Sri Lanka, Australia, Cambodia, Laos, and Vietnam. Table 3-7 lists insecticidal chemicals derived from plants.

Inert Dusts

Inert dusts, also called desiccants or sorptive dusts, are fine powders with low toxicity. Pest managers use them to control various insects and other invertebrates. These dusts kill pests through a physical, rather than chemical, action. Some are abrasive and scratch the pests' waxy body coverings, causing them to lose water. Other dusts remove (adsorb) this protective waxy coating (Fig. 3-12). Manufacturers sometimes combine inert dusts with aluminum fluosilicate. This gives the mixture an electrostatic charge and causes it to cling to surfaces, including the pest's outer body covering.

Because some inert dusts are low in toxicity, pest managers use them in locations where other pesticides are unsafe. Since the killing action is physical rather than chemical, these dusts do not lose their effectiveness over time. However, inert dusts are not effective once they become wet.

TABLE 3-8

Insect growth regulators

Compound*	Brand name*	Uses
diflubenzuron	Dimilin	controls leaf-eating insects
hydroprene	Gentrol	controls bed bugs
methoprene	Tango, Extinguish	controls ants and fleas
pyriproxyfen	various	controls flies, mosquitoes, midges and fleas

Note: *Some a.i.'s or products listed may not be currently registered as pesticides or may have had their registration cancelled.

Diatomaceous earth, silica gel, and boric acid powder are some of the materials used as desiccants. These pesticides leave highly visible residues on all treated surfaces. Boric acid powder is toxic to people if ingested, so do not use it around young children. Although most inert dusts are low in toxicity, avoid inhaling them because they can cause serious lung irritation.

Insect Growth Regulators

Insect growth regulators (IGRs) are chemicals that control insects by altering their normal development (Table 3-8). Natural growth hormones produced by insects regulate how long individuals remain in each of their larval or nymphal stages. They also control when the insects become reproductive adults. Synthetically produced IGRs mimic or interrupt the action of natural growth hormones. Some prevent insects from changing into adults, while others force insects to change into adults before they are physically able to reproduce.

Microbials

Manufacturers produce microbial pesticides by combining certain microorganisms with other ingredients. Various strains of the bacterium *Bacillus thuringiensis* control species of moth larvae, mosquito larvae, and black fly larvae (Fig. 3-13). *Agrobacterium radiobacter* controls the bacterium that produces crown gall in trees, shrubs, and vines. Certain fungi kill some pest mites; other fungi control the northern jointvetch weed in rice and soybeans. Some viruses effectively control several moth pests, including the codling moth. The plant disease caused by *Phytophthora palmivora* controls milkweed vine in citrus.

The use of microbial pesticides is growing in popularity because of their extremely low hazards to people and nontarget organisms and their specificity to target pests. Besides naturally occurring microbial organisms, manufacturers are researching uses for genetically altered organisms as pest control products.

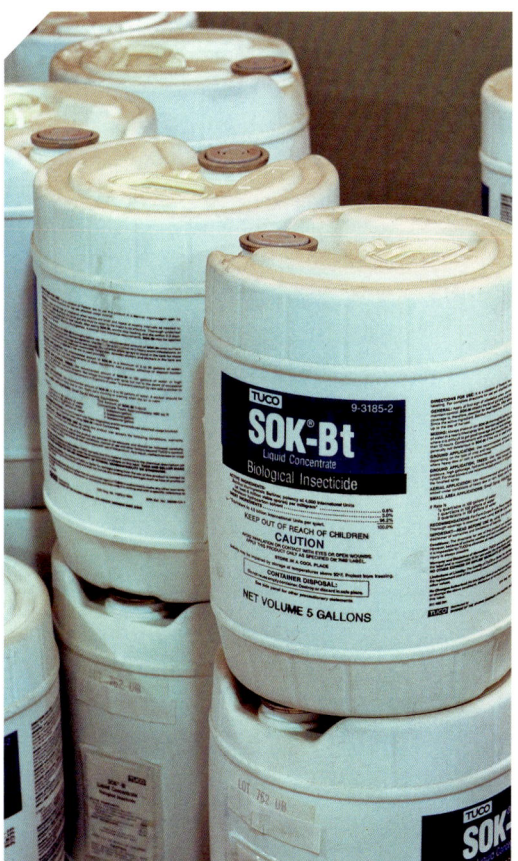

FIGURE 3-13

Microbial pesticides contain microorganisms that kill other living organisms. The insecticide shown here contains spores of the bacterium *Bacillus thuringiensis*.

Petroleum Oils

Some highly refined petroleum oils are lethal to certain invertebrates. Pest managers use them to control aphids, scales, mealybugs, eggs of these insects, and mites and mite eggs. Petroleum oils destroy these plant-feeding pests through suffocation. They can be used in combination with other insecticides to improve efficacy of treatment. Oils are effective against fungal diseases such as powdery mildew and in preventing virus transmission (both mechanical and by aphids). Less-refined petroleum oils have uses as nonselective herbicides. They destroy weeds by injuring cell membranes.

Refined oils used as pesticides can be classified based on timing of application (e.g., dormant or summer oils) or by other properties (e.g., narrow-range, superior, or supreme). Each type has certain features important for controlling pests and reducing injury to treated plants (phytotoxicity). Characteristics that influence the safety and effectiveness of oils are the
- unsulfonated residue (UR) rating
- distillation temperature and range
- hydrocarbon composition

Pheromones

Pheromones are unique chemicals produced by animals that stimulate behavior in other animals of the same species. Many insects depend on pheromones to locate mates. Synthetic insect pheromones are useful tools for monitoring insect activity, timing insecticide applications, and attracting insects to poisoned sprays. For monitoring, pest managers use synthetic pheromones with sticky insect traps. Pest managers use certain pheromones to disrupt mating activity of some insects and reduce pest populations (Fig. 3-14).

Plant Growth Regulators and Plant Hormones

In nature, hormones and growth regulators produced by plants control functions such as flowering, fruit development, nutrient storage, and dormancy. Manufacturers either derive plant growth regulators and plant hormones from plants or synthesize them. These synthesized

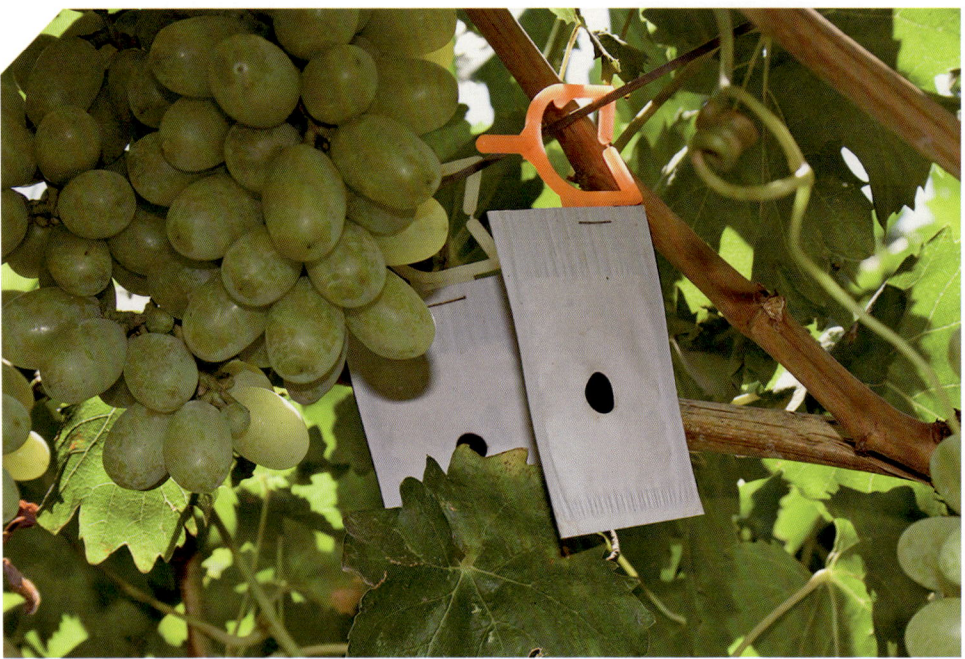

FIGURE 3-14

Pheromones are unique chemicals that attract certain species of insects. Synthetic pheromones are useful tools in a pest management program. This photograph shows pheromone dispensers placed for mating disruption of vine mealybug, *Planococcus ficus*.

TABLE 3-9

Materials with plant growth regulator and plant hormone activity

Compound*	Brand name*	Uses
carbaryl	Sevin	Thinning agent on apples. (Also used as an insecticide.)
chlorpropham	Sprout Nip	Inhibits potato sprouting.
cytokinin	Mepex	Promotes cell division, stimulates bud break, increases fruit set and size, and reduces plant size in cotton.
daminozide	Dazide 85 WSG	Controls plant height and promotes flowering of a broad variety of flowering ornamentals.
ethephon	Prep, Ethephon 6, Super Boll, Florel	Hastens maturity, harvest aid on cotton and walnuts, controls mistletoe in trees.
gibberellic acid	ProGibb, Gibgro, N-Large	Increases fruit set, size, and yield. Controls fruit maturity, slows aging in citrus.
1-naphthaleneacetamide (NAD)	Amid-thin	Thinning agent on some apple varieties.
mefluidide	Embark	Regulates growth of turfgrass, broadleaf vegetation, and ornamentals in landscaped areas.
mepiquat chloride	Compact	Improves yield, shortens plant height, accelerates maturity, and opens canopy of cotton plants.
naphthalene acetic acid (NAA)	Fruitone, Fruit Fix, Liqui-Stik	Thinning agent on some apple varieties, olives, and citrus. Controls sucker growth in citrus.
N6-benzyl adenine	Configure	Improves growth and fullness of white pine grown for Christmas trees. Promotes uniform flowering in ornamentals and plants in containers.
2,4-D	2,4-D	Increases fruit size and reduces drop in citrus. Intensifies color and improves skin appearance in potatoes. (Also used as an herbicide.)
abscisic acid (ABA)	ProTone	Inhibits growth. Causes dormancy of seeds and buds.
ethylene	Ethylene	Promotes fruit maturation and ripening.

Note: *Some materials listed here may not be registered for use as plant growth regulators or plant hormones. Check current labels before use.
Source: Adapted from Lovatt n.d.

materials mimic naturally occurring plant chemicals or induce abnormal growth changes in plants. They regulate plant growth, enhance fruit production, remove foliage for ease in harvesting a crop, or destroy undesirable plants. Table 3-9 lists some of the chemicals that have hormonelike action.

Soaps

Pesticide soaps control insects, mites, mosses, liverworts, algae, and lichens by interfering with the cellular metabolism of the target pest. Insecticidal soaps are most effective on soft-bodied insects such as aphids, scales, psyllids, and some larval stages of other insects. Pesticide soaps have the advantage of being nearly nontoxic to vertebrates, including people. Soap sprays might damage some nontarget plants, so before using them, check the label for any restrictions. Use only soaps labeled for pest control.

ADJUVANTS

Explain the role of adjuvants in pesticide applications.

Adjuvants are materials you can add to the spray tank to improve pesticide mixing and application or enhance performance. Manufacturers formulate pesticides to be suitable to many types of application conditions. However, they cannot formulate them for all possible situations. Use adjuvants to customize the formulation to specific needs and compensate for local conditions. Adjuvants are used to

- improve the wetting ability of spray solutions
- control evaporation of spray droplets

- improve weatherability of pesticides
- increase the penetration of pesticides through plant or insect cuticles
- adjust the pH of spray solutions
- improve spray droplet deposition
- increase safety to target plants
- correct incompatibility problems
- reduce spray drift

Familiarize yourself with adjuvant types to understand where and how to use them (Table 3-10). When selecting adjuvants, outline the effect you wish the adjuvant to have. Next, check pesticide and adjuvant labels to make sure these materials are compatible as well as suited to the application site, target pest, and application equipment.

Often, a single chemical will accomplish two or more adjuvant functions. Examples of these are spreader-stickers, spreader-activators, or spreader-sticker drift retardants. Some manufacturers also produce blends of chemicals to accomplish multiple functions. The effectiveness of most adjuvants is proportional to their concentration in the spray tank mixture, however. Therefore, ready-mixed

TABLE 3-10

Comparisons of adjuvants

FUNCTION	TYPE OF ADJUVANT											
	Surfactant	Sticker	Spreader-sticker	Extender	Activator	Compatibility agent	Buffer	Acidifier	Deposition aid	De-foamer	Thickener	Attractant
reduce surface tension	●		●		●							
improve ability to get into small cracks	●		●									
increase uptake by target	●		●		●			●				
improve sticking	●	●	●									
protect against wash-off/abrasion	●	●	●	●								
reduce sunlight degradation		●	●	●								
reduce volatilization	●	●	●									
increase persistence				●	●				●		●	
improve mixing						●	●	●				
lower pH							●	●				
slow breakdown							●	●				
reduce drift									●		●	
eliminate foam										●		
increase viscosity									●		●	
increase droplet size									●		●	
attract pests to pesticide												●

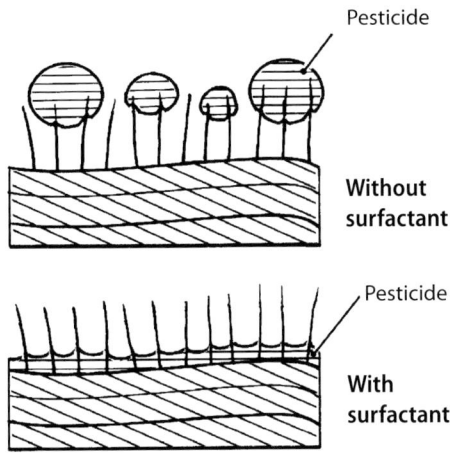

FIGURE 3-15

Surface tension prevents spray droplets from spreading out over waxy or hairy leaf or insect surfaces. Adding a surfactant, however, lowers surface tension, which allows droplets to spread out and come in contact with the cuticle of the leaf or insect.

blends may limit your ability to achieve the proper concentration of a component for your application requirements unless the requirements are identical to the ratio of components in the adjuvant mixture. It is often better to use several single-active-ingredient adjuvants rather than one multiple-function adjuvant. Add these at the appropriate concentrations for your specific needs.

Surfactants

Surfactants are surface-active agents, also known as wetting agents or spreaders. They enhance spray coverage by reducing the surface tension of spray droplets. Sometimes vegetable oils such as cottonseed oil and soy oil are used as surfactants. Surfactants allow better coverage on waxy or hairy surfaces, such as leaves of many plants or the outer coverings of insects and mites (Fig. 3-15). They also help to get sprays into small cracks or openings.

The amount of surface tension reduction is proportional, to an extent, to the amount of surfactant used. Surface tension is measured in dynes/cm. Water has a normal surface tension of about 72 dynes/cm. Optimal spreading occurs by lowering this to about 30 dynes/cm. At this point, spray droplets are able to penetrate the small openings in leaf surfaces or insect cuticles. Increasing surfactant concentration any more than this usually causes spray materials to run off treated surfaces. Pesticide runoff results in reduced effectiveness and a waste of materials, as well as increasing the chance of environmental contamination. Mix surfactants according to directions on their labels to achieve the appropriate surface tension reduction.

Three types of surfactants are available. Nonionic surfactants do not react in water. Anionic surfactants ionize into negatively charged ions in water. Cationic surfactants ionize into positively charged ions in water. The surfactant's charge or lack of charge is important to pesticide applications. The charge affects how the spray material will react after application, drying, and exposure to environmental conditions. Emulsifiers used in the formulation of many pesticides are usually a blend of anionic and nonionic surfactants. This enables petroleum or other solvent-based chemicals to break up into droplets and suspend in water.

Anionic surfactants (negative electrical charge) help prevent pesticides from washing off sprayed plants due to rain, dew, or irrigation. They prevent pesticides from being readily absorbed through plant cuticles because plant surfaces have a negative charge and like charges repel each other. Use anionic surfactants when the pesticide must remain on the outer surface of plants, even during adverse weather or environmental conditions. Also use them to increase the effectiveness of insecticides and miticides that are stomach or contact poisons. These surfactants keep more active ingredient on leaf surfaces rather than allowing them to be absorbed by the plant.

Nonionic surfactants (no electrical charge) increase pesticide penetration through plant cuticles. Labels recommend their use with systemic herbicides such as glyphosate and oxyfluorfen to improve target plant uptake. They also work with insecticides and fungicides that have systemic action. They improve the absorption of translocated pesticides into plant tissues. Rainfall, dew, or irrigation may wash pesticides mixed with nonionic surfactants off treated surfaces.

Cationic surfactants (positively charged) are strongly attracted to plant surfaces. Although they aid in getting pesticides through cuticles, they are highly phytotoxic when not blended with other types of surfactants. Pure cationic surfactants are not used as pesticide adjuvants.

Some surfactants are a blend of anionic and nonionic surfactants and may also contain cationic surfactants. Blends are general-purpose surfactants and usually have a wider range of applications.

Selecting Surfactants. When selecting surfactants for pesticide application, consider several factors:
- the nature of the target surface
- the physical and chemical nature of the pesticide
- whether the pesticide has contact or systemic action
- weather conditions and cultural practices
- the biology or habits of the pest

Consider also the cost of the surfactant compared with the cost per unit area of treatment. Surfactants are not always pure active ingredient; most contain an alcohol solvent. The percentage of alcohol varies from one brand of surfactant to another. You will need to use more surfactant if it contains a higher percentage of alcohol.

Stickers

Stickers are substances such as latex or other adhesives that improve pesticide attachment to sprayed surfaces. They protect pesticides from washing off due to rainfall, heavy dew, or irrigation. They also help prevent pesticide loss from wind or leaf abrasion. Many stickers incorporate ultraviolet inhibitors to slow pesticide breakdown by sunlight. Follow label directions carefully to avoid using too much sticker. Excess sticker binds the pesticide so well that it may be unavailable to react with target organisms. If the pesticide formulation already contains stickers, do not use additional amounts. Always read the pesticide label in case there are recommendations against using a sticker.

Spreader-Stickers

Spreader-stickers are mixtures of surfactants and latex or other adhesive stickers. These general-purpose adjuvants are used for many types of pesticide applications. When using a spreader-sticker, be certain that the surfactant is compatible with the type of pesticide being used. Also, check the pesticide formulation to see if it already contains a sticker.

Extenders

Extenders are chemicals that enhance the effectiveness or effective life of a pesticide. Some extenders function by screening out ultraviolet light, which decomposes many pesticides; others slow pesticide volatilization. Use stickers as extenders to slow the loss of pesticide from surfaces due to irrigation, rainfall, and abrasion. Remember that extenders may make sprayed areas toxic longer than expected because they slow pesticide breakdown.

Activators

Activators increase the activity of a pesticide. Some surfactants are activators because they reduce surface tension and allow greater pesticide contact. Activators also include chemicals that speed pesticide penetration through insect or plant cuticles. Use activators carefully because they may increase risk to nontarget organisms by making pesticides more toxic.

Compatibility Agents

When physical incompatibility occurs among pesticides, compatibility agents may reduce or eliminate separating or clumping. For example, one type of compatibility agent, an emulsifier, is a soaplike material that combines with oil to make the oil disperse in a water solution. When

SIDEBAR 3-1

TESTING AND ADJUSTING pH OF WATER USED FOR MIXING PESTICIDES

You can measure pH with an electronic pH meter, a pH test kit such as those used for testing swimming pool water, or pH test paper available from a chemical supply dealer.

TEST WATER

1. Using a clean container, obtain a sample of water from the same source that will be used to fill the spray tank.
2. Measure exactly 1 pint of this water into a clean quart jar.
3. Check the pH of the water using a pH meter, test kit, or test paper.

pH LEVEL

- 3.5–6.0: Satisfactory for spraying and short-term (12- to 24-hour) storage of most spray mixtures in the spray tank.
- 6.1–7.0: Adequate for immediate spraying of most pesticides. Do not leave the spray mixture in the tank for more than 1 to 2 hours, to prevent loss of effectiveness.
- Above 7.0: Add a buffer or acidifier.

ADJUST pH

1. Using a standard eyedropper, add 3 drops of buffer or acidifier to the measured pint of water.
2. Stir well with a clean glass rod or other clean, nonporous utensil.
3. Check pH as above.
4. If further adjustment is needed, add 3 drops of buffer or acidifier, stir well, then recheck pH. Repeat until pH is satisfactory. Remember how many times 3 drops were added to bring the solution to the proper pH.

CORRECT pH IN SPRAY TANK

1. Before adding pesticides to the sprayer, fill the tank with water.
2. For every 100 gallons of water in the spray tank, add 2 ounces of buffer or acidifier for each time 3 drops were used in the jar test above. Add buffer or acidifier to water while agitators are running. If tank is not equipped with an agitator, stir or mix well.
3. Check pH of the water in the spray tank to be certain it is correct. Adjust if necessary.
4. Add pesticides to spray tank.

TABLE 3-11

Effect of water pH on the chemical stability of selected pesticides

Compound	Brand name	Half-life at selected pH values*
carbaryl	Sevin	24 hours at pH 9.0, 2.5 days at pH 8.0, 24 days at pH 7.0
chlorothalonil	Bravo	38.1 days at pH 9.0, stable below pH 7.0
chlorpyrifos	Dursban, Lorsban	1.5 days at pH 8.0, 35 days at pH 7.0
diazinon	Diazinon	37 hours at pH 6.0, hydrolysis very rapid in strongly acidic or strongly alkaline solutions
dimethoate	Cygon	12 hours at pH 6.0, maximum stability between pH 4.0 and pH 7.0, unstable in alkaline water
ethoprop	Mocap	stable in acidic solutions, hydrolyzes rapidly in alkaline solutions
formetanate	Carzol	3 hours at pH 9.0, 14 hours at pH 7.0, 4 days at pH 5.0
malathion	Malathion	stable in neutral or moderately acidic solutions, undergoes rapid hydrolysis at pH above 7.0 or below 3.0
methomyl	Lannate	stable in slightly acidic water, slight hydrolysis after 6 hours in pH 9.1 solution
naled	Dibrom	undergoes 90 to 100% hydrolysis in 48 hours in alkaline water
phosmet	Imidan	4 hours at pH 8.0, 12 hours at pH 7.0, 13 days at pH 4.5

Notes: Some a.i.'s or products listed may not be currently registered as pesticides or may have had their registration cancelled.

*These figures are generalized estimates and reflect trends, but half-life periods may vary considerably. Hydrolysis depends on other factors besides the pH of the solution, including temperature, other pesticides and adjuvants in the spray tank, and formulation of the pesticide.

---

trying to correct an incompatibility problem with a compatibility agent, mix small quantities of the pesticides and compatibility agent in a jar. Add all components in your test in the same order that you mix them in the spray tank. Unless pesticide or compatibility labels require a specific mixing order, follow the technique described in Sidebar 10-1.

Buffers and Acidifiers

pH is a measure of the hydrogen ion activity of a solution: a neutral solution has a pH of 7; a solution with a pH of 6 is slightly acidic, while one with a pH of 8 is slightly alkaline. Because higher pH indicates higher alkalinity, it can be helpful to think of pH as a measure of alkalinity. Many pesticides are unstable in alkaline solutions but quite stable if the solution is slightly acidic. The optimal pH for most pesticides is about 6, although solutions in the range of pH 6 to 7 are usually satisfactory. Some pesticides are most effective when the solution is acidified to a pH of 3 to 3.5. High pH often causes accelerated pesticide breakdown. Table 3-11 shows some of the effects of water pH on the activity of pesticides. Sidebar 3-1 describes how to measure and alter the pH of the spray solution should this be necessary.

Buffers. Buffers are capable of changing the pH of a water solution to a prescribed level. They keep this level relatively constant, even though conditions such as water alkalinity may change.

Acidifiers. Acidifiers (also called acidulators) are acids that neutralize alkaline solutions and lower the pH. Acidifiers do not have a buffering action like buffers. Therefore, alkaline or acidic compounds added to the spray solution after the acidifier may change the pH of the solution.

Deposition Aids

Deposition aids are adjuvants that improve the ability of pesticide sprays to reach surfaces in a treatment area. Different types of products work as deposition aids. Inverting agents, for instance, encapsulate the pesticide, forming oil droplets of uniform size. These suspend in larger water droplets to form an invert suspension. Encapsulation prevents evaporation or volatilization of the pesticide before it reaches the target surface. Drift control agents increase droplet size by altering shear forces of the liquid spray emitted from a nozzle. Because larger droplets have more momentum, they travel farther and are influenced less by wind. The result is that more pesticide reaches target surfaces in the treatment area. Surfactants that alter the surface tension of the spray solution also improve deposition. They do this because they influence droplet size as well as distribution on sprayed surfaces.

Defoaming Agents

Many pesticide mixtures produce copious amounts of foam as a result of the action of hydraulic or mechanical agitators. Foaming in the spray tank introduces air into the pressure system. This makes it difficult to maintain the even pressure required for proper mixing and uniform pesticide application. Defoaming agents eliminate foam in the spray tank.

Thickeners

Thickeners increase the viscosity of spray mixtures. Although thickeners work as drift retardants, they also assist in keeping spray mixtures in suspension. In addition, they slow the separation process once these materials reach the target. They help to slow evaporation, extending pesticide activity and reducing drift. Sometimes regulations require the use of a thickener as a drift control agent when applying phenoxy herbicides such as 2,4-D.

Attractants

Attractants are food or bait, such as sugar, molasses, protein hydrolysates, or insect pheromones, that attract specific pests, usually insects. These combine with a pesticide to form a lethal mixture. Attractants allow spot applications of pesticides to localized areas within the treatment site. They often enhance pesticide specificity to target pests.

Spray Colorants

Spray colorants are dyes you add to the spray tank to be able to see areas you have sprayed. Use colorants in backpack sprayers when applying herbicides to turf or a landscaped area. Also use them in rangeland areas and when spraying fencerows. Spray colorants are not suitable for use on food crops; the dyes may remain on produce and there may not be an established residue tolerance.

Pesticide Mixtures

Combining two or more pesticides and applying them at the same time is convenient and cost effective. Only a few pesticide manufactures sell their products as premixed combinations. Usually, you must combine the pesticides at the time of application. When you combine mixtures of two or more pesticides or pesticides and fertilizers at the time of application, you create a tank mix. A common tank mix involves combining fungicides with insecticides as a dormant

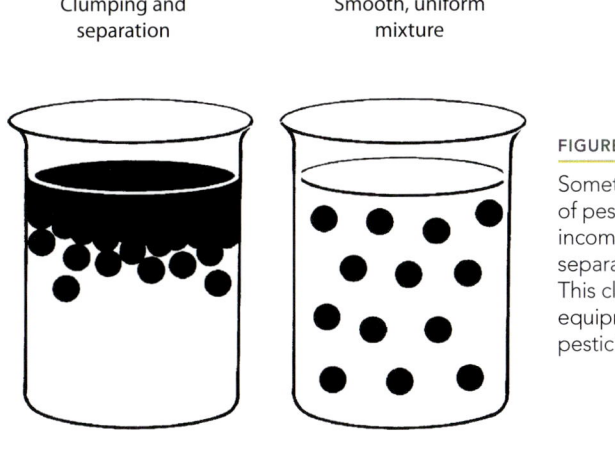

FIGURE 3-16

Sometimes mixtures of pesticides are incompatible and may separate or curdle. This clogs spray equipment and wastes the pesticide material.

Incompatible Compatible

spray in deciduous tree crops. Another involves combining two or more herbicides to increase the number of weed species controlled. Some people mix pesticides with micronutrients or fertilizers. This saves money by reducing the time, labor, and fuel required for multiple applications. Tank mixes reduce equipment wear and decrease labor costs. They also lessen the mechanical damage done to crops and soil by heavy application equipment. Drawbacks of using a tank mix have to do with chemical compatibility and the problems that arise from unexpected reactions among chemicals added to the tank. Chapter 10 describes in detail the problems that can occur when combining two or more pesticides.

If you mix DANGER pesticides with WARNING or CAUTION pesticides, treat the mixture as a DANGER pesticide. Required safety equipment and all other label restrictions must comply with the label having the greater restrictions.

INCOMPATIBILITY

Incompatibility is a physical condition that prevents pesticides from mixing properly to form a uniform solution or suspension. Precipitation of flakes, crystals, oily clumps, or severe separation is unacceptable (Fig. 3-16). Such incompatible mixtures clog application equipment and limit even distribution of the active ingredient in the spray tank, which prevents good pesticide coverage. If you can mix the incompatible mixture thoroughly and keep it in that condition with agitation, however, the mixture is probably suitable to use.

The cause of incompatibility may relate to the chemical nature of the materials you are mixing. Impurities in the spray tank or water may also affect compatibility. Even the order in which you mix pesticides in the spray tank is important. Sometimes the types of formulations being mixed influence compatibility. Pesticide formulations of the same type are rarely incompatible with each other because they usually contain the same inert ingredients and solvents. Methods used to test two or more ingredients for incompatibility can be found in Sidebar 10-1, along with a short explanation of where to find compatibility information prior to mixing two or more pesticides.

In some cases, chemicals appear to mix properly in solution, but instead they react with one another, altering their chemical makeup, and thus their effectiveness. For more on the chemical changes that can occur when combining pesticides, see "Chemical Changes with Pesticides and Pesticide Combinations" in Chapter 10.

Chapter 3 Review Questions

1. In the state of California, a pesticide is defined as _____ .
   - ☐ a. any substance used to control pest organisms in any situation
   - ☐ b. only those chemicals registered for pest control in California
   - ☐ c. chemicals derived from natural and organic sources only

2. How do we determine a pesticide's toxicity category (DANGER, WARNING, CAUTION)?
   - ☐ a. Scientists measure the time it takes a pesticide to kill pests after application to determine how toxic it is.
   - ☐ b. Scientists record the number of times a pesticide is misused by handlers to determine how toxic it is.
   - ☐ c. Scientists expose animals to doses of pesticide and observe how much causes injury to determine how toxic it is.

3. Match the pesticide group to the pest it controls.

1. acaricide	a. snails
	b. little mallow
2. herbicide	c. ground squirrels
	d. persea mites
3. molluscicide	e. yellow nutsedge
	f. webspinning spider mites
4. rodenticide	g. slugs
	h. roof rat

4. Match the signal word with its oral LD_{50}.

1. DANGER	a. from 50 to 500 mg/kg
2. CAUTION	b. below 50 mg/kg
3. WARNING	c. over 500 mg/kg

5. Match the chemical family with its unique hazard.

1. organochlorines	a. Some pesticides in this family are considered to be among the most acutely toxic chemicals known.
2. organophosphates	b. Toxic levels of pesticides from this chemical family have been found in waterway sediment throughout California.
3. carbamates	c. Most of the chemicals in this family persist for a long time in the environment.
4. triazines	d. Many weeds have developed resistance to herbicides from this family.
5. neonicotinoids	e. This family is highly toxic to fish and marine invertebrates.
6. pyrethroids	f. Chemicals in this family are highly toxic to mammals, although their effects are often short-lived.
7. sulfonylureas	g. When using pesticides in this family, applicators must check first to see if the site is in a Ground Water Protection Area.
8. strobilurins	h. Residues left by pesticides in this family may accumulate in pollen and nectar.

6. **Which of the following is a preemergent herbicide's general mode of action having contact action?**
   ☐ a. contact
   ☐ b. systemic

7. **Which of the following represents a mode of action of pesticides having contact action?**
   ☐ a. clogging an insect's air passages
   ☐ b. inhibiting seed germination
   ☐ c. root applications that translocate through a plant

8. **A pesticide's mode of action is _____.**
   ☐ a. how the chemical breaks down once it is released into the environment
   ☐ b. a descriptor that defines how abrasive the pesticide will be after mixing
   ☐ c. the method by which it kills or adversely affects the target pest

9. **Match the situation with the appropriate mode of action used to address it.**

1. A fungus has invaded and has begun to damage plant tissues.	a. desiccant
2. You need to keep weed seedlings from sprouting.	b. protectant
3. You need to cause a certain amount of leaf drop.	c. eradicant
4. Disease inoculum has been detected near valuable plants, and conditions are right for infection.	d. sterilant
5. Insect populations are breeding rapidly.	e. growth inhibitor

10. **A pesticide formulation is a mixture of _____.**
    ☐ a. concentrated pesticide and adjuvants or other ingredients you have added to a tank mix
    ☐ b. active ingredients and substances that improve application effectiveness, safety, handling, and storage
    ☐ c. water-soluble packaging and a concentrated chemical that makes mixing less hazardous

11. **Match the pesticide formulation with its primary benefit.**

1. wettable powder (WP)	a. This formulation is not abrasive to spray nozzles or pumps.
2. dry flowable (DF)	b. It is among the safest formulations to use if phytotoxicity is a concern.
3. soluble powder (SP)	c. This formulation is ready to use right out of the package and requires no dilution.
4. emulsifiable concentrate (EC)	d. Measuring and mixing is simple because this formulation is packaged in easy-to-pour plastic containers.
5. low-concentrate solution (S)	e. It is among the most versatile of all formulations and has many applications.

12. Which of the following should you consider when selecting pesticides for a job?
- ☐ a. the advice of your local pest control adviser, a farm advisor, and the county agricultural commissioner
- ☐ b. target pests, conditions at the application site, and the pesticides' hazards and mode(s) of action
- ☐ c. degree-day calculations, UC IPM's *Pest Management Guidelines*, and the application equipment available

13. Why are adjuvants used?
- ☐ a. They make mixing and loading safer, even when using DANGER pesticides.
- ☐ b. They prevent the contamination of groundwater in a Ground Water Protection Area.
- ☐ c. They customize formulations to specific needs and compensate for local conditions.

Chapter 4
Environmental Hazards Associated with Pesticide Use

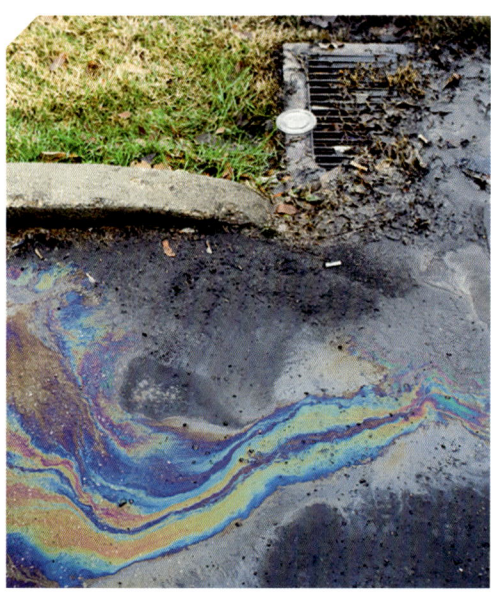

The Environment 100
Pesticide Characteristics 100
How Pesticides Move in the Environment 102
Sources of Pesticide Contamination 105
Environmental Impacts of Pesticide Application 110
Chapter 4 Review Questions 117

Knowledge Expectations

- Explain the potential environmental hazards associated with pesticides.
- Describe pesticide chemical and physical characteristics and how these characteristics indicate the potential for pesticides to move offsite.
- List the types of offsite movement of pesticides.
- Describe factors that influence offsite movement of pesticides.
- List features of a given site, including soil type and geology, that influence the potential for a pesticide to reach surface water or groundwater.
- Distinguish between point sources and nonpoint sources of environmental contamination by pesticides.
- Define pesticide residue, identify conditions that affect the buildup of residue, and explain how to avoid creating hazardous residues.
- Describe ways that pesticides can impact nontarget organisms.

Governmental agencies as well as the general public are becoming increasingly concerned about the harmful effects of pesticides on the environment. Initially, hazards to humans were the primary reason for the U.S. EPA to classify a pesticide as a restricted-use product. Now, more and more pesticide labels list environmental effects such as contamination of groundwater or toxicity to birds or aquatic organisms as reasons for restriction. The U.S. EPA requires extensive environmental testing when it evaluates applications submitted by manufacturers for the registration of new pesticides. The agency is also taking a close look at environmental effects when it reevaluates existing pesticide registrations.

Explain the potential environmental hazards associated with pesticides.

California has been active in pesticide regulation since passing its first pesticide law in 1901. California's Department of Pesticide Regulation (DPR) and county agricultural commissioners work with the U.S. EPA to regulate pesticide use. These agencies face an increasing challenge: protect the public, workers, and the environment while allowing the use of chemicals to manage pests. In California, regulators make sure we have safe and sensible pesticide rules, and they also make sure pesticide users follow those rules (DPR 2014).

The environmental hazards covered in this chapter include the contamination of surface water and groundwater, the damage to nontarget organisms (e.g., pollinators, endangered species, wildlife in natural habitats), and the contamination of sensitive areas (e.g., schools, wildlife habitat, apiaries, domestic animal habitat, public gardens). Related to these topics are the various ways pesticides escape from treated areas and enter the environment, such as drift, leaching, runoff, and residues that move into the environment before the pesticide breaks down. In addition, the factors that influence offsite movement of pesticides will be covered.

The Environment

The environment is made up of everything around us. It includes not only the natural elements that the word *environment* most often brings to mind, but also people and the manufactured components of our world. Neither is the environment limited to the outdoors—it also includes indoor areas where we live and work. The environment is much more than the oceans and the ozone layer. It is air, soil, water, plants, animals, houses, restaurants, office buildings, and factories and all that they contain. Anyone who uses a pesticide—indoors or outdoors, in a city or on a farm—must consider how that pesticide affects the environment (Fig. 4-1).

The applicator must ask two questions (Randall et al. 2008):
1. Where is the pesticide going to go in the environment after it leaves its container or application equipment?
2. What effects can this pesticide have on those nontarget sites it may reach in the environment?

Describe pesticide chemical and physical characteristics and how these characteristics indicate the potential for pesticides to move offsite.

Pesticide Characteristics

To understand how pesticides move in the environment, you must first understand certain physical and chemical characteristics of pesticides and how they determine a pesticide's interaction with the environment. These characteristics are solubility, adsorption, persistence, and volatility.

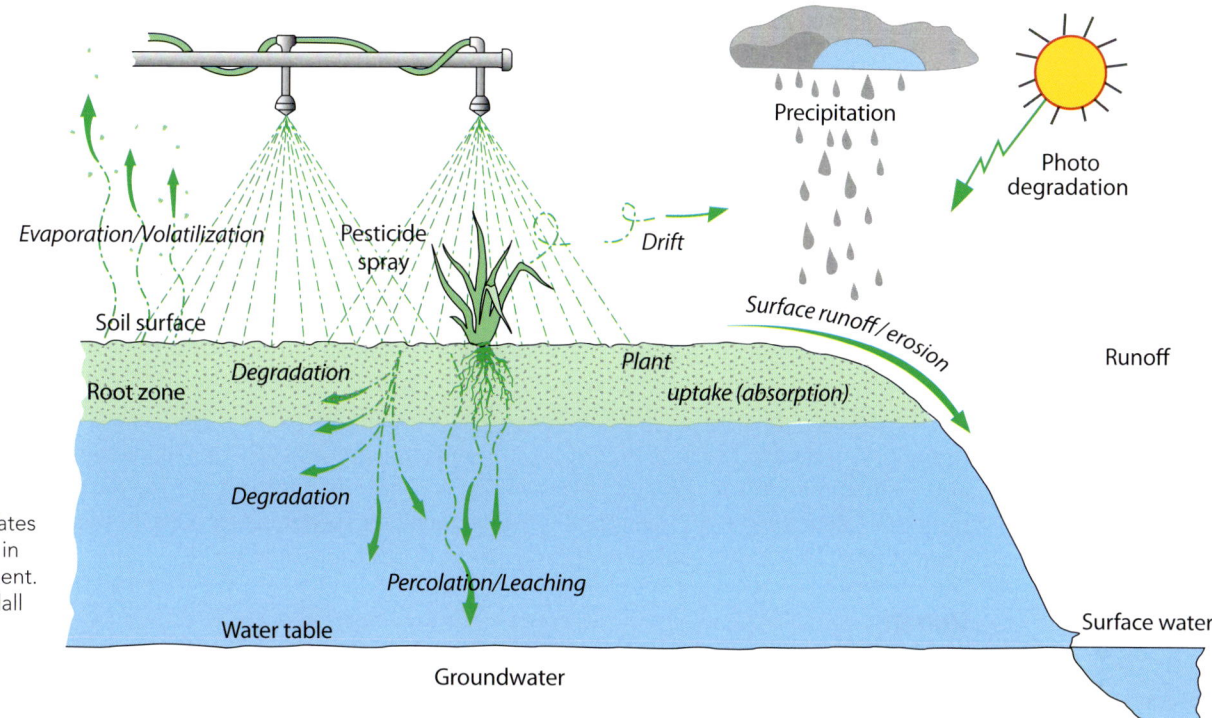

FIGURE 4-1
The various fates of pesticides in the environment. *Source:* Randall 2008.

SOLUBILITY

Solubility is a measure of the ability of a pesticide to dissolve in a solvent, usually water. Pesticides highly soluble in water dissolve easily. These pesticides are more likely to move with water in surface runoff or by movement through the soil water (leaching) than are less water-soluble pesticides, like those that dissolve in oil. For more information on the solubility of various formulations, see Chapter 3.

ADSORPTION

Adsorption is the process whereby a pesticide binds to soil particles. Adsorption occurs because of an attraction between the chemical and soil particles. Typically, oil-soluble pesticides are more attracted to clay particles and organic matter in soil than are water-soluble pesticides. Also, pesticide molecules with positive charges are more tightly adsorbed to negatively charged soil particles. A pesticide that adsorbs to soil particles is less likely to move from the spray site than a chemical that does not adsorb tightly to the soil.

PERSISTENCE

Persistence is the ability of a pesticide to remain present and active in its original form for an extended period before breaking down. A chemical's persistence is described in terms of its half-life, a comparative measure of the time needed for the chemical to break down—the longer the half-life, the more persistent the pesticide. For more on persistence and its benefits and drawbacks, see "Residues" later in this chapter.

VOLATILITY

Volatility is the tendency of a pesticide to turn into a gas or vapor. Some pesticides are more volatile than others. The chance of volatilization increases as temperatures and wind increase. Volatility is also more likely under conditions of low relative humidity (Randall et al. 2008). For more about the volatility of various pesticide formulations, see Chapter 3. For more about the hazards associated with volatility, see "Vapor Drift" in Chapter 10.

How Pesticides Move in the Environment

Pesticides that move away from the targeted application site, either indoors or outdoors, may immediately harm people and animals, damage objects, and cause environmental contamination. Pesticides move in several ways—in water, in air, attached to soil particles, and on or in objects. For techniques that help you reduce or avoid offsite movement of pesticides, see "Preventing Offsite Movement of Pesticides" in Chapter 10 and Randall et al. 2008.

List the types of offsite movement of pesticides.

MOVEMENT IN WATER

Pesticides can move into surface water or groundwater in the following ways:
- runoff (when rain or irrigation practices wash pesticides off treated surfaces)
- leaching (when rain or irrigation practices cause pesticides to move downward through soil)
- direct channels (when spillage/dumping occurs near or directly in a well)

In addition to these primary sources of surface water and groundwater contamination, drift can also result in the contamination of water sources. For more on how drift impacts the environment, see "Movement in Air" later in this chapter. Look for special instructions on the label that warn of pesticide hazards caused by the movement of pesticides in water.

Runoff

Runoff moves water from plant and soil surfaces into drainage systems, streams, ponds, or other surface water, where pesticides can be carried great distances (Fig. 4-2). Factors affecting runoff and erosion rates include slope, vegetative cover, soil characteristics, volume and rate of water moving downslope, temperature, and rainfall amount and intensity. These factors influence how much water runs off and how much moves into the soil (infiltration). Certain persistent pesticides bind to soil, which can then be washed away in water. In addition, a pesticide's solubility in water contributes to the contamination of surface water, as runoff can easily carry soluble pesticides away from the application site.

Describe factors that influence offsite movement of pesticides.

In an indoor environment, water contaminated with pesticides can flow into floor drains and contaminate water systems. A careless act such as dumping pesticide or rinsate down a sink or toilet can contaminate an entire sewage or water-treatment facility.

Surface water is a source of drinking water. Therefore, pesticide contamination of surface water (ditches, streams, rivers, ponds, and lakes) is a health concern. Pesticides that move in runoff water or with eroded sediment may contaminate and possibly harm plants and animals located downslope and may reach sources of surface water.

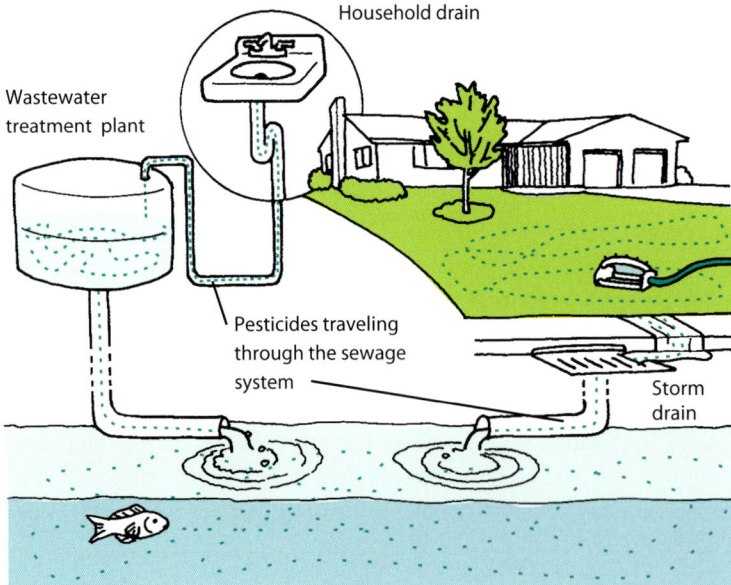

FIGURE 4-2

Irrigation or rain can wash pesticides applied on landscapes into storm drains that lead to creeks and rivers. Pesticides poured down indoor or outdoor drains also ultimately end up in surface water because water treatment plants cannot remove them.

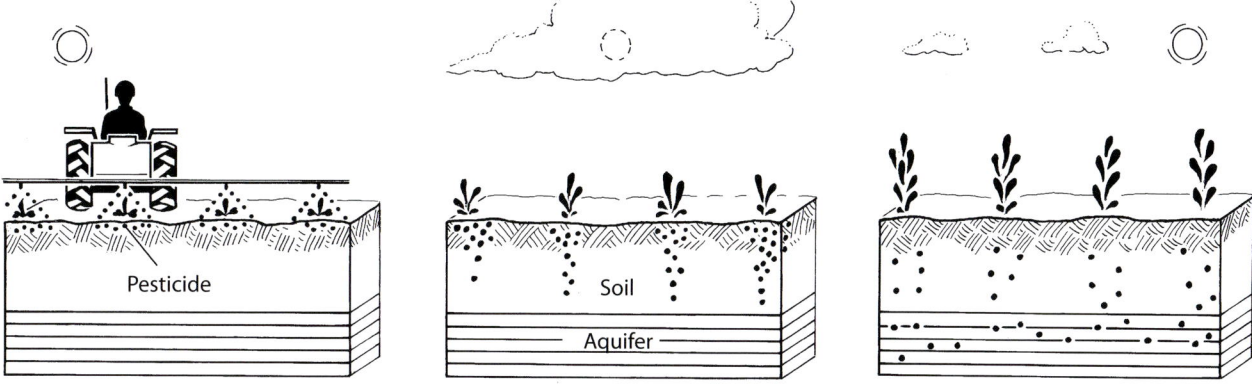

FIGURE 4-3

Water enters aquifers by percolation through the soil. As water passes down through the soil it may dissolve some pesticides and carry them into the aquifer. This process is called leaching.

Leaching

Some pesticides contaminate groundwater by moving through the soil in a process called leaching (Fig. 4-3). For a pesticide to leach into groundwater, it must move down through the soil in water and resist binding to soil particles and breaking down into nontoxic compounds. The movement of water down through the soil is sometimes referred to as percolation. A pesticide's chemical and physical characteristics (such as its persistence in soil) influence its ability to leach into groundwater. Persistent pesticides are likely to leach and contaminate groundwater. Pesticides having high solubility, low adsorption, or high persistence typically have a label statement informing the applicator of leaching concerns. A pesticide that adsorbs or binds itself strongly to soil particles will not leach as easily. In addition to the characteristics of the pesticide, soil properties and environmental conditions also affect the likelihood and extent that a pesticide will leach.

Some pesticides can leach in indoor environments. In a greenhouse, for example, pesticides may leach through the soil or other planting medium and contaminate other greenhouse surfaces.

Groundwater is a source of drinking water. Therefore, pesticide contamination of areas where groundwater accumulates (aquifers, as in Fig. 4-3) is a health concern. Pesticides that leach through soil may reach these underground sources of drinking water.

> List features of a given site, including soil type and geology, which influence the potential for a pesticide to reach surface water or groundwater.

Soil Properties

Four soil properties influence a pesticide's potential for leaching: texture and structure, organic matter, depth to groundwater, and geology.

Texture and Structure. Soil texture is how we describe the relative proportions of sand, silt, and clay-sized particles. Percolating water moves faster in sandy soils, and fewer binding sites are available for the adsorption of dissolved chemicals when compared with clay or silt soils. Though sandy soils are more prone to pesticide movement, leaching may also occur in clay or silt soils.

Soil structure is the shape or arrangement of soil particles—how they clump or bind together and form pores through which water moves. Small amounts of pesticide may also move through soil cracks, worm holes, and root channels, features referred to as macropores.

Organic Matter. Organic matter consists of decaying plant material. The higher the soil organic matter content, the greater the soil's ability to hold both water and adsorbed pesticides. Pesticides held in the root zone are less likely to leach into groundwater and may be taken up by plants.

Depth to Groundwater. Areas with a shallow water table have a greater chance for groundwater contamination because less soil is available to act as a filter, resulting in fewer opportunities for the pesticide to be degraded or adsorbed. When you must use pesticides in areas where the groundwater is close to the surface, select a pesticide with a low leaching potential and take extra precautions during mixing, application, and cleanup.

Geology. The permeability of the geologic layers lying between the surface of the soil and the groundwater is also an important factor. Highly permeable materials such as gravel deposits allow water and dissolved pesticides to move downward to groundwater freely. Layers of clay, which are much less permeable, can inhibit and slow the downward movement of water.

Direct Channels

Wells are direct channels into an aquifer—an area where groundwater accumulates—and may provide a connection between several such areas (Fig. 4-4). Careless or improper pesticide handling near wells has a high risk of contaminating groundwater. Examples include
- spilling pesticides near a well while filling a spray tank
- filling pesticide application equipment from a well without using backflow protection
- injecting pesticides into an irrigation system without using backflow protection
- disposing of surplus pesticides or washing contaminated equipment near a well

Improperly sealed, abandoned wells provide possible routes for pesticides and other contaminants into aquifers. Occasionally, pesticide waste or runoff may enter groundwater through direct channels such as sinkholes or exposed shallow aquifers.

MOVEMENT IN AIR

Pesticide movement away from the application site by wind or air currents is called drift. Outdoors, wind and temperature are easily felt by people applying pesticides, but applicators also experience drift situations indoors due to air currents created by ventilation systems and by forced-air heating and cooling systems. Pesticides may be carried away from a site in the air as spray droplets, vapors, or solid particles, even on blowing soil particles.

Factors that influence pesticide drift include spray droplet size, release height, wind direction and speed, temperature and humidity, potential for temperature inversions, and rain. For more information about factors that influence a pesticide's likelihood to drift, see "Spray Drift," below.

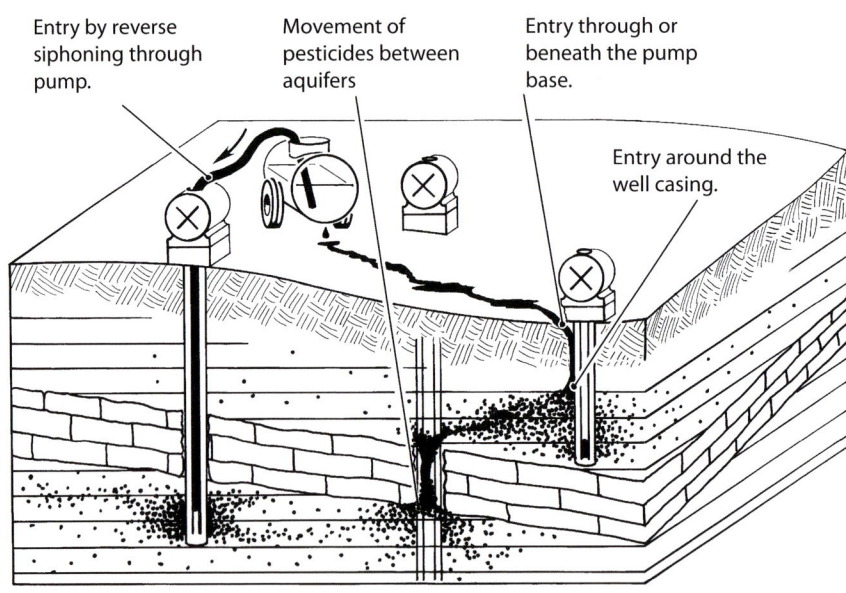

FIGURE 4-4

Water wells are direct channels into an aquifer and may provide connections between several aquifers. Pesticides and other contaminants can enter groundwater directly through wells.

Applicator Responsibility. The applicator is legally responsible for preventing drift. Applicators must assess the vulnerability of neighboring properties and areas downwind of the application site. Evaluate weather conditions for temperature inversions, wind direction, and wind speed before making the all-important decision about whether to spray. You may have to make adjustments to the application equipment to reduce spray drift. Consider using low-volatile formulations or adding a drift-control additive or thickener to help minimize drift. (For further discussion on equipment designed to minimize drift, see Chapter 8.) A good drift management program includes a combination of all drift-reducing techniques available for a particular application.

Applicators who apply pesticides indoors are also responsible for preventing drift. They must ensure pesticides do not move beyond the target site and that all people and animals are kept out of the treatment area according to label instructions. For more information on pesticide movement in air, see Randall et al. 2008.

Movement on or in Objects, Plants, or Animals

Pesticides can move away from the application site when they are on or in objects or organisms that move or are moved offsite. When pesticide handlers bring home or wear home contaminated personal protective equipment (PPE), work clothing, or other items, residues can rub off on carpeting, furniture, and laundry items, and onto pets and other people. For more information on residues, see "Residues" later in this chapter and Randall et al. 2008.

Sources of Pesticide Contamination

Pesticide contamination can come from several different sources, including drift, pollution, and residues. The following sections define each source of pesticide contamination and the factors that influence the potential of pesticides to contaminate the environment. For more information about the sources of pesticide contamination discussed below, see Randall et al. 2008.

DRIFT

Drift can be defined simply as the airborne movement of pesticides to nontarget areas. Off-target movement can be in the form of spray droplet drift, vapor drift, or particle (dust) drift. Significant drift can damage or contaminate sensitive crops, poison bees, pose health risks to humans and animals, and contaminate soil and water in adjacent areas. Applicators are legally responsible for the damages resulting from offsite movement of pesticides. You must make sure that no people or animals remain in the area where you are applying pesticides.

Spray Drift

Spray drift refers to the movement of a pesticide away from the treatment area in the air during a liquid application. Spray drift is the most frequent type of drift, because almost all spray applications result in some movement. Factors that influence or increase the likelihood of spray drift include
- spray droplet size
- release height
- formulation viscosity
- weather conditions

For methods used to avoid the conditions that contribute to spray drift, see "Preventing Pesticide Drift" in Chapter 10.

Spray Droplet Size

Spray droplet size is measured in microns and is controlled by a combination of sprayer pressure and nozzle size. Table 10-5 in chapter 10 shows standard droplet sizes and compares them to illustrate their capacity for drift. Fine droplets are able to drift farther than coarse droplets.

Release Height

Droplets that are released closer to their target are less likely to drift. You should carefully consider the distance between the spray nozzles and the target prior to any application to reduce drift potential.

Formulation Viscosity

The thickness, or viscosity, of the formulation you choose is a factor in spray drift. The more viscous the formulation, the less likely it is to move offsite. For example, an invert emulsion will drift less than a wettable powder.

Weather Conditions

Wind Speed, Humidity, and Temperature. Winds greater than 8 miles per hour can contribute to spray drift by blowing droplets away from the target site. However, some wind can help distribute spray more evenly across an application site, so not all wind conditions are to be avoided (see Chapter 7 for advice about safe wind conditions for pesticide applications). Conditions of low relative humidity, high temperatures, or both can also increase the potential for spray drift. During these times, evaporation rates rise, creating small droplets that drift more easily.

Temperature Inversions. Applications made under certain low-wind conditions can sometimes result in drift. Drift that occurs over long distances (over a mile) is most often the result of applications made under stable atmospheric conditions such as temperature inversions.

A temperature inversion exists when the air at ground level is cooler than the temperature of the air above it. Under these conditions, the air is considered stable because there is little or no vertical air movement. Almost all air movement associated with inversions is sideways (lateral), which results in a high concentration of small spray droplets suspended in the layer of cool air near the ground. These droplets can then be carried long distances, especially if wind speeds increase. When the spray droplets settle to the ground, they are still concentrated enough to cause potential damage or harm.

Inversions can occur at any time of the day and at any height above the ground, but they most often develop during the early evening hours as the ground temperature begins to cool and the warm air has already risen. They intensify during the night and may persist until midmorning, when the ground has warmed sufficiently to start the vertical mixing of air, causing a dilution and separation of suspended spray droplets. Consequently, applications made during early evening, night, or morning hours under what appear to be ideal conditions can result in highly damaging drift that can move long distances. This outcome is especially likely when humidity is high.

Vapor Drift

Vapor drift refers to the movement of pesticides as gaseous vapors from the target area. Some pesticides are volatile and can change readily from a solid or liquid form into a gas under the right conditions, especially when the air temperature is high and soil is dry and sandy. Pesticides that have volatilized may drift farther and for a longer time than they would have as spray droplets. Only those pesticides that are able to volatilize are susceptible to vapor drift. The likelihood that these pesticides will volatilize and drift increases as air temperatures increase.

Particle Drift (Dust Drift)

Particle drift refers to the movement of solid particles from the target area by air during or just after an application. These solid particles may include pesticides formulated as dusts or soil particles to which pesticides are attached. Some pesticides are persistent, remaining active on soil particles for long periods after they are applied. If particles are blown off the target area, contamination or damage to sensitive areas can occur.

Point Source, Nonpoint Source, and Direct Channel Pollution

> Distinguish between point sources and nonpoint sources of environmental contamination by pesticides.

Surface-water or groundwater contamination can result from point source, nonpoint source, or direct channel pollution (see Figs. 4-4 and 4-5). Nonpoint source pollution from pesticide applications has most commonly been blamed for pesticide contamination in the outdoor environment, but studies are revealing that water contamination also results from point source pollution. Point source pollution comes from a specific, identifiable place or location, such as

- a pesticide spill entering a storm sewer
- back-siphoning of pesticides
- contaminated surface water entering sinkholes
- repeated spilling of pesticides at mixing and loading sites
- careless spilling of wash water at equipment cleanup sites
- improper handling of spills and leaks at storage sites
- improper disposal of containers, rinsate from containers, and excess pesticides

Nonpoint source pollution comes from a widespread area. The movement of pesticides into streams or groundwater following a broadcast application to an agricultural field, large turf area, or right-of-way is an example of nonpoint source pollution. Indirect or nonpoint source contamination of groundwater can occur when contaminated surface streams interact with shallow groundwater through subsurface flow, such as tailwater entering a stream that disappears underground. Normally, surface water becomes contaminated when water runs off treated fields. Runoff risk is greatest when heavy rains immediately follow a pesticide application.

Direct channel pollution occurs when pesticides are handled, sprayed, or dumped near wells, sinkholes, or exposed shallow aquifers. Examples of direct channel contamination are provided in "Direct Channels" earlier in this chapter.

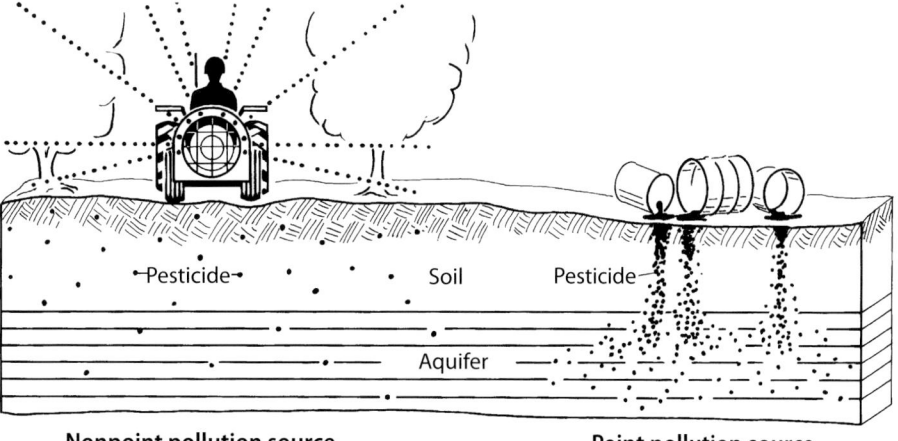

FIGURE 4-5

Point pollution sources are areas where large quantities of pesticide or other pollutants are discharged into one location. Nonpoint pollution sources arise from normal application of pesticide or other material over a large area.

Define pesticide residue, identify conditions that affect the buildup of residue, and explain how to avoid creating hazardous residues.

RESIDUES

Whenever you apply a pesticide, it remains as residue on treated surfaces for a time. The chemical nature of the pesticide or the persistence of the formulation affects the amount of residue. The frequency and amount of pesticide used (accumulation) also determine the amount of residue present. Finally, residues are subject to interaction with the environment (breakdown or recombination).

Residues are important and necessary because they provide the continuous exposure that improves the chances of controlling certain pests. However, residues are undesirable when they expose people, domestic animals, or wildlife to unsafe levels of pesticides. Pesticide materials that miss the treatment surface can remain as residues in soil, water, or on surfaces in nontarget areas. Also, empty pesticide containers hold small amounts of residues that require proper disposal to prevent environmental contamination (Fig. 4-6).

Pesticide Persistence

The amount of time from application until a pesticide breaks down is known as its persistence. Chlorinated hydrocarbon insecticides and certain classes of herbicides do not break down rapidly in the environment. These pesticides are considered highly persistent. Toxic effects against insects or weeds remain for as long as several years while the pesticide is present in the soil.

Pesticide persistence is a benefit in situations where you want or need long-term pest control. These situations include treating building foundations to prevent termite entry or treating soil for season-long weed control. A highly persistent material has some drawbacks, however, including
- increased chances of accidental poisoning
- increased restricted-entry intervals
- increased chances of offsite movement through runoff, leaching, human activities such as landscaping and construction, and wind and rain erosion

Plant-Back Restrictions. Persistence may, for a specified time, restrict the crops that a grower may plant in the treated area. Regulations establish plant-back restrictions, also called rotational crop restrictions, to prevent injury or residues in subsequent crops. When plant-back restrictions apply, the pesticide label specifies which crops a grower can or cannot plant. It also states how long after application a grower must wait before planting other types of crops. Plant-back restrictions are another important reason for keeping accurate pesticide application records.

FIGURE 4-6

Pesticide wastes include partially full containers of pesticide that have not been used, leftover mixtures in spray tanks, rinse water from pesticide containers, rinse water from inside and outside of spray equipment, and, as shown here, empty pesticide containers.

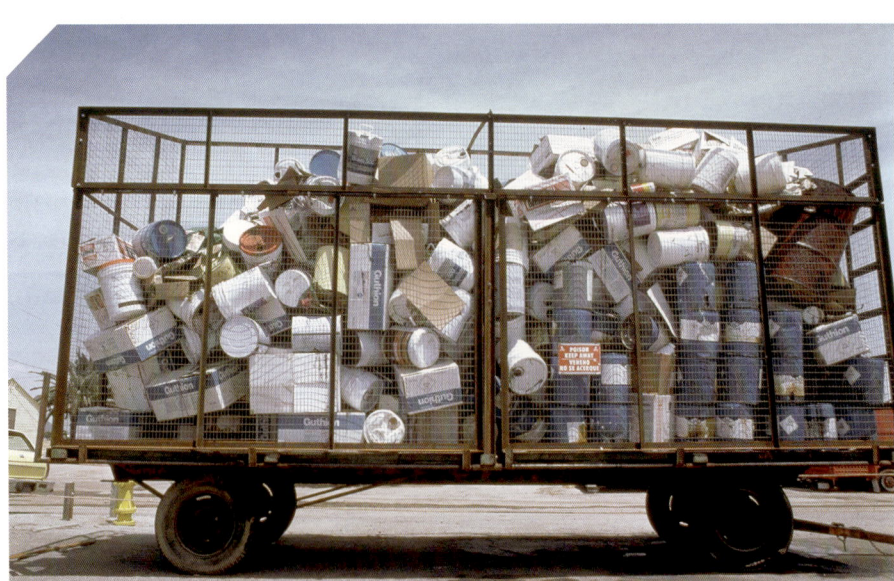

Accumulation

Accumulation is the buildup of a persistent pesticide resulting from repeated applications or exposures. Accumulation may occur in the soil, in groundwater, in plant and animal tissues (called bioaccumulation, which is covered in "Impact on Nontarget Organisms" later in this chapter), or in ponds and lakes. An example of pesticide accumulation is illustrated by copper compounds used as fungicides. These pesticides have been used for over 100 years in deciduous fruit and nut orchards. Because copper degrades very slowly, constant use over time means it accumulates in the soil. In some areas the concentration of copper in the soil has become toxic to organisms living or growing there.

Breakdown and Recombination

Special hazards may exist when pesticides break down in the environment. Some break down into different toxic compounds before breaking down further. Others fail to break down properly due to unusual environmental conditions. Occasionally some pesticides recombine with other chemicals in the environment and produce unforeseen compounds. Each location in the environment has unique characteristics that may influence the way chemicals break down. These factors also influence how they react with target and nontarget organisms.

Several variables influence chemical breakdown and recombination. These include
- soil type and moisture
- soil organic matter content
- airflow, temperature, sunlight, and rainfall
- the presence of plants and animals

For example, soil texture and organic matter content influence the activity and breakdown of some herbicides. Application rates, therefore, must be adjusted to correspond to the type and organic matter content of soil where you will apply these herbicides. In addition, microbes in the soil can hasten breakdown of pesticides, so you must know not only the soil type but also exactly what lives in the soil where pesticides are applied.

Weather also affects the breakdown and recombination of pesticides. Sunlight and heat, for example, contribute to the degradation of some pesticides but can increase their toxicity when chemicals break down and react with other substances in the environment.

Avoiding Hazardous Residues

Reduce chances of creating hazardous pesticide residues by taking the following steps.
- Comply with label restrictions on timing, placement, and rate of application, using the lowest effective rate whenever possible.
- Perform compatibility tests before tank-mixing two or more pesticides.
- Apply pesticides during dormant or fallow periods to prevent spraying edible produce whenever possible.
- Avoid pesticide spills.
- Fill application equipment in ways that prevent pesticide mixtures from siphoning back into wells.
- Calibrate application equipment properly and make an accurate measurement of the area you plan to spray.
- Select pesticides that break down rapidly when possible and use formulations that reduce the likelihood of drift.

For outdoor applications, reduce pesticide residues in the environment by using cultural practices such as managing soil and water movement. Control the amount and timing of irrigation water to eliminate runoff and slow the rate of percolation. In agriculture, reduce soil erosion by using practices such as reduced tillage, contour farming, terracing, grass-lined waterways, and subsurface drainage. Collect and reuse tailwater (the water that runs off the low end of a field) from irrigated fields to keep residues within the treatment site.

Environmental Impacts of Pesticide Application

Some types of pesticide you use may be harmful to nontarget organisms at the application site and in the surrounding environment, including nearby sensitive areas such as rivers, lakes, and aquifers. Before making a pesticide application, become familiar with the treatment area and its surroundings. Avoid using pesticides that disrupt natural enemies and other beneficial organisms, are likely to make their way into freshwater supplies, or harm wildlife or nontarget plants.

Remember that the result of unintended pesticide exposure is not always immediately apparent. Long-term consequences of offsite movement may include accumulation of pesticides in animals and soil, problems with wildlife breeding and offspring, and the development of diseases in otherwise healthy organisms long after the initial exposure.

The following sections discuss the effects of pesticides on surface water and groundwater; nontarget plants; bees and other beneficial insects; and fish, wildlife, and livestock.

IMPACT ON WATER SUPPLIES AND SENSITIVE AREAS

Groundwater. Potential contamination of groundwater with pesticides is a serious concern. About 97% of the total water in the world is salt water in the oceans. This water is unsuitable for most uses. Less than 1% of all the water on the planet is freshwater in an available form. People use this water for drinking, irrigation, and household and manufacturing purposes. Two-thirds of the freshwater (or about 2 million cubic miles) is groundwater trapped beneath the soil. The rest is surface water in lakes, ponds, streams, and rivers. Frozen water in polar ice caps and glaciers is also freshwater, but it is unavailable for use. Groundwater provides 40% of California's water needs. Cities obtain almost half of their water, including drinking water, from these groundwater sources. Most of the water used in rural areas is groundwater. Groundwater, therefore, is our most important freshwater source.

Researchers and regulators recognize that the potential for groundwater contamination from pesticides is very great. In the past, people thought pesticides did not threaten groundwater. However, this was only because available testing techniques were unable to detect contamination. At the time, studies suggested that microorganisms, environmental factors, and soil degraded or adsorbed most pesticides before they reached groundwater. Researchers suspected that the pesticides that did enter groundwater decomposed rapidly. More recently, however, newer detection methods have proved earlier assumptions to be inaccurate. The new equipment shows that small amounts of chemicals, including certain pesticides, exist in some groundwater locations. Environmental monitoring reports have prompted lawmakers to develop stringent laws to protect this resource. These laws regulate pesticide use and disposal.

Groundwater in California is especially vulnerable to contamination because it is directly below so much cultivated, industrial, and residential land. Contamination, when it occurs, may be difficult or impossible to contain. Because the water flows so slowly, it takes hundreds of years to remove contaminants from groundwater.

Surface Water. Surface water (ditches, streams, rivers, ponds, and lakes) is also an important source of drinking water. Therefore, pesticide contamination of surface water is a health concern. Pesticides that move in runoff water or with eroded sediment may reach sources of surface water, creating a health hazard for people and wildlife in the area.

Factors affecting runoff and erosion rates include slope, vegetative cover, soil characteristics, volume and rate of water moving downslope, temperature, and rainfall amount and intensity. For instance, runoff is much less likely to occur in sandy soils, where infiltration happens more readily than in clay soils.

Sensitive Areas. In addition to water sources, sensitive areas include sites where living things could easily be injured by a pesticide. Outdoor sensitive areas include

- schools, playgrounds, recreational areas, hospitals, and similar institutions

- habitats of endangered species
- apiaries and honey bee habitat, wildlife refuges, and parks
- areas where domestic animals and livestock are kept
- ornamental plantings, public gardens, and sensitive food or feed crops

Sensitive areas indoors include places where
- people live, work, shop, or are cared for
- food or feed is processed, prepared, stored, or served
- domestic or confined animals live, eat, or are otherwise cared for
- ornamental or other sensitive plants are grown or maintained, such as in malls and buildings

Sometimes, pesticides must be deliberately applied to a sensitive area to control a pest. Only applicators who are competent in handling pesticides should perform these applications. At other times, the sensitive area may be part of a larger target site. Whenever possible, take special precautions to avoid application to the sensitive area. Leaving an untreated buffer zone around a sensitive area is a practical way to avoid contaminating it.

In still other instances, the sensitive area may be near a site used for pesticide mixing and loading, storage, disposal, or equipment washing. You must take precautions to avoid accidental contamination of the sensitive area. Check the label for statements that alert you to special restrictions around sensitive areas. For more information on impacts on water supplies and sensitive areas, see Randall et al. 2008.

IMPACT ON NONTARGET ORGANISMS

Describe ways that pesticides can impact nontarget organisms.

Pesticides may affect nontarget organisms directly, causing immediate injury, as happens when broad-spectrum (nonselective) pesticides are applied in areas where natural enemies also live. When a pesticide is nonselective, it will kill the pest as well as many of the pest's natural enemies. Sometimes when you apply a more selective chemical, your application may still affect natural enemies by destroying the pest they depend on for food. After natural enemies die off or leave because of the lack of prey, they often require more time than the pest to increase their population size. Because the area lacks natural enemies that normally keep the pests in check, pest populations can grow rapidly and sometimes become bigger than before the pesticide treatment. This phenomenon is known as pest resurgence.

Another problem associated with pesticide use is that of secondary pest outbreak. Secondary pests are normally controlled by natural enemies or competition from the primary pest. Eliminating natural enemies or primary pests often results in an increase in secondary pest populations that can cause economic damage. For more on pest resurgence and secondary pest outbreaks, see Chapter 1.

Pesticides can also produce long-term damage in nontarget species through environmental pollution, as when pesticides accumulate in the bodies of animals or in the soil. For instance, if you use the same mixing and loading site or equipment cleaning site over a long period, pesticides are likely to accumulate in the soil. Harmful accumulation can also occur if you apply the same pesticide to the same location over and over again. When this occurs, plants and animals that come into contact with the soil may be harmed.

Bees and Other Beneficial Insects

Bees are an important part of our ecosystem, pollinating many fruit, seed, vegetable, and field crops. Without pollinators, many of the plant species we rely on for food and pleasure would die out. Other beneficial insects keep destructive pest populations in check and are needed to provide the balanced environment necessary for the production of food, the enjoyment of recreational areas, and plant health in suburban and urban areas. Many studies have shown a link between pesticides and harmful effects on beneficial insects, such as colony collapse disorder (CCD) in honey bees, even well after an application is complete. Generally, dusts, powders, and microencapsulated pesticide formulations are the most harmful to honey bees, and aerial spraying is the most hazardous method of application. Liquid solutions and granules are the least detrimental to pollinators. California regulations require that all pesticides sold in the state be tested for their toxic effects on honey bees, so check the label to ensure that you are using the pesticide in a way that minimizes harm to these important pollinators (Sidebar 4-1). See Chapter 10 for more information about how to protect pollinators and other beneficial insects during and after pesticide applications. The University of California IPM website, ipm.ucanr.edu, provides toxicity tables (see Table 4-1 for a sample) that indicate pesticides' effects on honey bees and other beneficial insects. Also, check the U.S. EPA website, epa.gov/pesticides/ecosystem/pollinator, for the most updated information on CCD and other effects of pesticides on beneficial insects.

SIDEBAR 4-1

SAMPLE U.S. EPA BEE LABEL, "PROTECTION OF POLLINATORS"

PROTECTION OF POLLINATORS

APPLICATION RESTRICTIONS EXIST FOR THIS PRODUCT BECAUSE OF RISK TO BEES AND OTHER INSECT POLLINATORS. FOLLOW APPLICATION RESTRICTIONS FOUND IN THE DIRECTIONS FOR USE TO PROTECT POLLINATORS.

Look for the bee hazard icon in the Directions for Use for each application site for specific use restrictions and instructions to protect bees and other insect pollinators.

This product can kill bees and other insect pollinators.
Bees and other insect pollinators will forage on plants when they flower, shed pollen, or produce nectar.

Bees and other insect pollinators can be exposed to this pesticide from:

- Direct contact during foliar applications, or contact with residues on plant surfaces after foliar applications
- Ingestion of residues in nectar and pollen when the pesticide is applied as a seed treatment, soil, tree injection, as well as foliar applications.

When Using This Product Take Steps To:

- Minimize exposure of this product to bees and other insect pollinators when they are foraging on pollinator attractive plants around the application site.
- Minimize drift of this product on to beehives or to off-site pollinator attractive habitat. Drift of this product onto beehives or off-site to pollinator attractive habitat can result in bee kills.

Information on protecting bees and other insect pollinators may be found at the Pesticide Environmental Stewardship website at:
http://pesticidestewardship.org/PollinatorProtection/Pages/default.aspx.

Pesticide incidents (for example, bee kills) should immediately be reported to the state/tribal lead agency. For contact information for your state, go to: www.aapco.org/officials.html. Pesticide incidents should also be reported to the National Pesticide Information Center at: www.npic.orst.edu or directly to EPA at: beekill@epa.gov

TABLE 4-1

Relative toxicities of insecticides and miticides used in alfalfa to natural enemies and honey bees

Common name (trade name)*	Mode of action[1]	Selectivity[2] (affected groups)	Predatory mites[3]	General predators[4]	Parasites[4]	Honey bees[5]	Duration of impact to natural enemies[6]
Bacillus thuringiensis ssp. *aizawai*	11.B1	narrow (caterpillars)	L	L	L	IV	short
Bacillus thuringiensis ssp. *kurstaki*	11.B2	narrow (caterpillars)	L	L	L	IV	short
carbaryl (Sevin)	1A	broad (insects, mites)	L/H	H	H	I	long
chlorantraniliprole (Coragen)	28	narrow (primarily caterpillars)	L	L	L/M	IV	short
chlorpyrifos (Lorsban)	1B	broad (insects, mites)	M	H	H	I	moderate
cyfluthrin (Baythroid)	3	broad (insects, mites)	H	H	H	I	moderate
dimethoate	1B	broad (insects, mites)	H	H	H	I	long
flubendiamide (Belt)	28	—	L	L	L/M	I	short
indoxacarb (Steward)	22A	narrow (caterpillars, lygus)	—	L	L	I	moderate
lambda-cyhalothrin (Warrior)	3	broad (plant bugs, beetles, caterpillars)	H	H	H	I	moderate
malathion	1B	broad (insects, mites)	H	H	H	II	moderate
methomyl (Lannate)	1A	broad (insects, mites)	H	H	H	III	moderate
methoxyfenozide (Intrepid)	18	narrow (caterpillars)	L	L	L	IV	short
neem oil (Trilogy)	—	broad (soft-bodied insects)	L	L	L	III	short
permethrin (Pounce, Ambush)	3	broad (insects, mites)	L	H	H	I	long
phosmet (Imidan)	1B	broad (insects, mites)	H	H	H	I	moderate to long
zeta-cypermethrin (Mustang)	3	broad (insects, mites)	H	M	M	I	moderate

Key:
H = high
M = moderate
L = low
— = no information

*Note: *Some a.i.'s or products listed may not be currently registered as pesticides or may have had their registration cancelled.*

1. Rotate chemicals with a different mode of action group number, and do not use products with the same mode of action group number more than twice per season to help prevent development of resistance. For example, the organophosphates have a group number of 1B; chemicals with a 1B group number should be alternated with chemicals that have a group number other than 1B. Group numbers are assigned by IRAC (Insecticide Resistance Action Committee). For more information, see their website, irac-online.org.

2. Broad: material affects most groups of insects and mites; narrow: material affects only a few specific groups.

3. Generally, toxicities are to western predatory mite (*Galendromus occidentalis*). Where differences have been measured in toxicity of the pesticide-resistant strain versus the native strain, these are listed as pesticide-resistant strain/native strain.

4. Toxicities are averages of reported effects and should be used only as a general guide. Actual toxicity of a specific chemical depends on the species of predator or parasite, environmental conditions, and application rate.

5. Ratings are as follows: I = do not apply to blooming plants; II = apply only during late evening; III = apply only during late evening, night, or early morning; and IV = apply at any time with reasonable safety to bees. For more information, see Hooven et al. 2013.

6. Short: hours to days; moderate: days to 2 weeks; long: many weeks or months.

Fish, Wildlife, and Livestock

Pesticides can be harmful to all kinds of animals. Most injuries occur from the direct effects of acute poisoning, but pesticides can also cause indirect harm by altering animals' food sources or habitats. Vertebrates, including birds, often feed or nest in areas where people apply pesticides. Sometimes animals are the unintended victims of baits used to control target pests. In addition, pesticides present in flooded fields or irrigation water may poison waterfowl. Although a pesticide dose may not directly cause death, its effect might weaken a nontarget animal enough so that it cannot get sufficient food or water or protect itself from natural enemies. Some pesticides may have an impact on the ability of wildlife to reproduce.

Bird kills resulting from pesticide exposure can occur in a number of ways. Birds may ingest pesticide granules, baits, or treated seeds; they may be exposed directly to sprays; they may consume treated crops or drink contaminated water; or they may feed on pesticide-contaminated insects and other prey.

It may be several years after a problem arises before a cause and solution can be identified. For example, dormant sprays of the organophosphate parathion were commonly applied in California orchards in the 1980s. Early reports from the Department of Fish and Game suggested these sprays might have adverse effects on raptors. After several years of research, these suspicions were confirmed, and mortality of hawks was directly related to dormant applications of parathion in 1989. Hawks absorbed the pesticide through their feet when landing on treated trees. These findings led to regulatory changes and changes in pest management practices. Use of reduced rates and alternate materials in the 1990s solved the problem.

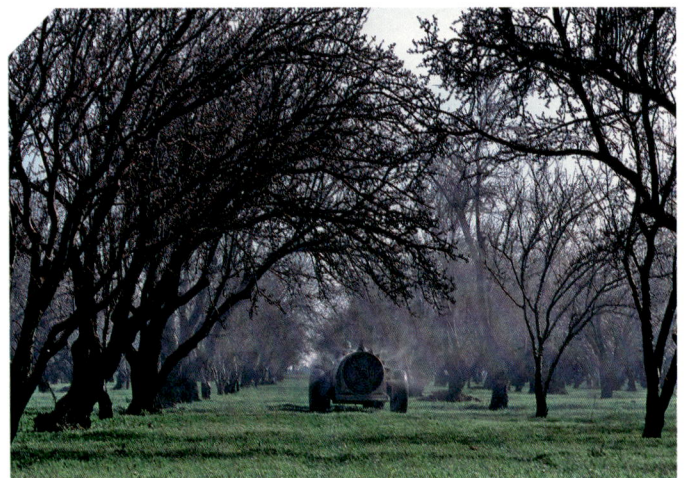

Runoff from pesticide applications into nearby ponds, streams, and lakes can harm aquatic animals and plants. For example, dormant spray applications of certain organophosphate or pyrethroid insecticides are typically made to stone fruit orchards during January and February, often the wettest time of the year. When it rains soon after an application, higher concentrations of organophosphate insecticides have been detected in storm drains, rivers, and other waterways. Finding more of these insecticides in waterways is a concern because of potential toxicity to some aquatic organisms at relatively low concentrations. From 1992 to 1995, the U.S. Geological Survey found that concentrations of diazinon in the Merced, Tuolumne, and San Joaquin Rivers frequently exceeded levels that are toxic to

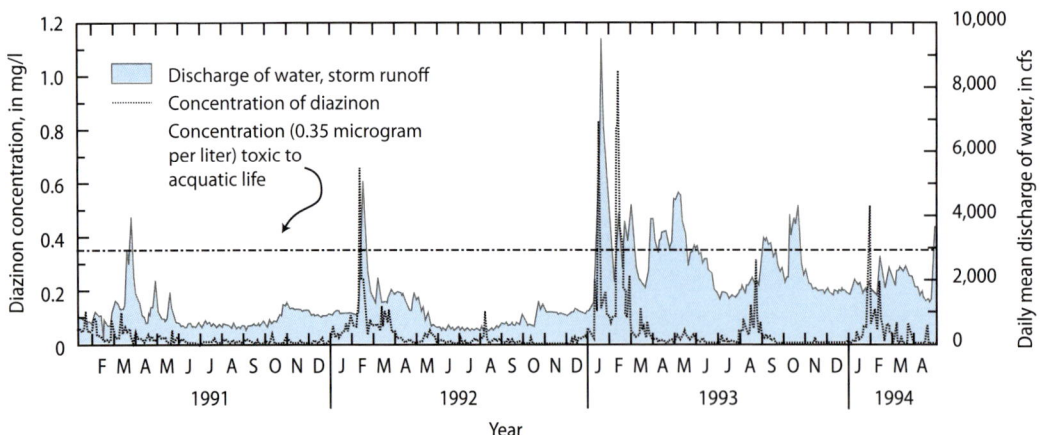

FIGURE 4-7

Applications of pesticides during the dormant spray season may run off the orchard floor into creeks and rivers, resulting in toxicity to aquatic invertebrates. This graph shows total discharge of water into the San Joaquin River and concentrations of diazinon measured near Vernalis in the years 1991 to 1994. *Source:* Dubrovsky et al. 1998.

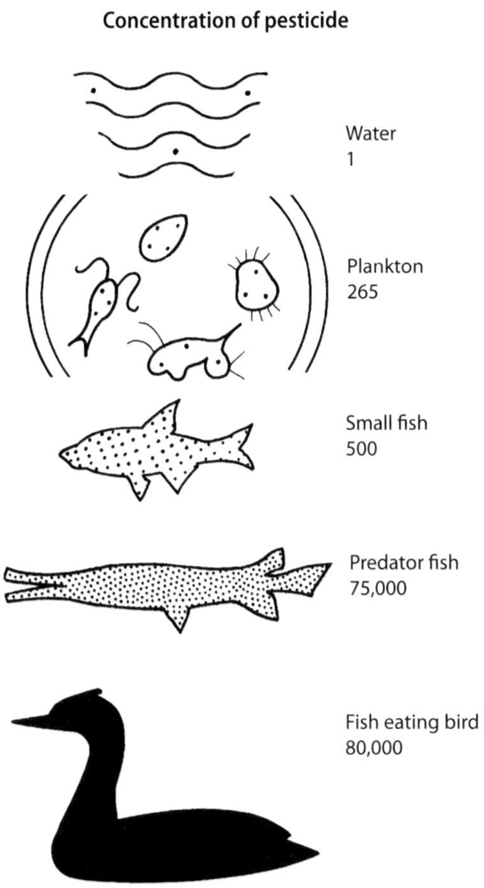

aquatic life after winter storms (Fig. 4-7). People reduced pesticide runoff in orchards in the 2000s by treating later in the year and/or switching to sprays of reduced-risk materials (*Bacillus thuringiensis* or spinosad) that do not run off into water or pose threats to aquatic invertebrates. Pesticide runoff continues to be a threat to aquatic wildlife, however, especially when people apply pesticides indiscriminately in urban areas.

Pesticide applications can destroy habitat and food sources on which nontarget organisms depend. For example, the use of herbicides to keep soil vegetation-free has in some cases resulted in soil eroding into creeks and rivers. Herbicides can also reduce plant diversity and remove food and shelter necessary for the survival of some wildlife. Preserving wildlife habitat should be a consideration whenever pesticides are used.

Applications of persistent pesticides can also lead to secondary poisoning of nontarget organisms. This phenomenon, called bioaccumulation (Fig. 4-8), occurs when certain pesticides gradually build up within the tissues of living organisms after feeding on other organisms (pest or nontarget) that have eaten or absorbed smaller amounts of these pesticides. Animals higher up on the food chain accumulate greater amounts of these pesticides in their tissues as time passes. Although this phenomenon is mostly associated with long-banned organochlorine insecticides, recent studies show that DDT, toxaphene, and chlordane continue to accumulate and build up in tissues of clams, fish, and other aquatic organisms. These sediment-bound organochlorine insecticides continue to arrive in rivers through soil erosion. Secondary kill may also occur when carnivores feed on dead or dying rodents that have consumed rodenticide baits.

Livestock can also be poisoned by pesticides, most commonly by eating contaminated feed and forage and by drinking contaminated water. Contamination can occur as a result of improper or careless transportation, storage, handling, application, or disposal of pesticides.

Endangered Species. An endangered species is on the brink of extinction throughout all or a significant portion of its range. A threatened species is likely to become endangered in the foreseeable future. The reasons for a species' decline are usually complex, and thus recovery is difficult. A major problem for most wildlife is the destruction of habitat, usually the result of industrial, agricultural, residential, or recreational development. Make every effort to avoid causing harm to threatened and endangered populations. Because all living things are part of a complex, delicately balanced network, the removal of a single species can set off a chain reaction that affects many others. The full significance of an extinction is not always readily apparent, and the long-term effects are often difficult to predict.

Each state is responsible for implementing the federal Endangered Species Protection Program in cooperation with the U.S. EPA to protect endangered and threatened species from the harmful effects of pesticides. Under this program, pesticide products that might adversely affect an endangered species carry a label statement instructing applicators to consult a county bulletin to determine whether they must take any special precautionary measures when using the product. The U.S. EPA develops these bulletins, which identify precautionary measures required in each county where one or more pesticides could affect an endangered or

Concentration of pesticide

Water — 1
Plankton — 265
Small fish — 500
Predator fish — 75,000
Fish eating bird — 80,000

FIGURE 4-8

Bioaccumulation is the way pesticides are accumulated through the biological food chain. Microorganisms and algae containing pesticides are eaten by small invertebrates and hatching fish, and larger fish and birds eat these organisms in turn. Each passes greater amounts of pesticide to the larger animal.

threatened species. Precautionary measures may include buffer strips, reduced application rates or timing restrictions, or a prohibition against using the pesticide within the identified habitat.

Enforcement agencies restrict the use of certain pesticides in areas where endangered species exist. For further information, consult your local University of California Cooperative Extension office. Farm advisors in these offices can also provide you with information on nonchemical pest control methods and information on how to integrate these into existing pest management plans. Try implementing an IPM program that emphasizes nonchemical control in areas where endangered species live. For more information on how to create an IPM program, see Chapters 1 and 10.

For information on endangered species laws and ways to protect these plants or animals, check with the U.S. EPA Endangered Species Protection Program, the local or regional office of the California Department of Fish and Wildlife, or DPR's online resources at cdpr.ca.gov/docs/endspec/index.htm, including the PRESCRIBE database at cdpr.ca.gov/docs/endspec/prescint.htm.

Nontarget Plants

Pest managers use herbicides to control weeds and undesirable plants in forests, along roadsides, and on rangelands. However, some of these herbicides may have detrimental effects on nontarget plants. These chemicals are phytotoxic, meaning they cause damage to whatever part of a plant they touch. Many plant species are important in natural and undeveloped areas. They protect the watershed, reduce erosion, provide food and shelter for wildlife (including bees), and are part of the native flora. Plants in natural areas are usually part of an ecological balance. Disrupting this balance in any way favors the increase of undesirable plants or plants having minimal benefit.

Phytotoxicity. Phytotoxicity is the toxic effect of a pesticide on a plant. It can be caused by any pesticide, even when that pesticide is applied as directed. Phytotoxicity can occur on any part of a plant—roots, stems, leaves, flowers, or fruits—and is especially problematic when pesticides are applied at too high a rate. The pesticide active ingredient is not always what causes phytotoxicity. It may result from solvents in the formulation or impurities (such as salts) in the water mixed with the pesticide. Excessive application rates, inadequate mixing, or improper pesticide dilution can contribute to phytotoxicity. Environmental conditions, such as temperature and humidity at the time of application, can also influence phytotoxicity. Plants stressed for water or nutrients may be more susceptible to injury from pesticide applications. Phytotoxic effects of pesticides on nontarget plants can also result from offsite movement via drift or runoff. For more about offsite movement of pesticides, see "How Pesticides Move in the Environment" in this chapter. For more information on the impacts of pesticides on nontarget organisms, see Randall et al. 2008.

Damage to Treated Surfaces

Pesticides may sometimes spot or damage treated surfaces or surfaces exposed to pesticide drift. The pesticide, solvents, or salts in the water used with the spray mixture may be responsible for this damage. Application rates and the concentration of the spray mixture can influence spotting, pitting, or staining. Follow label instructions for mixing and application. When in doubt, apply a small amount to a test area to be sure no damage occurs.

Chapter 4 Review Questions

1. True or false?
   - ☐ a. Groundwater contamination is a problem when using persistent pesticides.
   - ☐ b. Pesticides that drift from the target site can cause injury to nontarget organisms.
   - ☐ c. Applying pesticides to an unfamiliar site can result in contamination of nearby sensitive areas.
   - ☐ d. Point source pollution comes from pesticides that have been spilled over a wide area.
   - ☐ e. Nonpoint source pollution comes from pesticides that move into streams or groundwater following a broadcast application to a large area.
   - ☐ f. Direct channel pollution can come from washing equipment and dumping the rinse water close to a well.

2. Match the term with its definition.

1. solubility	a. The ability of a pesticide to remain present and active in its original form for an extended period before breaking down.
2. adsorption	b. The tendency of a pesticide to turn into a gas or vapor.
3. persistence	c. A measure of the ability of a pesticide to dissolve in a solvent.
4. volatility	d. The process whereby a pesticide binds to soil particles.

3. Match the type of offsite movement with its main cause.

1. spray drift	a. Volatile pesticides applied when air temperatures are high and soil is dry and sandy.
2. vapor drift	b. Soluble pesticides applied just before a heavy rain.
3. particle drift	c. Persistent pesticides applied to the soil.
4. runoff	d. Pesticides applied as small droplets when nozzles are too far from the target.
5. leaching	e. Dust formulations applied just before or during windy conditions.

4. Under what soil conditions are pesticides more likely to leach through soil?
   - ☐ a. a heavy clay soil, low in organic matter, where groundwater is shallow
   - ☐ b. a heavy clay soil, high in organic matter, where groundwater is deep
   - ☐ c. a sandy soil, low in organic matter, where groundwater is shallow

5. Which of the following may produce a pesticide residue on a crop that exceeds legal tolerances?
   - ☐ a. avoiding applications close to or during harvest times
   - ☐ b. allowing pesticide residue to drift onto the crop from a nearby area
   - ☐ c. using the lowest effective rate of pesticide active ingredient

6. **What is the definition of pesticide residue?**
   - ☐ a. what remains on treated surfaces for a time after application
   - ☐ b. the unsightly and unnecessary by-product of a pesticide application
   - ☐ c. how a pesticide kills the target pests upon application

7. **Which of the following conditions can contribute to the buildup of pesticide residues?**
   - ☐ a. misinterpreting the weather forecast and making your application just before a heavy rain
   - ☐ b. agitating a pesticide mixture too much before and during your application
   - ☐ c. failing to account for organic matter content of soil before determining the correct application rate

8. **What practice can cause pesticide residues to accumulate in an area?**
   - ☐ a. applying pesticides over a large application site
   - ☐ b. applying the same pesticide for many years to the same site
   - ☐ c. applying several different pesticides in a short time to the soil

9. **Which of the following site characteristics makes it more likely that a pesticide will contaminate groundwater?**
   - ☐ a. Geological layers at the site are made up of permeable gravel deposits.
   - ☐ b. Aquifers are located several miles away from the application site.
   - ☐ c. Groundwater is far from the surface under many layers of thick clay.

10. **Pesticides can cause indirect harm to nontarget organisms by _____.**
    - ☐ a. leaving unsightly residues on surfaces
    - ☐ b. altering their food sources or habitats
    - ☐ c. increasing secondary pest infestations

Chapter 5
Human Hazards Associated with Pesticide Use

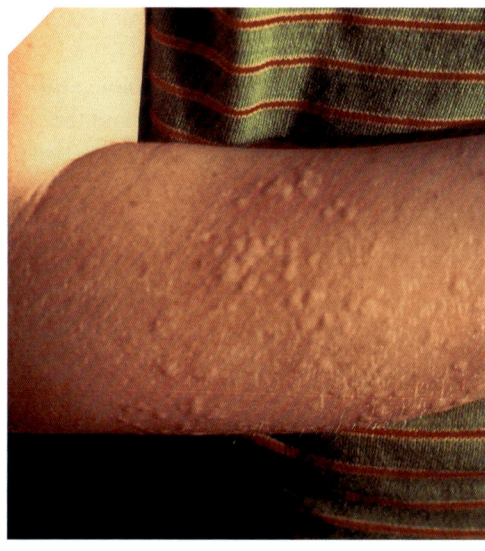

Potential for Human Injury 120
Other Effects on People 127
Pesticide Toxicity and Health Concerns 128
Delayed Effects 129
Chapter 5 Review Questions 129

Knowledge Expectations

- Describe the ways people get exposed to pesticides and the routes of entry.
- List the tasks most often associated with accidental pesticide exposure and explain why these tasks are hazardous.
- Name conditions at the application site that may change and influence the hazards associated with pesticide application.
- Describe how offsite movement of pesticides endangers human health.
- Explain how each of the following can contribute to human hazards associated with pesticide use:
    - a. incorrect dosage
    - b. incorrect application timing
    - c. incorrect pesticide product application
- Explain the human hazards associated with pesticides.
- Describe the potential effects on people of acute and chronic pesticide exposure.
- Define heat stress and describe how people develop heat stress.

Potential for Human Injury

Pesticides, like other poisonous chemicals, injure people by interfering with biological functions. The nature and extent of injury depend on the pesticide's toxicity and the amount entering the tissues. Some pesticides are very toxic and produce injury at low doses. A few drops of these might cause severe illness or death. Other pesticides are so mildly toxic that a person would have to consume several pounds before experiencing any effect.

However, because potential hazards exist with all pesticides, anyone working with these chemicals must avoid exposure. Treat all pesticides with respect. It is impossible to accurately predict what effects can result from long-term repeated exposures to even the least-toxic pesticides.

Pesticide poisoning symptoms can vary widely. If you suspect you have been exposed to pesticides, seek medical attention and be prepared to describe the pesticide and how you might have been exposed to it.

HOW PEOPLE GET EXPOSED TO PESTICIDES

People can come in contact with pesticides in several ways. However, the most serious exposure incidents occur when pesticide containers are mishandled during the transportation and storing of pesticides. Mixing and application are also frequent causes of injury due to pesticide overexposure. To greatly reduce exposure risks, secure pesticides correctly for transport, store pesticides in proper containers and in properly equipped facilities, wear proper work clothing, and use required personal protective equipment (PPE) during all handling tasks. In addition, following label requirements for restricted-entry and preharvest intervals, as well as guidelines for cleaning and storing PPE, protects workers and consumers.

Poisoning symptoms or injuries can result from a single exposure to a large quantity of pesticide. In other cases, illness might occur after exposure to repeated small doses over time. For example, about 12% of reported pesticide exposures involve children who were exposed to a single pesticide during a drift incident. About half the incidents occurred in industries that do not manufacture, sell, or transport pesticides and may have involved exposure to multiple pesticides at low doses over time.

It is common for individuals to vary in their sensitivity to the level of pesticide exposure. Some people show no reaction to a dose that might cause severe illness in others. A person's age and body size often influence his or her response to a given dose. Thus, smaller doses often have more impact on infants and young children than they do on adults. Also, adult females can be more sensitive to lower doses than adult males.

Describe the ways people get exposed to pesticides and the routes of entry.

List the tasks most often associated with accidental pesticide exposure and explain why these tasks are hazardous.

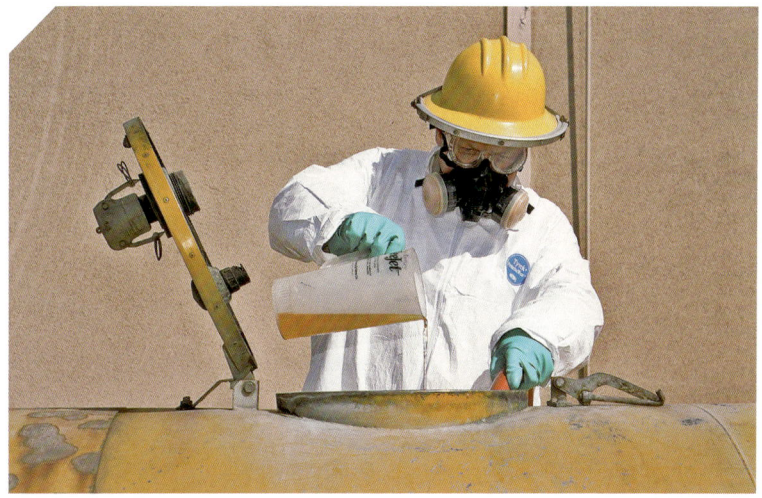

FIGURE 5-1
Accidents that result in pesticide injury or poisoning occur mainly during transportation and storage of pesticides, as well as when mixing or making an application. These accidents are often the result of carelessness, lack of safety training, or improper handling techniques. This person is wearing personal protective equipment that protects against injury or poisoning in case of an accident.

Accidents

The most harmful pesticide exposure risks occur during accidents that involve spills, splashes, or equipment failure. Usually these accidents happen while transporting or storing pesticides, and they can also occur during mixing and loading, or while making an application (Fig. 5-1). Carelessness is sometimes the cause, though a lack of training in proper transportation, handling, and storage techniques coupled with poor driving skills contribute to the problem. Accidents can happen anywhere pesticides are used, so be aware of your surroundings, read the label, and take all required safety precautions to minimize the likelihood of accidents.

Work-Related Exposure

Name conditions at the application site that may change and influence the hazards associated with pesticide application.

Pesticide applicators and handlers are most at risk from pesticide exposure because they work closely and frequently with these materials. Applicators are most at risk during mixing and loading. Laborers, tractor drivers, irrigators, and other employees risk exposure if they transport pesticides or work in recently treated areas. Restricted-entry intervals are important pesticide use restrictions designed to protect agricultural workers from exposure (Fig. 5-2). Techniques such as noting conditions at the application site that can change quickly and increase drift potential (such as weather conditions like wind speed and direction, temperature, cloud cover, etc.) and making spray applications when workers or the public are not present nearby also help. Another important step involves training employees on how to avoid contact with pesticide residues. For more information about variables that can affect hazards at application sites, see Chapter 4.

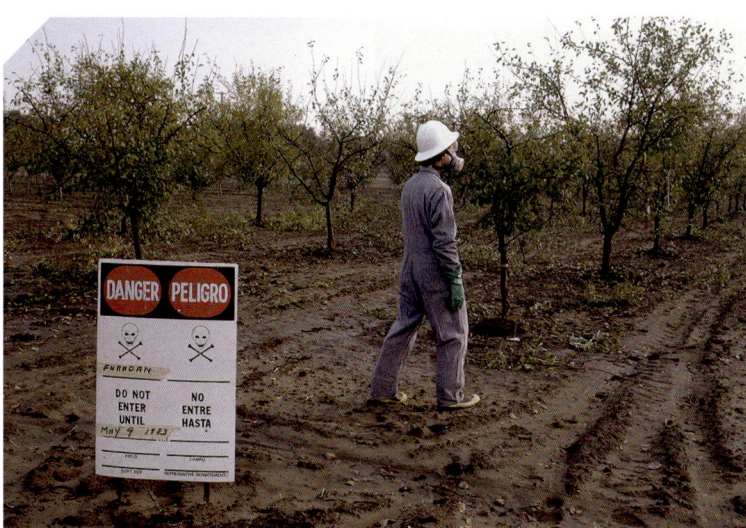

FIGURE 5-2
Restricted-entry intervals following agricultural pesticide applications have helped to reduce farmworker injury. Growers often post treated fields, like the one shown here, to warn workers not to enter during the restricted-entry interval.

People who maintain or repair application equipment may contact pesticide residues on that equipment. Oil-soluble pesticides are a major concern. These accumulate in grease deposits and on oily surfaces and may be difficult to remove. Frequent cleaning of the application equipment reduces pesticide residue and lowers risks to maintenance workers and operators. If equipment cleaning is impossible before repairs or maintenance, mechanics must wear required PPE to avoid unnecessary exposure. People who clean or repair pesticide-contaminated equipment are also considered pesticide handlers and must receive pesticide handler training.

Workers in packing sheds and food processing plants may also contact pesticide residues. When people use persistent pesticide materials or treat shipped produce with fumigants, accidental exposure to these materials can occur. Regulations establish preharvest intervals, (the fewest number of days before harvest a pesticide can be applied), for treated produce to protect consumers from pesticide exposure. These intervals also help reduce exposure to field, packing shed, and processing plant workers because the intervals provide more time for pesticide breakdown. These mandated intervals normally work for fumigants as well, except when they are used on produce shipped and stored in refrigerated containers or warehouses. The cold temperatures, limited ventilation, and inconstant shipping times associated with bringing large volumes of produce to market prevent fumigants from dissipating as expected. Because of this unexpected issue, people can be accidentally exposed to hazardous fumigant levels when working for hours in poorly ventilated cold storage areas. Extra ventilation can reduce worker exposure in this situation. In addition, if you are working with stored produce in low temperatures, take frequent outdoor breaks to limit exposure to these highly toxic pesticides.

It is difficult for greenhouse and nursery workers to avoid close contact with treated surfaces. This is due to the density of plants and limited space found in greenhouses. Also, most greenhouses have limited ventilation, which can increase the potential for breathing spray mists or vapors. It also increases the risk of getting dusts or mists onto the skin or into the eyes during applications. Similar conditions exist for pest control operators working in enclosed areas of dwellings, warehouses, factories, and offices.

Potential for Exposure in Residences

Excessive or improper use or storage of pesticides in and around residences subjects inhabitants to possible exposure. Even when household pesticides, such as mothballs, are stored in their original, properly labeled containers, small children may mistake them for food because of the way the pesticide looks. *Children who swallow pesticides account for many nonagricultural pesticide poisoning cases* (Fig. 5-3). Take care to keep all pesticides out of reach of small children. Accidental drift and other unintended offsite movement of pesticides also adversely affect people in and around the application site. Drift incidents can result in pesticide residues above legal

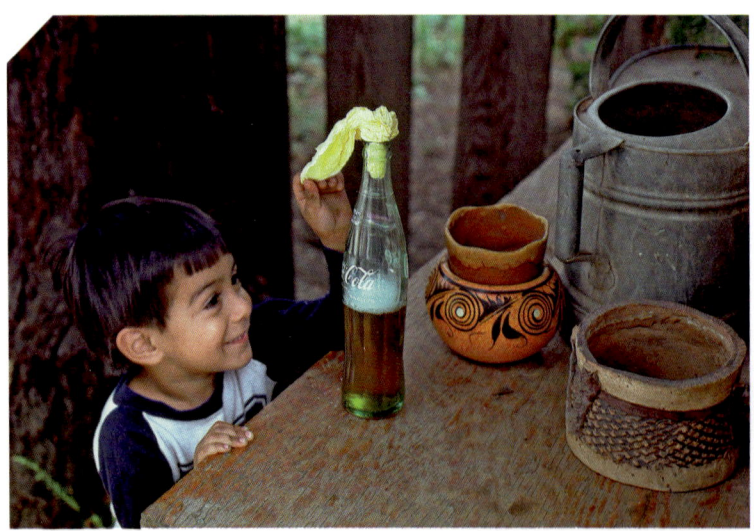

FIGURE 5-3

Children are the major group of nonagricultural pesticide poisoning victims. Improper storage of pesticides in the home is one of the primary ways children find and ingest pesticides.

Describe how offsite movement of pesticides endangers human health.

limits on fruits and vegetables harvested from people's backyard gardens. It can also contaminate laundry hanging on lines near application sites, land on toys left outside in nearby yards, or enter homes through open windows. Runoff and leaching can contaminate people's drinking water by polluting wells, lakes, streams, and aquifers. You must consider the location of people and the resources they rely on as you plan your application in order to avoid accidentally exposing yourself and others to pesticides. For more information about drift, see "Movement in Air" in Chapter 4.

Possible Food Contamination

Explain how each of the following can contribute to human hazards associated with pesticide use:
- incorrect dosage
- incorrect application timing
- incorrect pesticide product application

Illegal pesticide residues found on food are a rare but possible source of pesticide exposure. Incidents in which people have been poisoned by residues on food are few and have always been the result of pesticide misuse. Pesticide misuse occurs when an applicator applies a pesticide to the wrong crop, at the wrong time, or at the wrong rate (dose). Labels of pesticides registered for use in food production, storage, and handling areas specify how to avoid these mistakes. For instance, the pesticide label provides preharvest intervals to ensure that you do not harvest crops before they are safe to eat.

Government agencies establish acceptable pesticide residue tolerances, the maximum amounts of pesticide chemicals that may remain on or in raw agricultural commodities at the time of harvest. Researchers use laboratory and animal testing to establish tolerances, amounts of pesticide considered harmless to consumers. The U.S. EPA always includes a generous margin of safety in the tolerance level (see Chapter 3 for more about the testing that establishes these tolerances). During registration, the U.S. EPA establishes tolerances for each pesticide on each crop or commodity. When establishing tolerance levels, regulators consider the total diet of the consumer, plus their nonfood exposure, over a lifetime of 70 years. State and federal agencies monitor produce to ensure that growers do not exceed pesticide residue tolerances, and they usually seize any produce found having greater than maximum allowable pesticide residues. They may require growers to destroy this produce if there is no way to reduce residues to tolerance levels.

In the United States, pesticide misuse occasionally causes hazardous pesticide residues on produce. Residues exceeding tolerances can occur in the following ways during crop production.
- The crop can accumulate pesticides from the soil.
- A grower may apply a pesticide to an unregistered crop.
- The applicator may apply too much of a pesticide to the crop.
- The grower may apply the pesticide too close to harvest.
- A grower may not wait the appropriate amount of time between repeated applications.
- Drift from another area may contaminate the crop.

In addition, postharvest use of pesticides may leave residues on produce. Warehouse operators use certain pesticides to prevent damage to foodstuffs during storage. Food processors often must use some types of pesticides to protect produce and prevent pest problems in and around processing plants. Retail food store managers occasionally have pesticides applied to control pests that infest these facilities. Restaurants may need to control rodent or insect pests with pesticides to comply with health codes. Pesticides used in residences provide another possible source of food contamination. People who use pesticides in these circumstances must understand that their activities can pose a direct risk to human health. To keep from exceeding postharvest residue tolerances, you must follow pesticide label directions and, when using fumigants, use proper fumigation techniques.

Drinking water contamination offers another potential way for people to ingest pesticides. Improper use or disposal of pesticides has resulted in cases of groundwater contamination. Refer to "Impact on Water Supplies and Sensitive Areas" in Chapter 4 for ways you can protect groundwater from pesticide contamination.

124 CHAPTER 5

Explain the human hazards associated with pesticides.

Pesticide Exposure Through Other Sources

Contact with nonfood items may also expose people to pesticide residues. Entering treated residences or work areas too soon after application (before the end of the restricted-entry interval) could result in exposure. Entering a treated area after the expiration of the restricted-entry interval can also result in exposure if pesticides have been overapplied or if the interval is too short. Some manufacturers treat clothing, furniture, carpeting, and even some children's toys with certain pesticides. The pesticides protect these items from insect damage or reduce the buildup of fungi or bacteria. Another low-level source of exposure occurs if people come in close contact with pets that have been treated for fleas or ticks. Lawns, shrubs, and other residential, industrial, and public landscapes can also be sources of pesticide exposure.

How Pesticides Enter the Body

The tissues of an exposed person can absorb certain types of pesticides. These pesticides enter the body through the skin, eyes, lungs, or mouth (Fig. 5-4). A brief discussion of response to exposure is included below. You can find detailed emergency response and treatment techniques for all exposure types in Chapter 12.

Skin Exposure

Skin (or dermal) contact is the most frequent route of pesticide exposure. If certain pesticides contact the skin they may cause a skin rash or mild skin irritation (known as dermatitis). Other types of pesticides cause more severe skin injury, such as burns. Internal poisoning may also result if a pesticide absorbs through the skin: the blood carries these pesticides to other organs within the body.

The ability of a pesticide to penetrate the skin depends on its chemical characteristics and formulation. Oil-soluble pesticides pass through skin more easily than those that are soluble in water, for instance. The amount of pesticide absorbed by the skin also depends on which body parts are exposed. In a test using the organophosphate insecticide parathion (Fig. 5-5), for example, researchers found the forearm to be the least susceptible area for pesticide absorption. The palms of the hands and soles of the feet absorb parathion slightly faster than the forearm. The top of the hand is almost two and one-half times more susceptible to absorption than the forearm. The scalp, face, and forehead are four times more susceptible. The ear canal absorbs at a rate almost five

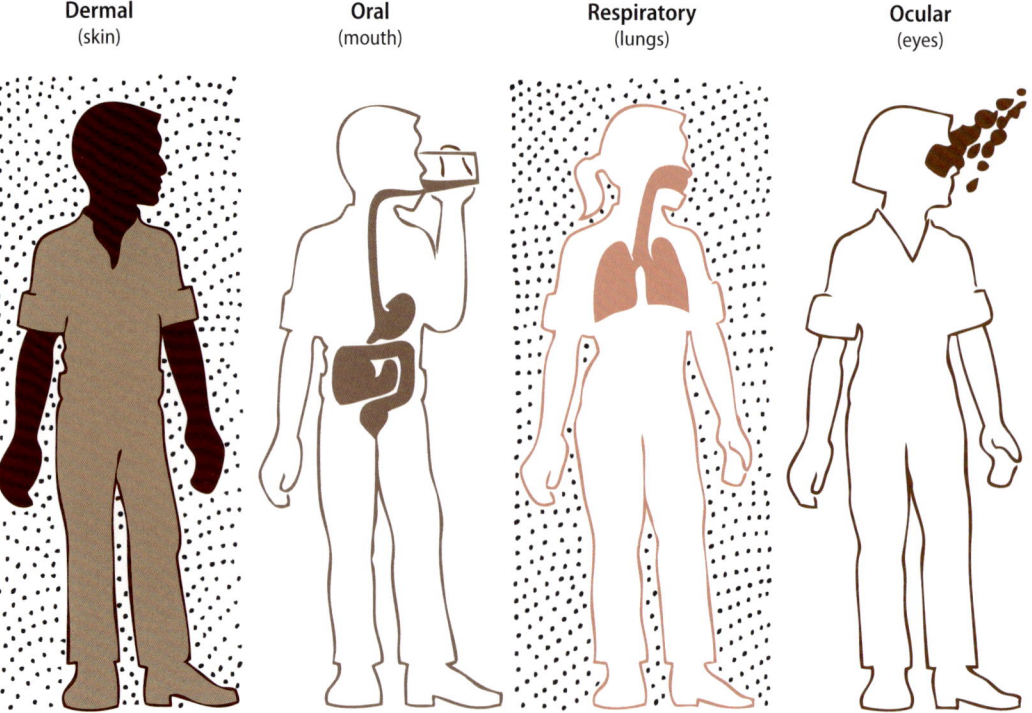

FIGURE 5-4

The most common ways for pesticide exposure to occur are through the skin (dermal), through the mouth (oral), through the lungs (respiratory), and through the eyes (ocular).

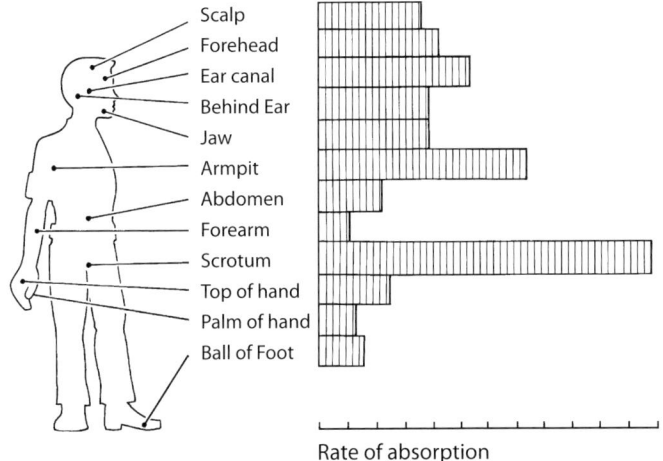

FIGURE 5-5

Different areas of the body absorb pesticides through the skin at different rates. This illustration shows the results of an early study in which researchers placed minute amounts of methyl parathion on body areas of various volunteers. They determined absorption rates by measuring the chemical in the volunteers' urine after a known period of time. (Testing pesticides on human subjects is not allowed in the United States.) *Source:* Feldmann 1967.

and one-half times faster than the forearm. Absorption in the armpit is nearly seven and one-half times greater. In this study, the genital area was the most susceptible area of the body to parathion absorption. This area was nearly twelve times more absorptive than the forearm.

To prevent skin exposure, always wear work clothing and the required PPE when working with pesticides, and be sure to wash your hands thoroughly before using the restroom when working with or around pesticides. See Chapter 6 for more about PPE. Also, avoid contact with recently treated plants, animals, and commodities. Remove contaminated clothing and wash thoroughly if you accidentally get a pesticide on your skin. However, *washing is not an alternative to preventing exposure.* Seek immediate medical attention if skin becomes irritated or other symptoms develop.

Eye Exposure

The active and other ingredients of some pesticide formulations can be caustic to the eyes. Besides their vulnerability to injury, the eyes provide another route for entry of certain pesticides into your body. California law requires that protective eyewear be worn
- during all mixing and loading activities
- while adjusting, cleaning, or repairing contaminated mixing, loading, or application equipment
- during most types of ground application

Protect your eyes by wearing a face shield, goggles, or safety glasses. For more about equipment that protects your eyes, see Chapter 6.

If pesticides get into your eyes, flush them with a gentle stream of clean water for 15 minutes. Hold the eyelids open during flushing. Seek immediate medical attention if irritation persists.

Respiratory Exposure

The lungs quickly absorb certain pesticides, and the blood transports these pesticides to other parts of the body. Some pesticides cause serious lung injury. Breathing dust or vapor during mixing or application is difficult to avoid unless one uses appropriate respiratory equipment. Always wear label-required respirators during mixing and application. Make sure any respirator you use fits properly and is in good condition. Fit testing must be performed prior to your first use of a respirator and annually thereafter. In addition to this yearly testing, you must fit check your respirator before each use to be sure it will protect you while you are handling pesticides. For more information about respirators, fit testing, and fit checking, see Chapter 6.

If you suspect that someone has experienced respiratory exposure to pesticides, be sure you wear appropriate safety equipment before moving the person away from the contaminated area into fresh air. Check the pesticide label for first aid instructions, monitor symptoms, alert a supervisor, and get medical attention quickly. Call 9-1-1 if the person is unconscious or symptoms are severe.

Exposure Through the Mouth (Oral)

It is extremely rare for someone to accidentally drink or eat a pesticide. The exceptions are when pesticides are improperly stored or negligently put into food containers. Pesticides stored in food containers can easily be mistaken for something safe to eat or drink. Improperly stored pesticides are especially dangerous if children are present nearby.

Exposure through the mouth occurs more commonly if spray materials or pesticide dusts splash or blow into your mouth during mixing or application. Ingestion occasionally happens by eating or drinking contaminated food or drinks. Smoking while handling pesticides increases your risk of ingesting pesticides.

Linings of your mouth, stomach, and intestines readily absorb some pesticides. If you swallow sufficient quantities, sometimes even small amounts, you may get sick. PPE, such as a respirator or face shield, minimizes the risk of pesticides getting into your mouth. See Chapter 6 for PPE that helps protect people from oral exposure.

Before eating, drinking, or smoking, be sure to wash your hands thoroughly. Keep food and drinks away from areas where pesticides are being applied or mixed. Never put pesticides into food or drink containers. Keep all pesticides in their original packages. Do not mix or measure pesticides with utensils that someone could use later for food preparation or serving, or use food containers to measure pesticides.

If you suspect oral exposure to pesticides, read the label for first aid. Call a poison control center or doctor for help immediately. Give medical personnel the pesticide's U.S. EPA registration number and the label's first aid statement, which provides specific instructions for treating pesticide poisoning (e.g., some chemicals require that you induce vomiting, and others prohibit it). Do not give anything by mouth to or induce vomiting if the person is unconscious.

Harmful Effects of Pesticides

Human pesticide injuries occur because products can
- cause damage when they contact the skin, eyes, mouth, or respiratory tract
- be absorbed by the body and cause systemic effects
- induce topical responses such as dermal irritation or allergic reaction

Any chemical can be harmful; some, even deadly. Many chemicals we are exposed to daily have risks associated with their use because of their toxicity and the chance for overexposure during their use. The likelihood that you will become ill or get injured through exposure to pesticides is determined by the dose (level of exposure) and the pesticide's toxicity. For more information, see Randall et al. 2008.

> Describe the potential effects on people of acute and chronic pesticide exposure.

Contact Effects

Contact symptoms include skin irritation (dermatitis), such as itching, redness, rashes, blisters, and burns. Skin discoloration may also occur. Many herbicides and fungicides cause dermatitis. Fumigants can cause severe blisters. Because herbicides are the most commonly applied pesticide group and they predominantly cause contact injury, contact skin effects are the most common form of pesticide injury or poisoning to applicators.

Herbicides, fungicides, insecticides, and fumigants may cause eye irritation or injury, sometimes resulting in irreversible damage. Swelling, stinging, and burning of the eyes, nose, mouth, or throat are relatively common contact symptoms. Permanent respiratory damage occurs less often.

Systemic Effects

Systemic effects in humans occur primarily when people are exposed to pesticides that target animals. For example, the nervous system of insects is very similar to that of humans. Thus, an insecticide targeting an insect nervous system often affects a human if the dose is sufficient. Likewise, the circulatory system in rodents is similar to that of humans. Therefore, rodenticides that target the blood system of rodents may also affect a human. Fumigants can cause systemic injury; the herbicide paraquat causes lethal systemic effects in humans.

Symptoms of systemic injury include
- nausea, vomiting, diarrhea, or stomach cramps
- headache, dizziness, weakness, or confusion
- excessive sweating, tearing, chills, or thirst
- chest pains
- breathing difficulties
- body aches and muscle cramps

Heat Stress

When you apply pesticides wearing any type of PPE, you may experience symptoms of heat stress. Heat stress develops when your body cannot cool down so that your core temperature rises. This condition can occur when the air temperature is close to or warmer than normal body temperature and humidity is high. Blood circulated to your skin cannot lose its heat, and so you begin to sweat as a way to cool off. But sweating is effective only if the humidity level is low enough to allow evaporation and if the fluids and salts that are lost are adequately replaced.

If your body cannot get rid of excess heat, it will store it. When this happens, your body's core temperature rises and your heart rate increases. As your body continues to store heat, you begin to lose concentration and have difficulty focusing on a task, may become irritable or sick, and often lose the desire to drink. The next stage is most often fainting. Heat stress can even lead to death if you are not cooled down.

Heat-related illness may mimic certain types of pesticide poisoning, so provide emergency or medical personnel with detailed information about the circumstances surrounding the incident. California regulations require that pesticide handlers receive training on recognizing, avoiding, and treating heat stress along with training on recognizing pesticide illness. For more information, see OSHA 2014.

Types of Injuries from Pesticide Exposure

A single massive dose absorbed during one pesticide exposure incident may cause an injury. Injury may also result from smaller doses absorbed during repeated exposures over time. The illness or injury may have a sudden onset and last a short while, but it also may continue for a long time. Injuries caused by pesticides are usually reversible. Either the body repairs itself or medical treatment cures the condition. Accidental exposure to a few types of pesticides, however, may cause irreversible, or permanent, damage, such as chronic illness, disability, or death.

For example, everyday handling of Category I or II organophosphate or carbamate insecticides can result in a drop in your levels of cholinesterase, the enzyme that helps regulate nerve impulses and muscle activity. That is why, as an employee who handles pesticides, you will be required to take a blood test to determine your unique baseline level of cholinesterase. If your cholinesterase level drops during the period when you are handling these pesticides, your physician will recommend that you stop handling them to avoid serious injury from continued exposure.

Other Effects on People

ALLERGIES

Certain individuals occasionally exhibit allergic reactions when exposed to some types of pesticides. The material causing the reaction may be the pesticide or one of the components of the pesticide formulation. Allergic symptoms often include breathing difficulties, sneezing, eye watering and itching, skin rashes, apprehension, and general discomfort. Sensitive people should avoid exposure to pesticides that produce allergic reactions. Try different types of pesticides or formulations or switch to nonchemical control methods to reduce allergy symptoms.

Define heat stress and describe how people develop heat stress.

Pesticide Toxicity and Health Concerns

Toxicity of a particular pesticide is estimated by subjecting test animals (usually rats, mice, rabbits, and dogs) to various dosages of the active ingredient and to each of its formulated products. Toxicity, measured for both short-term (acute) exposure and long-term (chronic) exposure, is evaluated at

- a range of doses that cause no immediate effects
- doses where there are some immediate effects
- doses where there are delayed or long-term effects
- the dose where death occurs

For a full treatment of pesticide toxicity, see Chapter 3.

Acute toxicity is the measure of harm (systemic or contact) caused by a single, one-time exposure event. Acute effects of pesticide exposure occur shortly after the event, usually within 24 hours. The following example of acute toxicity illustrates the problems that can occur when people are exposed to a harmful dose of alcohol.

Alcohol consumption is fairly common. Annually, only a few people die from lethal alcohol toxicity due to a single exposure event. Many people, however, have varying levels of harmful effects due to overexposure, such as headaches, digestive disorders, and disorientation. People's symptoms from drinking alcohol depend on the dose, the exposure period, and their own body chemistry and weight. Likewise, people's symptoms from an acute pesticide exposure event depend on the dose, the exposure period, and their own body chemistry and weight.

Some pesticides produce acute toxic effects because of their corrosive or irritant properties. These can result in respiratory, skin, or eye irritation or damage. Some can cause severe burns or permanent blindness. Chemicals with these irritant or corrosive properties need to be used with extra care. Fungicides, herbicides, and some insecticides pose contact injury concerns (Table 5-1). Manufacturers list systemic and contact effects in addition to the signal word. Systemic and contact acute toxicity concerns are indicated by the signal words and further explained in the "Precautionary Statements" portion of the product label under the "Hazards to Humans and Domestic Animals" section.

TABLE 5-1

Common pesticide poisoning symptoms related to contact with pesticide dust, liquid, or vapor

Type of contact	Symptoms*
skin	staining of the skin
	reddening of skin in area of contact
	mild burning or itching sensation
	painful burning sensation
	blistering of the skin
	cracking and damage to nails
eye	discomfort, including watering and slight burning
	severe, painful burning (permanent eye damage may occur)
inhaling or swallowing	sneezing
	irritation of nose and throat
	nasal stuffiness
	swelling of mouth or throat
	coughing
	breathing difficulties
	shortness of breath
	chest pains

Note: *Many of the symptoms listed in this table may also be caused by other factors such as irritating plants, allergies, colds, or flu. Usually, a medical examination is needed to determine the actual cause of such symptoms.

U.S. EPA and the manufacturer take into account both systemic and contact toxicity measures in assigning the product's signal word and toxicity category. These are assigned on the basis of the greatest concern, be it oral, dermal, or inhalation systemic effects, or skin, eyes, or respiratory tract contact effects. For more about signal words see "Pesticide Toxicity Categories" in Chapter 3.

The chronic toxicity of a pesticide is determined by subjecting test animals to long-term exposure to an active ingredient, typically 2 years. The harmful effects that occur from small, repeated doses over time are termed chronic effects.

A nonpesticidal example of chronic toxicity is the relationship between tobacco and lung cancer. Not everyone who smokes gets lung cancer; however, a significant number of people who smoke for years do get lung cancer. Another example of chronic toxicity is liver damage resulting from long-term exposure to moderate or high levels of alcohol.

The suspected chronic effects from exposure to certain pesticides include genetic changes, noncancerous or cancerous tumors, reproductive effects, infertility, fetal toxicity, miscarriages, birth defects, blood disorders, and nerve disorders.

If a product causes chronic effects in laboratory animals, the manufacturer is required to include chronic toxicity warning statements on the product label. This information is also listed on the Safety Data Sheet. The chronic toxicity of a pesticide is more difficult to determine through laboratory analysis than the acute toxicity. Remember that signal words for specific formulations are determined by using data from acute toxicity studies and do not take into account chronic, or long-term, effects. For more about how the label treats issues of toxicity, see "What Pesticide Labels Contain" in Chapter 11. For more about testing done to determine pesticide toxicity, see "Plant and Animal Testing" in Chapter 3.

Delayed Effects

Delayed effects are illnesses or injuries that do not appear immediately (within 24 hours) after exposure to a pesticide. They may be delayed for weeks, months, or even years. Whether you experience delayed effects depends on the pesticide, the extent and route of exposure, and how often you were exposed. Under "Precautionary Statements," the label states any delayed effects that the pesticide might cause and how to avoid exposures leading to them (see "What Pesticide Labels Contain" in Chapter 11 for details). Wearing extra protective gear and taking additional precautions may be necessary to reduce the risk of delayed effects. Delayed effects may be caused by either an acute exposure or chronic exposure to a pesticide. For more information on pesticide toxicity and health concerns, see Randall et al. 2008.

Chapter 5 Review Questions

1. The most frequent route of pesticide exposure is through the _____.
    - ☐ a. mouth
    - ☐ b. skin
    - ☐ c. eye

2. Pesticide drift can endanger human health in which of the following ways? Select all that apply.
    - ☐ a. It can cause residues to exceed legal limits on food crops.
    - ☐ b. It can contaminate fruits and vegetables in backyard gardens.
    - ☐ c. It can damage surfaces in and around homes.
    - ☐ d. It can contaminate laundry hung outside to dry.

3. **Which of the following conditions observed at a site can quickly change and affect the outcome of your pesticide application? Select all that apply.**
   - ☐ a. soil type and contents
   - ☐ b. wind speed and direction
   - ☐ c. temperature and cloud cover
   - ☐ d. presence of lakes or streams

4. **Why are mixing and loading considered among the most risky activities for pesticide handlers?**
   - ☐ a. PPE is rarely sufficiently protective during prolonged close contact with concentrated pesticides.
   - ☐ b. Label directions for measuring and mixing concentrated pesticides are often hard to follow precisely.
   - ☐ c. Spills and splashes are common when working with concentrated pesticides.

5. **What hazard does the preharvest interval help a pesticide applicator avoid? Select all that apply.**
   - ☐ a. exposing people to unsafe levels of pesticide residue on the food they eat
   - ☐ b. exposing fieldworkers to excessive pesticide residues on crops they harvest
   - ☐ c. exposing themselves to dangerous pesticide levels on plants they treat

6. **Which of the following could increase hazards to pesticide handlers and fieldworkers?**
   - ☐ a. applying the lowest effective rate of a pesticide
   - ☐ b. applying an oil-soluble pesticide
   - ☐ c. applying a highly selective pesticide

7. **Which of the following defines the difference between chronic and acute pesticide exposure?**
   - ☐ a. Chronic exposure is a result of short-term contact with any amount of pesticide; acute exposure is a result of long-term contact with a small amount of pesticide.
   - ☐ b. Chronic exposure results from a single low-dose incident; acute exposure results from a single high-dose incident.
   - ☐ c. Chronic exposure is repeated exposures to small amounts of pesticide; acute exposure is a short-term exposure to a large dose of pesticide.

8. **On a humid summer day, you notice that a co-worker has difficulty focusing on the job he is doing, is irritable, and starts to complain of feeling sick. When you offer him a cool drink, he shows no interest in it. Your co-worker is suffering from _____.**
   - ☐ a. heat stress
   - ☐ b. exhaustion
   - ☐ c. the flu

Chapter 6
Personal Protective Equipment and Personal Safety

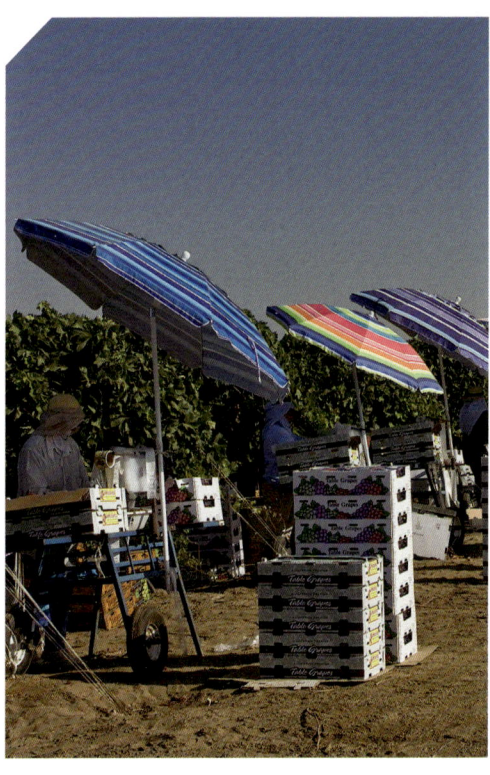

Worker Training and Personal Safety	132
Personal Protective Equipment	134
Engineering Controls	156
Chapter 6 Review Questions	158

Knowledge Expectations

- Explain how personal protective equipment (PPE) and engineering controls can protect a person from hazards associated with pesticides.
- Describe safety training provided to fieldworkers and pesticide handlers.
- Describe the employer's responsibility to provide employees with PPE for mixing, loading, applying, and storing pesticides.
- List various PPE and engineering controls that pesticide handlers use to protect themselves from pesticide exposure.
- Explain how to select the most effective PPE for the job.
- Describe how to wear, clean, maintain, and store reusable PPE and how to dispose of worn or single-use PPE.
- Describe how to prevent or mitigate heat stress.
- Explain the importance of selecting, fit testing, and wearing respiratory devices.
- Identify the limits of PPE to protect pesticide handlers.
- List the different kinds of engineering controls and explain when these are used.

Pesticides can pose hazards to humans. The hazard level depends on the product's toxicity, the length of exposure, and the knowledge and skill of the person working with the product. Therefore, both PPE and safety training are needed to reduce hazards to people and the environment associated with pesticide use. PPE includes clothing and devices worn to protect the human body from contact with pesticides or pesticide residues. Work clothing is not considered PPE unless it is listed as required on the label.

> Explain how personal protective equipment (PPE) and engineering controls can protect a person from hazards associated with pesticides.

The severity of a pesticide poisoning depends on the pesticide's chemical makeup and formulation, dose, and length of exposure. Following safety guidelines and wearing PPE can greatly reduce the potential for dermal, inhalation, eye, and oral exposure, thereby significantly reducing the chances of a pesticide poisoning.

All pesticide handlers—applicators, mixers, loaders, flaggers, etc.—and early-entry agricultural workers (those who enter an area before the restricted-entry interval has expired) are legally required to receive safety training and to follow all PPE instructions on the product label and in California laws and regulations. A pesticide label lists the minimum PPE that you must wear while performing handling or early-entry activities, and California regulations often require more than what appears on the label. You may decide to wear additional PPE for increased safety beyond what is required by regulation; however, you may not omit any equipment mentioned on the label or in regulation, and you must follow the most restrictive PPE requirements listed. Sometimes a label has different PPE requirements for pesticide handlers and early-entry workers, so read the label carefully (see Chapter 11 on how to find PPE requirements on pesticide labels).

The following sections describe required training for pesticide handlers and fieldworkers. They also define the types of PPE typically available for protection against pesticide exposure and discuss how to clean and maintain it so you stay safe on the job. For more information, see Randall et al. 2008.

Worker Training and Personal Safety

The State of California mandates that
- pesticide handlers receive annual pesticide safety training before they handle pesticides; and
- fieldworkers receive annual pesticide safety training before they enter a treated field

Certain classes of people who work with pesticides must take licensing exams in order to purchase, handle, and apply restricted materials; supervise pesticide handlers and fieldworkers; or advise others in the application of pesticides. Below you will find the types of training required by federal and California law for workers handling or otherwise directly contacting pesticides as part of their job.

> Describe safety training provided to fieldworkers and pesticide handlers.

TRAINING

California pesticide laws establish minimum standards of training for all employees handling pesticides as part of their work. This mandatory training must address the following topics.

Using Pesticides Safely
- Why you must wear clean work clothing daily.
- How to handle, open, and lift containers; how to pour; and how to operate mixing and application equipment.
- How to properly triple-rinse and dispose of containers.
- How to confine the pesticide to the application area or site.

- How to avoid contamination of people, animals, waterways, and sensitive areas.
- How and where to store containers; how to proceed when containers cannot be locked up.
- Why you must wash hands thoroughly before eating, smoking, drinking, or using the bathroom, and why you must shower thoroughly at the end of the exposure period.
- Why you must never take pesticides or pesticide containers home.
- How to read and understand pesticide labels and Safety Data Sheets, including the signal words, precautionary statements, first aid instructions, application rate, and mixing and application instructions.
- Why and when you must wear different types of PPE.
- How to fit and properly wear PPE, and how to inspect it for wear and damage.
- How to fit, use, and maintain respiratory equipment.
- When and how to use enclosed cabs, closed mixing systems, and other safety equipment and engineering controls.
- How to secure and safely transport pesticides in a vehicle.

Emergencies and Health
- How pesticides enter the body (skin, eyes, lungs, mouth).
- How to recognize pesticide poisoning symptoms.
- How to recognize chronic and acute effects of pesticides.
- How to administer first aid and implement decontamination procedures.
- How to handle nonroutine tasks or emergency situations such as spills, leaks, or fires.
- Where to find the name, address, and telephone number of the clinic, physician, or hospital emergency room that can provide immediate medical treatment.
- Where to find your company's policy for reporting injury or illness and obtaining medical treatment.
- When medical supervision is required and what medical supervision must be provided by your employer.
- How to recognize and avoid heat stress and what to do should it occur.

Legal Information and Worker Rights
- Which laws and regulations apply to you, and why it is important that you comply with them.
- How employees have the right to receive information about pesticides to which they may be exposed, and how employees are protected against discharge or other discrimination if they exercise these rights.
- How to locate and access documents pertaining to your company's hazard communication program, pesticide labels, pesticide safety information series sheets, Safety Data Sheets, pesticide use records, and other important documents.

Employer Responsibilities

Describe the employer's responsibility to provide employees with PPE for mixing, loading, applying, and storing pesticides.

Employers are responsible for providing the PPE and the training you need according to pesticide labels and California regulations. These regulations cover all employees tasked with mixing, loading, applying, storing, or otherwise handling pesticides. Employers must make this equipment easy to access and cannot force workers to purchase it for themselves. Employers are also responsible for ensuring that PPE is cleaned and maintained, either by an employee or a third party. If you are self-employed and require training information, contact your local agricultural commissioner's office.

In addition, all agricultural fieldworkers entering treated areas within 30 days of the expiration of any restricted-entry interval must receive pesticide-related training. Sidebar 6-1 lists

the information that fieldworker training must cover. Qualified trainers must train fieldworkers and pesticide handlers in agricultural areas. Qualified trainers include
- pest control advisers (PCAs)
- certified private or commercial applicators
- registered foresters
- University of California farm advisors
- certain county biologists
- people who have attended an EPA-approved train-the-trainer program

Continuing Education

Being certified or licensed as a pesticide applicator in California obligates you to keep current on new information by earning continuing education (CE) credits. CE class topics include issues of pesticide use, pesticide safety, and pest management. Keeping current is necessary because
- lawmakers change or revise pesticide laws and regulations from time to time
- pesticide chemicals are constantly being improved, with several new chemicals introduced each year
- pesticide use changes with increased knowledge of pests and their habits
- techniques of pesticide application often reflect new technologies in application equipment and formulation types
- researchers modify pest management techniques as they discover new information about pests
- pest managers discover new pests every year, and certain pests show resistance to pesticides used previously for their control

Without CE, a pesticide applicator can quickly lose touch with modern pest control practices and pesticide application techniques.

A good way to keep yourself current is to attend meetings of professional organizations affiliated with your work. Most occupational areas involved in pesticide use have one or more professional organizations. Several of these associations publish newsletters that contain new pest management and pesticide use information. In addition, the UC Cooperative Extension Service (county farm advisors' offices) sponsors workshops and seminars that focus on aspects of pest control, pest management, and pesticide use. Also, county agricultural commissioners' offices regularly conduct meetings to update people on pesticide laws and regulations. Special courses are also available through commercial continuing education providers, local community colleges, state colleges and universities, and the University of California. You can find a list of approved CE courses on the DPR website. Visit cdpr.ca.gov and enter "continuing education" in the search box.

Personal Protective Equipment

Personal protective equipment (PPE) helps protect your body and clothing from pesticide exposure. Some of this equipment also protects your eyes and prevents you from inhaling pesticide vapors. However, safety equipment is effective only if it fits correctly and you use it properly. Always keep it cleaned and maintained according to manufacturer's instructions.

The greatest risk of pesticide poisoning comes from pesticides contacting your skin. Oil-soluble pesticides pass through skin faster than water-soluble pesticides. In addition, some parts of your body absorb pesticide more quickly than other areas, and some application methods may expose you to more pesticide than others. Wearing the PPE required by pesticide labels helps protect the most vulnerable parts of your body from exposure (Fig. 6-1).

Follow the pesticide label and California regulations for the PPE you must use. In most instances, using additional equipment above what the label requires increases your protection. The only exception is with the use of certain fumigants. Protective clothing and gloves may trap certain fumigants close to your skin, which increases your exposure instead of lowering it. Follow label instructions strictly for the proper PPE when applying fumigants.

PPE offers various levels of protection, depending on the type of resistant material used. Some items of PPE simply act as barriers by keeping dry or liquid material off the skin. Others offer better protection against water-based products. Some offer protection from chemicals (solvent and active ingredient) that make up a concentrated pesticide product.

> **SIDEBAR 6-1**
>
> ## CRITERIA FOR FIELDWORKER TRAINING
>
> Worker Protection Standard (WPS) training for fieldworkers must include at least the following information. This training must be provided to any workers who enter pesticide-treated areas for the 30 days following expiration of a restricted-entry interval. Training must be provided to workers when an area has been treated with any type of pesticide, such as herbicides, fungicides, or insecticides. Training is required annually.
>
> **INFORMATION THAT MUST BE COVERED**
>
> - Where and how workers may come in contact with pesticides or pesticide residues during work, including hazards from chemigation and drift.
> - The routes by which pesticides can enter the body (skin, mouth, inhalation, and eyes).
> - Symptoms of acute pesticide poisoning or injury; long-term and delayed health effects from pesticide exposure, including sensitization.
> - First aid for pesticide injury and poisoning; emergency decontamination.
> - How workers can protect themselves from exposure (work clothing; avoiding skin, eye, and mouth contact; personal hygiene).
> - Obtaining medical help.
> - After-work care of pesticide-contaminated work clothes.
> - Potential hazards to children and pregnant women from pesticide exposure.
> - Warnings about taking home pesticides or pesticide containers.
> - An explanation of the WPS entry restrictions, application limitations, application exclusion zones, posting, oral warnings, access to pesticide use information, and protection from employer retaliation.
> - Their rights as an employee.
> - Their employer's responsibility to provide protections against pesticides.
> - Prevention, recognition, and first aid for heat-related exposure.
> - Information found on Safety Data Sheets (SOS).
> - How to report suspected violations.

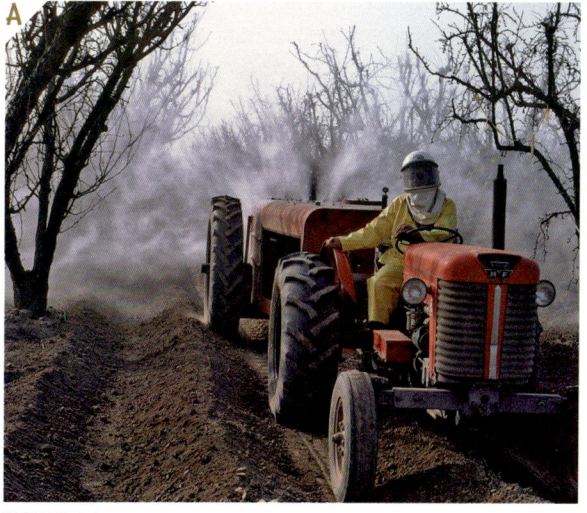
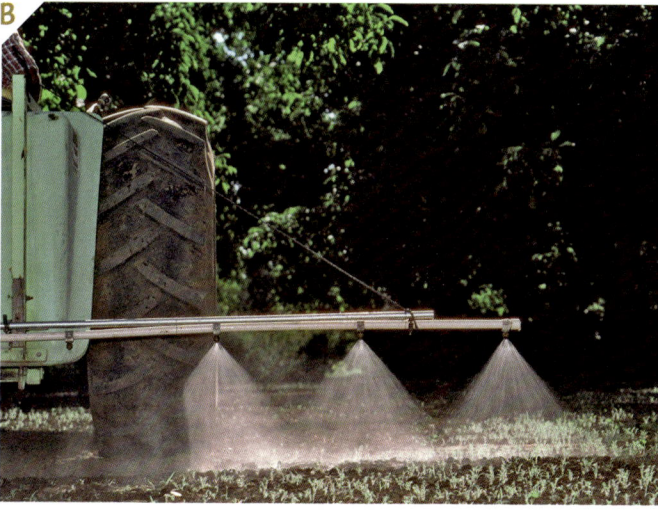

FIGURE 6-1

Pesticide labels tell you what personal protective equipment you must wear during pesticide applications. Some applications, such as spraying orchards (A), expose handlers to higher levels of pesticide than do low-volume applications (B).

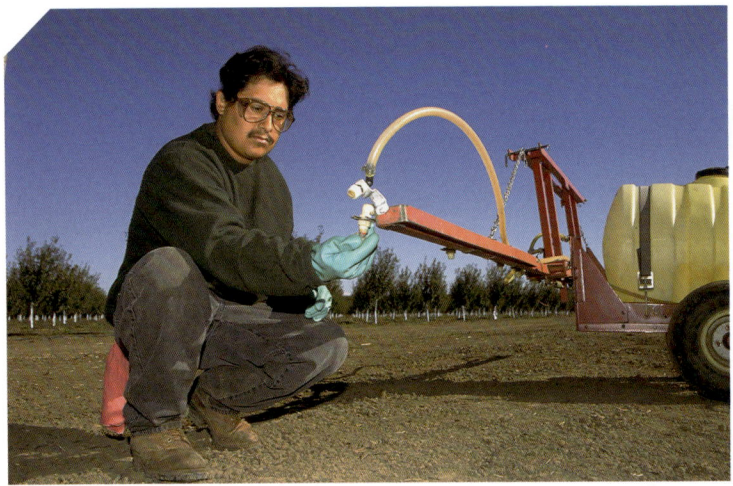

FIGURE 6-2

If you handle pesticides, you should wear a long-sleeved shirt, long pants, socks, and close-toed shoes, even if the label does not require these items. California regulations require employee handlers to wear eye protection and gloves when mixing and loading, even if the label does not require these items.

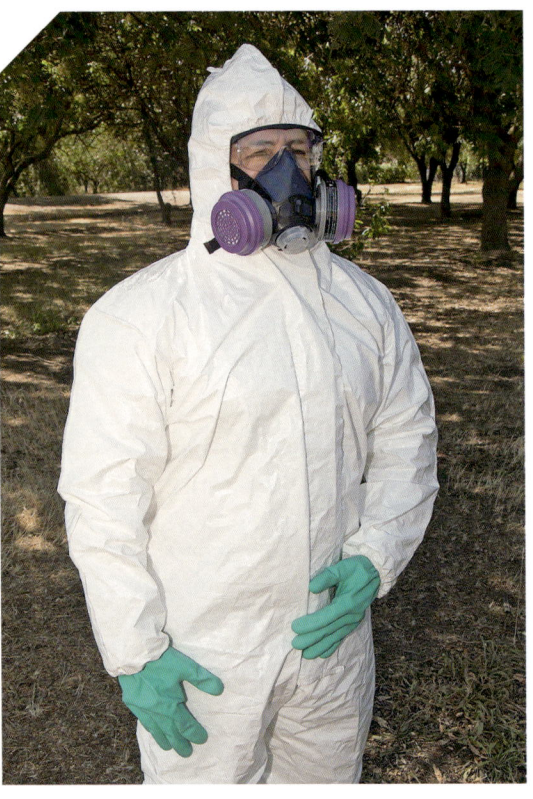

FIGURE 6-4

Chemical-resistant garments provide the maximum amount of protection from pesticide exposure.

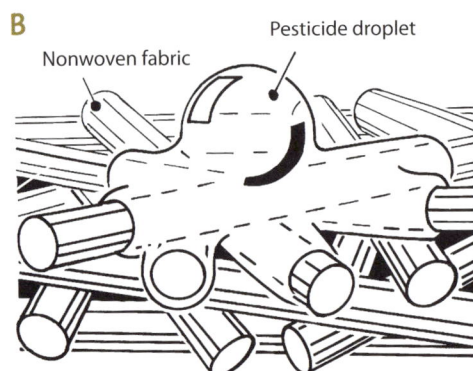

FIGURE 6-3

Woven fabrics promote wicking (A). It takes longer for pesticide droplets to pass through nonwoven fabrics (B).

WORK CLOTHES FOR HANDLERS AND FIELDWORKERS

Ordinary shirts, pants, shoes, and other work clothes are not considered PPE, even though pesticide labels often indicate that specific items of work clothing should be worn during certain activities. In California, if you handle pesticides you should wear a long-sleeved shirt, long pants, socks, and close-toed shoes, even if the label does not require these items (Fig. 6-2). Regulations require employee handlers to wear eye protection and gloves when mixing and loading, even if the label does not require these items. When using DANGER and WARNING pesticides, you must also wear coveralls. If you work in an area where you may contact pesticide residues, you should wear a long-sleeved shirt, long pants, socks, and close-toed shoes. Make sure the long-sleeved shirt and long pants are made of sturdy material and are free of holes and tears. Fasten the shirt collar completely to protect the lower part of your neck. Fabric with a tighter weave provides better protection, but it will still absorb liquids. Nonwoven fabrics take longer to absorb liquids, as shown in Figure 6-3.

List various PPE and engineering controls that pesticide handlers use to protect themselves from pesticide exposure.

In some instances, the product label requires that you wear a coverall, a chemical-resistant suit, or a chemical-resistant apron over your work clothes. If the label requires chemical-resistant PPE, you must observe certain temperature restrictions because of the potential for heat-related illness.

Explain how to select the most effective PPE for the job.

Chemical-Resistant Clothing. The term *chemical resistant* means that no measurable movement of the pesticide through the material oc-

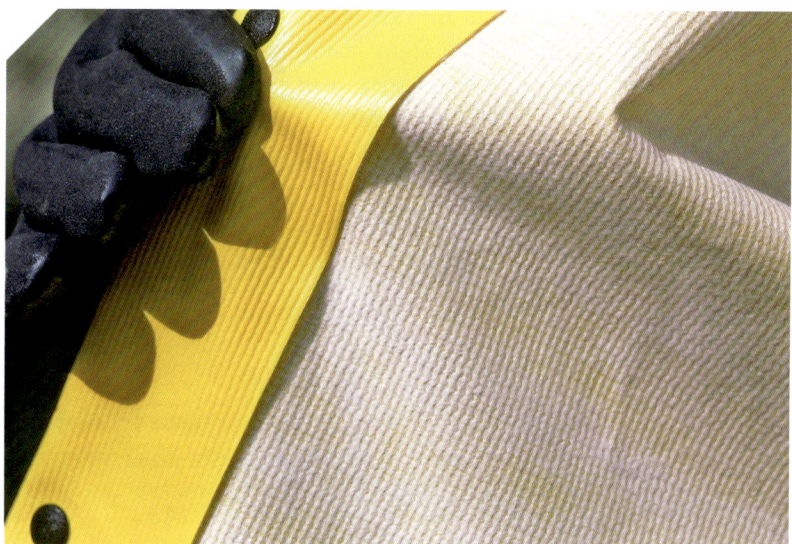

FIGURE 6-5

Be sure linings of protective clothing are made of nonabsorbent materials to prevent pesticide contamination.

curs during the period of use (Fig. 6-4). Some PPE is water resistant only. *Water resistant* refers to PPE that keeps a small amount of fine spray particles or small liquid splashes from penetrating the clothing and reaching the skin. Waterproof (liquid-proof) material keeps water-soluble materials out, but it may not necessarily keep out oil solvent–based products. Waterproof materials include items made of plastic or rubber. Some materials are actually chemically resistant, and, when worn correctly, can protect your skin from exposure to pesticides. The chemical resistance of a material is an indication of how strongly it resists chemical penetration by pesticide products during use. Read the PPE packaging carefully to determine whether the protective item is chemical resistant, liquid proof, or water resistant. Be sure linings of protective clothing are made of nonabsorbent materials to prevent pesticide contamination (Fig. 6-5).

When making a decision about which PPE to use, follow these general guidelines. Cotton, leather, canvas, and other absorbent materials are not chemically resistant even to dry formulations. Powders and dusts sometimes move through cotton and other woven materials as quickly as liquid formulations; they also may remain in the fibers even after several launderings. Do not use a hat that has a cloth or leather sweatband, and do not use cloth or cloth-lined gloves, footwear, or aprons. Cloth is difficult or impossible to clean after it becomes contaminated with pesticide, and it is usually too expensive to be disposed of and replaced after one use.

Gloves, boots, aprons, suits, and hoods come in a variety of chemical-resistant materials. Generally, the best choices of materials are plastics, such as polyvinyl chloride (PVC); rubber, such as butyl, nitrile, neoprene, or Viton rubber; or nonwoven fabrics coated with plastic or another barrier material such as Tyvek. Barrier laminate materials such as 4H or Silver Shield are resistant to most pesticides, but many pesticide handlers consider them uncomfortable to wear and difficult to use while performing many tasks.

The ability of a given material to protect an individual from a pesticide product is largely a function of the type of solvent used to formulate the pesticide product. Watch for signs that the material is not chemically resistant to the pesticide product that you are using. Sometimes it is easy to see when plastic or rubber is not resistant to a pesticide. The material may change color, become soft or spongy, swell or bubble up, dissolve or become like jelly, crack or get holes, or become stiff or brittle. If any of the changes occur, discard the item and choose another type of resistant material.

Always read the pesticide labeling to see if it states which materials are resistant to the pesticide product. In some instances, a pesticide label's PPE description lists a code letter

(A–H) developed by the U.S. EPA to help the user select suitable PPE. The U.S. EPA chemical resistance category selection chart is given in Table 6-1. DPR has also developed a glove key code chart printed on a wallet-sized plastic card (Fig. 6-6). You can pick one up at your local county agricultural commissioner's office or order one directly from DPR.

The chart's code letters are based on the solvents used in a pesticide product, not on the pesticide's active ingredient. By referring to this chart, a pesticide handler can determine how long a given material can be expected to withstand chemical exposure by a given solvent. For more information on PPE, see Randall et al. 2008.

TABLE 6-1

EPA Chemical resistance category selection chart for gloves

Selection category on label	Type of resistant material							
	Barrier laminate	Butyl rubber ≥14 mil	Nitrile rubber ≥14 mil	Neoprene rubber ≥14 mil	Natural rubber* ≥14 mil	Polyethylene	Polyvinyl chloride (PVC) ≥14 mil	Viton ≥14 mil
A (dry and water-based formulations)	high	high	high	high	high	high	high	high
B	high	high	slight	slight	none	slight	slight	slight
C	high	high	high	high	moderate	moderate	high	high
D	high	high	moderate	moderate	none	none	none	slight
E	high	slight	high	high	slight	none	moderate	high
F	high	high	high	moderate	slight	none	slight	high
G	high	slight	slight	slight	none	none	none	high
H	high	slight	slight	slight	none	none	none	high

Key: High: Highly chemically resistant. Clean or replace PPE at end of each day's work period. Rinse off pesticide at breaks.
Moderate: Moderately chemically resistant. Clean or replace PPE within an hour or two of contact.
Slight: Slightly chemically resistant. Clean or replace PPE within 10 minutes of contact.
None: No chemical resistance.
Note: *Includes natural rubber blends and laminates.
Source: EPA 2014.

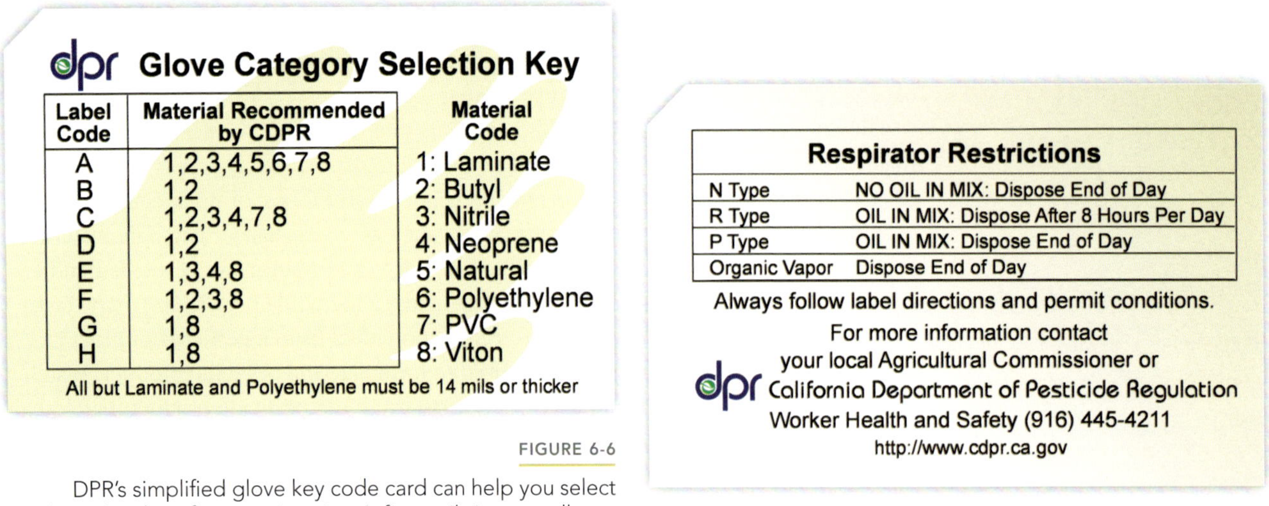

FIGURE 6-6

DPR's simplified glove key code card can help you select the right glove for your situation. It fits easily into a wallet or pocket and also contains respirator restrictions. You can get one at your local county agricultural commissioner's office or order one from DPR directly. *Source:* DPR.

PERSONAL PROTECTIVE EQUIPMENT AND PERSONAL SAFETY

Describe how to wear, clean, maintain and store reusable PPE, and how to dispose of worn or single-use PPE.

Reusables

Some PPE items, such as rubber and plastic suits, gloves, boots, aprons, capes, and headgear, are designed to be cleaned and reused several times. However, do not make the mistake of continuing to use these items when they no longer offer adequate protection. Wash the reusable items thoroughly between uses and inspect them for signs of wear or abrasion. Never wash contaminated gloves, boots, respirators, or other PPE in streams, ponds, or other bodies of water. Check for rips and leaks by using the rinse water to form a "balloon" (i.e., filling the PPE item with water) and/or by holding the items up to the light. Even tiny holes or thin places can allow large quantities of pesticide to penetrate the material and reach your skin. Discard any PPE item that shows signs of wear.

Even if you do not see any signs of wear, replace reusable chemical-resistant items regularly, since the ability of a chemical-resistant material to resist the pesticide decreases each time an item is worn. A good rule of thumb is to throw out gloves that have been worn for about 5 to 7 workdays. Extra-heavy-duty gloves, such as those made of butyl or nitrile rubber, may last as long as 10 to 14 days. Glove replacement is a high priority because adequate hand protection greatly reduces the pesticide handler's chance of exposure. The cost of frequently replacing your gloves is a wise investment. Footwear, aprons, headgear, and protective suits may last longer than gloves because they generally receive less exposure to the pesticides and less abrasion from rough surfaces. Replace them regularly and at any sign of wear. Most protective eyewear and respirator bodies, face pieces, and helmets are designed to be cleaned and reused. These items can last many years if they are of good quality and are maintained correctly.

Be sure to clean all reusable PPE items at the end of each exposure period, even if they were worn for only a brief period of exposure. Pesticide residues that remain on PPE are likely to penetrate the material. If you wear that PPE again, pesticide may already be on the inside of the material next to your skin. Also, PPE worn several times between launderings may build up pesticide residues. The residues can reach a level that can harm you, even if you are handling pesticides that are not highly toxic. After cleaning and drying reusable items, place them in a plastic bag or clothing hamper away from your personal clothes and away from the family laundry.

Disposables

Disposable PPE items are not designed to be cleaned and reused (Fig. 6-7). Discard them when they become contaminated with pesticides. Place disposable PPE in a separate plastic bag or container prior to disposal.

Chemical-resistant gloves, footwear, and aprons labeled as disposable are designed to be worn only once and then thrown away. These items often are made of thin vinyl, latex, or polyethylene. These inexpensive disposables may be a good choice for brief pesticide handling activities that require dexterity as long as the activity does not tear the thin plastic. For example, you might use disposable gloves, shoe covers, and an apron while pouring pesticide into a hopper or tank, cleaning or adjusting a nozzle, or making minor equipment adjustments.

Nonwoven (including coated nonwoven) coveralls and hoods, such as Tyvek, are usually designed to be disposed of after use. Most are intended to be worn for only 1 workday. The instructions with some coated nonwoven suits and hoods permit the user to wear

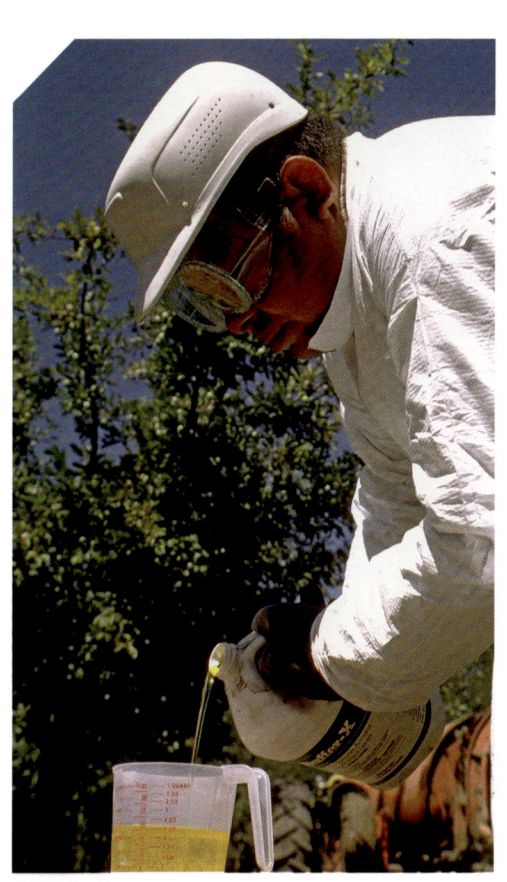

FIGURE 6-7

Disposable protective clothing is inexpensive and lightweight. Throw it away after use. Unless the fabric is specially coated, it is unsuitable for use when the label calls for a waterproof or chemical-resistant garment.

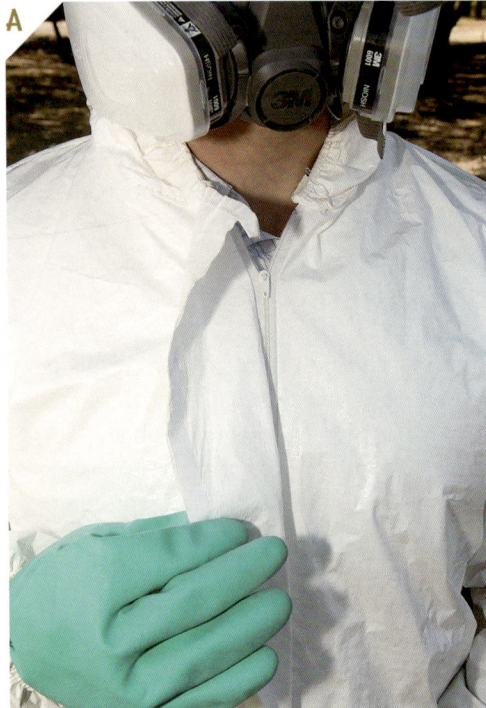

FIGURE 6-8

The protection offered by chemical-resistant coveralls depends on the fabric and design features such as flaps over zippers (A), elastic at the wrists and ankles (B), and seams that are bound and sealed.

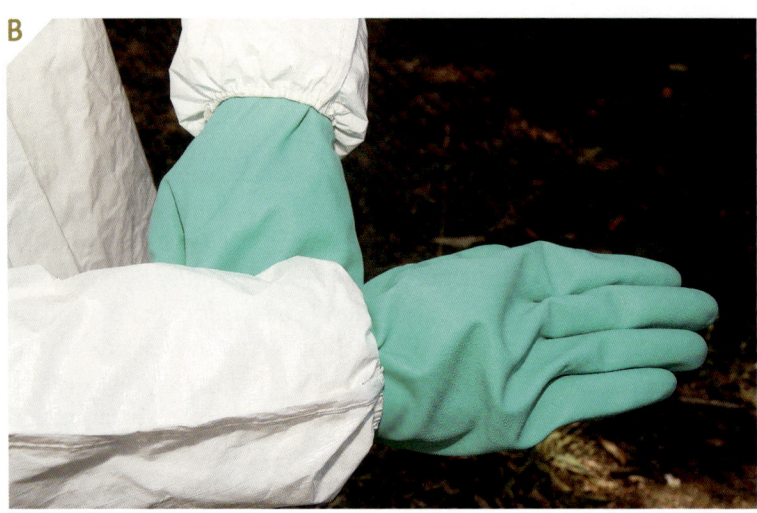

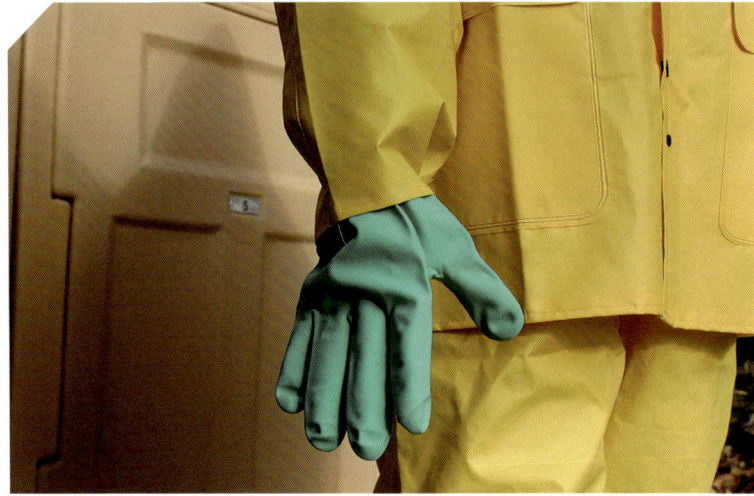

FIGURE 6-9

Two-piece chemical-resistant coveralls must have a jacket that falls below the waist to provide adequate protection during pesticide handling activities.

them more than once if each use period is short and not much pesticide gets on them. Pay close attention when reusing these items and be ready to change them whenever there are signs that pesticides could be getting through the material or that the inside surface is contaminated.

Dust and mist masks, prefilters, canisters, filtering and vapor-removing cartridges, and a few cartridge respirators are disposables. They cannot be cleaned. Dispose of used, damaged, or old items and replace them with new ones.

Coveralls

The protection offered by chemical-resistant coveralls depends on the fabric and design features such as flaps over zippers (Fig. 6-8A), elastic at the wrists and ankles (Fig. 6-8B), and seams that are bound and sealed. Make sure coveralls are made of sturdy material such as Tyvek or laminated Tyvek. When wearing a coverall, close the opening securely so your entire body (except the feet, hands, neck, and head) is covered. When wearing a two-piece outfit, do not tuck the shirt or coat in at the waist—have the shirt extend well below the waist of the pants and fit loosely around the hips (Fig. 6-9). You should wear coveralls over a long-sleeved shirt, long pants, and socks when handling pesticides that have moderate or high dermal toxicity or are skin irritants.

Several factors determine how well a coverall protects you. First, the coverall needs to fit loosely. Each layer of clothing and each layer of air between the pesticide and your skin provides added protection. That is why the coverall needs to fit loosely. If the coverall fits too tightly, there will not be a protective layer of air between it, your work clothes, and your skin.

PERSONAL PROTECTIVE EQUIPMENT AND PERSONAL SAFETY

The design and structure of the coveralls also affect how well they protect you. Well-designed coveralls have tightly constructed, sealed seams and snug, overlapping closures that do not allow gaps and do not unfasten readily. For example, many coveralls have zippers that are covered by flaps for added protection. This type of construction makes it harder for pesticides to get through these areas and come into contact with your inner clothing or skin. Some coveralls are designed for one-time use and should not be worn again after your work that day is complete. Your employer should provide a container or bag for used disposable coveralls and other disposable PPE.

Chemical-Resistant Suits

Some product labels require the handler to wear a chemical-resistant suit. This usually indicates the pesticide is very hazardous because of either acute or chronic effects. In these instances, take extra care to prevent the pesticide from getting on your skin.

If you expect that a large amount of pesticide could be deposited on your clothing over an extended period of time, wear a chemical-resistant suit even if the product label does not require it. Under these circumstances, even pesticides that are applied dry, such as dusts or granules, can get through ordinary fabric and may harm you.

Chemical-resistant suits made of rubber or plastic are sold as one-piece coveralls or as two-piece outfits consisting of a jacket worn over overalls. Chemical-resistant suits made of coated nonwoven fabric usually are sold as one-piece coveralls. Note that chemical-resistant PPE does not "breathe" like cotton or other fabrics, which may cause you to sweat excessively. In this case, you must take more care to protect yourself from exposure, since sweat can mix with the pesticide, soak through your clothing, and get on your skin.

The biggest drawback to chemical-resistant suits is they may make you uncomfortably warm. Unless you are handling pesticides in cool or climate-controlled environments, heat stress becomes a major concern. If a pesticide's label requires a chemical-resistant suit, you cannot apply the pesticide when the daytime temperature is above 80°F or the nighttime temperature is above 85°F. You can ignore these requirements if you make the application from an air-conditioned cab. You can also wear a body-cooling device, such as an ice vest, underneath your PPE. When temperatures will exceed the regulatory maximum, and any time they reach unsafe levels and cause symptoms related to heat illness, even if temperatures are below the regulatory maximum, take extra care to avoid heat stress. Drink plenty of water and take frequent rest breaks to cool down (Randall et al. 2008). For more information about heat stress and its effects, see "Heat Stress" in Chapter 5. For information about emergency first aid for heat stress, see "Recognizing and Responding to Heat Stress" in Chapter 12.

Describe how to prevent or mitigate heat stress.

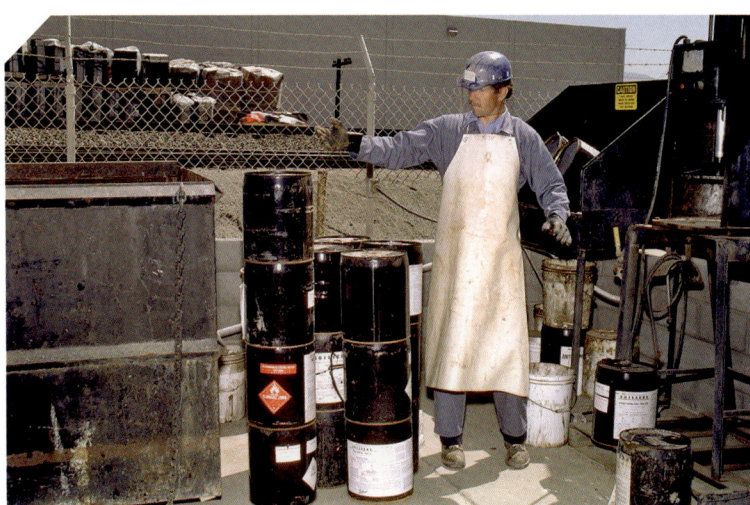

FIGURE 6-10

Follow label instructions for use of waterproof aprons. Select a style with a wide bib to provide added protection.

Chemical-Resistant Aprons

An apron protects you from splashes, spills, and billowing dust, and it protects your coveralls or other clothing. Consider wearing an apron whenever you handle pesticide concentrates. The product label may require that you wear a chemical-resistant apron when mixing or loading a pesticide or cleaning application equipment.

Choose an apron that extends from your neck to at least your knees (Fig. 6-10). Some aprons have attached sleeves and gloves. This style of apron protects your arms and hands and the front of your body by eliminating the potential gap where the sleeve and glove or sleeve and apron meet.

However, an apron can pose a safety hazard when you are working around equipment with moving parts. If an apron can get caught in machinery or get in your way, wear a chemical-resistant suit instead.

Disposable aprons made for one-time use are generally not suitable for pesticide handling. The thin plastic materials tear or puncture easily. Reusable aprons are more durable but require regular cleaning and decontamination. Discard them if they develop tears or holes.

Chemical-Resistant Headgear

For overhead exposure or exposure to a lot of airborne particles, wear something to protect your head and neck, such as a chemical-resistant wide-brimmed hat or hood. Plastic safari hats or bump caps with plastic sweatbands are a good choice because they are relatively cool in hot weather and are made with nonabsorbent material. More flexible hats and hoods are also available in chemical-resistant materials. Hats must not contain absorbent material such as cotton, leather, or straw. Many chemical-resistant jackets or coveralls can be purchased with attached protective hoods.

Gloves

The hands and forearms are the areas most likely to get exposed to pesticides when you are at work. Research shows that people who mix pesticides receive 85% of the total exposure to their hands and 13% to their forearms. Wearing chemical-resistant gloves, the study revealed, reduces exposure by 99%. Knowing this, chemical-resistant gloves are an essential part of your safety equipment. If you are an employee handler, regulations require you to wear gloves when handling most pesticides.

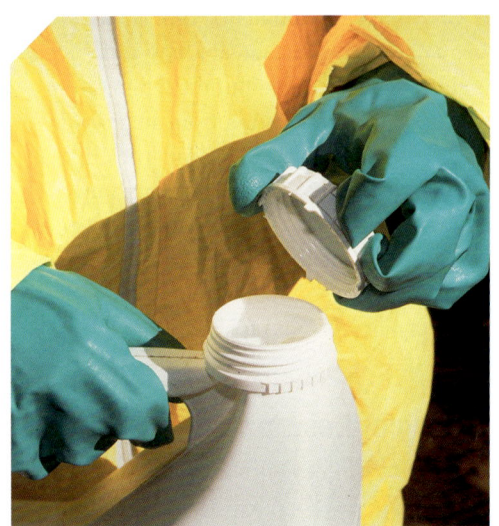

FIGURE 6-11
Use only unlined chemical-resistant gloves made of butyl, nitrile, neoprene or natural rubber, polyethylene, polyvinyl chloride (PVC), or Viton.

Never use leather or fabric gloves (unless specified on the pesticide label) because they absorb water and pesticides. Choose gloves made from natural rubber, barrier laminate, butyl, nitrile, polyethylene, PVC, Viton, or neoprene (Fig. 6-11). Select a material that offers the best resistance to the types of pesticide you are using. Some materials are suitable for total immersion in a liquid toxicant for extended periods. Other materials provide protection only against accidental splashes or occasional immersion. The thickness of the glove material also determines the amount of protection: thicker materials are better. Choose materials that resist puncturing and abrasion.

Wear unlined gloves, since fabrics used for linings may absorb pesticides. Linings make gloves dangerous to use and difficult to clean. If necessary, use woven, removable glove liners to insulate your hands from the cold or to absorb perspiration. California regulations prohibit laundering and reusing glove liners. You must discard glove liners immediately if they become contaminated or at the end of the workday regardless of their condition.

Make sure the cuffs of gloves are long enough to extend to the mid-forearm. Usually, wear the sleeves of your protective clothing on the outside of your gloves to keep out pesticides. Some special application situations, however, require holding one or both hands overhead while spraying liquids. In these cases, tuck the sleeve of the elevated arm inside the glove. Be careful when lowering your arm to prevent pesticides from entering the glove. If pesticide gets inside your gloves, take them off immediately, wash your hands, and put on clean PPE. You should keep several pairs of gloves nearby so you can change to a clean set as soon as your gloves become damaged or contaminated on the inside.

Check pesticide labels for special glove requirements. For example, certain fumigants specify that gloves made of cotton or a similar material be worn when handling the product, even though cotton is not recommended for most pesticide handling. Read all pesticide labels carefully to find the PPE that is required to protect you from exposure.

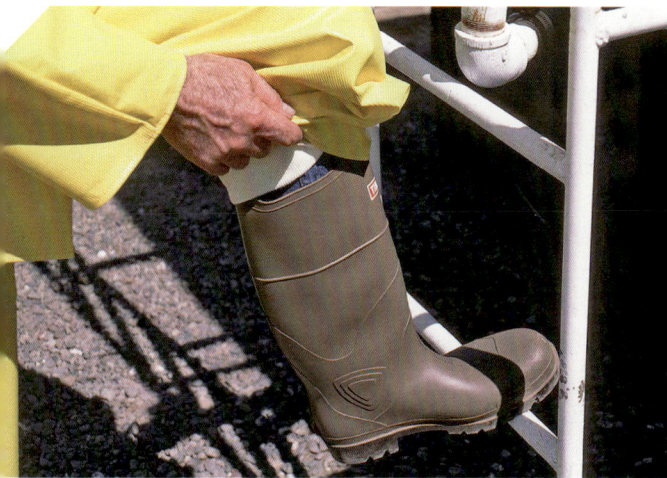

FIGURE 6-12

Chemical-resistant footwear protects your feet from pesticide exposure.

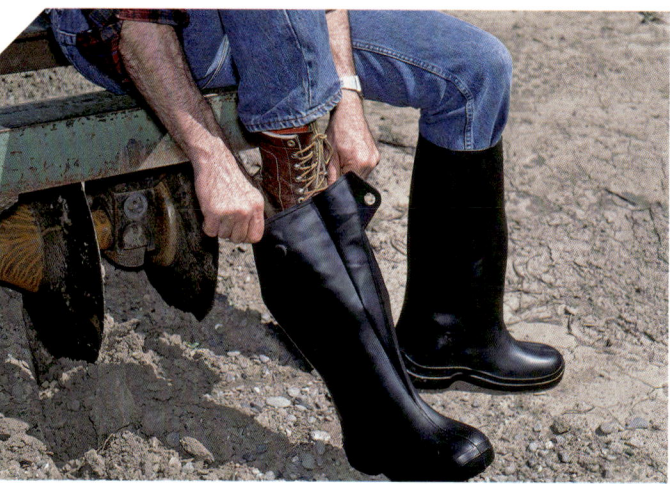

FIGURE 6-13

Protective footwear is also available in overshoe styles to wear over regular shoes or boots.

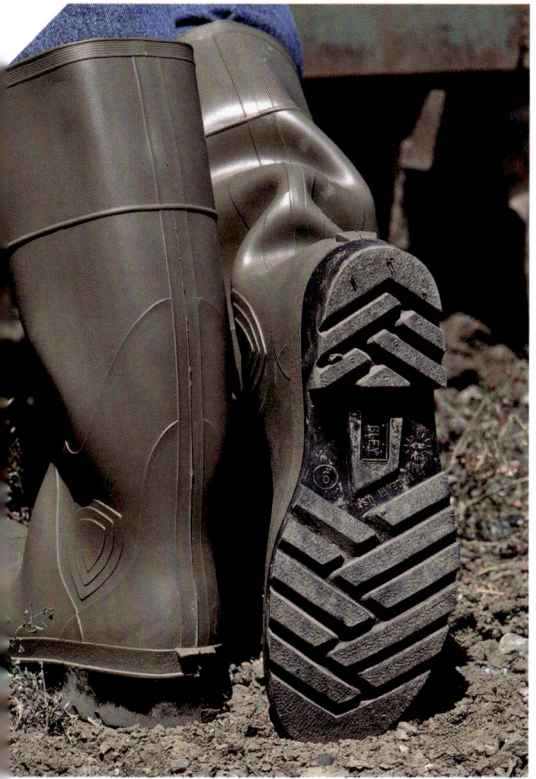

FIGURE 6-14

When choosing chemical-resistant boots, select a sole pattern that cleans easily and does not collect mud.

Footwear

Pesticide handlers often get pesticides on their feet, so you should always wear sturdy shoes and socks when you are around pesticides or pesticide residues. It is recommended that you wear waterproof or chemical-resistant footwear when handling pesticide concentrates or making applications or when residues pose a hazard to your feet. Canvas and leather shoes are not preferred when using pesticides because these materials absorb pesticides easily and cannot be decontaminated. Labels of some pesticides require the use of waterproof boots or boot coverings (Fig. 6-12). Select protective footwear made from rubber or synthetic materials such as PVC, nitrile, neoprene, or butyl. Choose the material based on its ability to protect you from the pesticides with which you work (Table 6-1). Some pesticides, such as 1,3-dichloropropene (Telone II), penetrate most protective waterproof materials.

If a pesticide might get on your feet or lower legs, wear chemical-resistant boots that extend past your ankle and at least halfway up to your knee (commonly known as irrigator boots). You should wear waterproof boots if you will be entering or walking through treated areas when surfaces are still wet with spray. Waterproof footwear is available in conventional boot and overshoe styles (Fig. 6-13). Some boots have internal steel toe caps to protect your toes against falling objects. Select footwear that fits well and is comfortable to wear. Wear the legs of your protective pants on the outside of the footwear to keep out any spray or spills. For increased protection, use rubber bands to seal pant legs tightly around the outside of the boots. Choose a sole design that is slip-proof on wet surfaces and easy to clean (Fig. 6-14).

Waterproof boots do not "breathe" like leather or fabric shoes, so you should wear clean cotton or wool socks to absorb perspiration. If pesticide gets inside your footwear, take it off immediately, thoroughly wash your feet, and put on clean PPE. Keep several pairs of footwear nearby so you can change to a clean set as soon as your boots become damaged or contaminated.

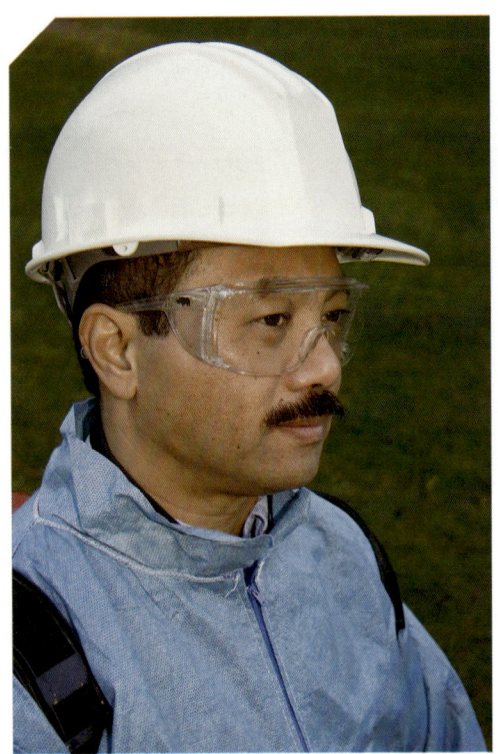

FIGURE 6-15

Unless the label specifies the type of eyewear, you may use safety glasses that have a brow piece and side shields when handling pesticides.

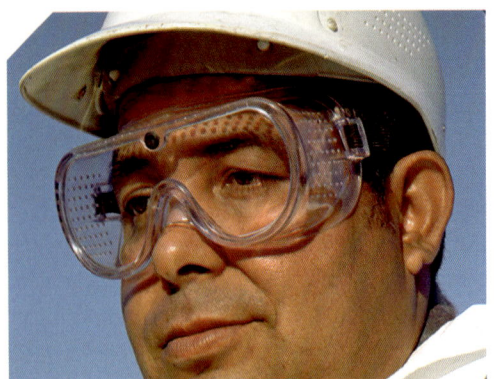

FIGURE 6-16

Protective goggles protect the eyes during mixing and applying pesticides. Some styles allow the user to wear prescription glasses.

PROTECT YOUR EYES

Eyes are extremely sensitive to certain pesticide formulations, especially concentrates. Eyes readily absorb pesticides, so always wear eye protection while handling them. It is essential during mixing and loading and while adjusting, cleaning, or repairing contaminated equipment. In California, regulations require protective eyewear during most pesticide handling activities performed by employee handlers, even if the requirement is not on the pesticide label. Situations in which eye protection is usually not necessary include when

- the operator is working in an enclosed cab.
- pesticides are being injected or incorporated into the soil.
- pesticides are being applied through vehicle-mounted spray nozzles that are located below and behind the operator with the nozzles directed downward.
- vertebrate pest control baits are being applied to vertebrate burrows using equipment that keeps people from touching the material.

Be sure to check California regulations to ensure that your situation does not require you to wear eye protection.

Goggles, a face shield, or safety glasses with shields at both the brow and sides are examples of protective eyewear. Some labels require a particular type of eye protection. If the pesticide label does not specify the type of eye protection, you must at least wear safety glasses that include a brow piece and side shields (Fig. 6-15). If you wear contact lenses, you should consult your eye doctor or physician before using pesticides, because contact lenses absorb pesticides and pass them through to the eye, making chronic exposure an issue.

Goggles and Safety Glasses. Goggles and safety glasses are the most common forms of eye protection. You must always wear the eye protection required by the pesticide label. In California, if specific protective eyewear is not mentioned on the label, you are still required to wear safety glasses, goggles, or a face shield when handling pesticides. To protect the eyes adequately, eyewear must have full side shields (Fig. 6-16). Goggles should either be indirectly vented or unvented, since direct venting allows pesticide entry. Nonfogging lenses are available for most styles, and you can buy solutions to reduce or eliminate fogging of ordinary lenses. You can wear some goggle styles over eyeglasses.

Elastic or synthetic rubber straps hold goggles in place when you wear them. Because elastic straps contain fabric, they easily absorb pesticide and possibly increase exposure to the back of the head. Avoid this problem by using a hood or protective headgear over the strap. Replace or thoroughly wash the elastic band if it becomes contaminated. Straps made of neoprene or other synthetic materials are safer because they are nonabsorbent and easy to clean.

The lenses of safety glasses or goggles may become coated with spray droplets during some pesticide applications. If this happens, carry cleaning supplies or an extra pair of safety glasses or goggles. Check and clean your safety glasses or goggles each time you stop to refill the

PERSONAL PROTECTIVE EQUIPMENT AND PERSONAL SAFETY   145

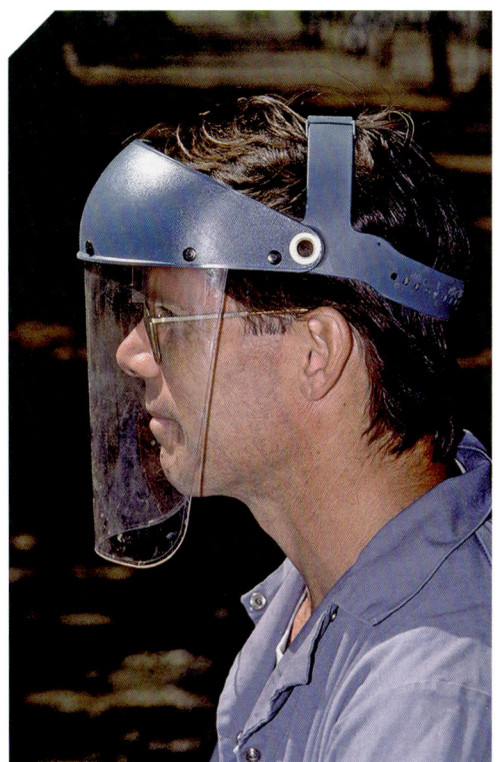

FIGURE 6-17

Face shields provide some eye protection and keep pesticides from splashing onto your face. Wear these with safety glasses or goggles for added eye protection.

spray tank. Use caution, however, to prevent scratching plastic lenses. Never wipe lenses to remove dirt—clean them with soap and water. Scratched lenses make safety glasses or goggles useless.

Face Shields. Face shields (Fig. 6-17) protect your eyes and prevent liquids from splashing onto your face while mixing pesticides. However, you should not use them without additional eye protection during application. This is because they do not prevent airborne sprays or dust from floating in around the edges of the face shield. Face shields are comfortable to wear, allow better air circulation, and provide a greater range of vision than goggles.

Plastic face shields require the same care as goggles to protect them from scratching. When not in use, face shields and goggles should be stored in plastic bags to keep them clean and prevent scratching.

In certain situations, under the California Code of Regulations, you must keep 1 pint of water (or eyewash) with you at all times. This regulation applies to employee handlers when the label requires protective eyewear. Water (or eyewash) can be carried on your person, or it may reside next to you in an enclosed cab or aircraft. If a pesticide gets past your eyewear's protection, you may not have time to look for clean water to flush your eyes because some corrosive and irritant products can cause injury within a few seconds. Therefore, carrying at least a pint of water or eyewash can make the difference for you or your co-workers in an emergency. See Chapter 12 for a detailed description of what to do if pesticide gets in your eyes.

PROTECT YOUR RESPIRATORY TRACT

The respiratory tract consists of the lungs and other parts of the breathing system. It is much more absorbent than the skin. Even if a pesticide label does not require it, consider wearing a respirator if you are handling any product for which the label states "do not breathe vapors or spray mist" or "harmful or fatal if inhaled." In addition, wear a respirator if you will be exposed to any pesticide that can potentially be inhaled.

Some fumigants and a few other pesticide formulations contain a chemical warning additive in the product formulation that alerts you when you begin to inhale the pesticide. Such warning agents are often used when the pesticide active ingredient is highly toxic but is not easily detected by smell. The additive may have a characteristic odor or be a mild irritant to alert you that you need to leave the area or put on a respirator, or it may warn you that your respirator is no longer protecting you.

If regulation, employer policy, permit condition, or the pesticide label mandates respirator use, you must be evaluated by a doctor and declared medically fit before you can wear a respirator on the job.

The State of California has regulations for a respiratory protection program. The following nine elements are required for all users of respirators, including pesticide handlers:
1. Procedures to select the proper respirator for your work site or job.
2. Medical evaluation to determine ability to use a respirator.
3. Fit testing for tight-fitting respirators.
4. Proper use of respirators.
5. Care and maintenance of respirators.
6. Breathing air quality and use for supplied air respirators.
7. Training on hazard recognition and dangers.
8. Training on proper use and care of respirators.
9. Program evaluation on respirator fit, selection, use, and maintenance.

Respiratory Equipment

Description

> Explain the importance of selecting, fit testing, and wearing respiratory devices.

Respirators protect the lungs and respiratory tract from airborne pesticides. You can choose from several types and styles suitable for mixing and applying pesticides. Select respiratory equipment based on the requirements listed on the pesticide label.

Two major groups of respirators are used when dealing with pesticides: air-supplying and air-purifying. Air-purifying respirators use physical and chemical filters to trap and remove contaminants as they pass through the respirator with the air being breathed by the wearer. The pesticide label provides guidance on which type of filters or cartridges to use. Adequate oxygen must be present in the air that is being breathed because an air-purifying respirator does not supply oxygen; it only filters the air that is being breathed. Air-supplying respirators provide clean, uncontaminated air from an outside source. They are used in low-oxygen environments and are generally more expensive. Often their big and bulky size puts a strain on the worker.

Air-purifying devices may be powered or nonpowered. The powered air-purifying respirators use a blower to move the contaminated air through a purifying filter and can be used with either a tight-fitting face piece or a loose-fitting hood. The nonpowered devices can be either half-mask or full-face devices that place a filtration unit between your breathing passage and the contaminated air source. Filters and cartridges are chemical-specific or dust/mist-specific. A combination chemical and dust/mist cartridge is also available. When handling some pesticides, an organic (OV) cartridge is required. The components of a typical nonpowered air-purifying respirator are a snap-on retainer, a prefilter, an air-purifying cartridge, a face piece that contains an exhalation valve, and a harness.

The National Institute for Occupational Safety and Health (NIOSH) is the federal agency responsible for testing and certifying respirators used in conjunction with pesticides (and other non-mining respiratory protection). Approval numbers beginning with the letters TC are assigned to all respirators reviewed by the agency and must be on the box containing the face piece. Pesticide product labels often specify the type of respirator required by listing its TC number. In addition, particulate filters are classified on the basis of oil degradation resistance and filter efficiency. The classification levels for oil degradation resistance are N, not oil resistant; R, oil resistant; and P, oil proof. The filter efficiency for each classification level may be 95, 99, or 100%.

The product formulation, toxicity, and type of application influence the type of respirator needed. Manufacturers use criteria approved by the U.S. EPA to assign PPE respirator requirements on labels (see Table 6-2). When a pesticide label requires a respirator, wear a NIOSH-approved respirator for use with that particular pesticide. Remember, a single type of respirator does not adequately protect you from every pesticide or formulation that you may use.

Respirators need to fit properly to be effective and safe. They should be in good working condition and be cleaned after each day's exposure period. Facial hair negatively affects the way most respirators seal around the face, which keeps them from protecting you adequately.

TABLE 6-2

Label examples based on the EPA respiratory protection criteria

EPA criteria	Vapor pressure (mmHG)	Label statement for respiratory protection	
		Oil in application mix	No oil in application mix
solid pesticides, any toxicity category	NA	Use a NIOSH-approved particulate respirator with any R or P filter with NIOSH approval number prefix TC-84A; or a NIOSH-approved powered air-purifying respirator with HE filter with NIOSH approval number prefix TC-21C.	Use a NIOSH-approved particulate respirator with any N, R, or P filter with NIOSH approval number prefix TC-84A; or a NIOSH-approved powered air-purifying respirator with HE filter with NIOSH approval number prefix TC-21C.
liquid pesticides, toxicity Category I	lower than 1×10^{-05}	Use a NIOSH-approved particulate respirator with an R or P filter with NIOSH approval number prefix TC-84A; or a NIOSH-approved powered air-purifying respirator with an HE filter with NIOSH approval number prefix TC-21C.	Use a NIOSH-approved particulate respirator with any N, R, or P filter with NIOSH approval number prefix TC-84A; or a NIOSH-approved powered air-purifying respirator with an HE filter with NIOSH approval number prefix TC-21C.
liquid pesticides, toxicity Category I	greater than 1×10^{-05}	Use a NIOSH-approved respirator with an organic vapor (OV) cartridge with a combination R or P filter, with NIOSH approval number prefix TC-84A; or a NIOSH-approved powered air-purifying respirator with organic vapor (OV) cartridge and combination HE filter with NIOSH approval number prefix TC-23C; or a NIOSH-approved gas mask with an organic vapor canister with NIOSH approval number prefix TC-14G.	Use a NIOSH-approved respirator with an organic vapor (OV) cartridge with any combination N, R, or P filter with NIOSH approval number prefix TC-84A; or a NIOSH-approved powered air-purifying respirator with organic vapor (OV) cartridge and combination HE filter with NIOSH approval number prefix TC-23C; or a NIOSH-approved gas mask with an organic vapor canister with NIOSH approval number prefix TC-14G.
organic gaseous products applied in enclosed areas	1×10^{-03} or lower	For handling activities in enclosed areas, use either a NIOSH-approved supplied air respirator with NIOSH approval number prefix TC-19C, or a self-contained breathing apparatus (SCBA) with NIOSH approval number TC-13F.	

Regulations prohibit pesticide applicators with facial hair from wearing tight-fitting respirators for this reason.

For more information on protecting your respiratory tract, see Randall et al. 2008.

Testing

California's pesticide regulations require that all respirators be fit tested to the actual wearer before use. Two types of fit tests can be performed: qualitative and quantitative.

A qualitative fit test involves exposing the person wearing the respirator to an irritating, flavored, or strong-smelling chemical (like saccharine, which has a sweet taste). After performing movement and breathing tests, the person reports whether he or she was able to detect any irritation, taste, or smell. Qualitative respirator fit test kits containing detailed instructions can be purchased, but you can also use the instructions for qualitative fit testing provided by OSHA in Title 29 of the Code of Federal Regulations Part 1910.134 (29 CFR 1910.134), Appendix A. Whether you use a kit or online information, you must be careful to follow the provided directions exactly.

One type of quantitative fit test device uses an electronic particle detector to measure the particles in the room and the particles present inside the respirator as the person performs movement and breathing tests. The ratio of these measurements will indicate whether the respirator fits properly. Another type draws a vacuum inside the mask and measures inward leakage. In both cases, these devices generate a fit factor value for comparison to the required fit factors found in the Title 29 regulations cited above.

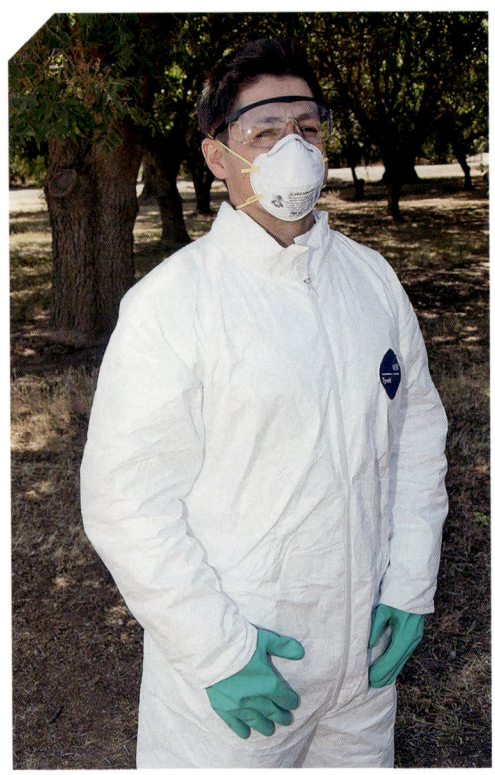

FIGURE 6-18

Some pesticide labels require the use of NIOSH-approved dust/mist filtering respirators.

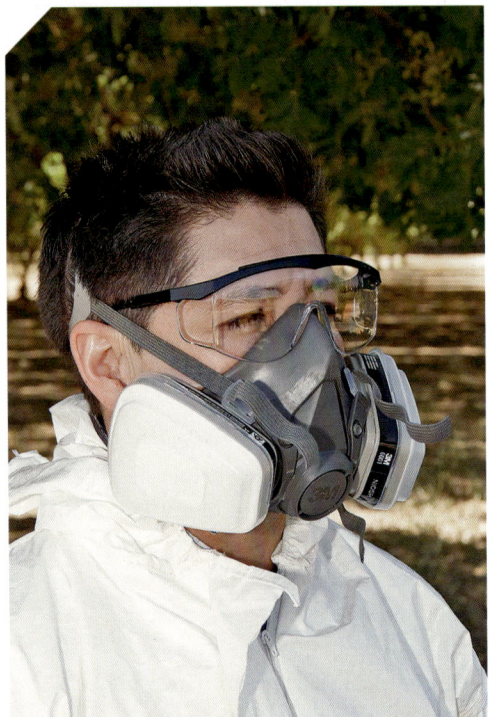

FIGURE 6-19

For certain pesticides, labels require that you wear an organic vapor-removing cartridge respirator with a prefilter approved for pesticides. These must be NIOSH approved.

A trained individual, following the appropriate directions, must perform a respirator fit test on each employee required to wear a tight-fitting respirator at least once per year. Additional fit testing must be performed if you undergo a physical change, such as extreme weight loss or dental work that alters the shape of your face. You should also perform a fit check (also called a user seal check) each time you use a respirator. This process, described in 29 CFR 1910.134 Appendix B-1, involves holding your hands or small plastic bags over the cartridges while wearing the respirator. Inhale to check for leaks around the face piece or exhalation valve. This procedure is known as a negative pressure check. Alternatively, you can perform a positive pressure check by covering the exhalation valve and gently exhaling to check for leaks. Repair or replace the respirator if you find any leaks.

Air-Purifying Respirators

Dust and Mist Masks (Filtering Face Pieces, Particulate Respirators). The simplest form of respiratory protection is a disposable dust and mist mask (Fig. 6-18). Disposable dust and mist masks are lightweight, soft, and fairly comfortable to wear. Two elastic straps hold them in place. Most have soft metal bands at the top edge. Shape this around the bridge of your nose for a better seal. All disposable masks used for pesticide handling must bear the NIOSH approval number TC-84A or indicate that it has been approved in accordance with part 84 of the Code of Federal Regulations (42 CFR part 84). NIOSH-approved respirators with R, P, or HE filters are suitable for products containing oil or products that have instructions that allow or require application with an oil-containing material. For products that do not contain oil and whose labels bear no instructions that allow or require application with oil-containing materials, NIOSH-approved respirators with N, R, P, or HE filters are suitable. The pesticide label refers to these approval numbers when it requires you to use this type of respiratory protection.

Cartridge Respirators. Some pesticide labels require the use of cartridge respirators with the NIOSH approval number TC-23C (Fig. 6-19) or indications that it has been approved in accordance with 42 CFR part 84. NIOSH-approved OV cartridge respirators with R, P, or HE prefilters are suitable for products containing oil or products that have instructions that would allow or require application with an oil-containing material. For products that do not contain oil and whose labels bear no instructions that allow or require application with oil-containing materials, NIOSH-approved OV cartridge respirators with N, R, P, or HE prefilters are suitable. The pesticide label refers to these approval numbers when it requires you to use this type of respiratory protection.

Cartridge respirators remove low levels of pesticide vapors, dusts, and mists from the air you breathe. Do not use these for protection against fumigants (gases). Never use cartridge respirators in atmospheres that pose an immediate threat to life or health. This includes atmospheres containing gases such as carbon monoxide or hydrogen sulfide or atmospheres with an oxygen level below 19.5%.

PERSONAL PROTECTIVE EQUIPMENT AND PERSONAL SAFETY 149

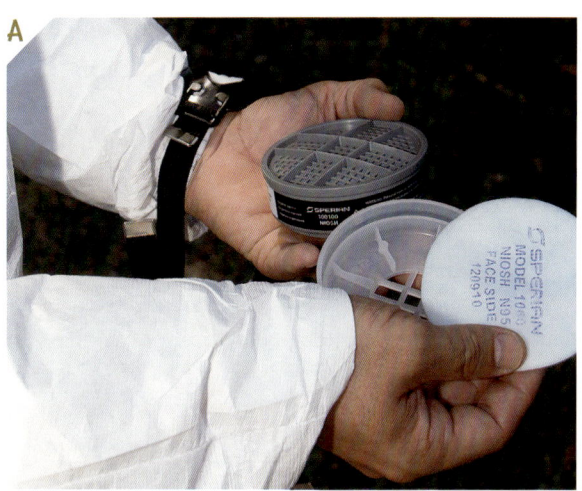
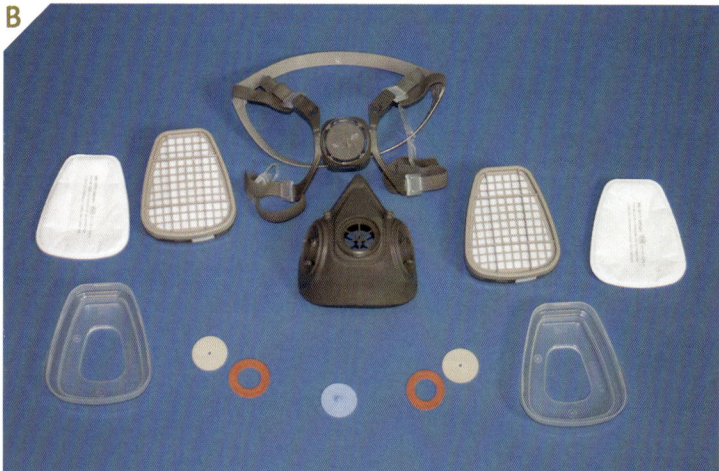

FIGURE 6-20

Many cartridge respirators have removable filtering cartridges. Be sure the cartridges you use are approved for the type of pesticide you are applying. For example, cartridges designated "OV" can be used to protect you from most pesticides.

Chemical cartridge respirators (TC-23C) and gas masks with canisters (TC–14G) absorb harmful vapors or gases. In addition, chemical cartridge respirators and gas masks with canisters usually have an external dust/mist filter. Chemical cartridge respirators come in both half-face mask and full-face mask styles. The cartridge must be appropriate for the particular contaminant (organic vapor, phosphine, etc.).

Cartridge respirators have fitted rubber face pieces and two-stage cartridge filters (Fig. 6-20A). In some models the filter cartridges are replaceable, while others require replacing the entire respirator. Cartridge respirators have a one-way exhalation valve. Inhaled air must pass through the cartridge filters, but the valve permits exhaled air to bypass the filters. At least two adjustable elastic headbands hold the face pieces in place (Fig. 6-20B). Cartridges made for pesticides include a particulate prefilter to mechanically trap airborne particles. They also have an activated carbon organic vapor cartridge to adsorb gases (Fig. 6-21).

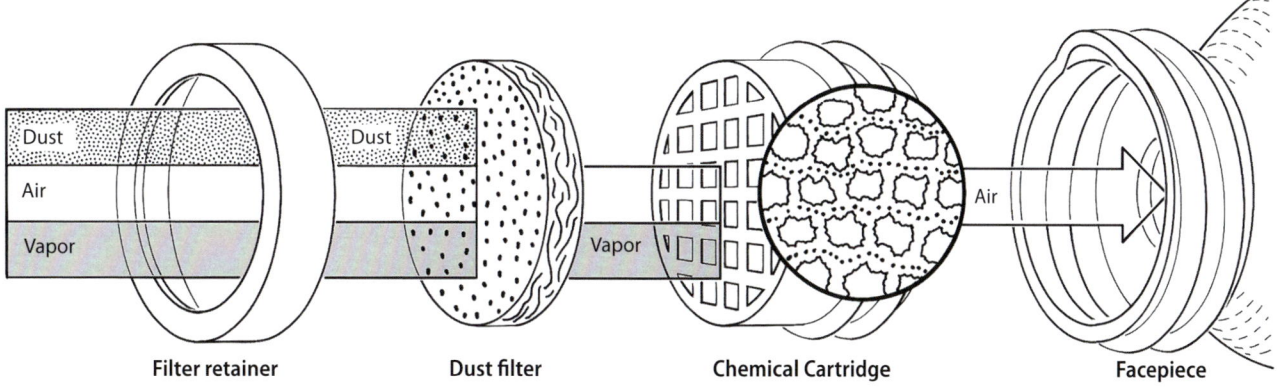

FIGURE 6-21

Respirator cartridges include a mechanical dust filter that removes dust and droplet particles and an activated charcoal chemical cartridge to remove vapors.

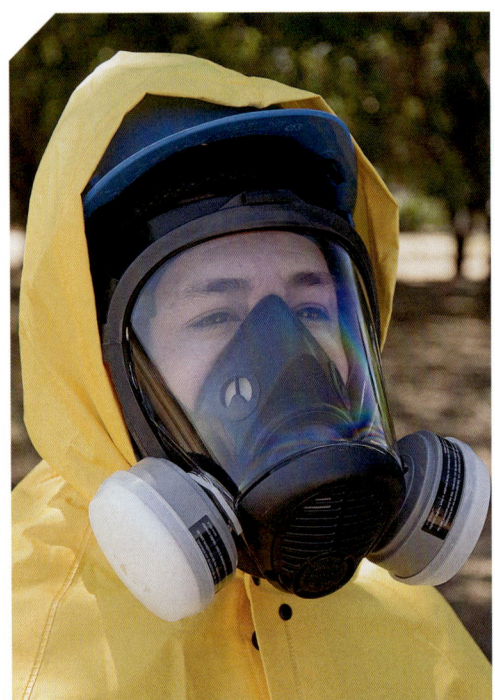

FIGURE 6-22

Some cartridge respirators have built-in eye protection.

The cartridges on respirators have a limited effective life. Replace the organic vapor cartridges if you
- have difficulty breathing
- begin to smell a pesticide odor
- detect any pesticide or pesticidelike taste
- experience any irritation

These signs may indicate that the organic vapor unit cannot absorb more pesticide and has reached the end of its service life. Besides the above guidelines, change cartridges following pesticide label requirements, equipment manufacturer's recommendations, or, lacking information to the contrary, at the end of each daily work period.

You need eye protection when using any respirator. Therefore, be sure you can wear the respirator comfortably with goggles, safety glasses, or a face shield. Some cartridge respirators include a full–face piece with built-in eye protection (Fig. 6-22). You must always wear all required PPE.

Powered Air-Purifying Respirators. A powered air-purifying respirator (TC-21C) forces filtered air through a hose to a hood, helmet, or face mask (Fig. 6-23A). You usually wear the motor, pump, batteries, and filters on a waist belt (Fig. 6-23B). These devices have large, efficient filters and provide comfortable protection for lengthy application jobs. Like other cartridge respirators, use these only when the atmosphere poses no immediate threat to life or health. Use them only when the oxygen level is 19.5% or greater.

These respirators often incorporate face shields for eye protection. They are comfortable to wear because the user does not actively force air through filters or valves. The constant supply of forced air around the user's face eliminates the need for a mask-to-face seal. A person with facial hair can wear this type of respirator as long as it has a hood, helmet, or other loose-fitting-type mask. Any tight-fitting mask must still have a face-to-face piece seal free of facial hair.

Air-Supplying Respirators

You can get maximum respiratory protection from an air-supply respirator (also referred to as an atmosphere-supplying respirator). Use this type of equipment when working in areas being fumigated. These also protect you when working with concentrated amounts of highly toxic pesticides.

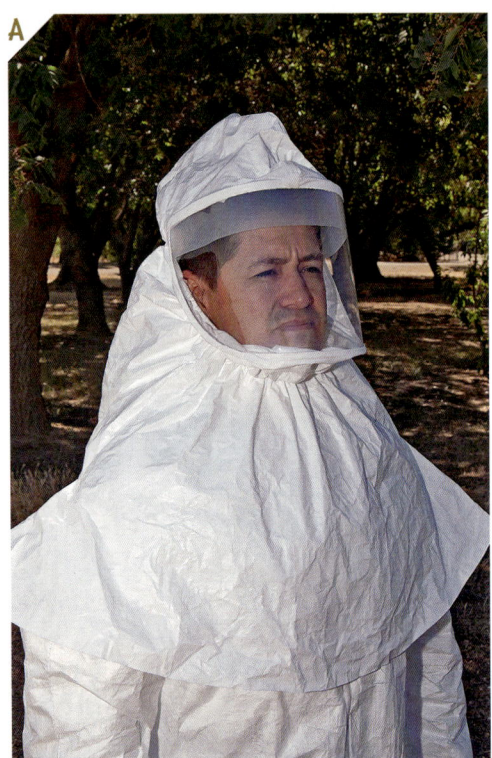

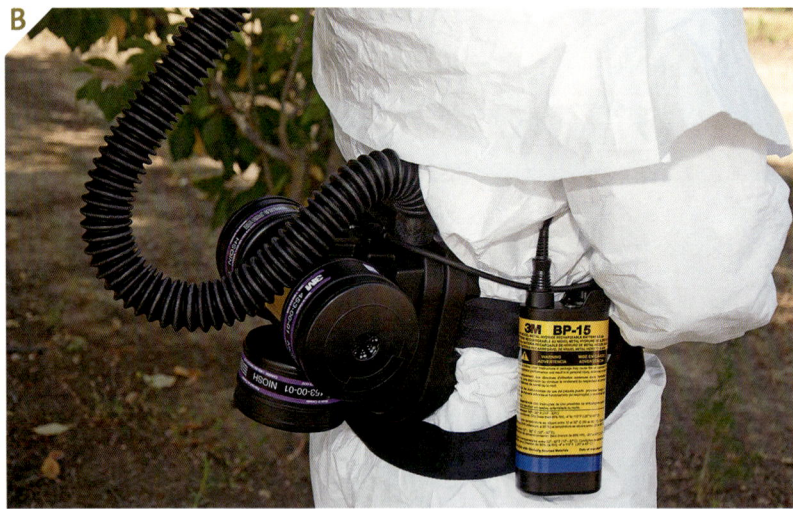

FIGURE 6-23

A battery-powered fan forces filtered air through a flexible hose into a hood (A) in this powered air-purifying respirator. This design allows you to wear eyeglasses. People with beards and long sideburns can use this style of respirator. The filters, motor, and battery pack are worn on a waist belt (B).

Wear this type of respirator if the atmosphere contains less than 19.5% oxygen. Emergency workers wear these when responding to toxic spills or fires or when rescuing injured people. Several styles and types are available. Supplied air respirators do not require filters or cartridges to remove toxic materials. This is because they provide an outside source of clean, uncontaminated air. There are two types of atmosphere-supplying respirators, as follows.

Self-Contained Breathing Apparatus. A self-contained breathing apparatus (SCBA) provides clean air from pressurized tanks that the user wears, similar to a scuba diver (Fig. 6-24).

The SCBA (TC-13F) uses a compressed-air tank and provides complete respiratory protection against toxic gases in an oxygen-deficient environment. It provides a limited quantity of air. Once you exhaust the air supply, the system cannot provide any protection. Therefore manufacturers equip these units with warning devices to alert users when the air supply is getting low. Air tanks may be heavy and bulky, but they give unlimited mobility.

Supplied Air Respirator. Supplied air respirators (TC-19C) use long hoses to supply air to a full–face mask, and may or may not have a blower or compressor. External air models connect the wearer to a distant air pump or stationary tank by means of a hose. If you are using an external air model, locate the air pump where safe, fresh air is available.

Hose-connected supplied air respirators provide a large or unlimited quantity of fresh air. However, the range of available hose restricts the wearer's mobility. The maximum legal hose length is 300 feet. Long hoses are cumbersome and awkward to handle: users must take precautions to avoid kinking, snagging, or damaging the hose.

Supplied air respirators use either half- or full-face pieces; full-face piece models provide eye protection. Other models attach to a hood or helmet that encloses the entire head and has a clear plastic face shield.

Face pieces use a pressure demand regulator that admits fresh air into the mask as the wearer begins to inhale. Airflow diminishes when the user exhales but never to the extent that the pesticide-laden atmosphere can enter the mask. Self-contained units use this method because of the limited air supply. Hoods provide a continuous flow of fresh air around the entire head, whether inhaling or exhaling. Hoods do not require critical sealing around the face and can be worn with beards, long sideburns, and eyeglasses. Hoods do not require fit testing. Use a hood when the air supply comes from an external source through a hose.

Cleaning and maintenance of air-supplying respirators are critical to their safe operation. Masks must fit properly and exhalation valves have to be in good working order to prevent any outside air from entering. Keep hoods free of holes or tears. Regularly inspect air hoses, from both self-contained tanks and from air pumps, and replace them if cracked or worn. Keep air pressure regulators clean, dry, and protected from damage. If the air-regulating systems on SCBA or supplied air respirators require repair, only factory-trained or authorized technicians should work on them.

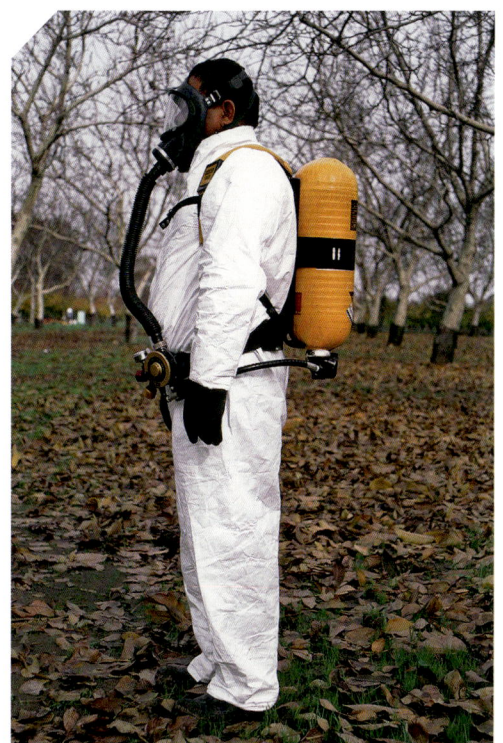

FIGURE 6-24

This self-contained breathing apparatus (SCBA) provides the wearer with uncontaminated air from a compressed air tank.

Cleaning and Maintaining PPE

Always keep PPE in good working condition. PPE is effective only as long as it is free from pesticide contamination and works properly. Therefore, you must frequently clean and inspect this equipment. Replace or repair equipment when you find a problem.

When you finish any work in which you are handling pesticides or are exposed to them, remove your PPE right away. Start by washing the outside of your gloves with detergent and water before removing the rest of your PPE. Wash the outside of other chemical-resistant items before you remove your gloves. This practice helps you avoid contacting the contaminated part of the items while you are removing them, thus keeping the inside surface from becoming contaminated. If any other clothes have pesticides on them, change them also. Determine whether contaminated items should be disposed of or cleaned for reuse. For more information, see Randall et al. 2008.

Respirators

Extend the life of cartridge or supplied air respirators through regular cleaning and safe storage. The ability of a respirator to protect you from harmful pesticides depends in part on how well you maintain it.

Inspection. You should inspect your respirator for wear and damage twice: once before using it for the first time each day and again before cleaning it at the end of each day. Check the headbands for fraying, tears, or loss of elasticity and replace them if necessary. Remove filters and replace the gaskets if they are defective (brittle, broken, or warped). Never use these types of cartridge respirators without gaskets since gaskets prevent contaminated air from bypassing the filter cartridge. Valve assemblies are essential parts of a cartridge respirator and must be in good working order. Disassemble and inspect valve flaps for wear, deformities, or punctures. Replace parts if you suspect they might leak. Check the threads of all valves and cartridge parts to make sure they are in good condition and that the valve seats are smooth. Look for cracks and scratches.

Examine the face piece for cracks, cuts, scratches, and any signs of aging. If you find damage, replace the defective parts.

When replacing items on a respirator, use only approved replacement parts for that specific brand and model. If you use unapproved parts, the respirator is not in compliance with the law and may be ineffective. If you keep a respirator for emergency use or as a backup, inspect it at least monthly.

Cleaning. After removing filters from reusable cartridge respirators, soak the face piece, gaskets, and valve parts in a solution of warm water and mild liquid detergent. Do not use abrasives or cleaning compounds containing alcohol or other organic solvents. You must use sanitizers if more than one worker wears the same respirator. Use a soft brush or cloth to remove any pesticide residue (Fig. 6-25). Rinse the respirator and valve parts in clean water. Air-dry your

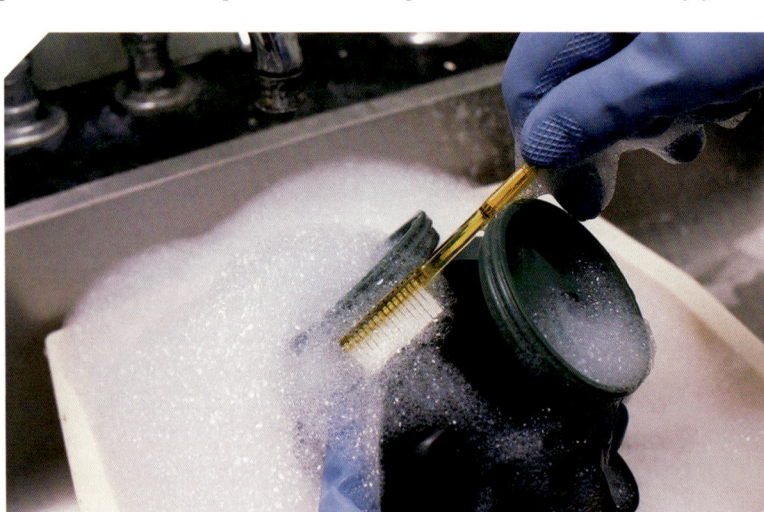

FIGURE 6-25

After use, remove cartridges and wash respirators in warm, soapy water. Use a soft brush or cloth to remove pesticide residue.

filters rather than leaving them in direct sunlight or using applied heat. Heat and sunlight can damage filters or cause them to wear out more quickly.

After it is completely dry, reassemble the respirator and store it in a clean plastic bag. This protects it from dirt and environmental deterioration.

Dispose of one-time-use cartridge respirators according to the manufacturer's instructions. Do not try to clean disposable cartridge respirators.

If you remove your respirator between handling activities, follow these guidelines:
- Wipe the respirator body and face piece with a clean cloth.
- Replace caps, if available, over cartridges, canisters, and prefilters.
- Seal the respirator in a sturdy, airtight container, such as a plastic bag with a zip closure. If you do not seal the respirator immediately after each use, the disposable parts will have to be replaced more often because cartridges and canisters continue to collect impurities as long as they are exposed to the air (Randall et al. 2008).

Boots and Gloves

Wash rubber boots and gloves under running water before you take them off to remove pesticide residues. Use a detergent solution and soft brush, then rinse with clean water (Fig. 6-26). Do not get the insides of the boots wet. At the end of each day, wash rubber gloves with soap and warm water. Inspect them for holes while washing and discard the gloves if you find any. You may wash gloves in a washing machine by placing them into a cloth net bag. Use warm water and wash according to the instructions given below for protective clothing. Turn gloves inside out for drying. Store dry boots and gloves in plastic bags to keep them clean and prevent deterioration. Remember that glove liners cannot be washed and reused. You must discard glove liners at the end of each pesticide handling activity.

Face Shields and Goggles

Wash goggles, face shields, shielded safety glasses, respirator bodies, and face pieces after each day of use. Use care when washing face shields and goggles to avoid scratching the plastic. Submerge them in warm, soapy water. If necessary, remove pesticide residue with a soft, wet cloth or soft brush (Fig. 6-27). Do not rub antifogging lenses, since this reduces their effectiveness. Rinse well with clear water and air-dry or blot with a soft cotton cloth; rubbing increases chances of scratching. Inspect goggles and face shields for excessive scratches and for cracks and loss of headband elasticity. You can replace scratched lenses on many styles without replacing the entire goggle. Store goggles and face shields in paper bags to keep them clean.

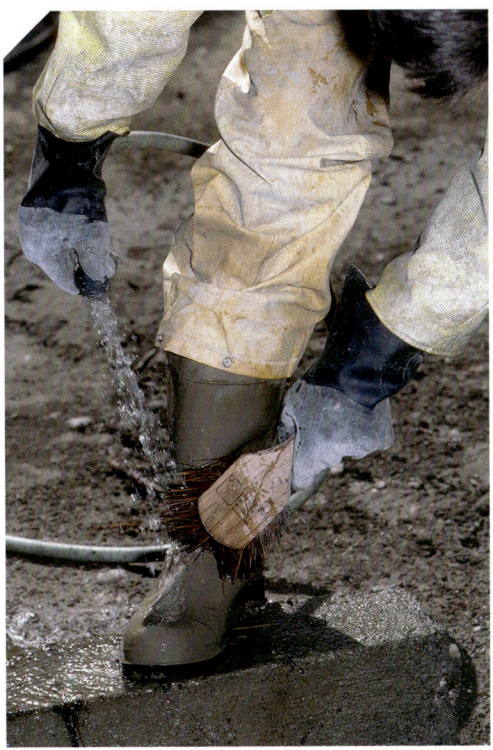

FIGURE 6-26

Wash boots before removing them. Use a brush and soapy water, then rinse with clean water. Do not get the boots wet inside. Let boots air out after washing; store them in a clean plastic bag once they dry.

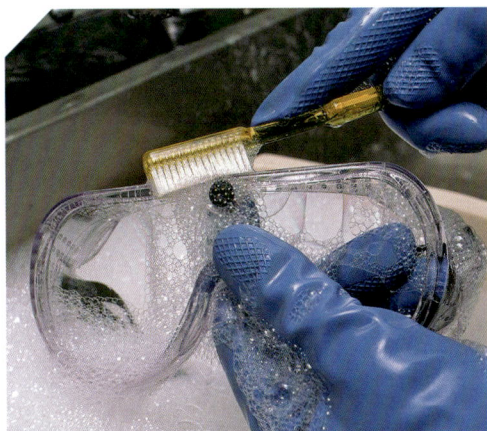

FIGURE 6-27

Wash safety glasses, goggles, and face shields in warm, soapy water. Use a soft brush or cloth to remove pesticide residue. Blot dry and store in a clean plastic bag.

> **SIDEBAR 6-2**
>
> ### TECHNIQUES FOR WASHING PESTICIDE-CONTAMINATED CLOTHING AND PPE
>
> **A. PROCEDURE FOR WASHING PESTICIDE-CONTAMINATED CLOTHING**
>
> 1. Keep pesticide-contaminated clothing separate from all other laundry.
> 2. Do not handle contaminated clothing with bare hands; wear rubber gloves or shake clothing from plastic bag into washer.
> 3. Wash only small amounts of clothing at a time. Do not combine clothing contaminated with different pesticides; wash these in separate loads.
> 4. Before washing, presoak clothing:
>   - a. Soak in tub or automatic washer or spray garments outdoors with a garden hose.
>   - b. Use a commercial solvent to soak product or apply prewash spray or liquid laundry detergent to soiled spots.
> 5. Wash garments in a washing machine using the hottest water temperature, full water level, and normal (12-minute) wash cycle. Use the maximum recommended amount of liquid laundry detergent. Never use bleach or ammonia to wash contaminated clothing—they do not remove most pesticides, and when mixed with pesticides, they release toxic vapors that can kill you.
> 6. If you notice pesticide odor, visible spots, or stains, repeat step 5 several times until clothing is fully clean.
> 7. Clean washing machine before using for other laundry by repeating step 5 using full amount of hot water, normal wash cycle, and laundry detergent, but no clothing.
> 8. Hang laundry outdoors on a clothesline to avoid contaminating automatic dryer.
>
> Do not attempt to wash heavily contaminated clothing; destroy it by transporting it to an approved disposal site. These suggestions will help you reduce the likelihood that your family's laundry will be contaminated by pesticides:
>
> 1. Whenever possible, wear disposable protective clothing that can be destroyed after use.
> 2. Always wear all required protective clothing when working with pesticides.
> 3. Wear clean protective clothing daily when working with pesticides. Wash contaminated clothing daily.
> 4. Remove contaminated clothing at work site and empty pockets and cuffs. Place clothing in A clean plastic bag until it can be laundered. Keep contaminated clothing separated from all other laundry.
> 5. Remove clothing immediately if it has had a pesticide concentrate spilled on it.
>
> **B. PROCEDURE FOR WASHING CONTAMINATED PPE**
>
> 1. Wash only a few items at a time so there is plenty of agitation and water for dilution.
> 2. Wash in a washing machine using a heavy-duty liquid detergent and hot water for the wash cycle. Set your washer to the longest heavy-duty wash cycle and two rinse cycles.
> 3. Use two entire machine cycles to wash items that are moderately to heavily contaminated. (If PPE is too contaminated, bundle it in a plastic bag, label the bag, and take it to a household hazardous waste collection site.)
> 4. Run the washer through at least one additional entire cycle without clothing using detergent and hot water to clean the machine before any other laundry is washed.

Chemical-Resistant Clothing

Do not re-wear contaminated chemical-resistant clothing until you have washed it. Wash contaminated garments at the end of each workday. Immediate washing reduces the chances of you or others being exposed to any residues. Throw away clothing that has been saturated with pesticides; send all contaminated clothing to a site approved for pesticide residues. Local agencies allow burning in some locations, but first check with the agricultural commissioner's office. Clean moderately or lightly contaminated clothing by washing. Throw away all single-use (disposable) chemical-resistant clothing at the end of each workday.

Change out of contaminated clothing at your work site if possible. Empty pockets and cuffs of garments to remove excess pesticide residue. Until they can be laundered, place contaminated garments into a clean plastic bag. Never reuse plastic bags, since they may acquire a buildup of pesticide residues. Do not combine contaminated clothing with any other laundry before, during, or after washing.

Work Clothing. Launder in a washing machine using hot water and liquid laundry detergent. Liquid detergent removes oil-based pesticides better than powdered detergent. Use the maximum amount recommended in the detergent instructions. Set the washing machine to its longest cycle (at least 12 minutes) and use the highest water level. Use household bleach if necessary but be aware that bleach does not contribute to the decontamination process (see Sidebar 6-2A). You may also wish to soak work clothing in hot, soapy water for at least half an hour. This includes long-sleeved shirts, full-length pants, cotton coveralls, socks, and underwear. To improve pesticide removal, apply a prewash product such as a solvent soak, prewash spray, or liquid laundry detergent. Add extra amounts to heavily soiled spots.

Always wash pesticide-contaminated items separately from the family laundry. Otherwise, pesticide residues may be transferred to the other laundry and may harm you or your family. Separate clothing contaminated with different types of pesticide. Do not combine these into one wash load. When putting clothing into the washing machine, protect your hands from exposure by wearing gloves (Fig. 6-28). Check for garments that have a pesticide odor or visible pesticide spots or stains. Rewash these one or two more times in the same manner.

After washing is completed, run the washer through another complete cycle using hot water and detergent but without any laundry. This step helps to remove pesticide residues left in the washer and prevents contaminating other loads of laundry.

Whenever possible, hang washed clothing outdoors for drying. The ultraviolet light in sunlight breaks down many pesticides, and air drying helps avoid contaminating the clothes dryer. If you use a clothes dryer, never combine the washed work clothing with other laundry.

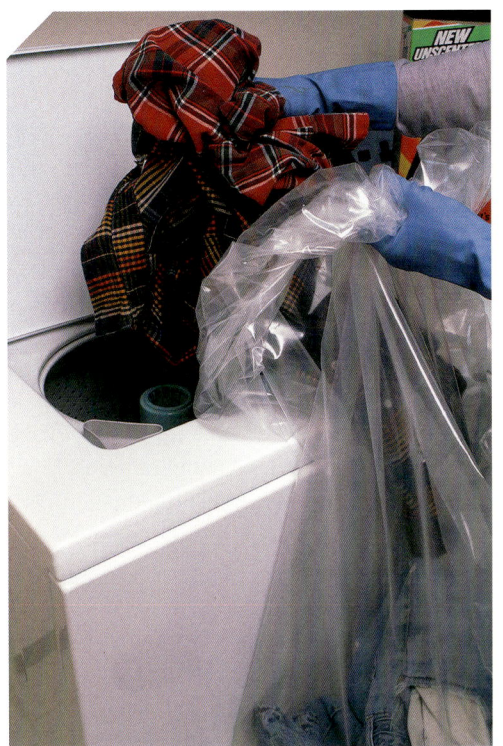

FIGURE 6.28

Avoid touching pesticide-contaminated work clothing with your bare hands. Wear rubber gloves or dump the clothing into the washer from the plastic bag. Do not combine contaminated clothing with any other household clothing.

Washing PPE

Be sure that the people who clean and maintain your PPE know that touching these pesticide-contaminated items can harm them. Instruct them to wear gloves and an apron and work in a well-ventilated area, if possible, and avoid inhaling steam from the washer or dryer.

Follow the manufacturer's instructions for cleaning chemical-resistant items. If the manufacturer instructs you to clean the item but gives no detailed instructions, follow the steps in "Procedure for Washing Contaminated PPE" in Sidebar 6-2B. Some chemical-resistant items that are not flat, such as gloves, footwear, and coveralls, must be washed twice—once to clean the outside of the item and a second time after turning the item inside out. Some chemical-resistant items, such as heavy-duty boots and rigid hats or helmets, can be washed by hand using hot water and a heavy-duty liquid detergent.

Storing PPE

Never use PPE for any other purpose. When not in use, keep it stored in a clean, dry place, protected from temperature extremes and bright light. If possible, store these items in sealable plastic bags. Light, heat, dirt, and air pollutants contribute to the deterioration of rubber, plastic, and synthetic rubber products. Never store any PPE in areas where you keep pesticides.

PROBLEMS ASSOCIATED WITH PPE

You may experience problems or occasional frustrations with PPE. Sometimes these problems cause applicators to become careless and stop wearing the required PPE. Fortunately, you can overcome most problems. First, select the right type of equipment for the job. Make sure equipment fits properly and is in good working order. Finally, if possible, avoid applications when the temperature is too warm.

Fitting

Accurate sizing helps to improve comfort by eliminating binding or slipping. Properly fitted respiratory equipment prevents unsafe air leaks. When selecting chemical-resistant pants and jackets for the correct size, try them on with the same weight of regular clothing you would wear during an actual pesticide application.

If weather is cold, wear a long-sleeved shirt and sweater or coat under the chemical-resistant jacket. Be sure you are comfortable and can move freely, without binding. During hot weather, wear lightweight cotton clothing under the PPE. This provides an absorbent layer and assists in cooling your body.

Discomfort and Inconvenience

Discomfort and inconvenience are the main reasons why people dislike wearing PPE. Eye protection fogs up, becomes covered with spray, and restricts the wearer's range of vision. PPE can be cold during cold weather and very hot in warm or hot weather. Heavy, stiff materials can restrict movement. Gloves impair feeling in the hands, promote sweating, and can be cold or hot, depending on the weather. Respirators are uncomfortable to wear if they restrict breathing.

Despite these problems, you must always wear required PPE during mixing and application. If you become uncomfortable, stop and make adjustments or replace the equipment with another style. Whenever possible, plan pesticide applications during times when the temperature is moderate. Take short breaks and get out of the PPE for a few minutes, especially if temperatures are high. If conditions are too extreme, trade off jobs with a co-worker to reduce problems associated with working in extreme temperatures.

Limits to Protection

PPE has limitations to the amount of protection provided: it never completely protects you. You still must prevent pesticides from being spilled, splashed, or sprayed onto your body. The equipment helps to reduce exposure, but you must do everything possible to prevent the exposure from happening. Some pesticides can penetrate protective materials, and pesticide solvents and adjuvants may enhance penetration.

Pesticides confined next to your skin cannot dissipate through air movement or volatilization. Therefore, if you get pesticides on your skin or clothing before putting on PPE, the equipment may increase the amount of pesticide absorbed. You will also contaminate the inside of the protective garment. Always wear clean PPE over clean clothing.

Engineering Controls

Engineering controls have been developed to protect people as they are mixing, loading, and applying pesticides in a variety of situations. These protective devices are considered PPE, even though they are not worn on the body, and employers are required to provide them if they are mandated by pesticide labels or California regulation. Engineering controls include enclosed cabs, closed mixing systems, pesticide packaging, and atmosphere-monitoring equipment.

Enclosed Cabs. Enclosed cabs installed on tractors protect you from exposure to pesticides (Fig. 6-29). Some types provide you protection from spray droplets and mists and offer a comfortable air-conditioned environment as well. These cabs, however, do not replace the label respirator requirements. Respirators, if required, must be worn while making an application from inside this type of cab. Using an enclosed cab does, however, eliminate the temperature restrictions on applications when applying pesticides that require the use of chemical-resistant PPE (above 80°F during the day and 85°F at night).

Other types of enclosed cabs are acceptable for respiratory protection. Properly designed and maintained cabs provide a high degree of protection. These work well in orchards and vineyards or other areas where pesticide exposure potential is high. Most models offer heating and cooling of the air forced into the cab for added operator comfort. Cab insulation reduces noise from the tractor and spraying equipment. Many have front and rear window washers and wipers.

Cabs acceptable for respiratory protection protect you only if you regularly clean and service them. Clean or replace pesticide filters whenever they exceed their filtering capacity. If you mix pesticides or get out of the cab during a pesticide application, put on PPE. However, be sure to remove contaminated PPE before getting back inside the cab. For maximum convenience and

PERSONAL PROTECTIVE EQUIPMENT AND PERSONAL SAFETY 157

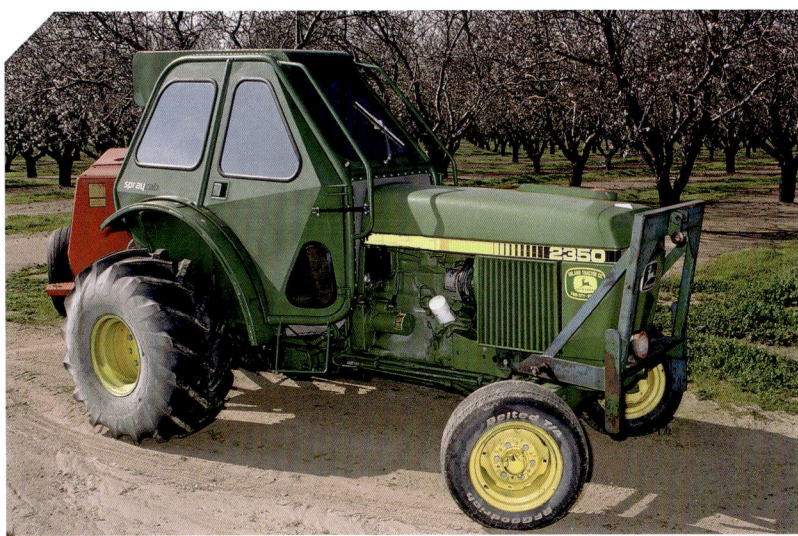

FIGURE 6-29

Enclosed cabs protect operators against pesticide exposure. This model includes a pesticide air filtering system that eliminates the need for the operator to wear a respirator while inside the cab.

protection, assign another person the duties of mixing pesticides and refilling the sprayer.

Select a respiratory-enclosed cab based on your needs and expectations. For example, consider the power source for the blower. Units that connect to the tractor hydraulic system move large volumes of air but may be noisy. Electric motor drives are quieter but may not have as much power because of the limitations of the tractor electrical system. The volume of air that the unit supplies influences the amount of protection provided.

Factors that contribute to the filtering ability of these cabs include
- size of the unit
- volume of air being moved
- number of filter stages
- type of filtering material used
- appropriateness of the filter media to the pesticides being used

Multiple-stage filters that include a prefilter, a high-efficiency particulate air filter (HEPA), and an activated carbon filter are the safest for reducing pesticide exposure. Blowers that move large volumes of air must have large-capacity filters.

Other features of enclosed cabs that might influence their function include
- the visibility afforded the operator
- how the height of the cab relates to application sites where it will be used
- the strength of the cab for protecting the operator from tree limbs or in case of tractor rollover
- the availability of heating and air-conditioning

Closed Mixing Systems. Employees must use a closed mixing system when mixing, loading, diluting, or transferring liquid formulations of pesticides with the signal word DANGER (Fig. 6-30) if these pesticides are being used for the production of an agricultural commodity. They must also use closed systems when loading or transferring dry formulations of pesticides with the signal word DANGER after mixing these with water or other diluent.

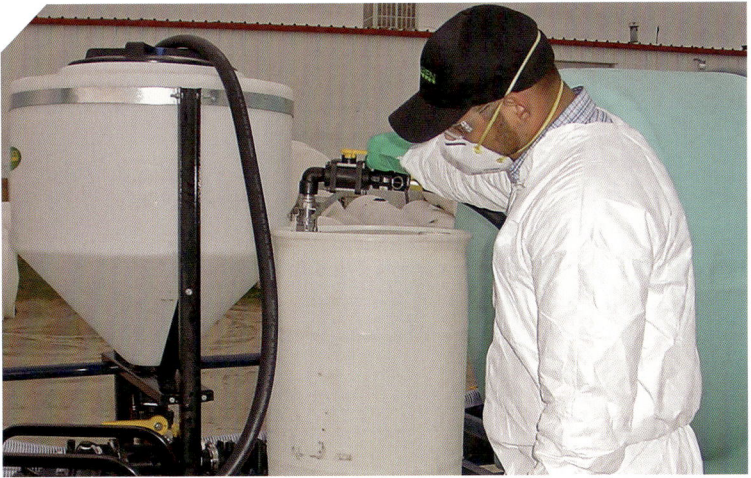

FIGURE 6-30

Closed mixing systems are required when mixing more than 1 gallon per day of liquid DANGER pesticides for the production of an agricultural commodity. These systems allow you to accurately measure the liquid pesticides. Most also rinse the empty containers.

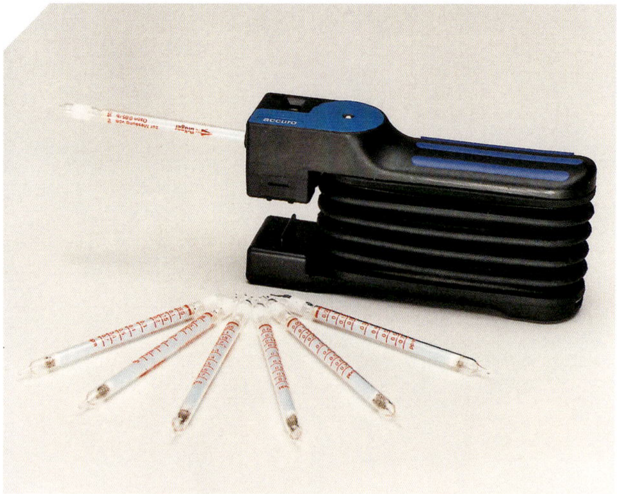

FIGURE 6-31
When working with fumigants, use an atmosphere monitoring device before entering treated areas. Color changes in the glass tubes indicate the concentration of a toxicant in the atmosphere. Specific types of tubes are used for different fumigants.

Closed mixing systems enable accurate and safe measuring of pesticides being put into the spray tank. Not all situations require closed mixing systems. To find out if your situation requires the use of a closed mixing system, review regulations on the DPR website, cdpr.ca.gov/docs/legbills/calcode. See the DPR Pesticide Safety Information Series A-3 for legal requirements of closed mixing systems.

Packaging. Special pesticide packaging helps to reduce exposure to concentrated pesticide active ingredients. This packaging includes preweighed water-soluble bags and packets of powdered formulations. These dissolve in the spray tank, reducing your exposure to the powder and dust. Pesticides packaged in this way constitute closed mixing systems according to regulations.

Atmosphere Monitoring Equipment. Never enter an enclosed fumigated area, even after venting, without measuring for toxic levels of pesticide vapors. Several different atmosphere monitoring devices detect and measure vapors (Fig. 6-31). When taking measurements, wear all required PPE or use remote sensing equipment. Take measurements in several locations within the enclosed space, since fumigant vapors sometimes become trapped in localized pockets.

Choose atmosphere monitoring equipment that is suitable to the type of fumigation work you perform. Be certain that the equipment provides accurate readings at the concentration levels you encounter. Learn about the shortcomings of these devices, since other contaminants in the atmosphere can produce erroneous readings. Get proper training on this equipment so you can reliably detect dangerous levels of pesticides.

Chapter 6 Review Questions

1. **PPE protects you from exposure to pesticides by _____.**
   - ☐ a. keeping dry and liquid material off your skin
   - ☐ b. covering only the most vulnerable part of your body
   - ☐ c. preventing you from having on-the-job accidents

2. **Which of the following is required training for fieldworkers who will enter treated areas within 30 days of the expiration of any restricted-entry interval?**
   - ☐ a. first aid for pesticide injury and poisoning and emergency decontamination instruction
   - ☐ b. posting requirements for sites that have been treated with DANGER or WARNING pesticides
   - ☐ c. proper use of a closed mixing system or other engineering control used to protect workers from exposure

3. **Pesticide handlers must be trained in which three subject areas?**
   - ☐ a. integrated pest management, pest identification, and application equipment maintenance
   - ☐ b. closed mixing systems, PPE requirements, and reading the pesticide label
   - ☐ c. using pesticides safely, emergencies and health, and legal information and worker rights

4. **Who is responsible for purchasing PPE required by pesticide labels and ensuring that it is properly cleaned and maintained?**
   - ☐ a. workers
   - ☐ b. employers
   - ☐ c. pest control advisers

5. **Match the PPE with the protection it offers.**

1. coverall	a. protects you from pesticides that have moderate or high dermal toxicity or are skin irritants
2. chemical-resistant suit	b. protects your coveralls and guards you from splashes, spills, and billowing dust
3. chemical-resistant apron	c. protects your lungs from pesticides in the air
4. chemical-resistant hat	d. protects you when a large amount of pesticide could be deposited on your clothing over an extended period of time
5. gloves	e. protects your eyes and prevents liquids from splashing onto your face during mixing
6. face shield	f. protects you from overhead exposure or exposure to a lot of airborne particles
7. respirator	g. keeps pesticides from contaminating your hands and forearms

6. **Match the situation with the most appropriate PPE.**

1. You are spraying a large volume of a DANGER pesticide that is likely to drift onto your clothing and may remain in the air as you make the application. Temperatures are moderate.	a. chemical-resistant headgear, goggles, gloves, and coveralls
2. You are spraying a CAUTION pesticide over your head into trees.	b. closed mixing system, coveralls, safety glasses, respiratory protection, and gloves
3. You are mixing and then loading a DANGER pesticide that will be sprayed on a field of tomatoes.	c. chemical-resistant suit, respirator, goggles, gloves, and a hat

7. **How often must you clean reusable PPE?**
   - ☐ a. at the end of each work period, before using the equipment again
   - ☐ b. at least once per week if the equipment is used more than 2 days
   - ☐ c. at the beginning of each spray season

8. **Which is true about disposable PPE?**
   - ☐ a. Nonwoven coveralls and hoods can be worn for as many as 7 workdays.
   - ☐ b. Use an employer-provided container or bag for discarding disposable PPE.
   - ☐ c. Dust/mist masks, prefilters, canisters, and filtering and vapor-removing cartridges can be cleaned and reused three or four times before disposing of them.

9. **What should you do to avoid heat stress during a pesticide application?**
   - ☐ a. Make the application as quickly as possible.
   - ☐ b. Use less than the recommended PPE if it will be very hot outside.
   - ☐ c. Drink plenty of water and take frequent rest breaks in a cool or shady place.

10. **California's pesticide regulations require that all respirators be fit tested to the actual wearer before use because _____ .**
    - ☐ a. people often won't wear ill-fitting devices, even when they are required.
    - ☐ b. they are impossible to clean when they are not custom fitted.
    - ☐ c. respirators must fit properly to be effective and safe.

11. **Which respirator types are suitable for use when applying pesticides that have instructions requiring application with an oil-containing material?**
    - ☐ a. NIOSH-approved organic vapor (OV) cartridge respirators with N, R, P, or HE prefilters
    - ☐ b. NIOSH-approved organic vapor (OV) cartridge respirators with R, P, or HE prefilters
    - ☐ c. NIOSH-approved respirators with N, R, P, or HE filters

12. **PPE can make pesticide exposure more hazardous in which of the following situations?**
    - ☐ a. when it restricts your ability to move freely during handling activities
    - ☐ b. when you get pesticides on your skin or clothing before putting on your PPE
    - ☐ c. when your goggles fog up or get coated with spray during an application

13. **Engineering controls that help protect you from pesticide exposure include which of the following?**
    - ☐ a. enclosed cabs and closed mixing systems
    - ☐ b. SCBA devices and water-soluble pesticide packaging
    - ☐ c. chemical-resistant materials and atmosphere monitoring devices

14. **When must you use a closed mixing system?**
    - ☐ a. mixing, loading, diluting, or transferring liquid formulations of DANGER pesticides intended for application in any situation
    - ☐ b. mixing, loading, diluting, or transferring liquid formulations of pesticides with any signal word intended for application to an agricultural commodity
    - ☐ c. mixing, loading, diluting, or transferring most liquid formulations of DANGER pesticides intended for application to an agricultural commodity

Chapter 7
Using Pesticides Safely

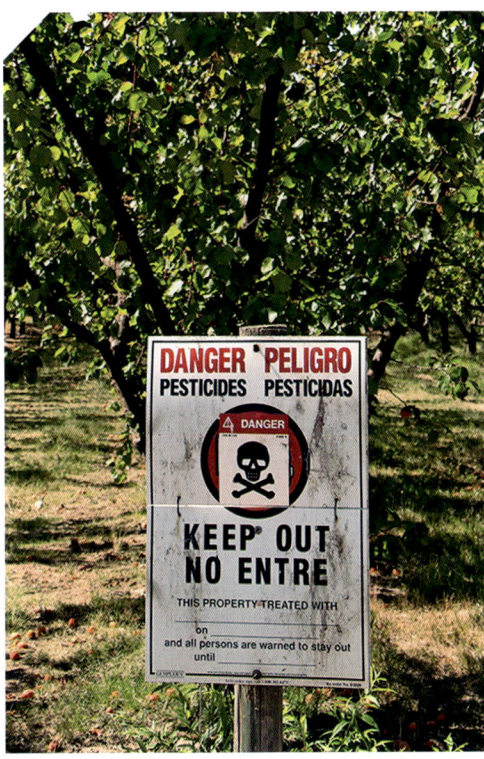

Pesticide Applicator Safety 162
Fieldworker Safety 166
Public Safety 168
Handling Pesticides Safely 168
Mixing Pesticides Safely 177
Applying Pesticides Safely 180
Cleanup and Disposal 187
Recordkeeping 188
Liability 190
Chapter 7 Review Questions 191

Knowledge Expectations

- Describe ways in which applicators ensure the public's safety before, during, and after pesticide applications.
- Explain why and in which situations it is important to communicate with neighbors and others in the area before making a pesticide application.
- Describe how to restrict access to areas where pesticides are in use or have been used.
- List procedures and safety precautions for transporting pesticides in a vehicle.
- List the components of a proper storage area.
- Describe techniques for mixing and loading pesticides safely, including the equipment, location, and procedures used in the process.
- Describe the proper weather conditions for the safe application of pesticides.
- Describe how to identify potentially sensitive areas that could be adversely affected by pesticide application, mixing and loading, storage, disposal, and equipment washing.
- Explain how to properly process all types of pesticide containers for disposal.
- Describe the procedures to follow for safe, effective cleanup after handling pesticides, including cleaning application equipment, as well as personal decontamination.
- Describe how pesticide records can contribute to pesticide safety.

Pesticide Applicator Safety

You are the key to preventing pesticide accidents. By following the pesticide label and complying with the laws and regulations dealing with pesticides, you can avoid most problems. In addition, when mixing pesticides together or with other materials, confirm that these combinations are safe. Also, check your equipment to be sure it is functioning properly. Remember, faulty, broken, or worn equipment causes accidents. Finally, never take alcohol or drugs before, during, or immediately after applying pesticides.

This chapter describes how to prevent occupational exposure to pesticides. Quite simply, you avoid pesticide-related problems by
- reading and following the requirements in the pesticide labeling and laws and regulations
- using safe work habits
- wearing the required personal protective equipment (PPE)
- protecting people from pesticide exposure
- avoiding practices that may harm nontarget plants and animals in the environment
- preventing pesticides from moving offsite
- complying with all laws, regulations, and restricted material permit conditions that apply to pesticide handling, storage, and application in your work situation

BLOOD TESTS FOR EXPOSURE MONITORING

California's pesticide worker safety regulations require a special blood test before employees can handle Category I or II organophosphate or carbamate insecticides. This test is mandatory if employees will handle these materials for more than 6 calendar days in any period of 30 consecutive days. Handling begins the moment you open a pesticide container for mixing or application. It continues until you have bathed and changed clothing after you are done handling the pesticide. In case of a spill or other emergency, exposure begins at the onset of the incident. Exposure continues until you have bathed and changed clothing.

The blood test you will take is called a red cell and plasma cholinesterase determination. It establishes a baseline for measuring exposure to organophosphate and carbamate insecticides. These insecticides interfere with your body's nervous system by blocking the production of cholinesterase, the enzyme that helps to regulate nerve impulses and muscle activity. It counteracts the effects of another chemical, acetylcholine, which normally transmits nerve signals (Fig. 7-1).

These insecticides have the potential to impair your nervous system if you should receive a sufficient exposure. Each person has a unique baseline level of cholinesterase in their blood and in their blood plasma. The lowering of a person's cholinesterase may indicate that exposure to one of these insecticides has occurred. (Other factors besides insecticides could also lower your cholinesterase.) If your cholinesterase level drops, your physician may advise you to stop handling this group of insecticides for a while. Your physician may then prescribe additional tests to determine when your cholinesterase level returns to normal.

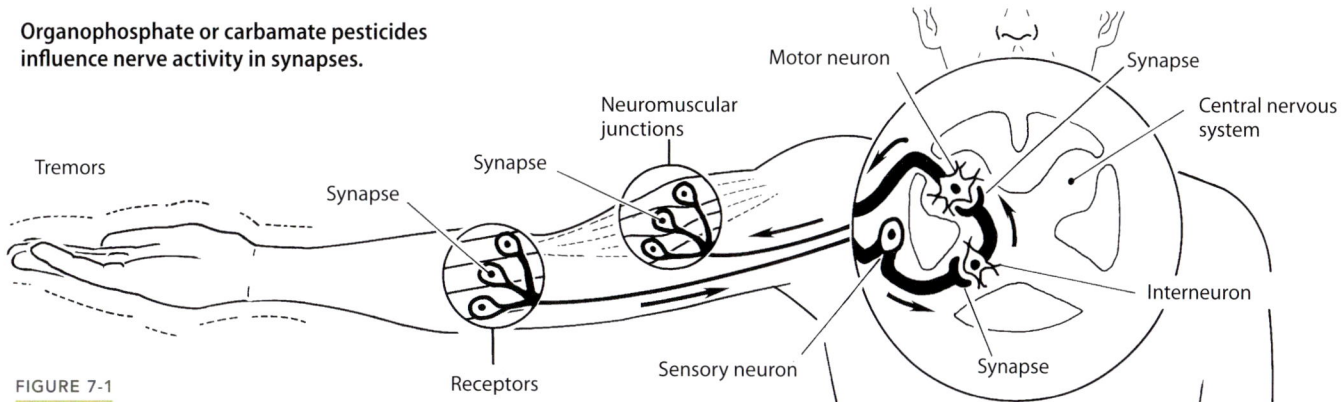

FIGURE 7-1
Organophosphate and N-methyl carbamate insecticides interfere with the transmission of nerve signals across a synapse.

PLANNING

Planning for pesticide applications helps to prevent accidents. Find out about the pesticides you use by studying Safety Data Sheets and pesticide labels. From these you will learn about the dangers and the precautions you should take to avoid exposure. Inspect areas where you will be working to locate potential hazards that can affect your safety. Finally, plan what you need to do if an accident happens. Use the checklist in Sidebar 7-1 for planning pesticide applications.

Pesticide Label. Thoroughly read and understand the entire pesticide label. The label gives specific information for each type of application. It is also the legal document that you must follow for any pesticide use. Look for signal words (DANGER/POISON, DANGER, WARNING, CAUTION) and required PPE. Make sure that you have and use this PPE and that it is in good condition. Review the label for any special environmental precautions as well as application rates. Applying more pesticide than is allowed on the label is illegal. Always be sure the label lists the intended application site or commodity. It is illegal to use a pesticide on sites or commodities not listed on the label. Finally, consult the label for restrictions on and requirements for disposal of unwanted pesticide and empty containers. For more about pesticide labels, see Chapter 11.

Safety Data Sheet. A Safety Data Sheet (SDS) provides detailed information about pesticide hazards. An SDS has sixteen sections, as follows:

1. Product Identification
2. Hazards Identification
3. Composition/Information on Ingredients
4. First Aid Measures
5. Fire-Fighting Measures
6. Accidental Release Measures
7. Handling and Storage
8. Exposure Controls/Personal Protection
9. Physical and Chemical Properties
10. Stability and Reactivity
11. Toxicological Information
12. Ecological Information
13. Disposal Considerations
14. Transport Information
15. Regulatory Information
16. Other Information

SIDEBAR 7-1

CHECKLIST FOR PLANNING A PESTICIDE APPLICATION

PERSONAL
- ☐ Medical checkup and necessary blood tests?
- ☐ Properly trained for this type of application?

PESTICIDE
- ☐ Read and thoroughly understood label?
- ☐ Checked to be sure use is consistent with target pest and application area?
- ☐ Read Safety Data Sheet for information on hazards?
- ☐ Obtained necessary permits?
- ☐ Know proper rate of pesticide to be applied?

EQUIPMENT
- ☐ Proper personal protective equipment (boots, gloves, respiratory equipment, protective clothing, eye protection, head wear)?
- ☐ Necessary measuring and mixing equipment?
- ☐ Suitable application equipment for this job (tank capacity, pressure range, volume of output, nozzle size, pump compatible with formulation type)?
- ☐ Application equipment properly calibrated?
- ☐ Emergency water and first aid supplies?
- ☐ Necessary supplies to contain spills or leaks (absorbent materials, cleaning supplies, holding containers)?

TRANSPORTING
- ☐ Safe transport of pesticides to application site?
- ☐ Pesticides and containers secured from theft or unauthorized access?
- ☐ Vehicles properly marked and permits obtained, if necessary, for transporting hazardous materials and hazardous wastes?

MIXING AND LOADING
- ☐ Safe mixing and loading site located?
- ☐ Clean water available for mixing?
- ☐ Water pH tested?
- ☐ Proper adjuvants obtained for correcting pH, preventing foaming, and improving deposition?
- ☐ Compatibility of pesticide tank mixes or fertilizer-pesticide combinations checked?
- ☐ Liquid containers triple-rinsed and rinsate put into spray tank?

TREATMENT SITE
- ☐ Boundaries of treatment site inspected?
- ☐ Environmentally sensitive areas within and around treatment area identified?
- ☐ In agricultural applications, people working or living in or near treatment area, including fieldworkers and their supervisors, notified?
- ☐ Treatment site properly posted with required signs?
- ☐ Soil types determined and noted, if these are factor in pesticide efficacy?
- ☐ Livestock, pets, honey bees, other animals properly protected?
- ☐ Aspects of groundwater determined, if applicable?
- ☐ Hazards within treatment site identified, including electrical wires and outlets, ignition sources, obstacles, steep slopes, and other dangerous conditions?
- ☐ Plants in treatment area in proper condition for pesticide application (correct growth stage, not under moisture stress, other requirements as specified on pesticide label)?

WEATHER CONDITIONS
- ☐ Weather suitable for application (low wind, proper temperature, lack of fog or rainfall)?

APPLICATION
- ☐ Application pattern established suitable for treatment area, hazards, and prevailing weather conditions?
- ☐ Application rate selected that will give most uniform coverage?
- ☐ Equipment frequently checked during application to ensure that everything is working properly and is providing a uniform application?

CLEANUP
- ☐ Application equipment properly cleaned and decontaminated after application?
- ☐ Personal protective equipment safely stored and cleaned or laundered according to approved methods?
- ☐ Disposable materials burned or disposed of in approved way?

DISPOSAL
- ☐ Paper pesticide containers burned or disposed of according to local regulation?
- ☐ Plastic and metal containers triple-rinsed?
- ☐ Plastic and metal containers properly stored until disposed of in suitable disposal area?

STORAGE
- ☐ Unused pesticides returned to supplier or stored in locked facility for later use?
- ☐ Storage facility suitable for pesticides?

REPORTS
- ☐ Necessary reports filed with requesting agency?

FOLLOW-UP
- ☐ Treatment areas inspected after application to ensure that pesticide controlled the target pests without causing undue damage to nontarget organisms or surfaces of items in treatment area?

DAMAGE
- ☐ Damage, if it occurred, promptly reported?

Manufacturers prepare these sheets and make them available to every person selling, storing, or handling pesticides. Ask your employer for them, or, if self-employed, obtain them from the chemical manufacturer or pesticide dealer. You can obtain SDSs for every labeled pesticide. A sample SDS with descriptions of each section can be found in Chapter 11.

Hazards. To increase your awareness of hazards, read the SDS and the pesticide labeling. These documents include important information about the dangers to you, to people and animals, and to the environment. Carefully inspect the treatment area to look for conditions or objects that may affect the safety of the application:

- Evaluate the weather and make sure it is suitable for an application. If appropriate, choose a time of day when the pesticide application will be least disruptive.
- Become familiar with the boundaries of the treatment site. When applicable, determine the soil type and variations in soil types. Soil type might influence the efficacy of herbicides or other soil-applied pesticides. It may also influence percolation into groundwater. Look for environmentally sensitive areas such as streams, irrigation ditches, ponds, lakes, homes, schools, or parks.
- Arrange to protect or remove people, pets, livestock, honey bees, or other animals in the area.

Special hazards may exist if you apply pesticides inside and around homes, businesses, offices, and other buildings. Be careful around food, food preparation areas and utensils, bedding, pets, and surfaces contacted by people. Find out if infants or toddlers live or play in the treatment area. For more about hazards to humans and the environment, see Chapters 4 and 5.

Planning for Accidents. Plan for the possibility of an accident. This process includes locating an appropriate medical facility before you need emergency care. Also, find out where to get assistance with spill cleanup. Post in your vehicle the name, address, and telephone number of a medical facility close to where you are working. Also, write down the telephone numbers of the local fire department, sheriff, and highway patrol (see Sidebar 7-2), and keep a copy of the label,

> Describe ways in which applicators ensure the public's safety before, during, and after pesticide applications.

SIDEBAR 7-2
EMERGENCY NUMBERS FOR PESTICIDE ACCIDENTS AND SPILLS

WHEN PEOPLE HAVE BEEN EXPOSED TO PESTICIDES

Dial 9-1-1 for emergency medical assistance. Notify the operator that the problem is a pesticide exposure. Provide an accurate location and information on the type of pesticide involved.

After obtaining medical treatment for exposed people, determine whether a spill has taken place. Follow instructions below for a spill.

1. If the spill is on private property, notify the property owner(s) or operator(s) so they can assist with contacting and evacuating people who may become exposed to the spilled material.
2. Whether the spill is on private property, public property, a local road, or a state or federal highway, contact appropriate law enforcement (police, sheriff, or highway patrol) or the local fire department.
3. Contact the nearest agricultural commissioner's office to report the incident. Find the commissioner's telephone number for the county where the accident occurred at cdfa.ca.gov/exec/county/countymap/.

FOR PESTICIDE SPILLS ON PUBLIC ROADWAYS

Notify the local office of the California Highway Patrol (for highways) or your local law enforcement agency (for other public roadways) and the local fire department (dial 9-1-1). Inform the emergency operator that a pesticide spill has occurred; provide accurate location and type of pesticide.

- Contact CHEMTREC at 800-424-9300 for assistance in cleaning up a pesticide spill.
- Contact the California Emergency Management Agency (CalEMA). Usually a written report will need to be filed. Call CalEMA at 800-852-7550, and to find out how to properly file a report with them, check calema.ca.gov/hazardousmaterials/pages/spill-release-reporting.aspx.
- Contact your local agricultural commissioner's office. Find the commissioner's telephone number for the county where the accident occurred at cdfa.ca.gov/exec/county/countymap/.

which you can bring with you if necessary. The emergency number 9-1-1 usually gives you immediate access to medical help, local fire services, and law enforcement agencies.

Plan what to do if there is a pesticide spill and be prepared to protect the public from danger. Know the proper first aid to administer to victims of pesticide exposure or heat stress. Understand the steps you must take to reduce injury to yourself and others in case of an accident. Be sure you have emergency water for washing your eyes and skin. For more about planning for and responding to emergencies, see Chapter 12.

PESTICIDE COMBINATIONS

Often, the toxicity, mode of action, or efficacy of a pesticide changes when you combine it with another material. Combinations can alter the toxicity of pesticides to people as well as to target pests. For instance, some combinations change the amount and speed at which certain pesticides enter your body. These changes could affect your body's ability to quickly deactivate the toxic material. Adjuvants that enhance penetration or toxic action sometimes increase hazards to people, as well. Read the pesticide label for important information and restrictions on pesticide combinations. For more about pesticide combinations, see Chapters 3 and 10.

AVOIDING MEDICATIONS, ALCOHOL, AND DRUGS

Alcohol, drugs, and certain medications cause drowsiness, impair judgment, and often influence your ability to apply pesticides safely. These substances may also alter the toxicity of pesticides in case of exposure. For example, a severe illness may result if a person consumes alcohol the day before or shortly after even minimal exposure to the fungicide thiram. If you are taking any medication, consult a physician before handling, mixing, or applying pesticides. Do not take alcohol or drugs before, during, or immediately after a pesticide application.

Fieldworker Safety

In agriculture, fieldworkers may be working near where you are making a pesticide application. You must protect these fieldworkers from any type of pesticide exposure. Do not allow workers into an area that is being treated with a pesticide. Also, workers are not allowed into treated fields during restricted-entry intervals unless they are trained as early-entry workers (workers who enter an area after the pesticide application is complete, but before the restricted-entry interval or other entry restriction has expired). Make pesticide applications at times when workers are not present in surrounding areas. These times may include very early morning, late afternoon, or during the night. Preventing drift also lessens exposure risks to fieldworkers in adjacent areas.

NOTIFICATION

In an agricultural situation, before applying any pesticide you must notify all employees of the farming operation who are working within $\frac{1}{4}$ mile of the treatment area. Do this orally or by posting warning signs unless the pesticide label specifies the method you must use. Inform workers when you plan to make the application so they will leave and then not reenter the treated area. Tell them what pesticides you will apply and describe the hazards if they should become exposed. Inform them when they can reenter the area.

In general, all pesticide applications require advance notification to the property operator, and in some cases agricultural pesticide applications require postapplication notification. These notifications are in addition to posted and oral warnings provided to employees.

Explain why and in which situations it is important to communicate with neighbors and others in the area before making a pesticide application.

Describe how to restrict access to areas where pesticides are in use or have been used.

RESTRICTED-ENTRY INTERVAL

A restricted-entry interval is the time that must elapse after a pesticide application before anyone can go back into the treated area. Pesticide labels and the California Code of Regulations (CCR) list restricted-entry intervals. Always review the pesticide labeling as well as Title 3 of CCR for the restricted-entry intervals that apply in your situation. Pesticide use recommendations written by licensed pest control advisers must indicate the required restricted-entry interval. The local agricultural commissioner is also able to provide this information. In all situations where the restricted-entry interval on the label differs from California requirements, the longest restricted-entry interval applies. In addition, when tank-mixing pesticides with different restricted-entry intervals, you must use the longest interval indicated. You should check with the county agricultural commissioner's office for special restricted-entry intervals when you apply mixtures of certain pesticides.

POSTING

Sometimes you must post treated areas and buffer zones with warning signs (Fig. 7-2). Posting is a way to notify employees about a treated area and its buffer zones. Regulations require posting signs to be made of a durable material and printed in English and and a non-English language that is read by a majority of workers. They must contain a skull and crossbones at the center of the sign and the word *DANGER* in letters large enough to be read from a distance of 25 feet. If the restricted-entry interval is greater than 7 days, the sign must also list

- the date the restricted-entry interval expires
- the property operator's name
- any field identification

Check pesticide labels and current federal, state, and local laws to determine requirements for posting. Local offices of county agricultural commissioners have this information.

To post a treated area, place signs at usual points of entry. If there are no clear points of entry, signs must be posted on corners of the treated area. Along unfenced areas next to roads and other public rights-of-way, signs should be no more than 600 feet apart. Post the area before you make an application (but no sooner than 24 hours before the application). Signs must remain in place throughout the restricted-entry interval. Remove them within 3 days after the end of the restricted-entry interval and before you allow workers to enter the treated area.

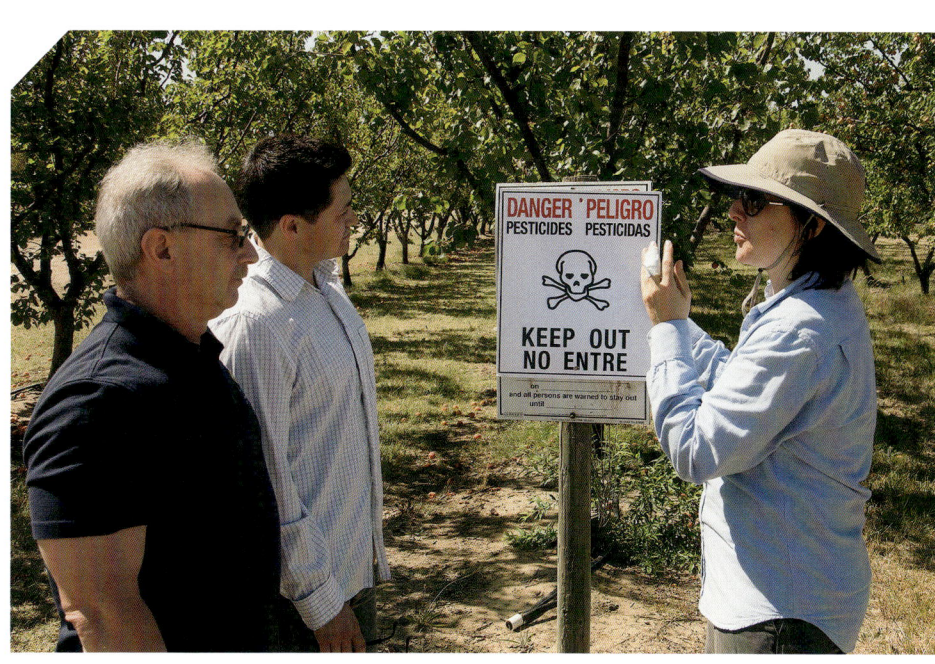

FIGURE 7-2

Some pesticide labels require treated areas to be posted. Also, an area must be posted if the restricted-entry interval is more than 48 hours. All greenhouse applications must be posted when the restricted entry interval is greater than 4 hours; unless access is carefully controlled throughout the restricted-entry interval.

Public Safety

Prevent the public from accidentally becoming exposed to pesticides during an application or from encountering treated areas after you make the application. Informing the public helps keep people from accidentally encountering hazardous situations during and after pesticide applications. The following actions can reduce the chances of exposure for people who live, work, or play near the application site.

- Notify people in the area about the planned pesticide application.
- Explain the potential hazards and possible exposure symptoms to people near the application site.
- Tell people what you are doing to reduce the possible hazards.
- Explain what people should do to avoid exposure before, during, and after the application.
- Apply pesticides at times when people are not present.
- Avoid accidental exposure by preventing offsite movement of pesticide materials.

Check pesticide labels and California regulations to be sure you have followed all requirements for the posting of warning signs in fields, buildings, parks, schools, and other areas where people might be present during or soon after a pesticide application. By law you must always notify workers of restricted-entry intervals. Sometimes you also must post this information, which helps keep people from entering treated areas prematurely.

Handling Pesticides Safely

Undiluted pesticides are a greater risk to people and the environment than diluted spray mixtures. The safe handling and transporting of undiluted pesticides can prevent many environmental and human health hazards. Along with toxic hazards, pesticides have a high dollar value and may be subject to theft. Part of your safe handling program should include security measures to reduce the risk of theft (for more on preventing pesticide theft, see "Stolen Pesticides" in Chapter 12).

MANUFACTURER'S PACKAGING

Manufacturers package pesticides in several different ways, depending on the formulation. The type of packaging and formulation affects the hazards of handling, transportation, and storage. Pesticides are available in paper bags, water-soluble bags, and plastic and metal containers (Fig. 7-3). Most packages are in convenient units of size for ease in measuring and mixing. Manufacturers usually pack quantities of these units in larger cardboard boxes for shipping and handling. The U.S. Department of Transportation (DOT) must approve these shipping containers.

Paper and plastic bags are common packages for powder and granule formulations. For safety, manufacturers package some highly toxic or otherwise hazardous powders in water-soluble plastic bags. However, if you do not handle them carefully, paper or plastic containers may tear or puncture. Opened paper and plastic bags may be difficult to reseal, presenting possible future problems with leaking. Spilled powders scatter easily and are difficult to clean up. To prevent

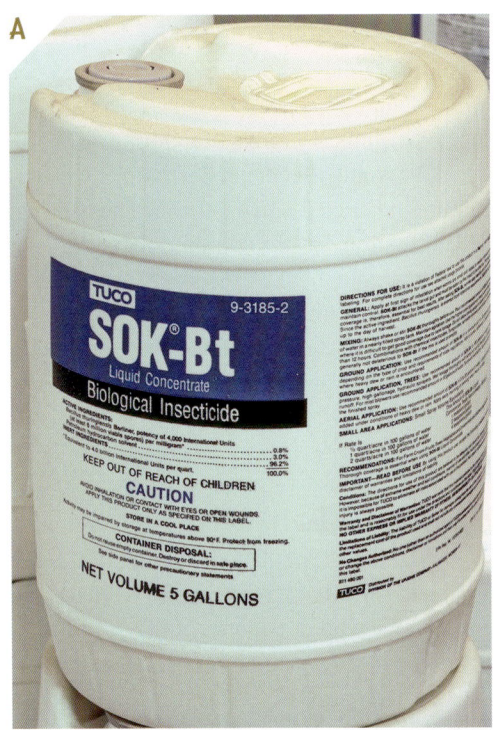
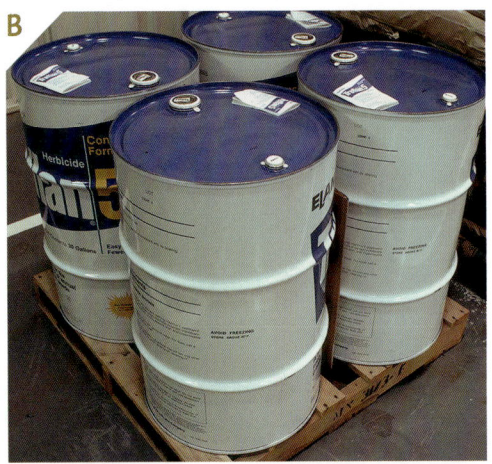
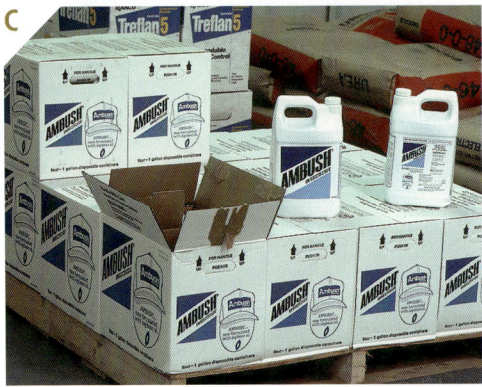

FIGURE 7-3

Pesticides are packaged in a variety of container types. Most packaging is in convenient units of size for ease in measuring and mixing.

tearing and reduce the danger of spilling, cut bags open with scissors or a sharp knife. This also makes the bags easier to close after use.

Manufacturers use plastic bottles and pails for packaging liquid and granular formulations. If improper handling results in one of these containers being punctured, there will be a pesticide spill. Uncapped containers are also subject to spilling. Spilled liquids are difficult to contain or clean up because they soak into wood, cloth, paper, and nearly everything else they contact. Granular formulations are easier to contain and clean up should a spill occur. Also, granules do not soak into porous surfaces.

Manufacturers use metal containers for liquid and dust aerosols and many liquid formulations. However, metal containers are not suitable for some corrosive chemicals. Manufacturers package fumigants (usually liquids under high pressure) in reusable steel cylinders (Fig. 7-4). Metal pesticide containers probably are the most resistant to damage because they are difficult to puncture and do not break. They are resealable and you can either recycle empty containers or dispose of them at an approved disposal site. However, take special precautions with metal aerosol containers. If you puncture, overheat, or burn them, they may explode or cause injury.

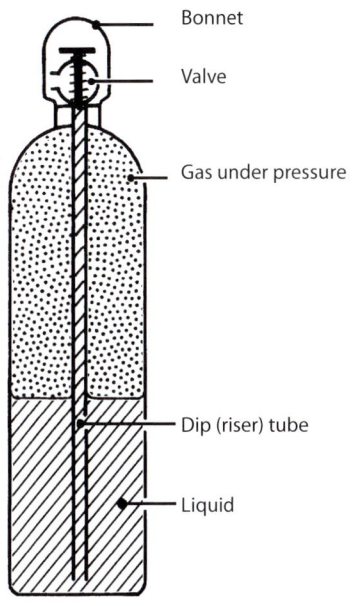

FIGURE 7-4

Most gas fumigants are supplied in large steel cylinders. These are capable of withstanding the high pressures of the gases they contain.

SERVICE CONTAINERS

Service containers are any container other than the original labeled packaging that holds pesticides. Manufacturers design these for applying, storing, or transporting pesticide concentrates or diluted preparations. If you are transporting a service container, label it with the following information:
- common name of the pesticide
- signal word
- name and address of the person responsible for the container

TRANSPORTING

Every pesticide user must understand possible hazards and the procedures for minimizing the risks associated with transporting pesticides. Careless handling of containers, incorrectly maintained equipment, and unforeseen accidents can lead to pesticide leaks and spills during transport. The fact that some pesticides are highly flammable increases the danger (fire and toxic fumes) while they are in transit. Another concern is that other vehicles could scatter pesticide products that are spilled on public roads. Such events have the potential to injure bystanders and animals. In addition, transportation-related pesticide spills and leaks can contaminate the environment, endanger residential areas, and lead to financial losses and legal actions.

Pesticides are transported from manufacturers to distributors and dealers, from retailers to end users, and from storage sites and mixing locations to application sites. Accidents can happen at any point in the distribution chain, even when transport distances are short. The first line of defense is knowing how to prevent transportation mishaps. When mishaps occur, however, initiating the appropriate response could mean the difference between a minor inconvenience and a community-wide disaster.

For information on transporting pesticides on public highways in California, contact the following agencies:
- California Highway Patrol
- California Public Utilities Commission

These agencies will provide you with current regulations and help you deter-

List procedures and safety precautions for transporting pesticides in a vehicle.

mine whether you need special licenses or permits. They will tell you whether these materials are subject to hazardous materials transportation requirements. Sidebar 7-3 lists places to get information and check regulations on transporting pesticides.

Transport Vehicle

Transport vehicles should be in good mechanical condition, including power train, chassis, and any onboard bulk tanks and associated fittings. In particular, make sure safety and control components such as brakes, tires, and steering are in good working order. A poorly maintained vehicle is, by itself, a safety risk; adding pesticides to the picture increases the potential risk of injury or contamination should a mishap occur. Regularly inspect application equipment being transported. Look for structural defects in the equipment such as cracks, punctures, and other causes of leaks or failure. Always carry equipment needed to make repairs in case a problem occurs while the vehicle is in transit.

Never carry pesticides in the passenger compartment of a vehicle because spilled chemicals and hazardous fumes can seriously injure the occupants. Spilled pesticides can be difficult or impossible to remove completely from the vehicle's interior, leading to long-term exposures. If pesticides must be carried in a station wagon, utility van, or similarly enclosed vehicle, ventilate the cargo and passenger compartments and keep passengers and pets away from pesticides during transport. Remember, cargo can shift during collisions and other sudden stops. Placing a safety barrier between the passengers and the cargo area is advisable.

The cargo area must be able to securely hold containers and provide protection from tears, punctures, or impacts that could lead to container damage (Fig. 7-5). Enclosed cargo boxes provide the greatest protection but are not always practical. Cargo boxes also offer the added benefit of security from curious children, careless adults, or vandals. Open truck beds are convenient for loading and unloading, but take precautions to minimize the possibility of theft or losing containers on sharp turns or bumpy roads. Never stack pesticide containers higher than the sides of the vehicle. Make sure flatbed trucks have side and tail racks and tie-down rings, cleats, or racks to simplify the job of securing the load. Before loading, inspect every cargo area for nails, stones, or sharp edges or objects that could damage containers. Steel beds are preferable to wood because they are more easily cleaned if a spill should occur. Devices are available for some vehicles that protect pesticide cargo in the case of a rear-end collision. In California, you are required to secure pesticides in a manner that will prevent spillage onto the vehicle or off the vehicle. Paper, cardboard, and similar containers must be covered (when necessary) to protect them from moisture.

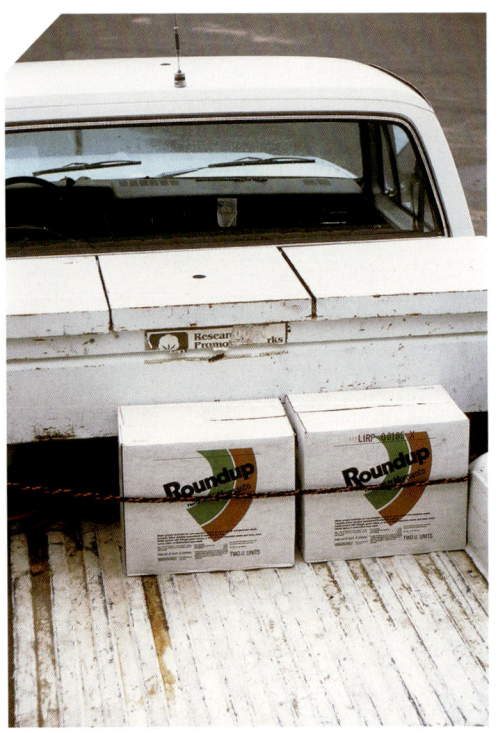

FIGURE 7-5

Transport pesticides in the cargo area of your vehicle, never in the passenger area. Secure containers in the cargo area and protect them from moisture and damage. Never carry people, animals, food, animal feed, or clothing in the same area.

Vehicle Operator

Both the owner and the operator of the transport vehicle can be held accountable for any injuries, contamination, or damage resulting from a chemical release that may occur. The vehicle operator may be the only person capable of reacting to a spill and in some instances may need to assist first-response emergency personnel as they arrive on the scene. In California, the vehicle operator is responsible for contacting emergency-response agencies and for ensuring the cleanup of spilled material if there is an accident. Who you should contact in an emergency, what to report to governmental agencies and emergency response personnel, and how to clean up (or who to contact to clean up) a pesticide spill should be determined in advance of transporting hazardous materials. Everyone involved in transporting pesticides should receive training in basic emergency response procedures, including spill control and emergency notification procedures. Refer to Chapter 12 for specific information on how to respond to a fire, spill, or leak involving agricultural chemicals.

If the person or company transporting the material cannot quickly and safely clean up a spill, municipal agencies may elect to take over a site and provide or contract for cleanup of roadways within their jurisdiction. These agencies include the California Department of Transportation (CalTrans) and designated city or county agencies, including some fire departments. If an agency does not elect to take over the site, however, the driver is responsible for ensuring that the site is properly cleaned.

Other Safety Precautions

Before departing with a pesticide cargo, make sure that the technical data for all pesticide products and emergency information for spill response are in the vehicle. A shipping paper, also called a vehicle manifest, may be required for certain products regulated as hazardous materials under DOT regulations. The regulatory section of a Safety Data Sheet lists whether the pesticide product is a DOT-regulated product.

Product labels and Safety Data Sheets contain information about the proper storage and handling of products, including acceptable storage temperatures, human and environmental hazards, PPE, and emergency telephone numbers. Keep this information in the vehicle to help the driver or emergency personnel properly respond to a pesticide release. It is also a good idea to have a phone number in the vehicle for 24-hour emergency assistance.

A mobile phone is strongly recommended for anyone routinely involved in the transport of pesticides or working alone in remote locations. Always carry a spill kit including a shovel and broom and PPE appropriate for the pesticides in transit, and know how to use these items. Be familiar with the travel route so you can anticipate and avoid problems such as construction delays. If a pesticide release occurs, a major traffic jam only further complicates cleanup.

Inspect containers before loading to be certain they are in good condition. Look for legible and attached labels, tight closures, and pesticide-free outside surfaces. Handle containers carefully during loading to avoid rips and punctures. Use packing or shipping containers to provide extra protection and secondary containment. Where practical, using a synthetic liner or tarpaulin large enough to cover the floor and sides of the cargo area (especially truck beds) can provide

---

SIDEBAR 7-3

WHERE TO GET INFORMATION AND REGULATIONS ON TRANSPORTING PESTICIDES

FOR INTERSTATE MOVEMENT OF PESTICIDES
U.S. Department of Transportation
California Field Office
1325 J Street, Suite 1540
Sacramento, CA 95814-2941
(916) 930-2760

FOR TRANSPORTATION OF PESTICIDES WITHIN CALIFORNIA
California Highway Patrol Motor Carrier Safety Unit
Division Offices

Northern Division
2485 Sonoma Street
Redding, CA 96001-3026
(530) 225-2715

Valley Division
2555 First Avenue
Sacramento, CA 95818
(916) 731-6300

Golden Gate Division
1551 Benicia Road
Vallejo, CA 94591-7568
(707) 551-4180

Central Division
5179 North Gates Avenue
Fresno, CA 93722-6414
(559) 277-7250

Southern Division
411 N. Central Avenue, Suite 410
Glendale, CA 91203
(818) 240-8200

Border Division
9330 Farnham Street
San Diego, CA 92123-1216
(858) 650-3600

Coastal Division
4115 Broad Street, #B-10
San Luis Obispo, CA 93401-7963
(805) 549-3261

Inland Division
847 E. Brier Drive
San Bernardino, CA 92408-2820
(909) 806-2400

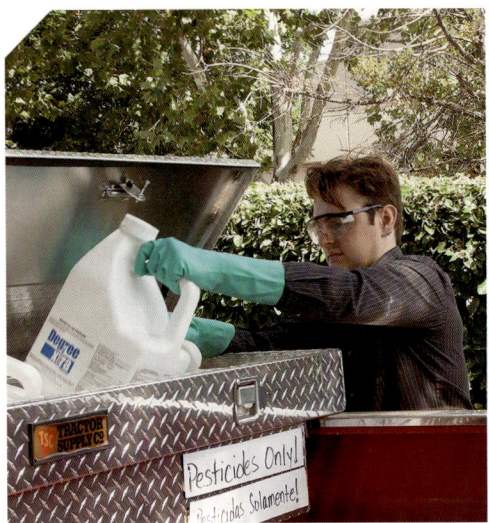

FIGURE 7-6

Keep pesticides in a lockable area of the vehicle to prevent unauthorized access while the vehicle is unattended.

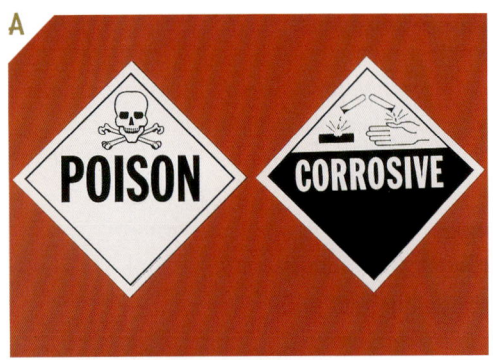

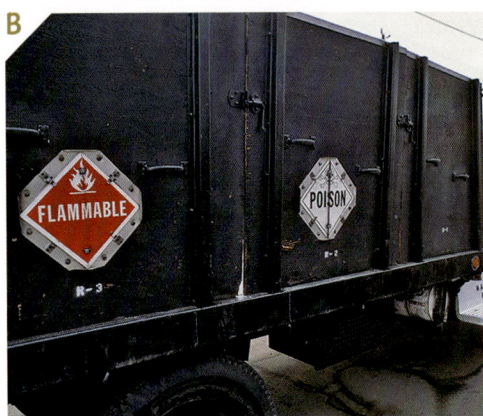

FIGURE 7-7

Sometimes the transporting vehicle must display specific placards when it carries certain quantities of pesticides. Check with local authorities for placarding requirements.

containment and easier cleanup of spilled materials. Organize the load to maximize stability while at the same time maintaining access to containers for ease of unloading. The less often you handle containers, the less likely they are to be damaged. Secure the load with tarps, ropes, brace bars, or other appropriate devices to prevent containers from shifting. Stabilize anything else that could move and damage a container during transport. Also, secure application equipment such as hand sprayers, backpack sprayers, spreaders, and spray tanks during transport.

Protect pesticides from temperature extremes and moisture during transit. Extremely low or high temperatures (below 40°F or above 110°F) can alter the stability or effectiveness of some pesticide formulations. Moisture can destroy paper and cardboard pesticide containers. Placing a waterproof cover over the load can provide protection from the elements, including the hot summer sun.

Never allow people, pets, or livestock to ride in a cargo area loaded with pesticides. Separate food, livestock feed, seeds, veterinary supplies, and plant materials from pesticides because contamination may render them unusable or result in a poisoning incident. Keep herbicides separate from other pesticides and fertilizers because of the potential for cross-contamination.

Transportation Security

Whenever possible, transport pesticides in a locked compartment or container (Fig. 7-6). If you must use an open vehicle to transport pesticides, never leave it unattended. Always secure your spray tank or mini-bulk container when it contains a pesticide mixture. Take all appropriate steps to reduce the chance of vandalism or theft.

The DOT requires diamond-shaped signs called placards on vehicles that transport certain types and quantities of hazardous materials (Fig. 7-7). Though few pesticides require placarding, you should always ask distributors whether what you are buying requires placarding. Most distributors furnish placards to you if you need to place them on your transportation vehicles. Hazardous materials include some pesticides; fertilizers such as anhydrous ammonia or ammonium nitrate; fuels such as gasoline, diesel, and propane; and explosives such as dynamite and detonators. Placards contain the information necessary to quickly assess an accident situation from a distance, reducing the possibility of someone approaching the accident site without wearing the proper PPE.

Persons, including farmers, who ship or transport materials in quantities that require placards are now required to develop and implement a transportation security plan. Vehicles must be placarded when transporting pesticides bearing a DOT poison label in containers larger than 119 gallons or in quantities greater than 1,000 pounds. Therefore, all operations that transport pesticides meeting these conditions must have a security plan. The security plan must include protection against unauthorized access, a security check of employees who pick up and transport placarded hazardous materials, and a security plan for the intended travel route. For further details on a transportation security plan, see the Hazardous Materials Information Center, phmsa.dot.gov. For more information, see Randall et al. 2008.

Handling

Handle bulk pesticide containers carefully. Do not drop or throw containers or packages, because this may cause damage and leaks. Check for contamination or leaks on all packages being handled. Do not let damaged packages or spilled pesticides contact your skin or clothing. Wear label-mandated PPE when handling pesticide packages. If a leak is present, you may also need respiratory and eye protection. Check the label for all precautions and required safety equipment. Never walk through a spilled pesticide. If you discover a damaged and leaking container, transfer the pesticide to another appropriate container. Use a container labeled for that pesticide or another properly labeled service container (see "Service Containers" earlier in this chapter for the information you need to label service containers properly).

Prevent theft or danger to children and animals. Never leave pesticide containers unattended or stored in unlocked areas. Always keep pesticides away from food and water and away from sources of heat and fire. Never allow paper containers to get wet.

Do not eat, drink, or smoke while handling pesticides or pesticide containers. Wash thoroughly when finished with handling duties and before eating, drinking, smoking, or using the bathroom.

Storage

Although many pesticide handlers use existing buildings or areas within existing buildings for pesticide storage, it is always best to build a separate storage facility just for pesticides. You should store pesticides in enclosed areas, on an impermeable (concrete) surface, and protected from rain.

A well-designed and maintained pesticide storage site
- protects people and animals from exposure
- reduces the chance of environmental contamination
- prevents damage to pesticides from temperature extremes and excess moisture
- safeguards the pesticides from theft, vandalism, and unauthorized use
- reduces the likelihood of liability

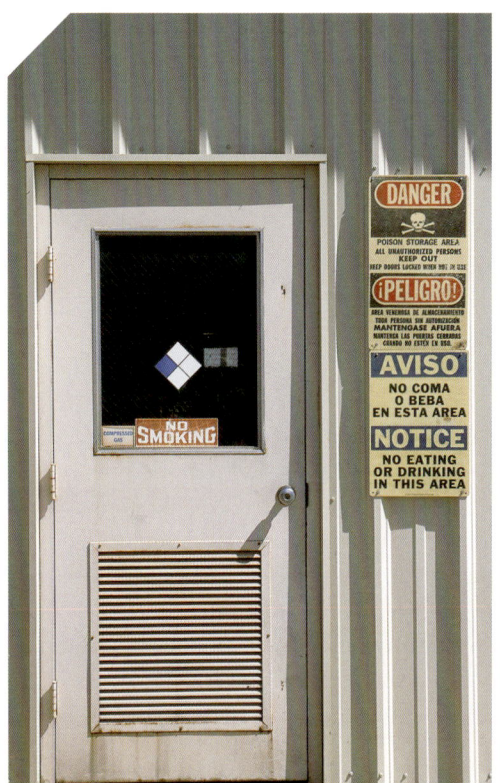

FIGURE 7-8

Store pesticides in a separate building, away from people, living areas, food, animal feed, and animals. Make sure the storage area is well ventilated, well lighted, dry, and secure. Securely lock doors and windows. Post the primary entrances with signs that warn that the building contains pesticides.

List the components of a proper storage area.

Secure the Site

Keeping unauthorized people, pets, and stray animals out is an important function of the pesticide storage site. Whether the designated area is as small as a cabinet or closet or as large as an entire room or building, keep it securely locked (Fig. 7-8). Post warning signs visible from at least 25 feet away on doors and windows to alert people that pesticides are stored inside. California regulations have specific requirements for the posting of these signs, so make sure you are familiar with them. In addition, you should post "No Smoking" warnings (not required by regulation)—many pesticides are highly flammable. Security of pesticides is covered in much more detail in Chapter 12.

Prevent Water Damage

Locate the pesticide storage facility where water damage is unlikely to occur. Carefully consider soil and land surface characteristics when selecting a storage site to prevent potential contamination of surface water or groundwater. Avoid locating the storage facility near a stream likely to flood or where runoff water can be a potential problem, such as at the base of a slope.

In extreme cases of flooding, all the pesticides from the storage site can move into surrounding areas. In certain situations, consider diking or constructing some other containment structure around the storage facility. A common recommendation is to set storage areas back at least 50 feet from a well to prevent groundwater contamination.

Water or excess moisture can damage pesticide containers and their contents. Moisture causes
- metal containers to rust
- paper and cardboard containers to split or crumble
- pesticide labeling to peel, smear, or otherwise become unreadable
- dry pesticides to clump, degrade, or dissolve
- slow-release products to release their active ingredients

Control the Temperature

Choose a cool, well-ventilated room or building that is insulated or temperature controlled. Exhaust fans directed to the outside of the building reduce temperatures and remove dust and vapors from the storage facility. Ventilation of the air from a pesticide storage area into other rooms is an unsafe practice. The pesticide labeling often specifies the temperature limits for storing a product. Temperature extremes can decrease the effectiveness of some pesticides. In addition, freezing temperatures can result in breakage of glass, metal, and plastic containers. Excessive heat can cause plastic containers to melt, some glass containers to explode, and a few pesticides to volatilize and drift from the storage site. Always store pesticide containers out of direct sunlight to prevent overheating.

Provide Adequate Lighting

Be sure the pesticide storage facility is well lighted. Pesticide handlers using the facility must be able to see well enough to read the pesticide label and notice whether containers are leaking or corroding. Without adequate lighting, pesticide handlers can have difficulty cleaning up spills and leaks. Because of the volatility of some pesticide formulations, use only spark-proof lighting fixtures and switches.

Use Nonporous Materials

Construct the floor of the pesticide storage area using sealed cement, glazed ceramic tile, no-wax sheet flooring, or other material that is free of cracks and easy to clean and decontaminate in the event of a spill or leak. Carpeting, wood, soil, and other absorbent floors are not suitable because they are difficult or impossible to decontaminate. A floor that slopes into a containment system or is recessed below the level of the doors helps to keep spilled or leaking pesticides within a confined area. For ease of cleanup, choose shelving and pallets made of nonabsorbent materials such as plastic or metal.

Maintain the Storage Site

Store only pesticide containers, pesticide equipment, and a spill kit at the storage site. Never keep food, drinks, tobacco, feed, medication, medical or veterinary supplies, seeds, clothing, or PPE at the site. These items could become contaminated by pesticide vapors, dusts, or spills, resulting in accidental exposure to people or animals.

Keep Labels Legible

Store pesticide containers with the labels in plain sight. Costly errors can result if the wrong pesticide is chosen. Be sure labels are always legible. If the label is destroyed or damaged, immediately mark the container as a service container with the following basic labeling information:
- name and address of person responsible
- name of the pesticide (both trade and common names are acceptable)
- signal word

It is also a good idea to record the U.S. EPA registration number, the percentage of each active ingredient, and the use classification. Then, request a replacement label from the pesticide dealer or the distributor to keep in the storage facility.

Store Pesticide Containers Safely

Store pesticides only in their original containers or an acceptable service container. You must follow California regulations pertaining to the labeling of service containers.

Never use milk jugs, soft drink bottles, fruit jars, medicine bottles, fuel cans, or other types of containers used for food, drink, or household products. Besides being illegal, switching containers has resulted in serious poisonings because children, as well as most adults, associate the shape, size, and color of a container with its usual contents. Never lend or borrow any pesticide product in an unmarked or unlabeled container.

Keep containers securely closed when not in use. Dry formulations tend to cake when wet or subjected to high humidity. Opened bags of wettable and soluble powders, dry flowables, dusts, and granules can be placed into sealable plastic bags or other suitable containers to reduce moisture absorption and to prevent a spill should a tear or break occur.

Place large drums and heavy bags on plastic pallets. Store other pesticides on metal shelving, placing the heaviest containers and liquids on the lower shelves. Do not allow containers to extend beyond the edge of shelving because they could easily be bumped or knocked off. Be sure the shelving is sturdy enough to handle the quantity and weight involved.

Store volatile pesticides separately to avoid possible cross-contamination of other pesticides, fertilizers, and seeds.

Place bulk or mini-bulk tanks on a reinforced concrete pad or other impermeable surface. Diking around a tank keeps spilled or leaking pesticides inside a restricted area and also helps prevent damage to the tanks from vehicles and equipment. Construct the area inside a dike large enough to contain the volume of the liquid in the tank plus at least 10%. Keep valves and pumps within the diked area. Make sure all drains within the dike connect to a holding tank. Outside, use fencing and locks to prevent tampering or unauthorized access to bulk tanks.

Look for Damage

Inspect pesticide containers regularly for tears, splits, breaks, leaks, rust, or corrosion. If you find a damaged container, immediately put on appropriate PPE and take action to prevent the pesticide from leaking or spreading into its surroundings. If a container is already leaking, take corrective action to prevent further leaking and immediately clean up any spilled pesticide. Be especially careful if the damaged container is an aerosol can or fumigant cylinder that contains pesticides under pressure.

Depending on the specific situation, consider the following actions:
- Use the pesticide immediately at a site and at a rate allowed by the label.
- Transfer the pesticide into another pesticide container that originally held the same pesticide and has an intact label.
- Transfer the contents to an appropriate service container that can be tightly closed. If possible, remove the label from the damaged container and place it on the new container. Otherwise, temporarily mark the new container with basic labeling information and get a copy of the label from the pesticide dealer or distributor as soon as possible.
- Place the entire damaged container and its contents into a suitable larger container.

Note Shelf Life of Pesticides

Keep an inventory of all pesticides in storage and mark each container with its purchase date. Be sure to note whether the product has an effective shelf life listed on its label. If you have questions about the shelf life of a product, contact the dealer or manufacturer. Signs of pesticide deterioration from age or poor storage conditions may appear during mixing. Watch for excessive clumping, poor suspension, layering, or abnormal coloration during mixing. Other times, however, the first indication of pesticide deterioration from age or poor storage conditions may be poor pest control and/or damage to the treated crop or surface.

To minimize storage problems, avoid storing large quantities of pesticides for long periods. Keep records of previous usage to make good estimates of future needs. Buy only as much as you need for the season.

Follow These Safe Storage Tips

The following safety tips help prevent pesticide accidents and exposures in storage areas and help people respond appropriately to pesticide spills and emergencies:

- Have duplicate copies of labels available in case of an emergency. Keep a Safety Data Sheet available for every chemical in the storage facility. The Internet or the pesticide dealer will have copies of current pesticide Safety Data Sheets and labels.
- Wear the appropriate PPE when handling pesticide containers.
- Label all items used for handling pesticides (measuring utensils, protective equipment, etc.) to prevent their use for other purposes.
- Keep a spill kit that contains clay, pet litter, fine sand, activated charcoal, vermiculite, or similar absorbent materials, as well as a shovel, a broom, and heavy-duty plastic bags in the storage area.
- Check the Safety Data Sheet for the types of materials that may be needed to deactivate spills.
- Treated seeds are usually colored with a bright dye to serve as a warning that the seeds have been treated with a pesticide. Unfortunately, the bright colors may be attractive to children. Never use treated seeds for feed or mix them with untreated seeds. Handle seeds with the same care as the pesticide itself and store in a locked storage facility away from feed, veterinary supplies, pesticides, other chemicals, equipment, pets, wildlife, and children.

Keep clean water for decontamination, an eyewash station, PPE, a fire extinguisher rated for chemical fires, first aid equipment, and emergency telephone numbers easily accessible at all times. In addition, keep plenty of soap, water, and paper towels available near (but not in) the storage facility.

Isolate Waste Products

Do not accumulate outdated or cancelled pesticide products; good recordkeeping can help you avoid this problem. Make every effort to use up what you purchase because leftover pesticides may become hazardous wastes. All of these materials could be subject to additional federal regulations on the storage, disposal, and reporting of hazardous materials. Outdated products—those whose shelf life has expired—may no longer be effective. Cancelled products often have a specified period beyond which they cannot be legally used. Use time-limited products according to the label directions before the expiration date to avoid generating hazardous wastes. Follow the status of products on the verge of cancellation and use these products before the deadline.

If you are holding pesticides or pesticide containers for disposal or recycling, store them in a special section of the storage site. Be sure to follow label directions for disposal of any excess or leftover product. Accidental use of pesticides meant for disposal can be a costly mistake. Make sure all empty containers are triple-rinsed or pressure-rinsed at the time of use, before storing for disposal or recycling. Refer to Sidebar 7-4 for an explanation of triple-rinsing procedures. Clearly mark properly rinsed containers. If possible, recycle these containers through a program supported by the Ag Container Recycling Council (ACRC) or contact your county agricultural commissioner's office to find out if container recycling is available in your area (see Randall et al. 2008).

USING PESTICIDES SAFELY 177

Mixing Pesticides Safely

Describe techniques for mixing and loading pesticides safely, including the equipment, location, and procedures used in the process.

Techniques for mixing pesticides safely are the same for large and small volumes. You must
- read the mixing directions on labels of all pesticides you will be using
- determine what PPE you need for mixing and application and acquire what you don't already have on hand
- check the spray equipment for cracked hoses or leaks and make sure the filters, screens, and nozzles are clean
- have a sufficient supply of fresh water nearby for eye flushing and washing your entire body in case of an accident
- choose the proper order to add chemicals, including adjuvants, to the spray tank (see "Testing for Incompatibility" in Chapter 10 for appropriate mixing order)

CLOSED MIXING AND LOADING SYSTEMS

Closed mixing and loading systems are designed to prevent pesticides from coming in contact with handlers or other persons during mixing and loading. The labeling of some pesticides, usually products with a high risk of causing human health effects, may require the use of a closed mixing and loading system. In California, you are required to use a closed mixing system when employees mix or load liquid pesticides with high acute dermal toxicity, which is indicated by any of the following precautionary statements on the label:

- Fatal if absorbed through skin.
- May be fatal if absorbed through skin.
- Corrosive, causes skin dam

There are two primary types of closed mixing and loading systems. One type uses mechanical devices to deliver the pesticide from the container to the equipment. The other type uses water-soluble packaging. For more about water-soluble packaging see "Water-Soluble Bags or Packets (WSB or WSP)" in Chapter 3.

MECHANICAL SYSTEMS

Mechanical systems often consist of a series of interconnected equipment parts that allow for the safe removal of a pesticide from its original container. These systems minimize exposure when rinsing the empty container and transferring the pesticide and rinsate to the application equipment (Fig. 7-9).

Closed mixing and loading systems are often custom-made with components from several commercial sources. Because pesticide container openings vary in shape and size, no single closed system can be used with all containers. Closed systems are available for containers as small as 2.5 gallons. Mechanical systems are now available to remove the pesticide concentrate from the original container either by gravity or by suction.

A mechanical loading system is often used with mini-bulk containers. Mini-bulk containers range in volume from 40 to 600 gallons and are adapted to closed systems. The applicator can use the closed system to attach the mini-bulk tanks to the sprayer without exposure to the chemical. Typically, pump and drive units deliver the product, and a meter

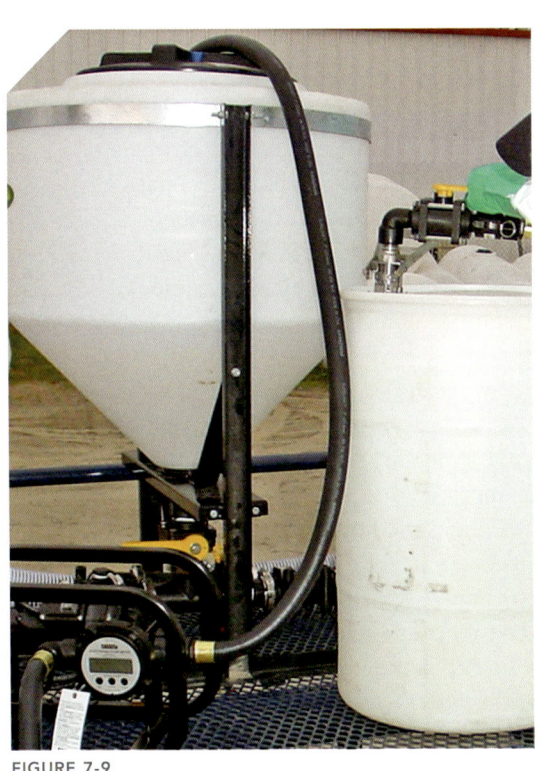

FIGURE 7-9

Closed mixing systems minimize exposure when loading a concentrated liquid pesticide into the tank, rinsing the empty container, and transferring the pesticide and rinsate to the tank.

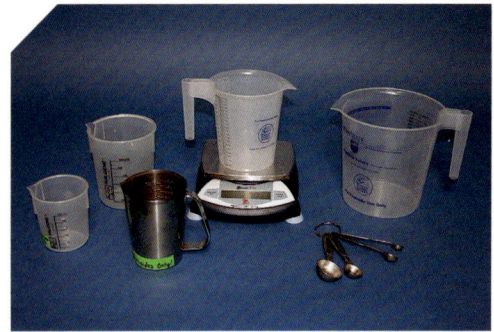

FIGURE 7-10

Measuring and weighing pesticides require a variety of calibrated utensils and an accurate scale.

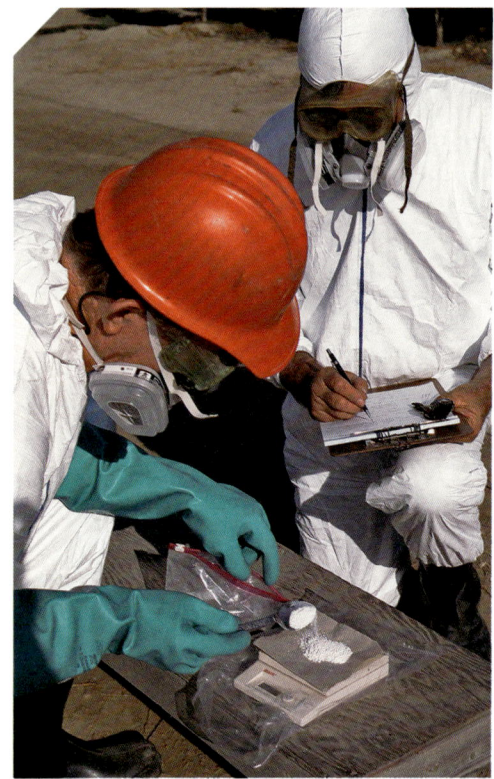

FIGURE 7-11

Always pour and measure pesticides below eye level. If measuring outdoors, stand upwind. Wear the label-mandated PPE for mixers when measuring pesticides.

allows accurate measuring from the mini-bulk tank to the sprayer. These meters require frequent calibration to be accurate. Mini-bulks must be returned to the dealer for refilling. This process eliminates the need to triple- or pressure-rinse multiple small containers and reduces the volume of used plastic containers.

WATER-SOLUBLE PACKAGING

Water-soluble bags are a simple type of closed mixing and loading system. The premeasured pesticide is contained inside a water-soluble bag or package. The pesticide bag is placed unopened into the mixing tank and dissolves in water or liquid fertilizer. Few manufacturers, however, provide water-soluble bags for small-volume applications (see Randall et al. 2008).

MEASURING PESTICIDES

You will be using an assortment of glass or plastic measuring utensils, including eyedroppers, for measuring small quantities (Fig. 7-10). To avoid mistaking your measuring equipment for kitchen utensils, identify these in a very obvious manner. For instance, paint handles with brightly colored waterproof paint or attach waterproof labels, and label them as "for pesticide use only." When not being used, keep all measuring and weighing equipment locked in a pesticide storage facility. This precaution prevents these items from being used for other purposes. Clean and dry utensils before storing them to prevent contaminating future mixtures.

Pesticide packages are available in different units of weight or volume. Whenever possible, plan a mixture that uses an even, preweighed amount of pesticide. The unit cost may be greater when you buy pesticides in smaller packages. However, this disadvantage can be minimal compared to the convenience and added safety of not having to weigh or measure. Do not open pesticides packaged in water-soluble packets, since these may contain highly hazardous formulations. Calibrate application equipment to use the whole packet or a number of whole packets.

Select a mixing location that you can clean easily should an accident occur. When not using premeasured packets, measure and weigh chemicals in a clear, open area. If outdoors, stand upwind to reduce chances of exposure. Wear an approved dust and mist respirator or cartridge respirator while weighing and mixing dry pesticides to prevent inhaling dust. Protect your hands and clothing with appropriate outerwear. Because liquids spill and splash easily, wear chemical-resistant gloves and a rubber apron or a waterproof suit. Refer to the pesticide label for specific PPE required for mixing and loading pesticides. Regardless of what the label says, you must wear a face shield, goggles, or other protective eyewear when performing mixing and loading activities. Reduce chances of spills or splashes into your face and eyes by always measuring and pouring pesticides below eye level (Fig. 7-11).

Open pesticide containers carefully to prevent spilling and to make resealing easier. Cut paper containers open with a sharp knife or scissors rather than by tearing. Metal and plastic containers have protective seals that you must break before use. Most of these containers have screw caps that allow you to easily reseal them.

After measuring or weighing the correct amount of pesticide, carefully pour it into the partially filled (no more than three-quarters full) spray tank (Fig. 7-12). Rinse the measuring container and pour the rinse solution into the spray tank. Use caution while rinsing to prevent splashing. Many closed mixing systems have container-rinsing devices that pump the rinse solution into the pesticide tank. Unless rinsed automatically, drain liquid containers into the

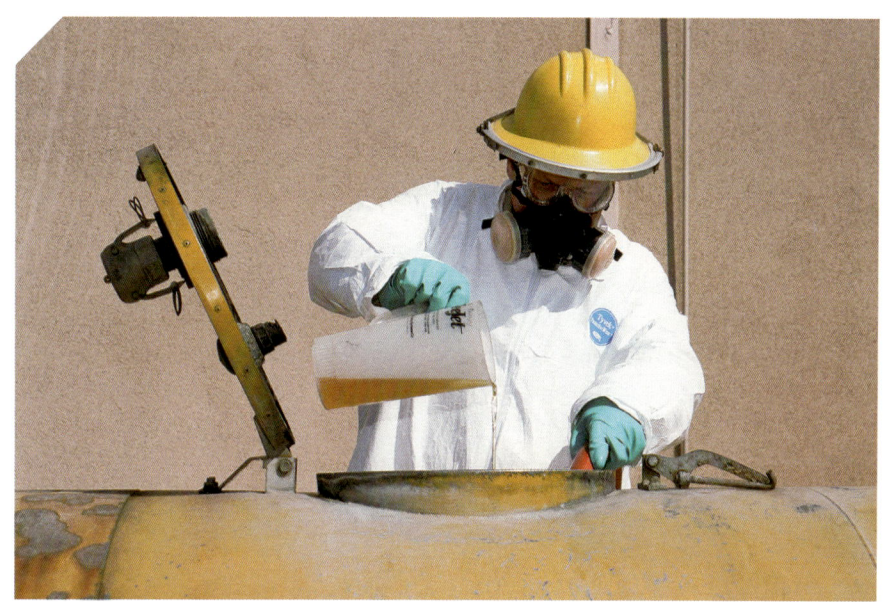

FIGURE 7-12
Carefully pour pesticides into the spray tank. Rinse measuring containers and empty and triple-rinse liquid pesticide containers. Pour the rinse solutions into the spray tank.

SIDEBAR 7-4

TRIPLE-RINSING PROCEDURES FOR PESTICIDE CONTAINERS

PROCEDURE

1. When container is empty, let it drain into spray or mixing tank for at least 30 seconds.
2. Add the correct amount of water to container as follows:

Container size	Rinse solution needed
5 gallons or less	¼ of the container volume
more than 5 gallons	⅕ of the container volume
28 gallons or more	does not require triple rinsing—return to dealer

3. Close container.
4. Shake container or roll to get solution on all interior surfaces.
5. Drain container into sprayer or mixing tank. After empty, let it drain for an additional 30 seconds.
6. Perform steps 2 through 5 two additional times.
7. Puncture container to prevent reuse.

AMOUNT OF ACTIVE INGREDIENT REMOVED FROM A 5-GALLON CONTAINER BY TRIPLE RINSING

Rinse step	Amount of active ingredient remaining*
drain	14.1875 grams a.i.
1st rinse	0.2183 gram a.i.
2nd rinse	0.0034 gram a.i.
3rd rinse	0.00005 gram a.i.

Note: *After draining, a 5-gallon container is assumed to still contain 1 ounce of formulated pesticide. This would amount to 14.1875 grams of a.i. if the formulation contained 4 pounds of a.i. per gallon.

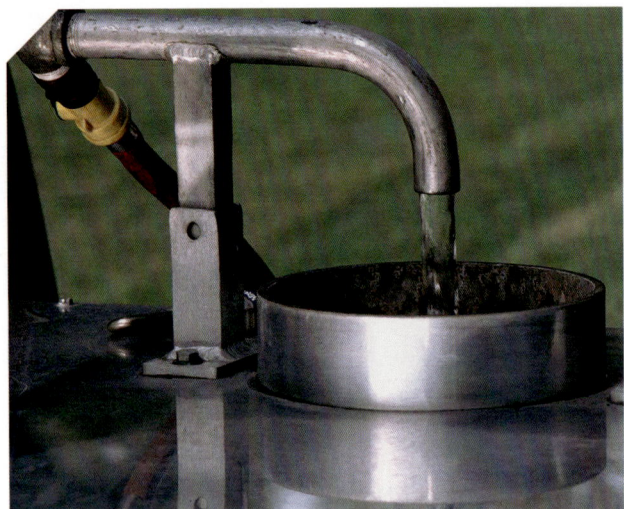

FIGURE 7-13
When filling a spray tank, be sure there is an air gap between the filler pipe and the top level of the water in the tank. This precaution prevents backflow of pesticide-contaminated water into the water supply.

spray tank for 30 seconds after you empty them. Rinse and drain the containers three more times (triple-rinse). After each draining, fill the container about one-quarter full of water and put the cap on again. Shake the container for several seconds to mix the residue with water. Pour each rinse solution into the spray tank. Sidebar 7-4 illustrates how much pesticide you can remove from the container by triple rinsing. You do not have to send containers that have been triple-rinsed to a Class I disposal site. Instead, take them to a pesticide container recycling center or a Class II disposal site.

For bags that hold dry pesticides, follow these emptying guidelines:
- Open and empty the bag so that no pesticide material remains in the bag that can be poured, drained, or otherwise feasibly removed.
- Empty the pesticide bag completely and hold the bag upside down for 5 seconds after continuous flow ceases.
- Straighten out the seams so that the bag is in its original "flat" position.
- Shake the bag twice and hold it upside down for 5 seconds after continuous particle flow ceases.
- Check with the county agriculture commissioner to find out if burning is allowed in your location. If so, obtain a burn permit and follow the guidelines in Sidebar 7-5 for burning empty pesticide bags.

Do not allow the spray tank to overflow during filling. Also, never let the hose, pipe, or other filling device come in contact with liquid in the tank. If you fill the tank through a top opening, leave an air gap between the spray tank and filling device for backflow prevention (Fig. 7-13). This space should equal at least twice the diameter of the filling pipe. It prevents siphoning of the spray mixture back into the water supply after you stop the water flow. Side- or bottom-filling systems require check valves to prevent backflow of pesticides into the water supply. For effective mixing techniques, see "Mixing Pesticides" in Chapter 10.

Applying Pesticides Safely

To use pesticides safely as well as effectively, confine them to the treatment area and apply them in the proper amounts. Avoid spills, leaks, and drift, which waste the pesticide and may leave residues in nontarget areas. Calibrate application equipment regularly, since improper equipment calibration can result in too little or too much pesticide reaching the target site. Safe pesticide applications require that you
- use proper equipment
- develop good application techniques
- reduce or eliminate drift
- be aware of all potential hazards

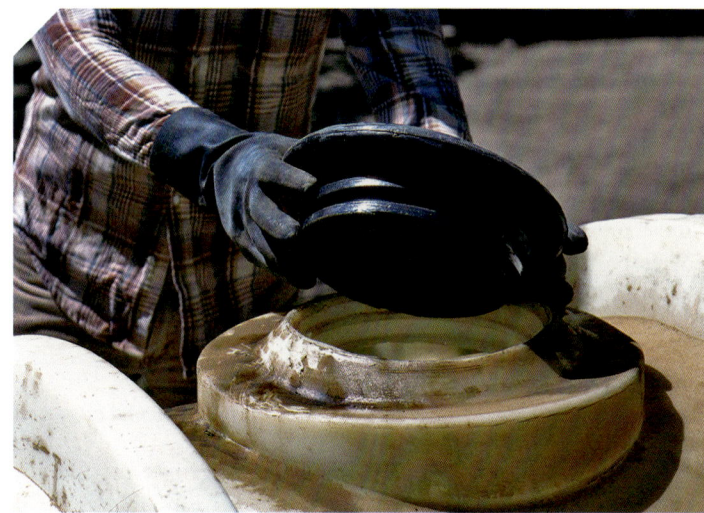

FIGURE 7-14

Be sure tank covers fit tightly to prevent pesticide mixtures from splashing out during operation or while transporting the equipment. If tanks are ever unattended, their covers must be lockable.

SELECTING APPLICATION EQUIPMENT

Be sure the equipment you use to apply pesticides is suited to the location and conditions of the treatment area. Equipment that is too big or powerful may be as much of a problem as equipment that is too small. Most pesticide application equipment works efficiently only in a limited number of situations. For example, some conditions require that spray be moved to target surfaces with a blast of air to improve accuracy.

Choose application equipment that is comfortable to work with and easy to use. Be sure the equipment is easy to repair and parts are readily available. Hand-held equipment must be lightweight so that it is convenient to use. Motor-powered units should be quiet enough to prevent operator stress yet powerful enough to do the job properly. Moving parts need shields and guards to prevent accidents and injuries. Powered equipment must have accurate gauges so you can monitor spray pressure and other functions.

Pesticide application equipment must be durable to withstand long hours of operation. Make sure that filler covers on spray tanks close properly, seal well, and are lockable (Fig. 7-14). Hoses and fittings should be strong, durable, and well maintained to prevent leaks and environmental contamination.

SAFE APPLICATION TECHNIQUES

Safe application techniques require that you
- work with the weather
- control droplet size and deposition
- know the application site and its hazards
- develop special application patterns for the site to accommodate hazards and environmental conditions
- leave buffer zones (strips) to protect sensitive areas

Describe the proper weather conditions for the safe application of pesticides.

Working with the Weather. Weather can significantly influence the safety and effectiveness of pesticide applications in outdoor areas. Its effect on pesticide applications in greenhouses and other confined spaces is more subtle. Temperature affects the phytotoxicity of certain pesticides. Label directions usually warn against using these products when temperatures are above or below critical limits. High temperatures accelerate pesticide degradation and volatilization. Clear, sunny weather produces warm temperatures. Ultraviolet light, which is most intense during these times, rapidly breaks down many pesticides.

Air temperature is responsible for the inversion phenomenon that can often cause pesticide drift. Inversions occur when the air 20 to 100 or more feet above the ground is warmer than the

FIGURE 7-15

A temperature inversion is caused by a layer of warm air occurring above cooler air close to the ground. This warm air prevents air near the ground from rising, similar to a lid.

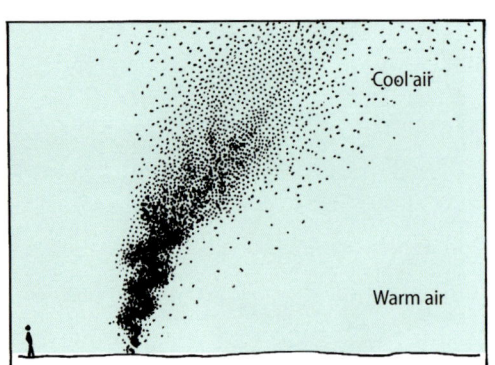
Normal condition—Smoke rises and disperses.

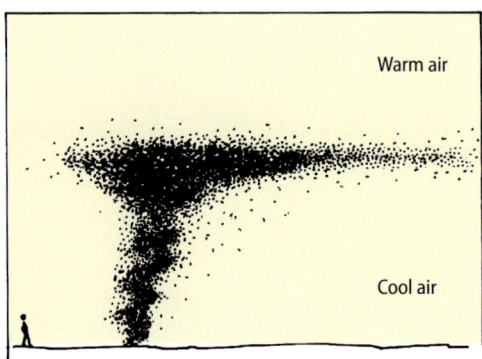
Inversion condition—Smoke concentrates.

air below it. The warm air forms a cap that blocks vertical air movement. To detect a temperature inversion, observe a column of smoke rising into the air. If the smoke begins moving sideways or collects in one area a few hundred feet above the ground, an inversion condition probably exists (Fig. 7-15). Inversion conditions are dangerous during a pesticide application. The inversion layer traps fine spray droplets and pesticide vapors. These become concentrated, similar to the smoke column. Rather than dispersing, the pesticide often moves as a concentrated cloud away from the treatment site.

Honey bees forage only during certain temperature ranges. Therefore, make applications when temperatures are not suitable for bee activity if you are using pesticides that might injure bees. Early mornings and evenings are times when bees are typically less active.

Rainfall, fog, and even heavy dew affect pesticide applications. The moisture dilutes and degrades pesticides and may wash the material off treated surfaces. Rainwater washes pesticides into the soil, producing possible groundwater and surface-water contamination. Water movement after heavy rains carries pesticides away from the application site. Fog also plays a role in offsite pesticide movement.

Wind influences pesticide drift and affects volatilization. Strong air movements are responsible for uneven pesticide deposition. However, some air movement has advantages in getting good coverage over treated surfaces.

Controlling Droplet Size and Deposition. The following factors influence how spray droplets cover the treated surfaces:
- droplet size
- pressure of the spray stream
- force and volume of the air used to distribute spray
- speed of travel of the application equipment

Droplet size is a result of nozzle size, style, and condition combined with spray volume, spray pressure, and weather influences. Most nozzles emit sprays in a wide range of droplet sizes. However, the best spray applications result from applying uniform-sized droplets evenly to all treated surfaces. Increase the uniformity of spray droplets by selecting nozzles designed for the working pressure and output volume of your sprayer. Inspect and replace worn or defective nozzles. The type of application equipment used must be suitable for the physical and environmental features of the location. Application speed and release height are critical. Adjust your speed and boom height to the type and size of the area and density of foliage being treated. For example, you must travel slowly and adjust nozzle height and direction when spraying an orchard with large trees, especially when they have dense foliage. However, the same orchard sprayed when no foliage is present could be treated at a higher equipment travel speed because bare branches allow easier coverage. Another consideration is the effect on the nozzle spray pattern of the nozzles' distance from the target site. If the target is too close, the spray pattern cannot fully develop to provide optimal coverage and rate distribution. If the target is too far away, there is risk of excessive overlap of the spray. Keeping the nozzles too far from the target also increases

USING PESTICIDES SAFELY

drift from ambient air movement and the air disturbance created by the moving application equipment. This is especially true when making applications with fine to very fine spray droplets, such as when applying fungicides and some insecticides.

Site Characteristics and Environmental Hazards. Carefully observe the site where a pesticide will be applied, noting the environmentally sensitive areas where pesticide drift, leaching, runoff, and residues will do the most damage. Sensitive areas include ponds, streams, or marshes and areas where water moves easily, such as watersheds. These are easy to see when observing an area targeted for pesticide application and should be avoided. Pesticide labels often indicate a minimum distance from surface water (a buffer zone) for safe application. Sensitive areas also include fields, buildings, or recreation areas above aquifers or near sinkholes or wells. Since some sensitive areas, such as aquifers, cannot be seen when observing an application site, it is best to check DPR's groundwater protection area (GWPA) maps (see cdpr.ca.gov/docs/emon/grndwtr/gwpamaps.htm) to find out whether leaching, runoff, or both are major problems.

Describe how to identify potentially sensitive areas that could be adversely affected by pesticide application, mixing and loading, storage, disposal, and equipment washing.

TABLE 7-1

Groundwater ubiquity score (GUS) and potential for groundwater contamination of selected pesticides

GUS value	Leaching potential
<0.1	extremely low
0.1–1.0	very low
1.0–2.0	low
2.0–3.0	moderate
3.0–4.0	high
>4.0	very high

Potential for groundwater contamination based on GUS* for selected pesticides					
Extremely low–low		Intermediate		High–very high	
Pesticide common name**	GUS value	Pesticide common name**	GUS value	Pesticide common name**	GUS value
bifenthrin	−2.72	2,4-D amine	2.70	atrazine	4.40
buprofezin	0.73	2,4-D ester	2.00	bentazon†	1.45 to 3.38†
chlorpyrifos	0.32	azoxystrobin	2.43	bromacil	4.44
cypermethrin*	−2.27 to −1.38†	diuron	2.58	clopyralid	5.46
diazinon	1.28	fipronil	2.13	dicamba	3.78
glyphosate	−0.69	norflurazon	2.70	imazapyr	3.91
iprodione	1.32			imidacloprid	3.76
malathion	0.00			prometon	4.95
mancozeb	1.29			simazine	3.35
oryzalin	1.59			sulfosulfuron	3.42
paraquat	−5.58			triclopyr	5.63
pendimethalin	0.59				
permethrin	−0.88 to −1.48†				
pyraclostrobin	−0.06				
pyrethrins	−1.08				
spinosyns*	−0.35 and 0.09†				
trifloxystrobin	0.56				

Notes: *The groundwater ubiquity score (GUS) is a methodology used to estimate the potential of pesticides to contaminate groundwater. Persistence of pesticides and binding ability of pesticides to soil particles are used to obtain GUS values.
**Some a.i.'s or products listed may not be currently registered as pesticides or may have had their registration cancelled.
†A range of values comes from a change in absorption rates and half-life based on conditions at the application site.
Source: Pfeiffer 2010.

Always check with the county agricultural commissioner if the property you're treating is near or in a GWPA to ensure that it is actually within the GWPA. Whenever groundwater is present, however, be sure to check the pesticide label to see whether the product is likely to leach (Table 7-1).

Sensitive areas also include dwellings, schools, hospitals, parks, playgrounds, commercial areas, and other places where people may work, live, or play. The location and type of crops, especially those next to the application site, must also be considered when you are selecting material. This is because of the possibility that material will drift onto crops that are not listed on the pesticide label, contaminating them.

Application Pattern. An application pattern is the route you follow while applying a pesticide. The purpose of any application pattern is to provide an even distribution of pesticide over the treated area. To do this, you must avoid overlaps or gaps. Pesticide application speed usually determines the uniformity of the application pattern. At higher speeds, the equipment bounces more. With air blast sprayers, as you increase travel speed you reduce the volume of displaced air. When establishing an application pattern, consider

- prevailing weather conditions
- what is being sprayed
- hazards in or near the application site

Design a pattern that eliminates the need to travel through airborne spray or walk or drive through freshly treated areas. Operating the application equipment (such as boom sprayers) during turns produces an uneven application. Figure 7-16 illustrates how to make a uniform application by shutting the sprayer off during turns. Watch for clogged nozzles that will also produce uneven applications.

Leave untreated buffer zones when a treatment area adjoins sensitive areas. Buffer zones are locations that provide untreated space to keep nontarget organisms, people, or structures from unnecessary exposure to pesticides (Fig. 7-17). As a general rule, the buffer should be no less than the width of one spray swath. The size of the buffer zone depends on the

- type of application equipment you are using

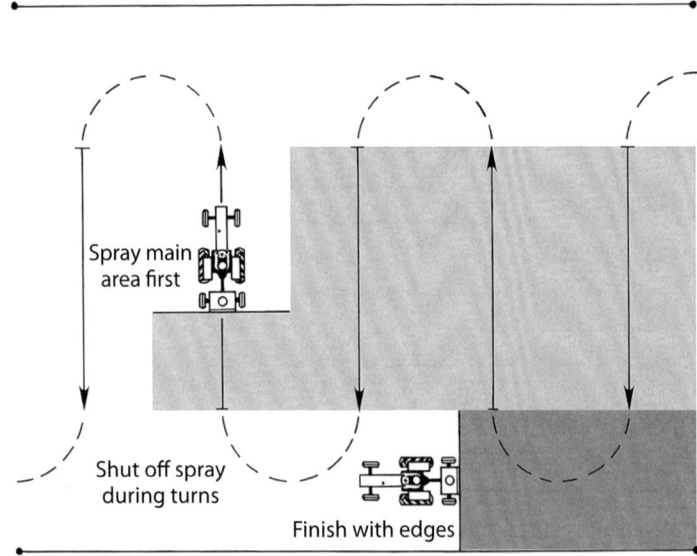

FIGURE 7.16

Shut off spray nozzles during turns to avoid uneven applications. After spraying the main part of the treatment area, finish by spraying the edges.

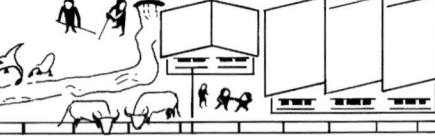

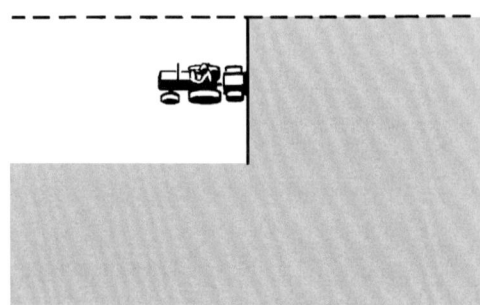

FIGURE 7.17

Leave untreated buffer zones when an application site adjoins sensitive areas. The buffer zone should be no less than the width of one spray swath.

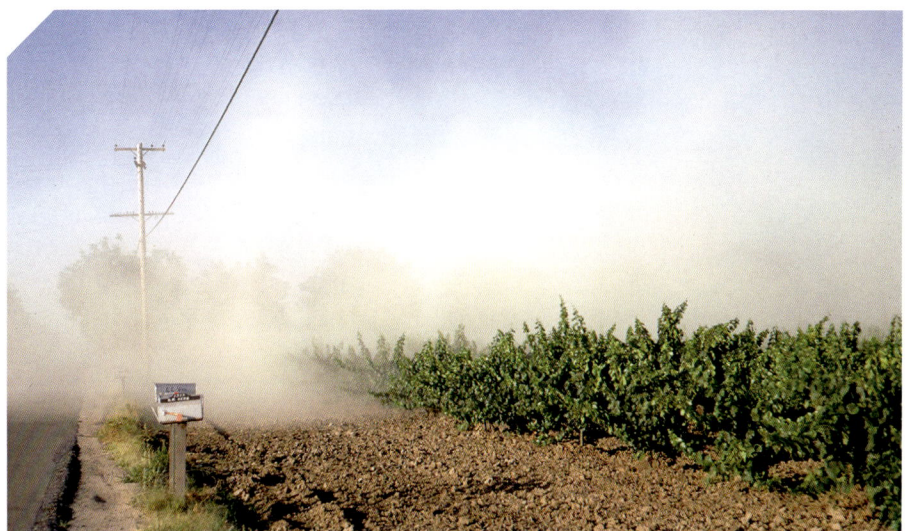

FIGURE 7-18

Pesticide sprays and dusts drift when you apply them during windy periods. Drift is also the result of small droplet size caused by high pressure and small nozzle orifices.

- prevailing weather conditions
- nature of pesticide being applied
- type of pest problem being treated
- sensitive nature of adjoining areas
- label directions

PESTICIDE DRIFT

Pesticide drift refers to the movement of pesticides away from the treatment site in air. Drift is most serious when you make applications during windy conditions, especially while using high pressure and nozzles that produce small droplets. Wind carries these spray droplets away from specified treatment areas (Fig. 7-18). Another form of drift occurs when sprayed pesticides partially evaporate before reaching the target. The resulting vapor can drift away from the treatment area through air movement, often traveling several miles. Pesticides can also move away from the application site in water through leaching or runoff, so be careful to avoid practices and conditions that influence all types of offsite movement (Table 7-2).

TABLE 7-2

Factors influencing pesticide leaching

Category	Factors
cultural practices	amount and type of pesticide used
	method of pesticide application

	irrigation practices at treatment site:
	  frequency of irrigation
	  timing of irrigation in relation to pesticide application

geologic conditions of treatment area	slope
	underlying formations
	proximity of surface-water channels such as ponds, lakes, rivers

interaction of pesticides in soils	properties of pesticides:
	  • water solubility
	  • volatility
	  • soil adsorption
	  • decomposition

	soil influence on pesticides:
	  • soil texture
	  • soil organic matter content
	  • soil water content

TABLE 7-3

Factors influencing pesticide drift

Category	Factors
pesticide	volatility of active ingredient
	solvent used to dissolve or suspend active ingredient (formulation)
	solvent used to dilute pesticide in spray tank
adjuvants	deposition aids, thickeners, and stickers (reduce drift by making droplets larger or less volatile)
application equipment	operating pressure of spraying system
	nozzle size
	distance from nozzles to target surface
	height from which spray is released
	speed of travel of application equipment
	application pattern and technique
target surfaces	size of target area
	location of target area
	nature of target surfaces
weather conditions	wind intensity
	wind direction
	air temperature
	humidity

Table 7-3 lists some of the factors that influence drift. You can take many steps to reduce this problem. Eliminating very small droplets significantly reduces drift. Increase droplet size by using larger nozzles and by lowering the output pressure of the sprayer. Certain adjuvants, called deposition aids, assist in increasing spray droplet size or reducing evaporation potential. Add one of these to the spray tank to help avoid drift, but only if the pesticide label permits adding this type of adjuvant.

Do not spray during windy conditions. Usually, winds between 2 and 5 miles per hour can help provide good pesticide distribution in trees and leafy plants. Stronger winds, however, increase drift potential. In some cases, spraying may be illegal if the wind speed is over a designated rate. Contact the local agricultural commissioner for information on pesticide application restrictions during windy conditions.

Other conditions, such as a temperature inversion, also promote drift of small droplets and vapors. High temperatures and low humidity increase the evaporation rate, which reduces the size of droplets before they reach their target. The resulting smaller droplets are much more likely to drift. For information on preventing pesticide drift, see "Preventing Pesticide Drift" in Chapter 10.

SPECIAL HAZARDS IN TREATMENT AREAS

Pesticides containing petroleum-based carriers may be flammable. Never use these in areas where open flames or other ignition sources are present. Gas-fired water heaters and electric motors may ignite flammable pesticides. When applying pesticides in areas where such hazards exist, use a nonflammable, water-based spray. Otherwise, shut off all ignition sources.

The spray from water-based pesticides usually conducts electricity. If the spray contacts an electrical source, you risk a potentially fatal electric shock. Never direct any spray onto power transmission lines, electrical cords, outlets, motors, or appliances. Disconnect motors and appliances and shut off electricity in areas where you are applying pesticides to prevent chances of electrocution.

> **SIDEBAR 7-5**
>
> **GUIDELINES FOR EMPTYING AND BURNING PESTICIDE BAGS**
>
> Obtain an agricultural burn permit from your local air pollution control district.
>
> **EMPTYING GUIDELINES**
>
> - Open and empty the bag so that no pesticide material remains that can be poured, drained, or otherwise feasibly removed.
> - Empty the pesticide bag completely and hold it upside down for 5 seconds after continuous flow ceases.
> - Straighten out the seams so that the bag is in its original flat position.
> - Again, hold the bag upside down for 5 seconds after continuous particle flow ceases; shake the bag twice and hold for 5 seconds or until continuous flow ceases.
>
> **PESTICIDE BAG BURNING GUIDELINES**
>
> - Burn pesticide bags only at the location specified on the agricultural burn permit.
> - Select a location that will minimize the amount of smoke blowing over areas where people or domestic animals may be located. To select a site, consider distances to homes, parks, schools, and businesses; wind speed and direction; inversions; and length of time to burn the bags.
> - Place a rock, brick, or similar noncombustible weight on top of the stack of bags to be burned.
> - Light the bag on the bottom of the stack.
> - Stand upwind of the burn site to avoid breathing the smoke.
> - Control the site until burning is completed and the fire is extinguished.

Cleanup and Disposal

DISPOSAL OF LEFTOVER PESTICIDE MIXTURES

To avoid problems associated with leftover pesticide mixtures, calculate the exact size of the treatment area, then mix only enough pesticide for the job. If you have some leftover spray mixture, use it in another appropriate location. Otherwise, you must send the leftover material to a Class I disposal site. Private companies specialize in collecting and transporting pesticide wastes to Class I disposal sites.

Never indiscriminately dump excess pesticide. Such dumping is a potential source of environmental and groundwater contamination. It is also illegal. People convicted of dumping are subject to large fines and possible jail terms.

PESTICIDE CONTAINER DISPOSAL

Explain how to properly process all types of pesticide containers for disposal.

Requirements concerning the disposal of pesticide containers vary from county to county. Obtain disposal information from your local county agricultural commissioner.

Some localities allow you to burn paper containers as part of an agricultural burn permit. For burning pesticide bags, follow the instructions in Sidebar 7-5. In nonagricultural areas, contact local authorities to work out arrangements for disposing of plastic and paper pesticide containers. Unrinsed empty containers are hazardous waste, so they should always be triple-rinsed at the time of use. Dispose of these according to provisions of State Water Quality Control Board and Department of Toxic Substances Control regulations. Address container disposal questions to your local county agricultural commissioner.

You can recycle triple-rinsed or pressure-rinsed metal and plastic containers or take them to an approved Class II disposal site. Many counties participate in a pesticide container recycling program. Contact your local agricultural commissioner's office for information on container recycling opportunities locally. If these containers have not been triple-rinsed, or if used containers cannot be rinsed, you must send them to a Class I disposal site. Check with the Water

Quality Control Board or agricultural commissioner in your area for the locations of approved disposal sites.

CLEANING APPLICATION EQUIPMENT

After each use, you must clean and decontaminate application equipment. Otherwise, residues remaining in tanks may contaminate a subsequent pesticide mixture and alter its toxicity. Pesticide residue on the outside of application equipment can be hazardous to people who must operate or repair this equipment. Therefore, wash the outside of spray equipment with water, using a small amount of detergent if necessary. Clean equipment in an area where you can contain runoff. Otherwise, clean the equipment at the application site. For a more detailed treatment of this subject, including what should be done with rinsates, see "Application Equipment Maintenance" in Chapter 8.

PERSONAL CLEANUP

After using pesticides, clean your PPE, shower thoroughly, and change into clean, uncontaminated clothing. When showering, take special care to wash your hair and clean your fingernails. Place clothing that you wore during the pesticide application into a plastic bag until you can launder it. Never eat, drink, smoke, or use the bathroom until you have thoroughly washed. Always wash your work clothing separately from other clothing, especially if you bring it home to launder. See Chapter 6 for additional information on cleaning and maintaining PPE.

Recordkeeping

Maintain records of every pesticide application you make and other activities associated with your use of pesticides. Keep records of the following pertinent information.

THE PESTICIDE APPLICATION

- name, manufacturer, and U.S. EPA registration number of the pesticide
- total amount of pesticide used
- amount of water used
- date and time when the application was completed

OTHER RECORDS

- posting requirements
- pesticides handled by employees
- handler training specific to classes of pesticides handled
- fieldworker training
- pesticide storage inventory

Also note temperature and general weather information at the time of application. Write down any other conditions that might have an influence on the effectiveness of the pesticide. Keep a record of the names of people you spoke to regarding each pesticide application. Include any follow-up information and notes of application results. See Figure 10-21 in Chapter 10 for a pesticide application follow-up checklist. Figure 7-19 is an example of a pesticide application record. Keep copies of written recommendations with your application records.

Application records are helpful as a history of pesticide use, especially when plant-back restrictions (also called rotational crop restrictions) exist. Even more important, this information is vital in case problems associated with the application should develop. Good records may also be important to your defense in any legal action. In addition, recording the delivery date, quantity, and expiration date of pesticides purchased can help ensure you use them while they are still effective. For more information about the importance of recordkeeping, see Chapter 10.

	Date:	Applicator:
APPLICATION SITE	Owner/Responsible Party:	Location:
	Size of Treatment Area:	Plant Age and Condition:
	Description (Turf, Ag Crop, etc.):	Soil Conditions:
	Surrounding Sensitive Areas:	
	Previous Pesticides Used:	
PEST PROBLEM	Primary Pest:	Damage Observed:
	Other Pests Present:	Location of Damage:
	Beneficials Present:	
	Severity of Pest Problem:	
PESTICIDE(S) USED	Pesticide(s): Formulation: Rate:	Total Amount Used:
	(1)	
	(2)	
	(3)	
	Adjuvants	Total Gallons of
	Type: _____ Amount: _____	Diluted Spray Used:
APPLICATION	Date(s) of Application:	Weather Conditions
		Temperature:
	Equipment used:	Cloud Cover:
		Wind Speed:
		Wind Direction:
	Equipment Calibrated By:	Other:
	Pesticides Mixed By:	Travel Speed:
	Pesticides Applied By:	Total Hours for Application:
	Persons Notified or Spoken to Regarding Application:	
	(1)	
	(2)	
	(3)	
FOLLOW-UP	Effectiveness of Application: Beneficials Present: Pest Resurgence Noted:	
	Injury to Nontarget Plants or Surfaces:	
COMMENTS		

FIGURE 7-19

Pesticide application record.

Liability

You assume personal responsibility for accidents and injuries that arise as a result of each pesticide application. You may be subject to fines, jail sentences, and loss of your applicator certificate or license if you are negligent in your application of pesticides or have broken state or federal laws. Also, courts may hold you responsible in lawsuits for personal injury or damages. If you are working for someone else, your actions may result in lawsuits against and fines to your employer. Should someone bring a claim of negligence against you, accurate records of all your pesticide applications will help in your defense.

Should the pesticide you are applying drift and damage plants, animals, or someone's belongings or cause human injury, you may incur personal liability. The pesticides you apply can potentially damage the intended crops or surfaces. Situations that might cause damage include but are not limited to
- improper mixing
- using the wrong adjuvants
- improper application
- applying the wrong pesticide
- poor timing
- using a pesticide that has been contaminated with impurities
- failing to notify people in and around the treatment area

Someone may sue you for destroying beneficial insects such as honey bees. If the bees are essential for pollinating a crop, you could be liable for the loss of the crop as well. There have been instances where applicators were sued because they applied pesticides to the wrong location.

Pesticides and pesticide application equipment are attractive nuisances. Children, fascinated with what you are doing, may be injured or even killed by chemicals and equipment if you leave these unattended.

Often, taking prompt action greatly reduces the extent of damage (and therefore liability) from a pesticide accident or application error. See Chapter 12 for information on how to deal with pesticide emergencies.

LIABILITY INSURANCE

Commercial pesticide applicators must buy liability insurance or a surety bond to protect themselves from claims associated with pesticide use. Proof of financial liability, either from insurance or a surety bond is a licensing requirement in the state of California. Clients of professional applicators may require the applicators to have liability insurance. Policies cover the costs of damages from accidents and improper use. This type of insurance is often expensive and sometimes difficult to obtain due to the nature of pesticide injury claims. Insurance companies consider as better risks applicators who maintain complete records and are conscientious in their efforts to use pesticides responsibly.

Some professional organizations representing pesticide applicators have information on insurance companies and policies. Some provide opportunities to participate in group policies. Select insurance suitable to your operation and specialty. Be sure you understand the extent of coverage and policy liability limits.

Chapter 7 Review Questions

1. In which of the following situations must you notify people in the area of your pesticide application? Select all that apply.
   - ☐ a. when fieldworkers or other employees are within ¼ mile of the treatment site
   - ☐ b. when people have hung laundry to dry outdoors in homes nearby
   - ☐ c. when people near the site have fruits or vegetables growing in gardens
   - ☐ d. when beekeepers have hives close to the treatment site
   - ☐ e. when the application site is near a school or park

2. Which of the following is considered a good way to keep the public from encountering hazards during your pesticide application?
   - ☐ a. Pass out wallet-sized cards listing emergency contacts, including poison control, to everyone within ¼ mile of the application site.
   - ☐ b. Notify people in the area and provide them with information about how to avoid exposure to the pesticide you're applying.
   - ☐ c. Notify all area emergency response agencies of your pesticide application and provide them with all labeling for the product you will apply.

3. The restricted-entry interval (REI) for the pesticide you are applying is 8 days. How will you keep people out of the treated field during that period?
   - ☐ a. Place warning signs at usual points of entry, or in the case of an unfenced field, at the corners of the treated area.
   - ☐ b. Notify fieldworkers of the REI orally before the application and remind them again after the application.
   - ☐ c. Erect a temporary barrier around the treated area that remains locked for the duration of the REI.

4. When transporting pesticides in a vehicle, you should _____.
   - ☐ a. secure the packages inside the passenger compartment
   - ☐ b. carry them in the cargo area of a truck, but have someone ride in that area to make sure containers remain undamaged in transit
   - ☐ c. secure containers in the vehicle's cargo area after checking it carefully for anything that might damage containers in transit

5. A proper pesticide storage facility should be _____.
   - ☐ a. protected by a security system and equipped with a telephone for emergencies
   - ☐ b. securely locked and clearly identified as a pesticide storage facility
   - ☐ c. well lighted and supplied with plenty of sturdy wooden storage shelves

6. True or false?
   - ☐ a. You can find mixing directions for any pesticide on its label.
   - ☐ b. PPE is optional during mixing and loading activities, especially if you use a closed mixing and loading system.
   - ☐ c. If you mix and load more than 1 gallon of Category I (DANGER) liquid pesticides in California, you must use a closed mixing and loading system.
   - ☐ d. You can use any type of measuring utensil (plastic, glass, or metal) when measuring pesticides.
   - ☐ e. It is always safest to create mixtures using even, premeasured amounts of pesticide, rather than having to hand-measure it.
   - ☐ f. You should always mix pesticides in an area that is easy to clean in case of an accident.

7. High temperatures during or soon after a pesticide application can cause which of the following problems?
   - ☐ a. increased phytotoxicity and accelerated chemical breakdown
   - ☐ b. increased absorption and faster translocation
   - ☐ c. increased leaching potential and a loss of potency

8. Match the sensitive area with the steps used to preserve it.

1. lakes, ponds, or streams	a. Choose pesticides that are less likely to drift and are less toxic to people and animals. Leave a buffer strip adjoining these features of the landscape.
2. aquifers, sinkholes, or wells	b. Check the label for the proper distance to maintain from these features of the landscape and use a formulation less likely to have problems with runoff.
3. parks, schools, playgrounds, or recreational areas	c. Check DPR's Ground Water Protection Area (GWPA) maps and avoid using pesticides that leach to protect these features of the landscape. Read the label to find out about a pesticide's leaching potential.

9. Which statement about triple rinsing pesticide containers is true?
   - ☐ a. You must wear extra PPE for triple rinsing with a closed system.
   - ☐ b. Triple-rinsed containers can be taken to a Class II disposal site.
   - ☐ c. Triple rinsing is not necessary if you intend to recycle the container.

10. Which of the following is the BEST place to clean your application equipment after use?
    - ☐ a. on a paved surface near the application site
    - ☐ b. at a do-it-yourself car wash
    - ☐ c. at the application site

11. Keeping accurate application records can prevent problems associated with which of the following?
    - ☐ a. increased volatility
    - ☐ b. plant-back restrictions
    - ☐ c. expiration date

Chapter 8
Pesticide Application Equipment

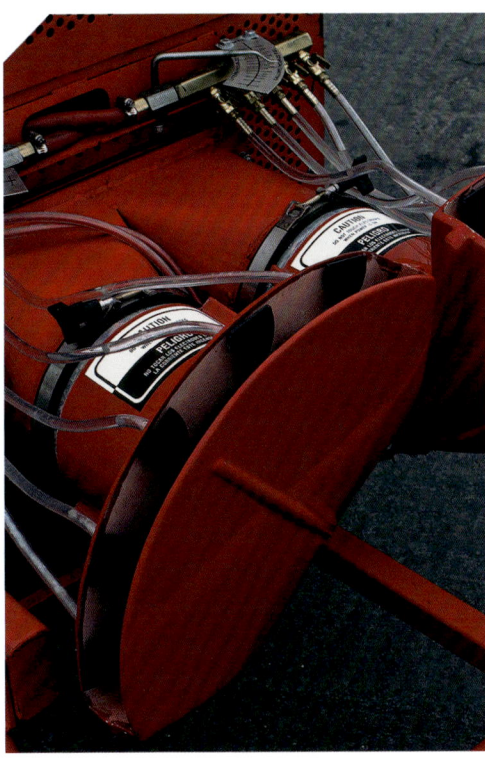

Application Methods	194
Liquid Application Equipment	195
Dust and Granule Application Equipment	231
Livestock and Poultry Application Equipment	233
Bait Application Equipment	234
Application Equipment Maintenance	235
Chapter 8 Review Questions	240

Knowledge Expectations

- List components of liquid application equipment, explain how they work together, and identify which components work best with which pesticide formulations.
- Name the parts of application equipment that can be switched out or adjusted to accommodate changing conditions and formulations.
- Describe how to recognize wear in various components.
- Describe the various nozzles available, including design, size, angles, and output.
- List the important factors to consider when selecting nozzles for a given application.
- List the types of application equipment and describe the advantages and limitations of each type.
- List the types of application equipment used to apply liquids and describe the situations in which each should be used.
- List types of chemigation systems and describe the situations in which they can be used.
- List the types of application equipment used to apply dusts and describe the situations in which each should be used.
- List the types of application equipment used to apply granules and describe the situations in which each should be used.
- List types of bait application equipment and explain how they work.
- Describe how to maintain different kinds of application equipment.
- Describe safe and effective practices for cleaning application equipment.
- Describe how to properly store application equipment.

Pesticide application equipment ranges from simple devices attached to garden hoses to elaborate machines mounted on self-propelled ground applicators, fixed-wing aircraft, or helicopters. Some equipment specifically applies dusts, while other types apply granules. You can select from many different types of equipment designed for applying liquids. Special equipment is available for many purposes, including

- controlling weeds
- applying pesticides to orchards, vineyards, row crops, and field crops
- injecting pesticides into the soil
- applying pesticides to animals
- controlling aquatic pests
- controlling pests in buildings and residences

Application Methods

The pesticide application method you choose depends on the nature and habits of the target pest, the characteristics of the target site, the properties of the pesticide, the suitability of the application equipment, and the cost and efficiency of alternative methods. Your choice will often be predetermined by one or more of these factors. Following are some common application methods.

- **Band application** involves applying a pesticide in parallel strips or bands, such as between rows of crops rather than uniformly over the entire field.
- **Basal application** directs herbicides to the lower portions of brush or small trees to control vegetation.
- **Broadcast application** is the uniform application of a pesticide to an entire area or field.
- **Crack and crevice application** is the placement of small amounts of pesticide into cracks and crevices in buildings, such as along baseboards and in cabinets, where insects or other pests commonly hide or enter a structure.
- **Directed-spray application** specifically targets the pests to minimize pesticide contact with nontarget plants and animals.
- **Foliar application** directs pesticide to the leafy portions of a plant.
- **Rope-wick or wiper treatments** release pesticides onto a device that is wiped onto weeds taller than the crop or wiped selectively onto individual weeds in an ornamental planting bed.
- **Soil application** places pesticide directly on or in the soil rather than on a growing plant.
- **Soil incorporation** is the use of tillage, rainfall, or irrigation equipment to move the pesticide into the soil.
- **Soil injection** is the application of a pesticide under pressure beneath the soil surface.
- **Space treatment** is the application of a pesticide in an enclosed area.
- **Spot treatment** is the application of a pesticide to small, distinct areas.
- **Tree injection** is the application of pesticides under the bark of trees.

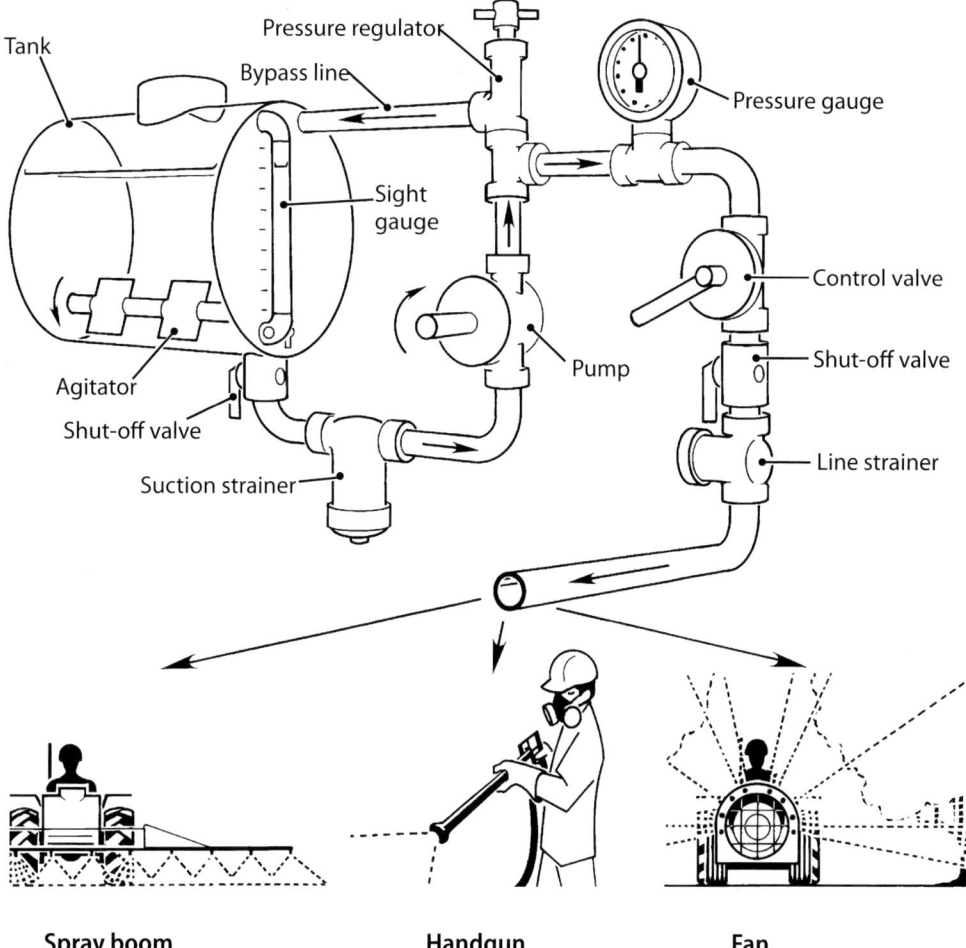

FIGURE 8-1

Liquid application equipment usually includes a tank for mixing and holding pesticides (often equipped with an agitator) and a pump for creating hydraulic pressure, and it may also include a pressure regulator, pressure gauge, control valve, and several types of strainers. Spray is emitted through nozzles on a spray boom, manifold, or hand spray gun, and may be dispersed by a fan.

List components of liquid application equipment, explain how they work together, and identify which components work best with which pesticide formulations.

Each method requires the use of specific application equipment. This chapter describes a variety of pesticide application equipment and baiting devices, except those used with aircraft. It explains and illustrates components such as tanks, pumps, and nozzles. It also discusses maintenance, cleaning, and storage procedures for some equipment types (for more information, see Randall et al. 2008).

Liquid Application Equipment

Most liquid application equipment uses hydraulic pressure or air to generate pesticide droplets and propel them to the target. This equipment is either hand-operated or powered by mechanical sources such as a tractor power take-off (PTO) or an electric, gasoline, or diesel engine. Liquid application equipment consists of several components, including

- a tank for mixing and holding the pesticide
- a pump or other device for creating pressure to move the liquid
- one or more nozzles for breaking the spray up into small droplets and directing it toward the target
- on some equipment, fans, pressure regulators, filter screens or strainers, control valves, agitators, booms, hoses, and fittings to improve pesticide handling, mixing, and application (Fig. 8-1).

Components of Liquid Application Equipment

Before considering a pesticide application machine as a whole unit, look at all the individual components. Make sure they meet your application needs by assessing the application site and customizing the sprayer to best target the pest, accommodate plant structures and sizes, and apply pesticides uniformly. Some components, such as nozzles, are easy to replace when worn or damaged or if your application requires a change. Other parts, such as tanks, are expensive to replace and may be difficult to repair if they become damaged. Select these with care to be sure they are compatible with the pesticides you plan to use.

Name the parts of application equipment that can be switched out or adjusted to accommodate changing conditions and formulations.

Pesticide Tanks

Manufacturers produce tanks for mixing and holding liquid pesticides from metal, fiberglass, and thermoplastic materials such as polyethylene and polypropylene. Choose a nonabsorptive material so you can easily clean the tank of pesticide residues. Tanks must be resistant to corrosion and rust to protect them from reacting with corrosive pesticides. They should have a large opening for easy filling and cleaning (Fig. 8-2). Table 8-1 is a guide for selecting tanks based on your pesticide application needs.

The tank should have a cover. A tight-fitting cover prevents pesticides from spilling or splashing. Many counties require that tank covers be lockable. Although not always required by law, a lockable cover may be a worthwhile safety feature. It prevents unauthorized or accidental exposure to the tank contents. Larger tanks need a bottom drain so you can completely empty them. All tanks 50 gallons or larger must have a sight gauge or

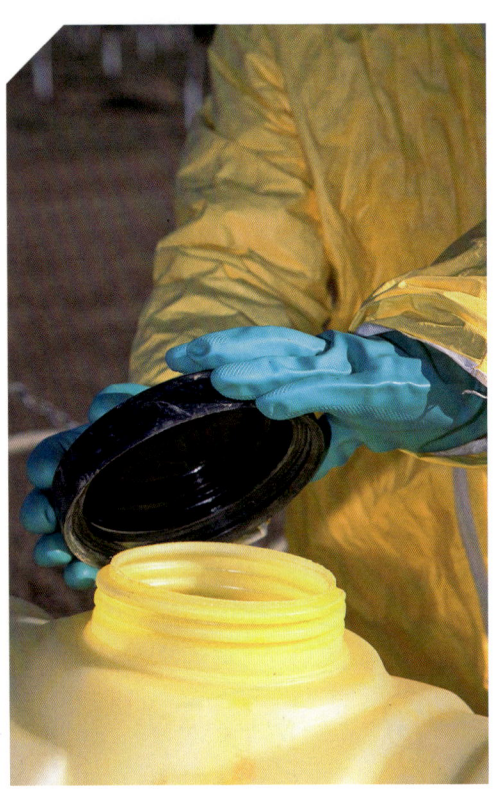

FIGURE 8-2

Pesticide tanks must have a large top opening for ease in filling. The opening should be fitted with a splashproof cover.

TABLE 8-1

Pesticide tank selection guide

Characteristics	Tank type				
	Coated metal	Stainless steel	Fiberglass	Polypropylene	Polyethylene
acid resistance	fair to good	depends on grade	fair to good	good	good
alkali resistance	excellent	excellent	fair	good	good
organic solvent resistance	excellent	excellent	poor to fair	good	fair
rust and corrosion resistance	fair to good	excellent	excellent	excellent	excellent
absorbs pesticides	if scratched	no	if scratched	no	no
easily cleaned	good	excellent	fair	excellent	excellent
easily repaired	yes	yes	yes	no	no
strength and durability	good to excellent	excellent	good	good	good
weight	heavy	heavy	medium	light	light
requires external reinforcement	no	no	no	yes	yes
cost	moderate	high	moderate	low	low

PESTICIDE APPLICATION EQUIPMENT

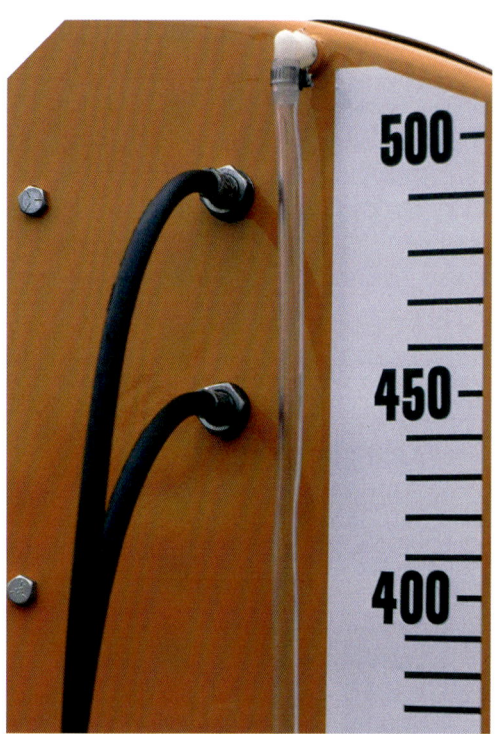

FIGURE 8-3

A sight gauge enables the operator to tell how much spray solution is contained in the tank at all times. External tubes must be equipped with a shut-off valve to prevent leaks if the gauge becomes damaged.

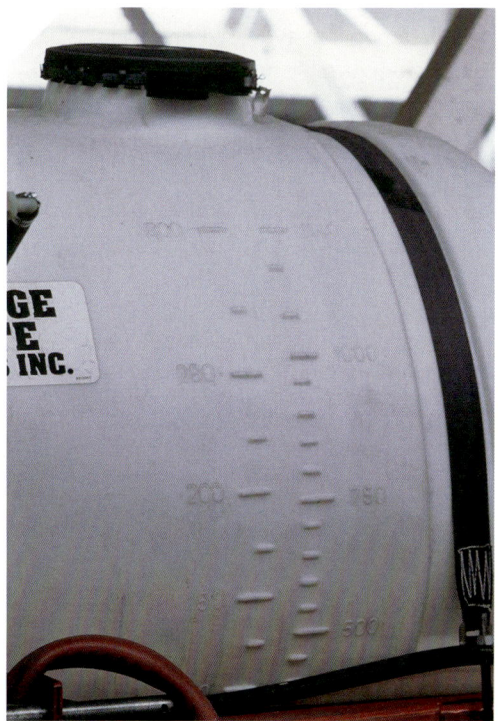

FIGURE 8-4

Manufacturers produce most thermoplastic sprayer tanks from either high-density polyethylene or polypropylene. Pictured is a polyethylene tank.

other accurate means to determine the amount of liquid in the tank. Equip external sight gauges with shut-off valves to prevent leaking if they become damaged (Fig. 8-3). Tanks are commonly available in capacities from 3 to over 1,600 gallons.

Metal Tanks. Manufacturers produce tanks from several different grades of stainless steel. They also make steel tanks with epoxy or other coatings to prevent them from rusting or corroding. Stainless steel has superior qualities for rust and corrosion resistance, so you can use most pesticides in them. Stainless steel cleans easily and is strong and durable, though you should still look for signs of rust or corrosion regularly. If damaged, you can repair stainless steel tanks, although repairs may require skill. These tanks are more expensive than tanks made from other materials, but they generally last longer.

> Describe how to recognize wear in various components.

Galvanized or coated metal tanks require more care and attention. Scratches or chips in the protective coating expose bare metal and may cause serious corrosion problems. You cannot use some pesticides in coated metal tanks. Glyphosate, for example, reacts with metal to produce hydrogen gas, resulting in an explosion hazard. Epoxy coatings have fair to good resistance to acids and excellent resistance to alkaline materials and organic solvents. You must inspect epoxy-coated metal tanks regularly and touch up chips and scratches to prevent corrosion.

Fiberglass Tanks. Fiberglass tanks are strong and durable and you can easily repair small damaged areas. They are lighter than metal tanks. Fiberglass is highly resistant to organic solvents. It has good to fair resistance to acids, but only fair resistance to alkaline materials. The fiberglass material absorbs pesticide liquids if the interior tank walls have scratches or abrasions. This absorption may cause contamination of future tank mixes. Therefore, you must repair scratched areas with resin to protect against this problem.

Thermoplastic Tanks. Most thermoplastic materials have good resistance to acids and alkalis. Polyethylene is a common material used for spray tanks, although low-density polyethylene does not resist organic solvents well. Manufacturers produce most thermoplastic sprayer tanks from either high-density polyethylene or polypropylene (Fig. 8-4). These plastics are lightweight and durable. However, when these plastics get warm, they become flexible and will deform unless they are reinforced or supported. Minor scratches or abrasions do not cause absorption problems. However, polyethylene and polypropylene are difficult to repair if they become punctured or cracked. They may also be degraded by long-term exposure to sunlight and weather. If you see spiderwebbing (small, interconnected cracks) on any surface of the thermoplastic tank, it means that the tank is beginning to weaken and should be replaced.

Pumps

Most liquid sprayers use pumps to move the pesticide from the tank to the nozzles. The pump must create adequate flow to build the pressure needed for generating spray droplets and propelling them to the target. A range of pump sizes is available, depending on your task and budget.

Selecting the appropriate pump for a particular application depends on a number of factors. The formulations of pesticides you use are a factor in pump selection. You must also consider the volume and pressure needed to apply these pesticides. Water-soluble and emulsifiable concentrate pesticide formulations are less abrasive to pumps than wettable powder, flowable, or dry flowable formulations. Construction materials and type of pump also affect how well pumps perform and wear. When choosing a sprayer pump, consider the following features.

Output capacity. The pump must supply enough volume (or flow rate) for all nozzles under every use condition. If the sprayer has hydraulic agitation, the pump must have sufficient output to recirculate liquid in the tank while spraying. Pump output capacity is given in gallons per minute (gpm).

Pressure. A pump must operate with the desired capacity at a pressure suitable for the work you perform. Some high-capacity pumps are able to work only at low pressures. You can regulate most high-pressure pumps so they are suitable for low-pressure work as well. Pressure is measured in pounds per square inch (psi).

Resistance to corrosion and wear. The materials used to construct the pump, as well as pump design, affect its ability to resist corrosion and wear. Pumps with the fewest parts contacting spray chemicals are the most suitable for corrosive pesticides. Pump design is also important in reducing the amount of wear due to wettable powder abrasion.

Ease of repair. An important feature of any pump is the ease with which you can repair it. Be sure the most commonly needed parts are readily available.

Type of drive. Pumps require different operating speeds depending on their design. Most PTO shafts rotate at 540 or 1,000 revolutions per minute (rpm). Gasoline and diesel engines and electric motors all have specific operational speed ranges. Because each pump also has particular horsepower requirements, match it with the speed and horsepower of the drive unit. If a pump needs to operate at higher speeds, you may need a special transmission or belt drive.

Table 8-2 is a guide for selecting common pump designs. Other types of pumps not included in this table may also be available and suitable for certain applications.

Diaphragm Pumps (Fig. 8-5). Diaphragm pumps are a popular style used on several types of spray equipment. Manufacturers produce these pumps from durable materials, including aluminum, steel, and high-impact plastic. You can use these for low- and high-pressure applications. Diaphragm pumps handle abrasive and corrosive chemicals well because only the chemical-resistant diaphragm contacts pumped liquids. They are also simple to maintain and repair.

Diaphragm pumps have a low- to medium-volume capacity of between 5 and 40 gpm. They can operate at pressures from 200 to 700 psi. These pumps operate in the range of 500 to 800 rpm, well matched to PTO speed.

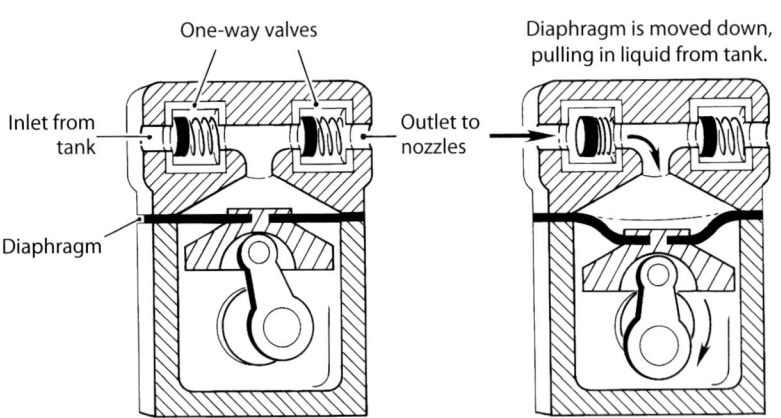
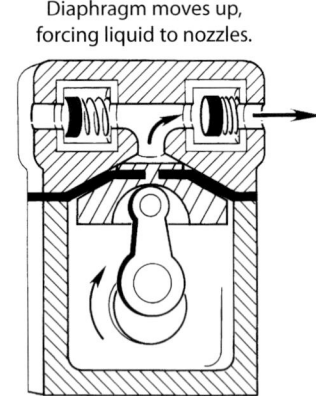

FIGURE 8-5

In a diaphragm pump, a flexible diaphragm is moved up and down by a cam mechanism. This oscillation moves liquid through one-way valves. Some diaphragm pumps incorporate two or three diaphragms moved by the same cam.

A cam that moves one to three diaphragms produces the pumping action. Moving a diaphragm in one direction creates a negative pressure inside the pumping chamber. This negative pressure forces open a one-way valve, pulling liquid pesticide from the tank into the chamber. As the diaphragm reverses direction, the one-way valve seals shut. Positive pressure in the chamber forces open a second one-way valve, pushing the liquid pesticide out another opening. Pressure in the system may pulsate due to this action. However, more expensive pumps have two or three diaphragms working opposite each other that minimize pulsating pressure. Manufacturers equip some diaphragm pumps with surge chambers or pressure dampers to reduce pulsating pressure.

Diaphragm pumps have only a few moving parts. Diaphragms usually wear out after a while, so you must replace them when they begin to leak. Replace the rubber valves when they fail to seal properly. The petroleum-based solvents in emulsifiable concentrate formulations accelerate the deterioration of these rubber components.

TABLE 8-2

Guide for selecting the proper pump for a pesticide sprayer

	Pump type	Pressure range (psi)	Output volume (gpm)	Operating speed (rpm)	Suitable pesticide formulations	Comments
	centrifugal	5–200	>200	1,000–5,000	all	Used on large, heavy-duty sprayers. Common on air blast sprayers. Best for high-volume uses.
	diaphragm	20–700	5–40	500–800	all (organic solvents may deteriorate some parts)	Often used on low-volume weed sprayers. Also used with some high-pressure equipment.
	gear	20–100	5–65	500–2,000	nonabrasive	Limited uses. Good for low-volume and low-pressure applications.
	piston	20–1,000	2–60	500–800	nonabrasive unless equipped with wear-resistant cups	Excellent for high-pressure applications. Very versatile.
	roller	10–300	8–40	300–2,000	nonabrasive only; may be damaged by organic solvents	Limited low-volume uses. Can produce moderate pressure.

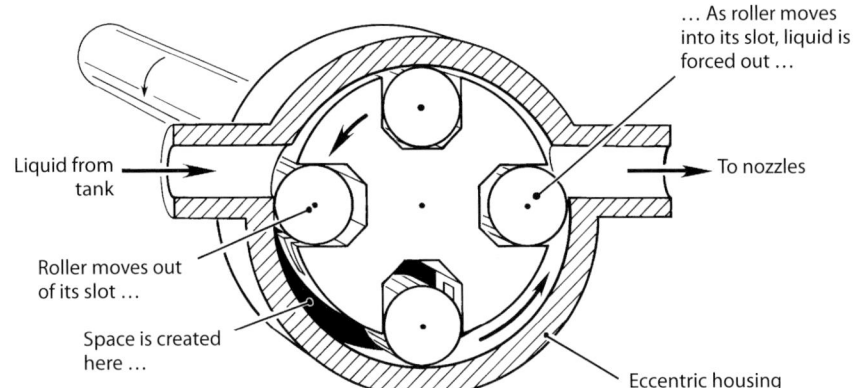

FIGURE 8-6

Roller pumps consist of cylindrical rollers that move in or out of slots in a spinning rotor. This action creates space for liquid during half of the rotor rotation and discharges the liquid out of the pumping chamber during the remainder of the rotor rotation.

Low-pressure diaphragm pumps are suitable for most herbicide applications. You can use the high-pressure styles in hydraulic and air blast sprayers.

Roller Pumps (Fig. 8-6). Roller pumps are among the least-expensive pump types. They are capable of producing moderate flow volumes from 8 to 40 gpm. Low to moderate pressures in the range of 10 to 300 psi are also possible with roller pumps. They operate in the speed range of 300 to 2,000 rpm. In these pumps, a series of rollers fit into slots around the circumference of a rotating disc, or impeller. The impeller spins off-center to its housing. This allows the rollers to move farther in or farther out of their slots. Liquid is picked up at the point where rollers are farthest out. The impeller rotation forces the rollers back into their slots and pressurizes the liquid.

Roller pumps are subject to considerable wear, especially from abrasive materials like wettable powders. Rollers made of rubber last longer. However, you must use nylon or Teflon rollers to pump petroleum-based pesticides such as oils or emulsions because petroleum-based pesticides deteriorate rubber. Usually, you can easily replace worn-out rollers. Roller pumps are most suitable for herbicide applications, especially if you use flowable, emulsifiable concentrate, soluble powder, or other nonabrasive formulations.

Gear Pumps (Fig. 8-7). Gear pumps are suitable for low-pressure applications from 20 to 100 psi. They can produce spray in a range of 5 to 65 gpm. They operate in the range of 500 to 2,000 rpm.

Manufacturers produce two types of gear pump designs. The external gear design has two identical gears that mesh with each other and move fluid through the pumping chamber. An internal gear design has a smaller gear meshing inside a larger gear, producing the pumping action.

Manufacturers build gear pumps from brass, bronze, or alloy steel. These usually are molded parts, making them difficult to repair. You can use lubricating liquids such as oil sprays or

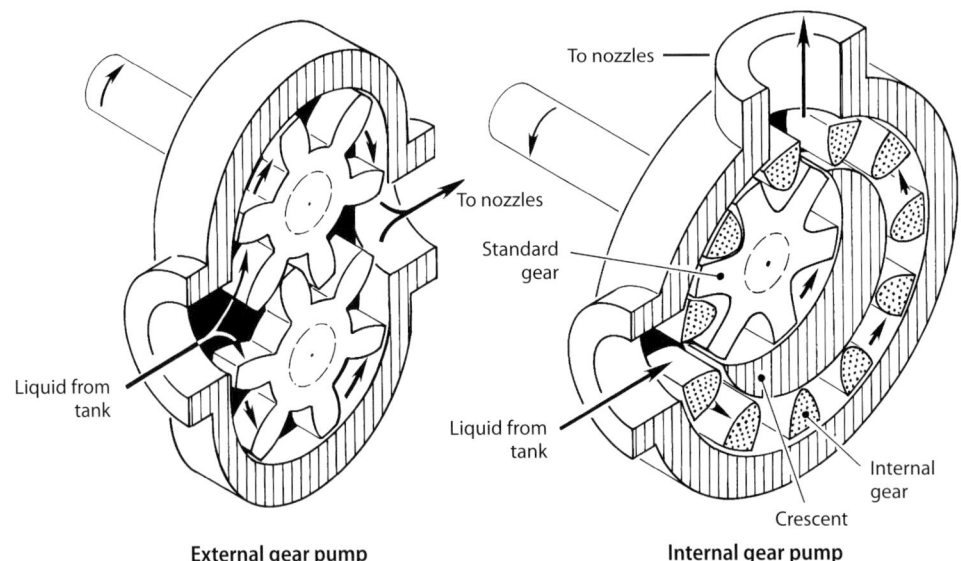

FIGURE 8-7

The external gear pump moves liquids by a meshing action of two identical gears. The internal gear pump consists of a standard gear that meshes with and drives an internal gear to move liquids. The close meshing of the gears in both of these designs forces fluids to move in only one direction through the pumping chamber.

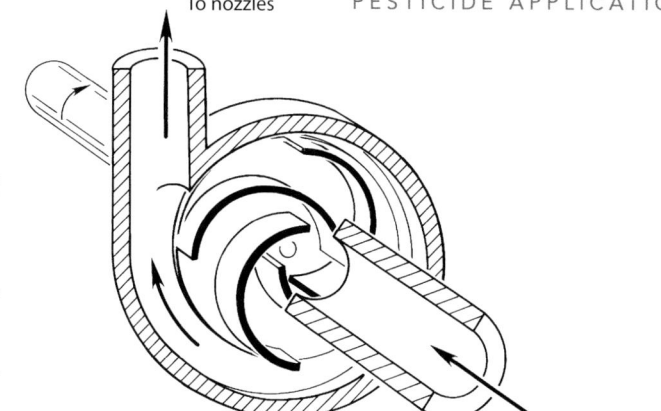

FIGURE 8-8

In a centrifugal pump, liquid enters near the center of a vaned rotor. As the rotor spins, the liquid is moved away from the center by centrifugal force. Rotors must turn at a high rpm in order to build up sufficient pressure for most spray applications.

emulsifiable concentrates in gear pumps. However, wettable powders and similar abrasive formulations create very fast wear in these pumps.

Centrifugal Pumps (Fig. 8-8). Manufacturers produce centrifugal pumps out of high-impact plastic, aluminum, cast iron, or bronze. These pumps are heavy-duty and adaptable to a wide variety of spray applications. They can produce volumes in excess of 200 gpm at pressures from 5 to 200 psi. Centrifugal pumps require operating speeds from 1,000 to 5,000 rpm. A high-speed impeller creates the pumping action that forces liquids out of the pump. Manufacturers produce high-pressure centrifugal pumps by adding one or more stages of impellers. In these, fluids pass from one impeller to the next.

Centrifugal pumps have a wide range of applications. You can use them for spraying abrasive materials because there is no close contact between moving parts. They are often easy to repair and work well for high-volume air blast sprayers.

Piston Pumps (Fig. 8-9). Piston pumps operate at pressures from 20 to 1,000 psi at volumes from 2 to 60 gpm. They operate at from 500 to 800 rpm. These are generally the most expensive pumps. However, you usually need this type for high-pressure applications or if you use both high and low pressures, for example, when using a sprayer equipped with a system or rate controller.

One or more pistons travel inside cylinders, forcing fluids through one-way valves. This action is similar to that of diaphragm pumps. However, piston displacement (or movement) is usually greater than diaphragm movement. Pulsating pressure may be a problem with piston pumps, as it is in diaphragm pumps. Abrasive chemicals cause wear in piston pumps, although most have easily replaceable cylinder liners and piston cups. More-expensive piston pumps have stainless steel or ceramic cylinder liners to resist wear.

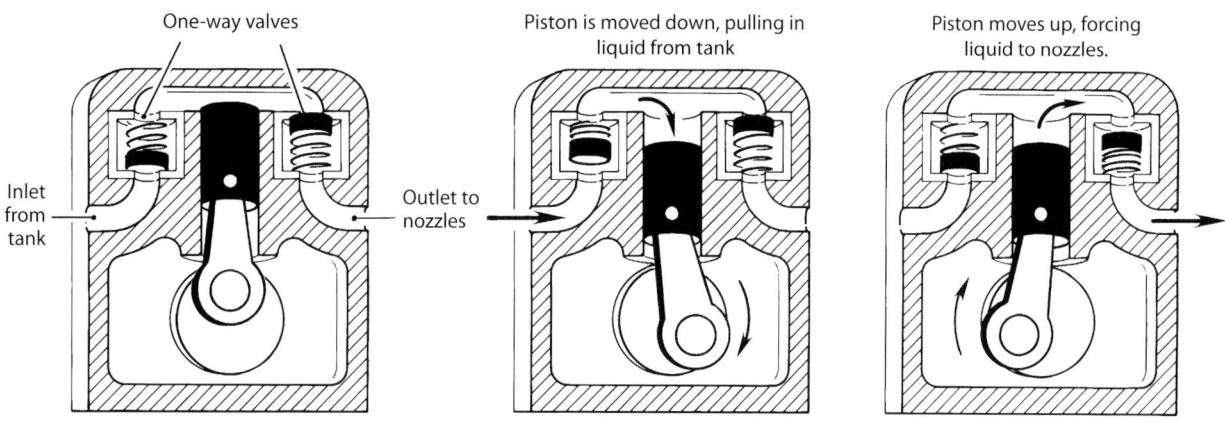

FIGURE 8-9

This sequence shows how a piston pump works. The downward movement of a piston draws liquid through a one-way valve into the cylinder. When the piston moves up, liquid is forced out through another one-way valve. Some pumps consist of several pistons working opposite each other.

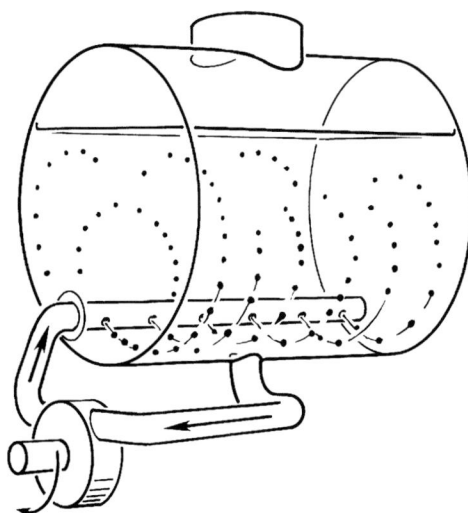

FIGURE 8-10

Hydraulic agitators recirculate spray material back into the spray tank, providing continual mixing of the solution.

Agitators

Spraying equipment needs an agitator for initial mixing of pesticides and to keep insoluble mixtures from settling inside spray tanks. Use a sprayer with an agitator whenever you use wettable powders, water-dispersible granules, flowables, or emulsions. Hydraulic and mechanical agitators are available.

Hydraulic Agitators (Fig. 8-10). Hydraulic agitators circulate spray material through jets located in the bottom of the spray tank. In most designs, this fluid comes from a bypass line on the pressure (outlet) side of the pump. Other sprayers have a separate pump to circulate fluid for tank agitation. Jets located in the bottom of the tank must be at least 1 foot from tank walls. This prevents the spray from weakening or making holes in the tank. The main disadvantage with hydraulic agitators is that they are not able to break up settled spray material when you shut the pump down for a while. Severe settling requires mechanical agitation to re-suspend insoluble particles.

Mechanical Agitators. Mechanical agitators are propellers or paddles mounted on one or more rotating shafts near the bottom of a spray tank (Fig. 8-11). The shaft passes through the tank wall and connects to the drive line by belts or chains. Mechanical agitators can provide constant mixing in the tank even if the sprayer pump is not running. They are usually effective in suspending settled formulations. Mechanical agitators require some maintenance, especially where shafts pass through tank walls. Packings and grease fittings prevent leaks but need periodic tightening and servicing. Be sure to use a marine-grade grease on bearings and seals exposed to liquids. Also, periodically tighten and service belts or chains.

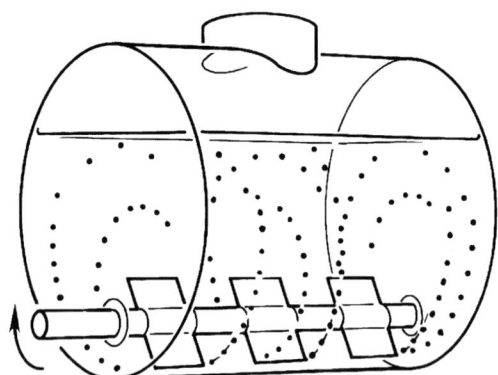

FIGURE 8-11

Mechanical agitators consist of paddles or propellers that continually stir the liquid in the spray tank.

FIGURE 8-12

Strainers hold filter screens and are located in different parts of the system. The suction strainer is positioned between the tank and pump. The pressure strainer is located between the pump and nozzles. Nozzle strainers are located adjacent to nozzles.

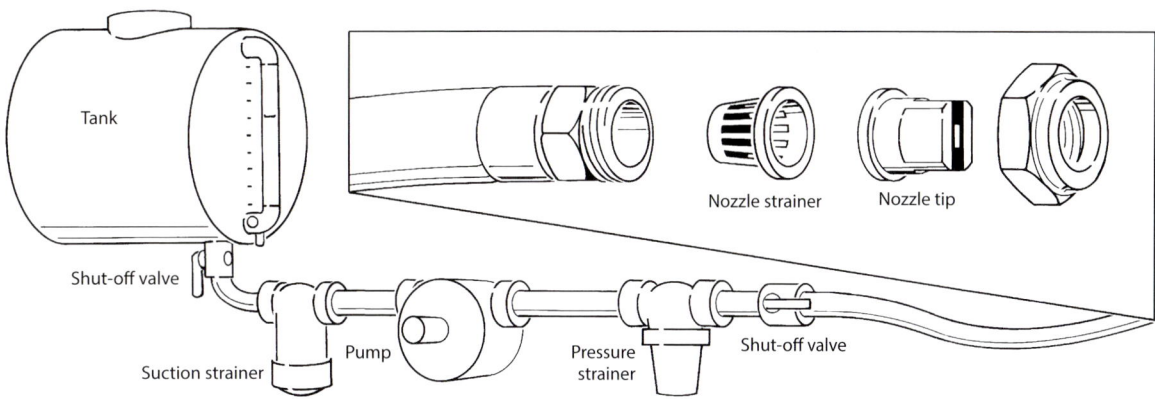

Filter Screens and Strainers

Filter screens and strainers protect pumps and prevent clogged nozzles. They remove undissolved clumps of pesticide formulation, sand, soil, and other debris from the spraying system. Filter screens and strainers help prevent clogged nozzles when using water that may contain small quantities of sand. Filters and strainers must be cleaned often because they collect and hold the materials they remove, such as pesticide clumps and debris containing pesticide residue.

Strainers. Strainers (Fig. 8-12) are devices containing filter screens that remove foreign particles that would otherwise clog nozzles or damage pumps and other sprayer components. Strainers can be placed between the tank and pump (suction strainer), between the pump and nozzles (pressure strainer), and at the nozzles (nozzle strainer).

A simple suction strainer connects to the end of the intake hose near the bottom of the spray tank. This type of strainer is used in low-capacity systems, usually with roller pumps. Other systems use low-capacity suction strainers sometimes called line strainers. Manufacturers install these into a section of the hose connecting the tank to the pump. Both the suction and low-capacity line strainers have an effective straining area of about 3 to 5 square inches.

Larger-capacity sprayers have a Y or T line strainer located between the tank and pump. These contain screens providing from 7 to 30 square inches of filter surface. A capped opening on the line strainer allows removing and cleaning of the filter screen. You do not have to disassemble any plumbing or disconnect hoses. Shut-off valves between the strainer and the tank prevent spray material leaks when you remove the filter for servicing.

A pressure strainer is similar to a suction strainer, but it is located between the pump and nozzles. It also contains a capped opening so you can remove the filter screen for cleaning. The sprayer should have a shut-off valve between the pressure strainer and the pump. This prevents leaks while cleaning filters.

Use nozzle strainers to protect nozzle orifices from smaller particles missed by the suction and pressure strainers. These go between the nozzle and nozzle retainer. Most spray nozzle manufacturer guides recommend a specific strainer size based on the nozzle you choose, typically 50 or 100 mesh.

Some nozzle strainers have spring-loaded check valves. These keep the nozzles from dripping when you shut off the spray. These check valves usually lower the pressure at the nozzle, however. You may need to increase the system pressure to accommodate them. Other nozzles have body assemblies with diaphragm regulators. These regulators allow the use of nozzle strainers without the need for a metal check valve.

Filter Screens. Filter screens range in size from 10 to 200 mesh. A 10 mesh size has 10 openings per inch; the larger the mesh number, the finer the screen. For most spraying equipment, the suction strainer should have a coarse screen in the range of 10 to 20 mesh. A smaller mesh restricts liquid flow to the pump and also plugs easily. Clogged filter screens can cause pressure to drop within the system and increases strain on the pump.

FIGURE 8-13

Spraying with worn or damaged nozzles causes unacceptable variations in the amount of pesticide deposited in an area. This graphic illustrates what can happen when output differs by more than 10% between nozzles on the same boom (CV = coefficient of variation). *Source:* TeeJet.

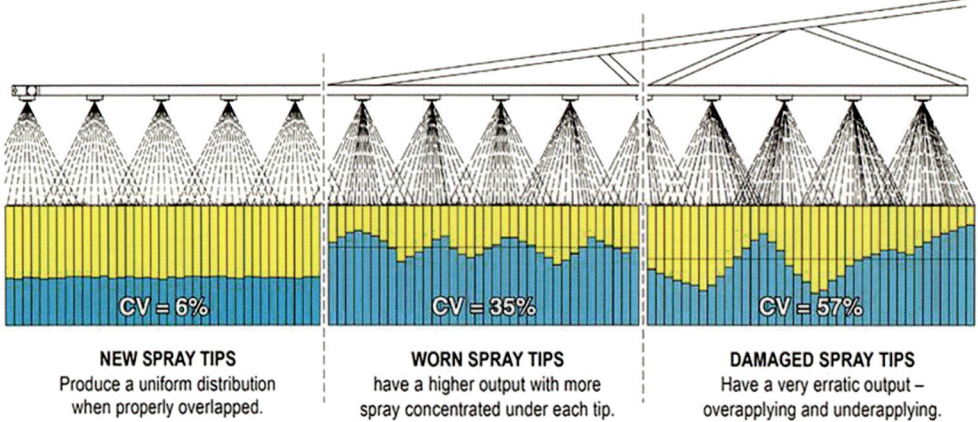

NEW SPRAY TIPS Produce a uniform distribution when properly overlapped.

WORN SPRAY TIPS have a higher output with more spray concentrated under each tip.

DAMAGED SPRAY TIPS Have a very erratic output – overapplying and underapplying.

For the pressure strainer, use a finer screen in the range of 40 to 50 mesh. This allows the pressure strainer to collect particles missed by the suction strainer.

Screens of nozzle strainers most commonly range from 50 to 200 mesh. Use smaller-mesh screens when equipping your sprayer with smaller nozzle orifices. Match filter screens with nozzle orifice dimensions to prevent clogging. However, the filter size should never be much smaller than the orifice. You do not need nozzle strainers if the nozzle orifice is larger than the pressure strainer screen mesh. Most nozzle manufacturers will list the proper nozzle screen size for the nozzle you choose.

Nozzles

Nozzles are one of the most important parts of the sprayer because they control a pesticide's application rate, droplet size, and spray pattern. Your choice of nozzle impacts the amount of potential drift that may occur as well as the effectiveness and efficiency of your application (Fig. 8-13). If you do not carefully select and maintain nozzles, you can waste all your pest control efforts.

Several different nozzle designs and construction materials are available, depending on the type of application. Base your nozzle selection on several criteria, including the

- material the nozzle is made of
- type of nozzle design
- nozzle orifice size
- pesticide formulation
- droplet size, pattern, or distribution
- drift risk

Nozzle Construction and Wear. In general, nozzles have five parts: the nozzle body, a strainer, a tip gasket or disc, a spray tip, and a cap. Manufacturers make nozzles out of various materials, all of which are subject to wear. Worn nozzles do not generate proper droplet patterns or regulate flow to the manufacturer's specifications, resulting in poor pesticide coverage and unpredictable droplet sizes. The design of the nozzle, the kinds of materials being sprayed, and the spray pressure influence nozzle wear. Flat-fan nozzle styles with sharp-edged orifices initially wear much faster than, for example, a flooding tip with a circular orifice. Also, as the spray pattern angle increases, the wear on the nozzle increases. Further, the size of the orifice affects wear: larger orifices wear more slowly than smaller ones.

Spray materials influence wear differently depending on the amount of dissolved or suspended solids in the liquid. True solutions (like mixtures made using soluble powder formulations) cause the least amount of wear, while suspensions (like mixtures made using wettable powders) cause different degrees of wear. Wear caused by suspended solids depends on

- particle size
- size distribution
- shape

- hardness
- concentration

The solids that influence wear may be the a.i. or may be an inert carrier in the formulation. Rate of nozzle wear, even when using the same type of pesticide over time, varies. Sometimes chemical companies make small changes in inert ingredients in their formulations; these have no effect on the performance of the pesticide but may influence nozzle wear. Also, formulations of the same pesticide can vary from one manufacturer to another. Some pesticides form crystals under certain conditions of water pH, water temperature, and the presence of other chemicals. These crystals often increase wear on nozzles. Higher liquid pressure increases the rate of nozzle wear, as well.

As a nozzle wears, the volume and pattern of spray change and affect the quality of application. Replace nozzles when they fail to deliver either accurate pesticide amounts or the desired spray pattern.

The output from nozzles of the same size, used together on a boom, should not vary from each other by more than 10%. If they do, it is an indication that your nozzles should be replaced. To ensure uniform wear, be sure to use nozzles made from the same material. Nozzles may be made from any of the following materials.

- Brass nozzles are moderately inexpensive but wear quickly from abrasion. Brass is an acceptable material if you do not use abrasive sprays or if you replace nozzles frequently.
- Stainless steel nozzles do not corrode, and they resist abrasion. Although hardened stainless steel wears exceptionally well, these nozzles are more expensive than most others. To address the issue of expense, some manufacturers produce plastic nozzles with stainless steel inserts, reducing the cost while increasing the life of the nozzle.
- Aluminum and monel (nickel alloy) nozzles resist corrosion but are highly susceptible to abrasion because they are made of such soft metals. Avoid using aluminum and monel nozzles unless you need specific corrosion resistance.
- Plastic nozzles are the least expensive. The plastic material resists corrosion, but nozzles made totally of plastic may swell if exposed to organic solvents. Plastics also have low abrasion resistance. Use solid plastic nozzles only with selected pesticides. Some plastic nozzles have stainless steel orifice inserts, making them much more resistant to wear. The inserts also reduce swelling problems.
- Tungsten carbide and ceramic nozzles are highly resistant to abrasion and corrosion. To reduce costs, manufacturers use tungsten carbide or ceramic inserts with brass or plastic nozzle bodies. Use these types of nozzles for high-pressure and abrasive sprays. Ceramic nozzles are usually affordable and last a long time.

Nozzle Types. Different applications require nozzles adapted to specific requirements. Nozzles used to apply herbicides in a field may be unsuitable for applying insecticides or fungicides to foliage. Spraying weeds along a roadside may require different nozzles than spraying weeds in a cornfield. Orchard sprayers have different nozzle requirements than row crop sprayers. Residential, industrial, and institutional applications need nozzles suitable for confined spaces.

Flat-fan nozzles (Fig. 8-14). Viewed from the front or back, flat-fan nozzles distribute pesticide in a flat fan shape, with fan angles ranging

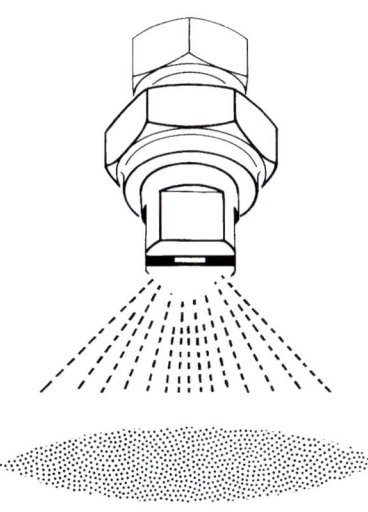
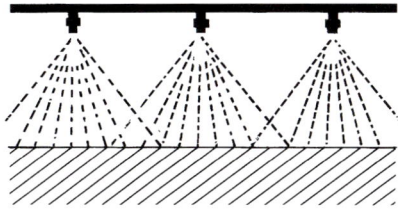

FIGURE 8-14

Flat-fan nozzles produce a fan-shaped pattern that has more droplets in the center part of the fan than at either edge. This configuration of droplets allows for overlap of the spray, eliminating gaps and providing an even pattern when multiple nozzles are used.

Describe the various nozzles available, including design, size, angles and output.

between 50 and 160 degrees. The most common angles are 65, 80, and 110 degrees. Flat-fan nozzles produce a pattern with more spray droplets in the center of the fan. The pattern tapers off at each end. This allows you to evenly space a series of flat-fan nozzles on a boom, allowing an overlap of the spray pattern of each nozzle. If you operate the nozzles at the correct height, the spray patterns combine into an even swath with nearly uniform deposits between nozzles. Use flat-fan nozzles for soil applications of herbicides, fungicides, and insecticides.

An off-center flat-fan nozzle emits a pattern of spray more to one side (laterally) than the other (Fig. 8-15). Use this nozzle on orchard and vineyard soil for applying herbicide to both sides of the plant row. When placed at the end of a boom it keeps herbicides from getting too close to the tree or vine.

Low-pressure flat-fan nozzles provide an acceptable spray pattern at pressures as low as 15 psi. Use these nozzles for the same types of applications as conventional flat-fan nozzles. This type of nozzle has fewer problems with drift because its large orifice produces bigger droplets at a lower pressure. However, contact and coverage of the spray can be limited with low-pressure nozzles.

There are also variable-pressure flat-fan nozzles that provide pressures somewhere between low-pressure nozzles and more typical flat-fan nozzles. These nozzles can be used to eliminate some of the problems associated with other flat-fan nozzle types.

Even flat-fan nozzles (Fig. 8-16). Manufacturers produce even flat-fan nozzles in angles of 40, 80, and 95 degrees. They are similar to flat-fan nozzles, except there is no tapering of spray volume at the pattern ends. Use even flat-fan nozzles when applying separate bands of spray that should not overlap.

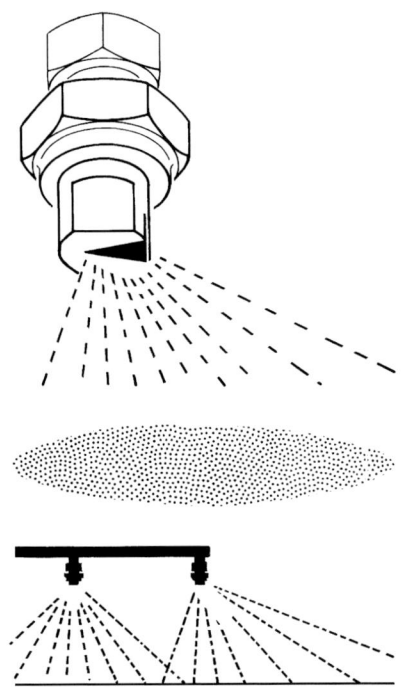

FIGURE 8-15

Off-center flat-fan nozzles emit a full pattern of spray to one side of the nozzle. These are used on the ends of spray booms to extend the reach of the nozzle.

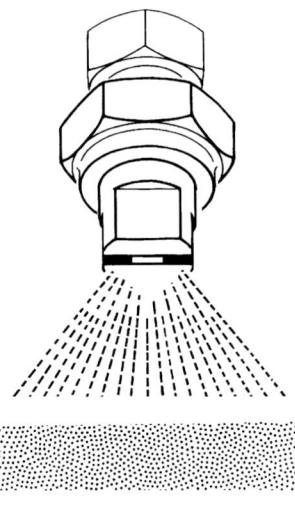

FIGURE 8-16

Even flat-fan nozzles provide a uniform distribution of spray throughout the fan pattern. The spray from these nozzles is not overlapped; these nozzles are used to apply separate bands of pesticide without overlap.

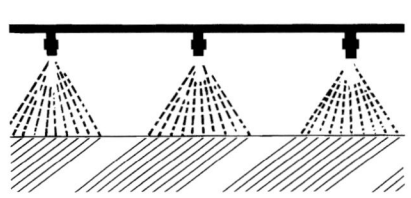

PESTICIDE APPLICATION EQUIPMENT   207

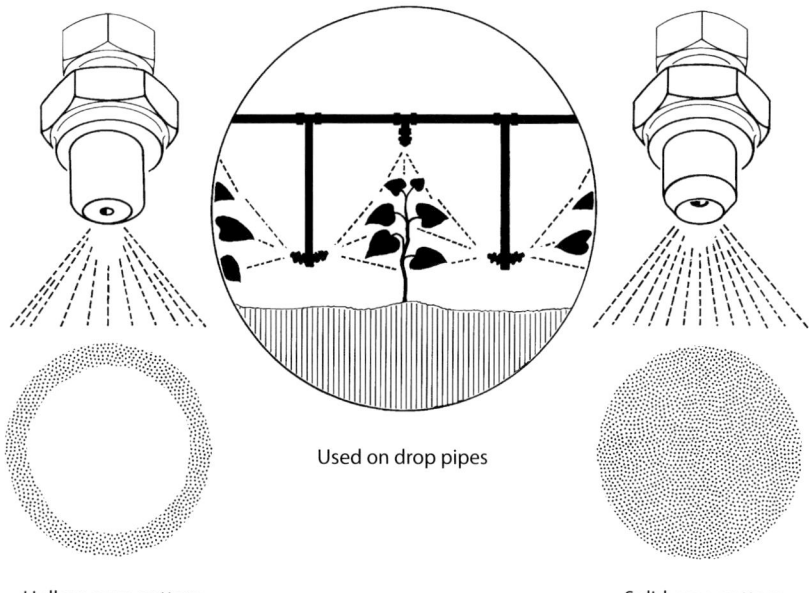

FIGURE 8-17
Cone nozzles are used for applying insecticides and fungicides to foliage, especially when larger volumes are required to ensure complete coverage.

Cone nozzles (Fig. 8-17). Use cone nozzles for applying insecticides and fungicides to dense foliage. These produce spray in either a hollow or solid cone pattern, with spray angles from 20 to 110 degrees. Use hollow cone nozzles for most applications. If you need larger, heavier droplets to reduce drift or if you require greater volume, use solid cone nozzles.

Disc-core nozzles (Fig. 8-18). A type of cone nozzle, disc-core nozzles are used in air blast sprayers. They are suitable for high-pressure and high-flow-rate application of insecticides and fungicides. Standard disc-core nozzles produce a hollow cone spray pattern, while full-cone spray patterns produce greater volume output. The orifice is in a disc made of brass, hardened stainless steel, ceramic, or tungsten carbide. Fitted behind this disc is a core, sometimes called a spinner plate. This core produces a high rotation speed of the liquid into the whirl chamber. Manufacturers make cores out of brass, aluminum, nylon, hardened stainless steel, and tungsten carbide. Using different combinations of discs and cores provides a wide range of volume output and droplet size. Because the flow rate and calibration of the spray is affected by the combination of the disc and core, you must carefully follow the manufacturer's nozzle tables in order to get the correct rate.

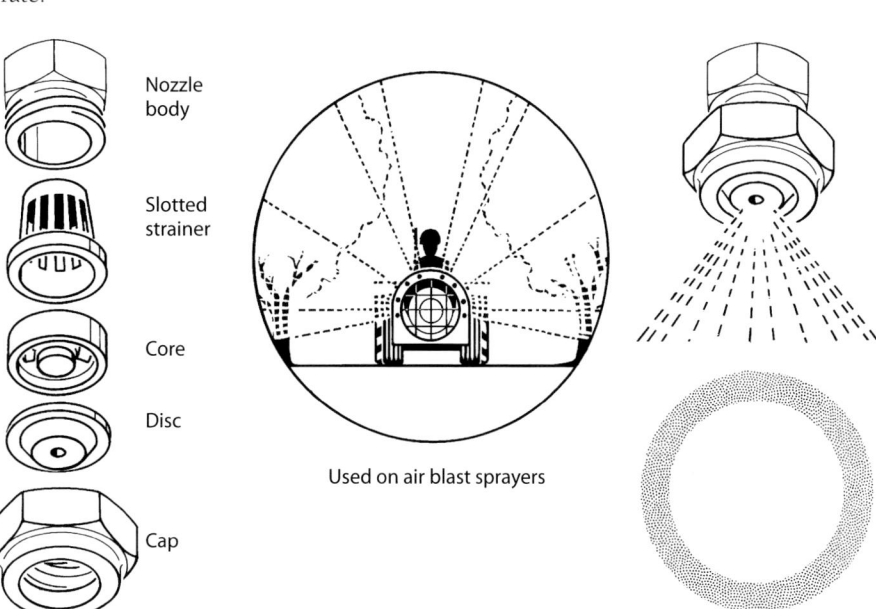

FIGURE 8-18
Disc-core nozzles are used in high-pressure applications that have a high flow rate, such as air blast sprayers. They are also used for some low-volume applications with air blast sprayers. Cores (or spinner plates) break up spray droplets and improve the deposition pattern.

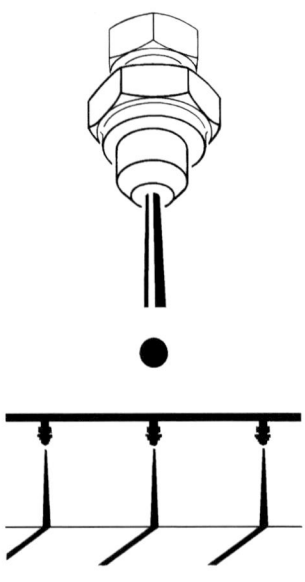
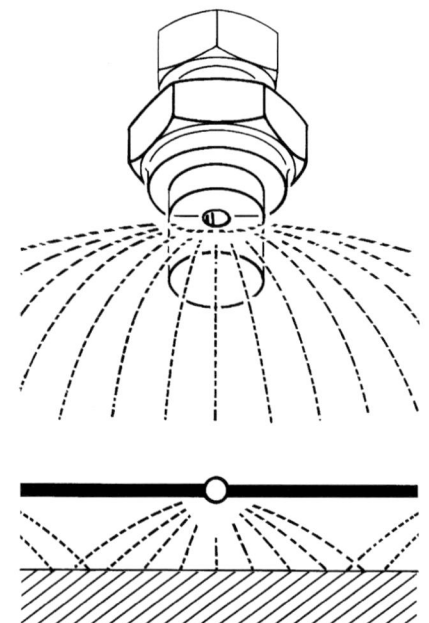
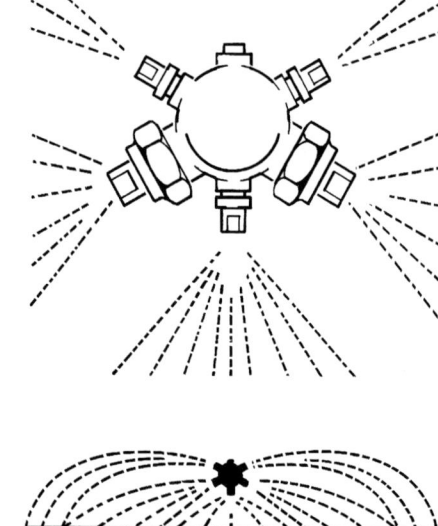
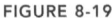

FIGURE 8-19

Solid stream nozzles are used in high-pressure hand spray guns and in low-pressure crack and crevice units. They are also used on boom sprayers for applying fluids in bands.

FIGURE 8-20

Flooding nozzles are used to apply large volumes of liquid under low pressure. They are occasionally used for pesticide application but are more commonly used for liquid fertilizers.

FIGURE 8-21

Broadcast nozzles enable a wide swath to be sprayed without using a series of nozzles on a boom. Swath widths from 30 to 60 feet can be produced.

Solid stream nozzles (Fig. 8-19). Solid stream nozzles produce a single solid stream of pesticide. Use these in hand spray guns for spraying distant objects. They are also suitable for crack and crevice treatments in and around buildings and for banding fluids in row crops. Different orifice sizes determine the volume of output.

Flooding nozzles (Fig. 8-20). Flooding nozzles produce a relatively wide fan angle of up to 160 degrees. Use these to apply large volumes of liquid at low pressure. People commonly use these for liquid fertilizers. Operators rarely use flooding nozzles for pesticide application because it is usually unnecessary to apply a large volume of liquid. Because of the large fan angle, use a wide spacing on the boom.

Broadcast nozzles (Fig. 8-21). Use broadcast nozzles on boomless sprayers. These sprayers have a cluster of nozzles attached at one point that produces a swath of 30 to 60 feet. Broadcast nozzles are useful where you cannot use a spray boom but need a wide swath. You can use broadcast nozzles, like flooding nozzles, when large volumes of liquid need to be applied. It is more difficult, however, to be accurate with broadcast nozzles than with a series of evenly spaced flat nozzles on a boom.

Bifluid nozzles. Bifluid nozzles break liquids up into extremely fine droplets, such as in a mist or fog. To do this, they use a high-velocity airstream. Use these on some types of aerosol generators for fogging enclosed areas such as greenhouses and warehouses. They also work for fogging confined outdoor areas.

Nozzle Tip Codes. Most manufacturers have a method of coding nozzle tips, and they print identification numbers on the face of the nozzle. For example, for flat spray nozzles, a common nozzle is number 8004. The first two digits indicate that the nozzle produces an 80-degree fan spray. The last two numbers indicate the volume of spray (0.4 gpm) output at 40 psi. Nozzle number 6515 is a 65-degree fan spray producing a volume of 1.5 gpm at 40 psi. Check the manufacturer's catalog to determine the rated operating pressure for the nozzles you use. Some nozzle styles operate at higher or lower pressures. For example, manufacturers commonly rate flood nozzles at 10 psi.

PESTICIDE APPLICATION EQUIPMENT

List the important factors to consider when selecting nozzles for a given application.

Manufacturers code solid stream, flood, broadcast, bifluid, and disc nozzles in a similar way. For example, some assign disc core nozzles numbers such as 4, 6, 7, and 10. Sometimes the letter "D" precedes this number to indicate a disc nozzle. The number represents the size, in sixty-fourths of an inch, of the orifice (except for the smallest sizes). For example, a D7 nozzle has an orifice diameter of $7/64$ inch. You can match several sizes of cores to discs to regulate the output capacity of the nozzle at different pressures. Follow the manufacturer's instructions for the proper installation of discs and cores.

When selecting nozzles, read the manufacturer's catalog. Learn about the nozzle sizing, its proper application, and the optimal pressure range. Manufacturers have charts for selecting spray volume or determining nozzle size. Table 8-3 is a guide for selecting nozzles.

TABLE 8-3

Guide for selecting nozzles

Style of nozzle	Suggested uses	Recommended pressure	Spray pattern	
flat-fan	Preemergent and postemergent herbicides, insecticides, and fungicides. Used on a boom.	20–60 psi. Keep pressure as low as possible when spraying weeds.	Fan-shaped pattern with fewer droplets at sides than in center of fan pattern. Suitable for overlapping with other nozzles to produce wide spray swath.	
off-center flat-fan	Used on ends of spray booms to extend reach of spray pattern.	Same as flat-fan nozzles.	Fan-shaped with angle to one side.	
even flat-fan	Preemergent and postemergent herbicides, insecticides, and fungicides. Use on boom. Do not overlap spray pattern.	20–40 psi. Keep pressure low when used for weed control.	Fan-shaped pattern with even distribution of spray across width of fan.	
cone	Insecticides and fungicides applied to foliage. Often used with air blast sprayers.	40–120 psi.	Hollow or solid cone pattern. Fine spray droplets, good penetration.	
solid stream	All types of pesticides. Used on booms and handguns.	5–200 psi.	Low- or high-pressure solid stream. High pressure breaks spray into fine to medium droplets.	
flood	Herbicides and fertilizers. High volume and low pressure reduce drift. Used on booms.	5–20 psi.	Wide, fan-shaped pattern of coarse droplets.	
broadcast	Weed and brush control in pastures and turf. Nozzles are clustered without boom.	10–30 psi.	Wide, fan-shaped pattern ranging from fine to coarse droplets.	
bifluid	Used for developing extremely fine, airborne droplets. Flying insect control in enclosed spaces.	None. Uses air pressure to move liquids.	Fog or mist.	

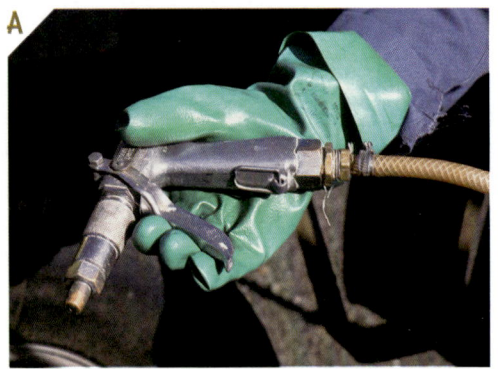
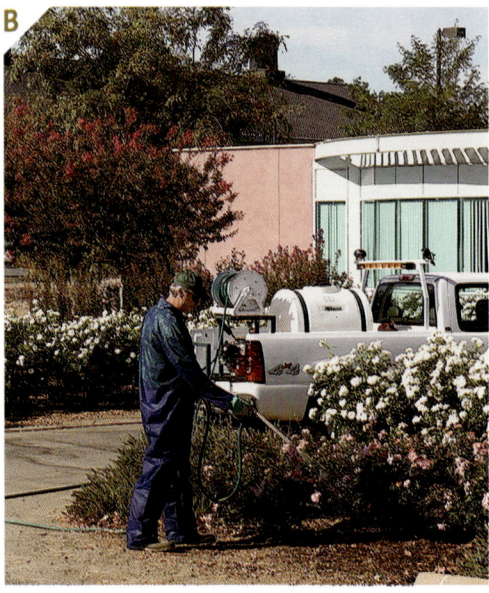

FIGURE 8-22

Hand spray guns usually produce high-pressure streams or sprays (A); they are used for applying insecticides and fungicides to trees and shrubs and are also used for spraying aquatic areas, livestock, buildings, and roadsides (B).

Hand Spray Guns

Use hand spray guns to apply a high-pressure stream or spray of pesticide to a targeted area (Fig. 8-22), such as when applying insecticides and fungicides to trees, vines, and shrubs in landscape, nursery, aquatic, and greenhouse settings. Also use hand spray guns to apply herbicides along roadsides, rights-of-way, aquatic areas, and fencerows. Applicators also use them to apply insecticides to livestock for control of external parasites.

You can attach hand spray guns to many different types of spraying equipment. Many orchard sprayers or low-pressure row crop sprayers have connectors for attaching a hand spray gun for occasional touch-up or specialized spraying. Operators of some greenhouses put pesticide pumps and tanks in a separate room. This equipment pumps pesticides through permanent plumbing to different outlets within the greenhouse. These provide convenient locations for connecting flexible hoses and hand spray guns. You can also connect hand spray guns to portable sprayers by a flexible hose. Long hoses let you spray areas farther from the pumping equipment. However, be sure the system accommodates the pressure drop due to the long hose.

A spray gun usually has a handle, a valve, and a nozzle (or a small boom with several nozzles). The valve can be part of a trigger mechanism or can connect to a knob at the end of the handle. Nozzles are usually interchangeable so you can use the hand spray gun for different types of applications. In some models, you can adjust the pressure and spray pattern with a valve mechanism.

Pressure Regulators

A pressure regulator is a spring-loaded valve that controls the pressure of liquid. In sprayers, pressure regulators are used between the pump and the nozzle, spray boom, or manifold (Fig. 8-23). To change the pressure, adjust the amount of compression on the valve by turning the pressure-

FIGURE 8-23

A pressure regulator is a spring-loaded valve that controls the pressure of fluid going to the nozzles. If pressure increases, excess pesticide is bypassed back into the spray tank.

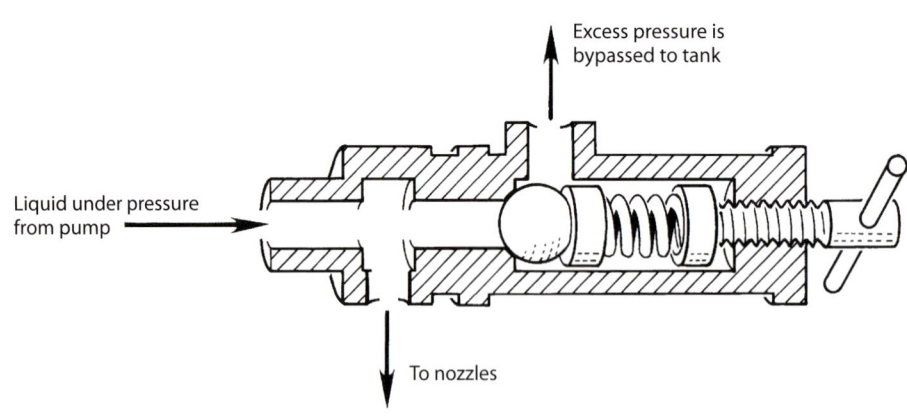

regulating screw or handle. Increasing the spring tension (turning the screw clockwise) increases the pressure going to the nozzles. When the pressure in the system exceeds the pressure of the spring-loaded valve, the valve opens. This allows some spray material to flow back into the tank and prevents pressure in the system from going any higher. Should the pump output pressure drop (by slowing the pump down, for example), the regulator reduces or stops the flow of liquid into the tank.

For an accurate reading, adjust pressure regulators while the system is operating and nozzles are spraying. When you shut off the nozzles, pressure in the system increases slightly and the pressure regulator sends all the liquid through the bypass.

Unloaders

An unloader senses pressure changes that occur when turning on or shutting off the flow of liquid to the nozzles. When you shut off the nozzles, the unloader returns all the pumped liquid into the spray tank. Once the flow to the nozzles starts, the unloader redirects the liquid at the pressure set by the pressure regulator. Unloaders are an important part of high-pressure systems because they protect pumps, valves, hoses, and other components from excessive, sudden pressure surges. They also reduce the power load on the sprayer engine.

Pressure Gauges

Equip your liquid sprayers with pressure gauges so you can monitor the fluid pressure in the system (Fig. 8-24). A change in pressure also warns you of potential malfunctions such as leaks or clogged nozzles. Usually, install the pressure gauge between the pressure regulator and the nozzles as close to the spray nozzle boom as possible to minimize pressure losses through tubing. In this position, it monitors pressure in the system while spray is being emitted through the nozzles.

Proper equipment calibration depends on an accurate pressure gauge. Recalibrate the gauge on your sprayer periodically by comparing its readings to another calibrated gauge. Also use this second gauge to measure pressure at the nozzles during calibration. (Chapter 9 describes methods of calibrating spray equipment.) A damaged pressure gauge, such as one with a bent indicator needle, should be replaced immediately.

You have a choice of gauges to measure different ranges of pressures. For example, some measure from 1 to 20 psi, while others measure from 1 to 200 psi, 1 to 500 psi, or 1 to 1,000 psi. Be sure the gauge you use is compatible with your sprayer pressure range. If your sprayer produces a maximum of 50 psi, a gauge with a range of 1 to 500 psi will be difficult to read and will have reduced accuracy. Use a gauge with a range of 1 to 100 psi for greater accuracy. The

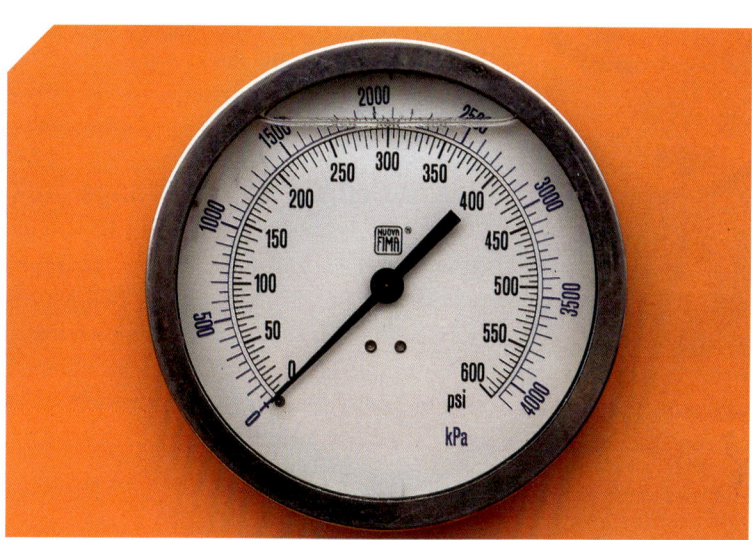

FIGURE 8-24

A pressure gauge is used to monitor the pressure of spray going to the nozzles and will alert the operator to problems in the system.

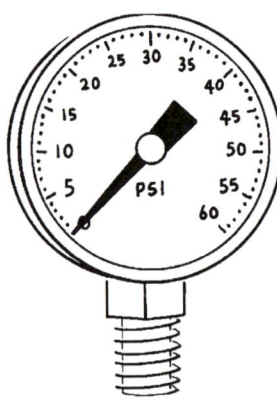

Suitable for 30 psi

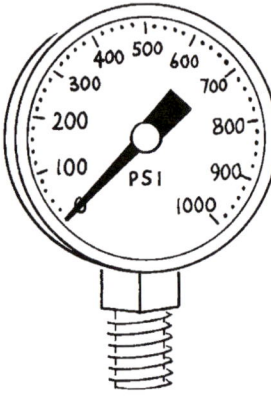

Suitable for 500–700 psi

FIGURE 8-25

Select a pressure gauge that is compatible with the pressure range of the sprayer. It should have a higher maximum pressure than the sprayer to prevent damage due to unexpected pressure surges.

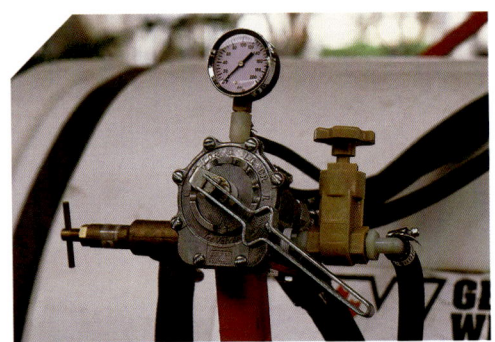

FIGURE 8-26

Control valves are used to turn on or shut off spray to nozzles. Multiple valves are often used to regulate spray to different nozzles, giving the operator options to adjust the application according to the characteristics of the location.

1 to 500 psi gauge works best on sprayers that operate at maximum pressures of 300 or 400 psi (Fig. 8-25). Gauges should operate at about 50% of their maximum pressure. This protects them against damage in the case of unexpected pressure surges.

When possible, use liquid-filled gauges on spray equipment. These last longer and can absorb the shock of rapid pressure changes and vibrations from the equipment. You can recognize these gauges by the clear liquid (glycerin) visible inside the face of the dial.

Control Valves

Use control valves to turn on and shut off liquid being pumped to the nozzles (Fig. 8-26). These may be trigger-type valves on hand spray guns or lever valves controlling spray to nozzles on a boom. You can operate other control valves by cables, such as on air blast orchard sprayers, or by electric solenoids. You can even set up your sprayers so that electric solenoids control each nozzle individually.

On air blast sprayers, manufacturers usually fit nozzles to two manifolds, each with a separate control valve. This allows you to spray from either side of the sprayer or from both sides at the same time.

Field and row crop spray booms often have two or three controllable sections and special valves for these sections. In one case, a control valve for a three-section boom has seven spray selections available to the operator. For a boom divided into left, center, and right sections, the valve supplies spray to the

- right section only
- left section only
- center section only
- right and left sections
- right and center sections
- left and center sections
- all three sections

Electronic Sprayer Controllers. Electronic sprayer controllers allow very accurate metering of pesticide sprays. They use microcomputers to monitor and regulate spray output and/or pressure at each nozzle. Some units warn you of malfunctions of nozzles or pumps. These controllers allow you to apply consistent and precise amounts of pesticide even if the travel speed of your equipment varies. Some controllers use sensing devices to regulate the spray according to target plant size or type. Other controllers use GPS navigation to automatically shut off nozzles and prevent respraying of areas in the field.

Hoses, Couplings, and Fittings

Hoses, couplings, and fittings must be strong and durable. They need to withstand the pressures produced by a spraying system and the corrosive action of spray material. Neoprene is the most common material used for sprayer hoses. Use reinforced hoses to reduce chances of bursting under the pressure of the system. Leaking or ruptured hoses expose you to pesticides and release unregulated amounts of pesticide into the environment.

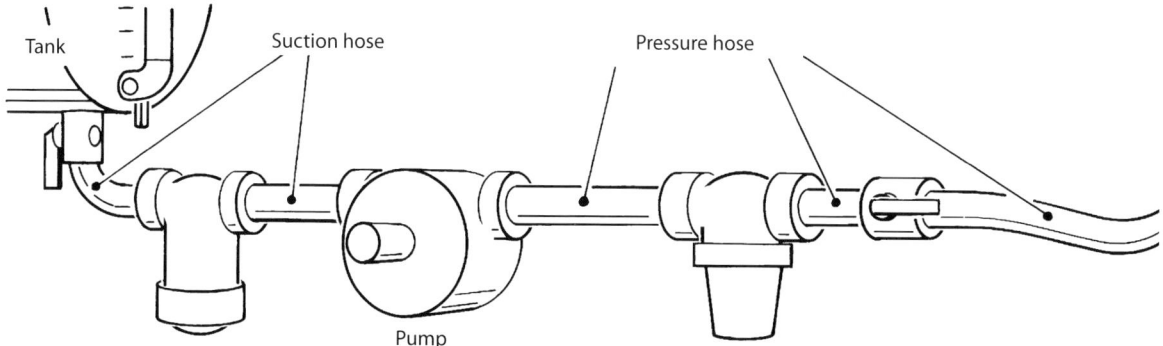

FIGURE 8-27

Suction hoses are used to connect the pump to the tank of the sprayer. Pressure hoses are placed between the pump and the nozzles. Suction hoses must be larger in diameter than pressure hoses and should be sturdy enough to prevent them from collapsing.

Two types of hose—pressure and suction—connect tanks, pumps, and booms or nozzles (Fig. 8-27). Use pressure hoses that can handle twice the operating pressure of your sprayer. For indoor uses, select a hose material that does not leave skid marks on floors or other surfaces.

Suction hoses that carry liquid from the tank to the pump must be larger in diameter than pressure hoses. Using hoses that are the same size or smaller than the pressure hose impedes liquid flow. This reduces the discharge rate at the nozzles and could damage the pump. Select suction hoses that are stiff enough to resist collapsing under the suction pressure of your sprayer's pump.

Fittings. Select noncorrosive couplings and fittings that can withstand the solvents used in pesticide formulations. Brass, stainless steel, and high-density plastic are common materials for these fittings. Use quick disconnect couplings and fittings in case you need to make repairs to the system. Be sure couplings or fittings do not reduce the internal diameter of the hoses they connect. This could cause a pressure drop at the nozzles and additional pressure on the pump.

If you need to attach or disconnect certain hoses during operation, use dry break couplings (Fig. 8-28). These prevent pesticide leaks when you disconnect the hoses. Dry break couplings have a spring-loaded check valve that automatically plugs the disconnected hoses and fittings.

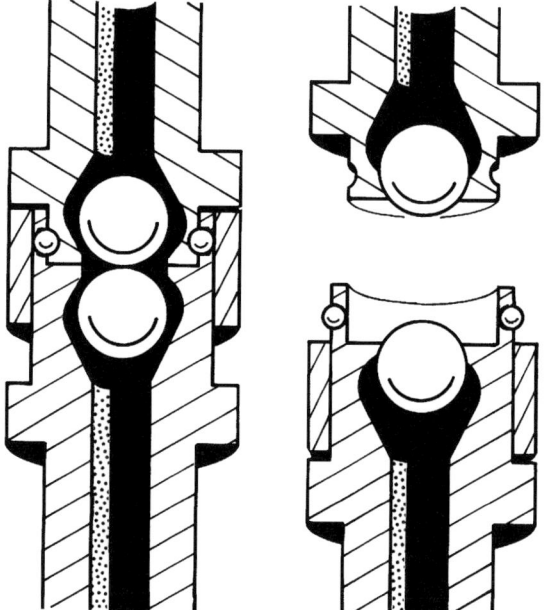

FIGURE 8-28

A dry break coupling allows hoses containing pesticides to be disconnected from equipment without spilling any material. Spring-loaded ball bearings seal the hose openings when dry break couplings are separated.

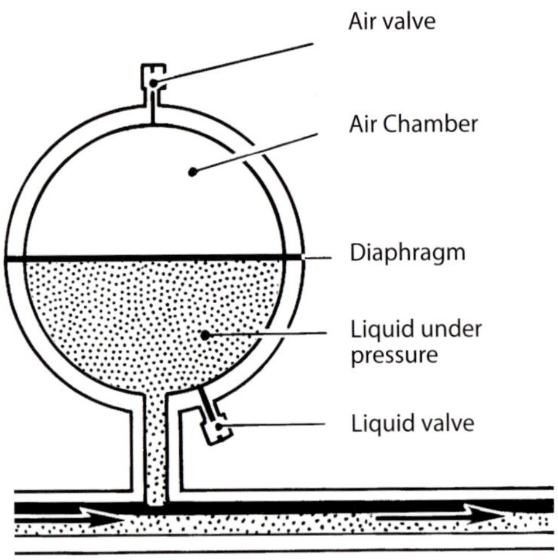

FIGURE 8-29

A surge chamber can be installed in the pressure system of a sprayer to minimize pressure fluctuations caused by the pumping action of piston and diaphragm pumps.

Labels: Air valve, Air Chamber, Diaphragm, Liquid under pressure, Liquid valve

List the types of application equipment and describe the advantages and limitations of each type.

List the types of application equipment used to apply liquids, and describe the situations in which each should be used.

Surge Chambers

You may need to install a surge chamber on the pressure line of your sprayer. This device minimizes pressure fluctuations caused by piston and diaphragm pumps (Fig. 8-29). One style of surge chamber consists of a hollow metal tank connected to the sprayer's pressure line. Air trapped in this tank compresses or expands according to changes in pressure of the pumped liquid. Compressing this air helps to minimize pressure variations.

Another type of surge chamber consists of a round tank separated by a diaphragm into two hemispheres. It has air on one side of the diaphragm and pumped liquid on the other. As pressure in the system increases, the pumped liquid distorts the diaphragm, compressing the trapped air. As a result, it moderates pressure peaks in the system. When the pumping cycle reverses, the compressed air forces liquid back into the system. This slows the rate of pressure drop. With some surge chambers, you can pump in compressed air to improve the dampening action at high pressures. You must drain liquid from some models daily to maintain air volume in the unit. If air volume in the surge chamber decreases too much, the surge chamber becomes less effective. In this case it will not adequately dampen high-pressure pulsations.

Spray Shields

When necessary, install spray shields on your boom sprayer to confine pesticide droplets and prevent drift. The shields consist of metal boxes or metal, plastic, or fabric shrouds. These surround the nozzles and confine the spray to a small area of ground or to specific plants. Attach these to the spray boom so they move with the tractor as a unit. Damaged spray shields should be replaced so that the crop is not harmed.

Closed-System Mixing Equipment

Closed-system mixing equipment allows you to handle toxic liquid pesticides more safely. These systems eliminate hand pouring, hand mixing, triple rinsing, and other handling activities. Sometimes containers must still be opened by hand and then resealed for storage, however. California regulations specify situations in which these systems must be used.

Some closed mixing systems use a transfer pump to move the pesticide from its original container to the sprayer tank. Other types attach to the pressure side of the sprayer; in these, the sprayer's pumping action sucks the pesticide from its container. Most devices have some type of metering device so you can measure the quantity of pesticide being transferred.

Many closed-system mixing units automatically rinse containers after they are empty. If the unit does not automatically rinse the container, use a separate rinsing device. Pump the rinsate into the spray tank.

Operators commonly install closed-system units on nurse tanks, a large tank with a pump and an agitator. Pesticides are mixed and held in the nurse tank, then fed to one or more sprayers for application.

Nonpowered, or Hand-Operated, Equipment

Nonpowered, or hand-operated, liquid spray equipment is comparatively inexpensive. It is also easy to use. These sprayers are usually simple to repair and maintain because they have only a few moving parts. You use these devices for applying pesticides to small areas or specific targets. They are handy for locations that are difficult to reach with larger equipment.

Nonpowered equipment is lightweight, so an individual can carry most models. Some are low-pressure sprayers with small tanks. Tanks usually do not have agitators, so they require occasional shaking when you use wettable powder, flowable, or emulsifiable concentrate formulations. Low-tech pressure regulators can be added to existing nonpowered equipment. Table 8-4 is a guide to selecting nonpowered devices suitable for different application needs.

TABLE 8-4

Guide for selecting nonpowered, hand-operated, application equipment for liquid pesticides

	Type	Uses	Suitable formulations	Comments
	aerosol can	Insect control on house plants or patio plants, pets, small areas, cracks and crevices, and confined spaces.	Liquids must dissolve in solvent; some dusts are available.	Very convenient. High cost per unit of active ingredient.
	hose-end sprayer	Home garden and small landscaped areas. Used for insect, weed, and pathogen control.	All formulations. Wettable powders and emulsifiable concentrates require frequent shaking.	Convenient and low-cost way of applying pesticides to small outdoor areas. Cannot spray straight up.
	trigger pump sprayer	Indoor plants, pets, and small home yard areas. Used for insect and pathogen control.	Liquid-soluble formulations are best.	Low cost and easy to use.
	compressed air sprayer	Many commercial and homeowner applications. Can develop fairly high pressures. Used for insect, weed, and pathogen control. Often used indoors for household pest control.	All formulations. Wettable powders and emulsifiable concentrates require frequent shaking.	Good overall sprayer for many types of applications. Needs thorough cleaning and regular servicing to keep sprayer in good working condition and prevent corrosion of parts.
	backpack sprayer	Same uses as compressed air sprayer.	All formulations. Wettable powders and emulsifiable concentrates require frequent shaking.	Durable and easy to use. Requires periodic maintenance.
	wick applicator	Applying contact herbicides to emerged weeds. Agricultural and landscape uses.	Only water-soluble herbicides.	Simple and easy to use. Needs frequent cleaning.

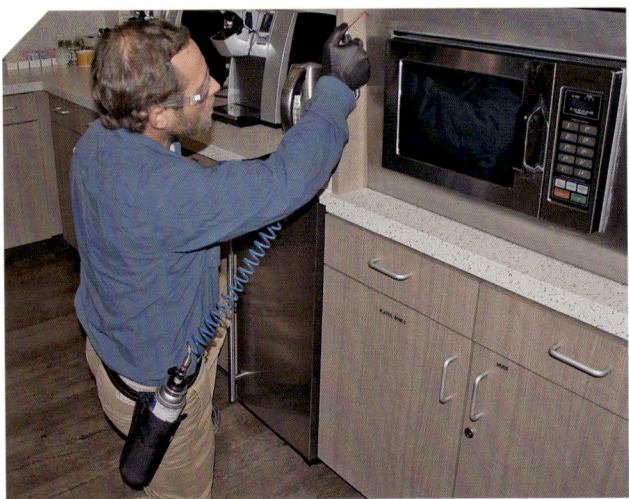

FIGURE 8-30

Aerosol dispensers used in commercial applications are attached to a hose and spray wand enabling the operator to inject liquids into cracks and crevices.

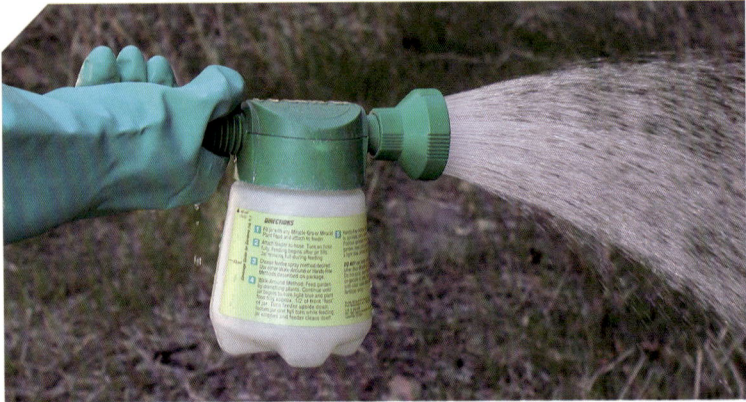

FIGURE 8-31

Hose-end sprayers are sometimes used to apply pesticides to lawns and shrubs. They apply high volumes of dilute pesticide.

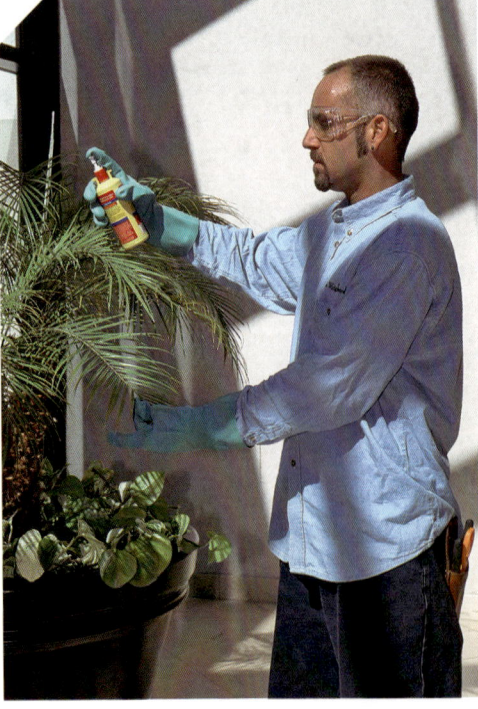

FIGURE 8-32

A trigger pump sprayer can be used to apply small quantities of diluted pesticide to surfaces such as houseplants or pets. It can also be used to apply some types of pesticides to confined areas.

Aerosol Cans. Pressurized spray applicators and aerosol foggers expel a fine spray of premixed pesticide through a nozzle at the top of the can. The propellant is an inert compressed gas. Some aerosol cans allow intermittent uses as needed, but aerosol foggers are one-time, total release units. Aerosol cans with a capacity of 1 quart or less are not reusable. Pesticides packaged this way are popular because of their convenience.

Pest control operators use larger aerosol cans for structural and greenhouse applications. Some types are refillable. Applicators can carry these on a waist belt and attach the can to a hose and spray wand (Fig. 8-30). Sometimes they connect two or more cans to a single wand, allowing them to select different pesticides during the same operation. Sprays packaged in aerosol cans offer convenience and portability to professional applicators and eliminate the need for chemical mixing.

Hose-End Sprayers (Fig. 8-31). Hose-end sprayers are commonly used to apply pesticides to lawns, flowers, and shrubs, usually in small areas. The sprayer combines concentrated pesticide mixtures with water from a garden hose and expels it through a high-volume nozzle. A 1- or 2-quart plastic or glass container holds the concentrated pesticide. One filling of the container can produce about 20 gallons of dilute spray. Nozzles adjust for droplet size and for aiming the spray in different directions. These sprayers generally have a valve to start and stop the flow of pesticide in the stream of water. Some have another valve to regulate and shut off the water flow from the garden hose.

Trigger Pump Sprayers (Fig. 8-32). In a trigger pump sprayer, squeezing the trigger forces a pesticide mixture through a nozzle, producing a fine spray. Some have an adjustable nozzle for controlling droplet size. You put a diluted pesticide in the plastic jar, which ranges in capacity from 1 pint to 1 gallon. Use this type of applicator to apply small amounts of pesticide to houseplants or pets and confined areas such as closets or cabinets.

PESTICIDE APPLICATION EQUIPMENT

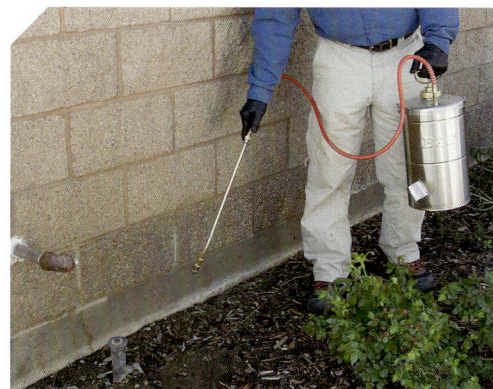

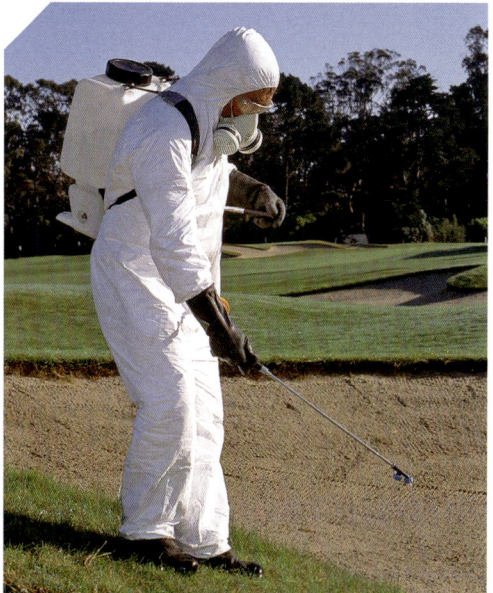

FIGURE 8-34

This type of hand-operated backpack sprayer usually requires continuous pumping action to maintain pressure for spraying. These units hold from 3 to 5 gallons of spray mixture; most have adjustable nozzles.

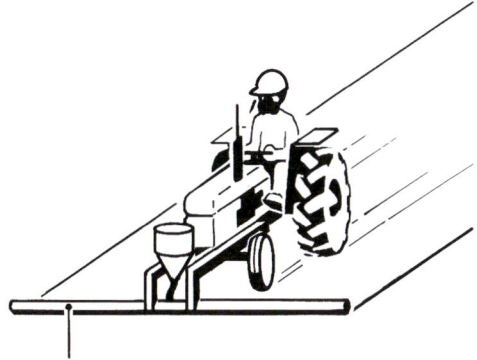

Pesticide saturated pad or rope

FIGURE 8-35

Wick applicators are used for application of contact herbicides. They can be used in areas where weeds are taller than the crop plant. Wick applicators reduce problems of drift and waste of herbicides.

FIGURE 8-33

Compressed air sprayers usually hold from ½ to 5 gallons of spray mixture. Air inside the tank is compressed with a self-contained pump or a carbon dioxide cartridge. Pesticide under pressure is forced through a hose attached to an adjustable nozzle at the end of a hand-held wand.

Compressed Air Sprayers (Fig. 8-33). Compressed air sprayers hold a diluted pesticide mixture in a small, airtight tank. You use a hand pump to compress air inside the tank. The compressed air forces the liquid through a hose and nozzle when you open a valve. Some models use compressed carbon dioxide cartridges as the propellant, eliminating the need for hand pumping. Metal or plastic tanks have a capacity of less than 5 gallons. Conventional tank sizes include ½, 1, 2, and 3 gallons. You should clearly mark these smaller tanks "for pesticides use only" to prevent their accidental use for other purposes. Some compressed air sprayers have harnesses for backpack use. Larger compressed air sprayers have separate air tanks that you fill from an air compressor or portable hand pump. Hoses or pipes connect these tanks to an airtight chamber containing the diluted pesticide mixture.

Use these sprayers for treating small areas and for applying liquid pesticides indoors. Most have adjustable nozzles to control droplet size and spray pattern. For indoor applications, you can use adapters to inject liquid spray into small cracks and crevices.

Backpack Sprayers (Fig. 8-34). Backpack sprayers have a hand-operated hydraulic pump that forces liquid pesticides through one or more nozzles. You operate the pump by moving a hand lever up and down. Some pumps create pressures of more than 100 psi. The tanks, usually made of plastic, have a capacity of around 5 gallons. These sprayers are useful in small areas where there is no access for larger equipment. Some backpack sprayers are also known as knapsack sprayers.

Wick Applicators (Fig. 8-35). Use wick applicators, or rope wick applicators, to apply contact or systemic herbicides. Their basic design consists of a cloth, carpeting pad, rope, or wick that is saturated with herbicide. You wipe this wick onto the leaves of target weeds. A simple hand-held model holds liquid herbicide in its hollow handle. Liquid feeds to the pad through a series of small holes. Other types of wick applicators incorporate a boom and herbicide reservoir attached to a tractor. More elaborate versions mechanically wind ropes through the herbicide reservoirs. This ensures a constant and more uniform herbicide distribution.

For controlling weeds that are taller than the crop, adjust the wick applicator height to contact just the weeds. Wick applicators waste little or no pesticide. Also, very little environmental contamination takes place as a result of the application process.

Powered Application Equipment

Many pesticide applications require powered equipment capable of applying high volumes of pesticide mixtures to large areas. Some units have self-contained motors, while others are powered by tractors or similar external sources. Manufacturers equip these machines with hydraulic or mechanical agitators and pressure regulators. They also come with a variety of spray booms, hand-held spray guns, and other nozzle arrangements. Powered equipment is more complex than hand-operated equipment and often requires considerable maintenance and servicing to keep it operating properly. Table 8-5 is a guide to help you select powered liquid application equipment.

TABLE 8-5

Guide for selecting powered liquid pesticide application equipment

	Type	Uses	Suitable formulations	Comments
	powered backpack sprayer	Aquatic, landscape, right-of-way, forest, and agricultural applications.	All. Some may require agitation.	May be heavy for long periods of use. Requires frequent maintenance.
	controlled droplet applicator	Application of contact herbicides and some insecticides. Some are hand-held while others are mounted on spray booms. Maybe also be used with air blast sprayers. Produces uniform droplet sizes.	Usually water-soluble formulations.	Plastic parts may break if handled carelessly.
	low-pressure sprayer	Very common sprayer used in commercial applications for weed, insect, and pathogen control. Used with spray booms or hand-held equipment.	All. Equipment may include agitator.	Frequent cleaning and servicing is required. Powered by own motor or external power source.
	high-pressure hydraulic sprayer	Landscape, right-of-way, and agricultural applications. Use on dense foliage and large trees or shrubs.	All. Equipment may include agitator.	Important to clean and service equipment frequently. Requires own motor or external power source. Abrasive pesticides may cause rapid wear of pumps and nozzles.
	air blast sprayer	For application of insecticides, fungicides, and growth regulators to trees, vines, and shrubs. Sometimes used on row crops and with livestock. Also used in aquatic areas.	All. Equipment may include agitator.	Frequent service and maintenance are required. High-horsepower motor is often needed to power pump and fan. Attachments available to help direct spray.
	ultra-low-volume applicator	Primarily used in agricultural and aquatic situations. Used with insecticides, fungicides, and growth regulators.	Usually only pesticides that dissolve in water or organic solvents.	Requires extreme care in calibration. Applies highly concentrated pesticides. Often used with a blower.
	electrostatic sprayer	Agricultural uses for applying insecticides, fungicides, and growth regulators to trees, vines, and row crops.	All. Requires agitation of some formulations.	Usually equipped with blower. Maintenance and frequent cleaning are required. Electronically charged spray droplets are attracted to target surfaces.
	aerosol generators and foggers	Mainly used to apply insecticides in confined areas. Used in aquatic areas for airborne insects.	Requires water- or solvent-soluble formulations.	Emitted spray is highly subject to drift. Keep equipment clean.
	chemical injection pump	Injects concentrated pesticides into spray boom or irrigation water. May be used with all classes of pesticides.	Requires liquid formulations.	Accurate metering is necessary to ensure proper calibration. With irrigation systems, must have backflow protection to prevent contaminating water supply.

PESTICIDE APPLICATION EQUIPMENT 219

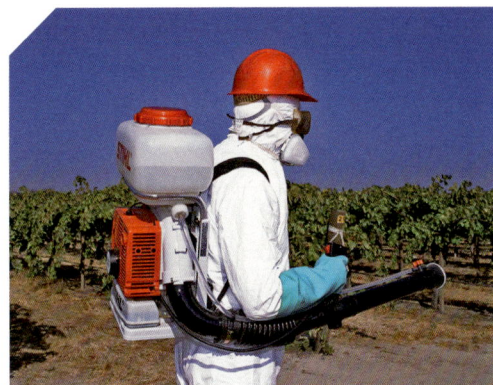

FIGURE 8-36
Powered backpack sprayers have small tanks and compact gasoline engines.

Powered Backpack Sprayers (Fig. 8-36). The smallest powered sprayer consists of a backpack unit with a compact gasoline engine. The engine drives a pump that forces diluted or concentrated liquid pesticide through one or more nozzles. Air blowers, also driven by the engine, help propel spray droplets. Backpack sprayers work best for low-volume applications because of their small tank size and inability to produce high pressure.

Controlled Droplet Applicators (Fig. 8-37). Controlled droplet applicators (CDAs) apply low volumes of specific types of pesticides (usually herbicides). Rather than passing through a nozzle, the liquid pesticide mixture drops onto a spinning disc or cup. This disc has serrated edges to distribute the spray by centrifugal force. Under optimal conditions, this equipment produces droplets of a more uniform size than is possible with pressure or hydraulic spray nozzles. Droplet size depends on the rotation speed of the disc and the nature of the pesticide being used: more-viscous liquids produce larger droplets. Rotation speed is adjustable from 1,000 to 6,000 rpm. As speed increases, the droplets become smaller. The size range of droplets produced by CDAs is 100 to 400 microns.

In most units, the pesticide mixture flows from a reservoir tank to the spinning disc or cup by gravitational force. This eliminates the need for a pump. An orifice in the pesticide hose controls the flow rate. In most models you can change this orifice size. Variable speed, low-voltage DC electric motors or hydraulic motors power CDAs. In some units you control the speed by changing drive belts on pulleys. Other units have electronic speed controllers. Hydraulic units accomplish speed control by adjusting the flow rate of the hydraulic fluid.

Some CDAs are inexpensive, self-contained, hand-held units. Others connect to a backpack tank by a flexible hose. You will commonly find one or more CDAs mounted on tractors or all-terrain vehicles (ATVs). Sometimes CDAs replace nozzles on air blast sprayers.

Uses for CDAs include applying contact, preemergent, and postemergent herbicides. You can also use them for some insecticide and fungicide applications. Because the rotational speed of CDAs controls droplet size, you can make very low-volume applications without excessive drift. CDAs apply from 1 quart to 3 gallons per acre per unit. However, some sprayers use multiple CDA "heads" to deliver a higher volume. In both cases, you need to perform accurate calibration. Keep low-volume applications consistent with pesticide label directions or current University of California recommendations.

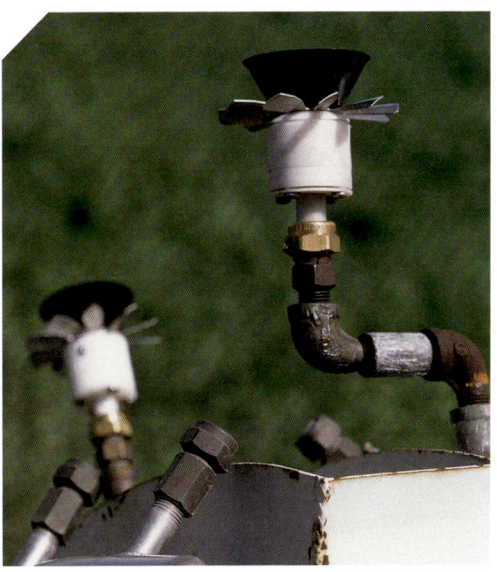

FIGURE 8-37
Controlled droplet applicators are designed to apply small volumes of uniform-sized droplets. These are available as hand-held units or can be mounted in groups on ATV-mounted spray booms or on air blast sprayers.

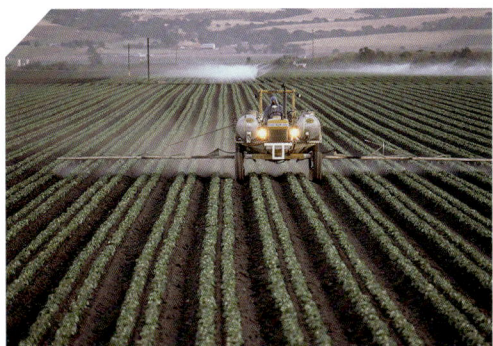

FIGURE 8-38
A common sprayer used for agricultural, right-of-way, forest, and landscape applications of pesticides is the low-pressure applicator like the one being used here to apply insecticides to lettuce. It applies sprays through a series of nozzles attached to a boom.

Low-Pressure Sprayers (Fig. 8-38). Low-pressure pesticide sprayers are useful tools in many different agricultural crop, turf, aquatic, and right-of-way settings. This equipment operates in the pressure range of 10 to 20 psi. You can also inject pesticides into the soil with low-pressure applicators by connecting them to soil shanks or chisels attached to a tractor tool bar. As shanks rip the soil, the unit pumps pesticide (or liquid fertilizer) below the surface. This is a common way of applying soil fumigants.

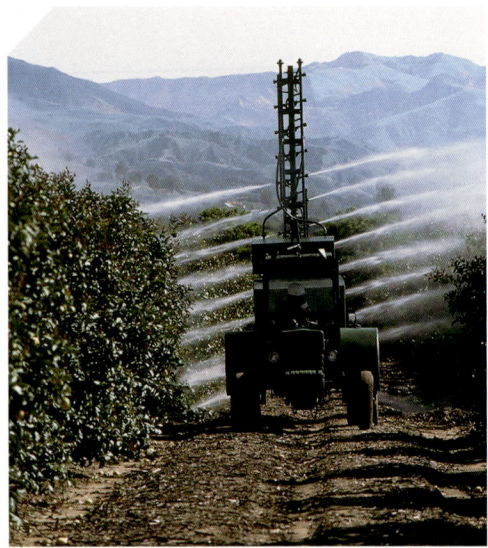

FIGURE 8-39

Oscillating boom sprayers, like the one being used here in citrus, are high-pressure units that direct large volumes of spray through dense foliage. They are used where thorough coverage is essential.

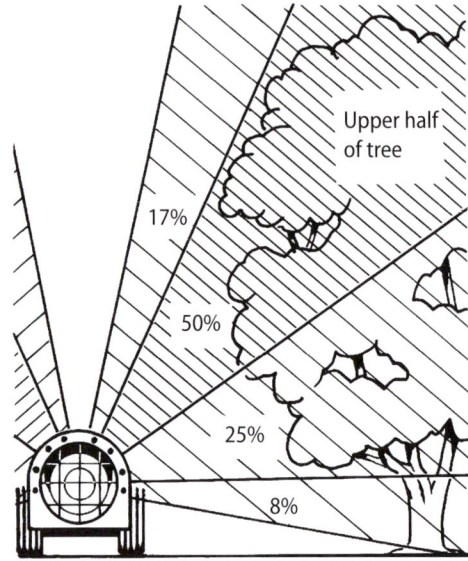

FIGURE 8-40

An orchard air blast sprayer may be adjusted to apply greater amounts of pesticides to some parts of the tree. This is done by using several different nozzle sizes or by using more nozzles in some locations. In most situations, two-thirds of the spray output is directed to the upper half of the tree. This drawing shows an ideal pattern for most mature orchards.

Users mount low-pressure sprayers onto trailers (tag-along models) or attach them to tractors or trucks. Some models are self-propelled. Electric motors or engines provide the power for pumps in some units, and others are PTO-driven or hydraulically powered. Occasionally, the wheels of the trailer power the pumps (ground wheel-driven) as you tow the unit. This method provides a relatively constant output rate even if the travel speed of the unit varies, because the pump speed is proportional to the travel speed.

Most low-pressure sprayers have tanks with a capacity of 100 gallons or more. Often, you can attach two or more tanks to a tractor to increase total capacity. Low pressure usually is not suitable when you need thorough coverage of dense foliage, however. It also does not work if the spray must travel any distance, unless you use a blower.

High-Pressure Hydraulic Sprayers (Fig. 8-39). High-pressure sprayers work well when spraying large areas such as orchards and field crops. You can also use them for spraying turf and landscape and right-of-way trees and shrubs. In addition, they are useful in aquatic areas and for treating livestock. This equipment forces high volumes of dilute pesticide either through hand spray guns or nozzles mounted on booms. Special boom designs improve spray coverage to all sides of crop plants. For instance, oscillating booms provide good coverage on densely foliated trees, such as citrus, and on large vines. With an oscillating boom sprayer, several high-pressure spray nozzles rotate from side to side and up and down as the sprayer moves along. This oscillating action, coupled with high pressure and high volume, provides thorough spray coverage to all parts of target plants.

Pressures between 100 and 400 psi or more are common with high-pressure sprayers. Most have large-capacity tanks, up to 2,000 gallons. High-pressure hydraulic sprayers mount on trailers, trucks, or tractors and may have a self-contained engine for powering the pump. Some are powered by a tractor PTO. With PTO-driven models, you must be careful to maintain a constant tractor engine speed to ensure a uniform application rate. Many models have pressure regulators and bypass mechanisms so they work as low-pressure sprayers as well.

Air Carrier Sprayers. Air carrier sprayers use fans or blowers to generate airflow that assists in moving the spray to the target. There are two general types of air carrier sprayers:

- **air blast sprayers,** which deliver large volumes of air and pesticide mixtures into orchard or vineyard canopies using one or two large fans that propel spray through one or two outlets (Fig. 8-40)
- **air assist sprayers,** which are used in agronomic row crops or with smaller trees and vines (Fig. 8-41)

Proper use of air carrier sprayers eliminates leaf shingling and significantly improves pesticide coverage on foliage compared with sprayers operating without fans or blowers. Because air moves spray droplets to target surfaces, air carrier sprayers do not require extremely high liquid pressure. You usually operate these sprayers in a range from 10 to 150 psi, depending on the sprayer design.

Air carrier sprayers use either hydraulic or air-shear nozzles to generate spray droplets. Hydraulic nozzles use pump pressure and nozzle design to produce droplets, while air-shear nozzles use high-velocity airflow from the sprayer fan to atomize low-pressure liquid streams.

PESTICIDE APPLICATION EQUIPMENT 221

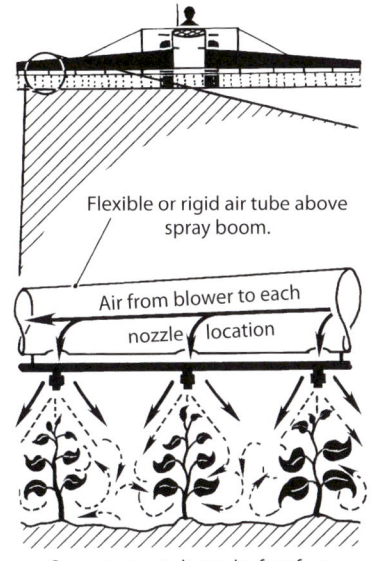

FIGURE 8-41

Air assist sprayers may also be used in row crops. As illustrated, air from a blower is carried to nozzles through a flexible or rigid tube. Pesticide droplets are distributed around the plant by the air turbulence, giving coverage to upper and lower plant surfaces.

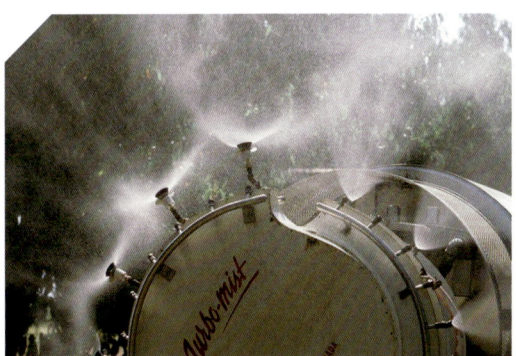

FIGURE 8-42

An ultra-low-volume sprayer produces low volumes of very small droplets; these are usually propelled by a fan or blower. Pesticide mixtures are much more concentrated than in higher-volume sprayers.

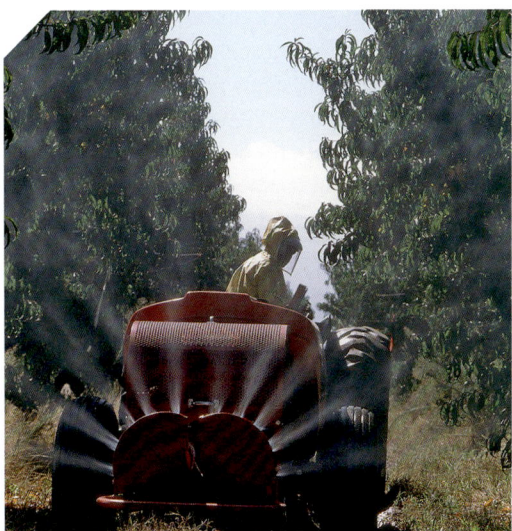

FIGURE 8-43

An electrostatic sprayer emits electrically charged spray droplets. These spray droplets are attracted to oppositely charged surfaces, increasing the pesticide deposition and target coverage.

Most air carrier sprayers have spray tanks ranging in capacity from 100 to 1,000 gallons. Low-volume or concentrate sprayers produce from 30 to 100 gallons of finished spray per acre. High-volume sprayers (dilute sprayers) have an output of 400 to 1,000 gallons per acre. Usually, you can convert a high-volume sprayer to low volume. To do this, change nozzle size(s), lower the pump output pressure, and adjust ground speed.

Air carrier sprayer nozzles discharge into the air stream produced by the sprayer's fan. Depending on air speed and spray release angle relative to airflow, spray droplets are further atomized and moved into dense foliage and treetops. Orchard and vineyard sprayers often use different-sized hydraulic nozzles at different locations on the manifold. Thus the sprayer applies different amounts of spray to different parts of the trees or vines (Fig. 8-40). Controlled droplet applicators sometimes replace nozzles on orchard, vineyard, row crop, and livestock air carrier sprayers.

Special attachments exist for air carrier sprayers: volutes direct the air and spray flow into tall trees, towers blow air around vines and trees, and cannons blow air across fields or into the dense foliage of vegetable crops. Many attachment designs are available, depending on the needs of the application.

The pumps and fans of air carrier sprayers are either self-powered by a gasoline or diesel engine or externally powered by a tractor PTO. Units with large fans require 50 to more than 100 horsepower to drive them. You can mount some smaller sprayers onto trucks or tractors, while larger ones are wheeled and designed for pulling behind tractors. Other variations include one that has the fan, pump, and spray nozzles attached to a tractor's three-point hitch and is connected by hoses to a wheeled tank pulled behind as a separate unit. Self-propelled spraying machines, including an enclosed operator cab, are also available.

Ultra-Low-Volume Sprayers (Fig. 8-42). Ultra-low-volume (ULV) sprayers apply from less than 1 quart to a few gallons of spray per acre. Low-volume nozzles (sometimes controlled droplet applicators) break up the spray into small droplets. Air from a fan or blower propels the droplets to the treatment surfaces. ULV sprayers apply highly concentrated pesticides. Mixing the pesticides with vegetable oil carriers reduces droplet evaporation. Vegetable oil also improves the spreading ability of droplets once they have contacted the target surface. ULV sprayers, powered by lightweight gasoline engines, usually have small tanks. These sprayers are smaller and much lighter than higher-volume machines. Because of the smaller droplet size and smaller blowers, ULV sprayers generally are limited to applications made during low winds to minimize drift and obtain satisfactory penetration and coverage.

Accurate calibration of ULV sprayers is critical because of the high concentration of pesticide being applied. There may be greater hazards to the operator with ULV sprayers because of the concentrated pesticides used.

Electrostatic Sprayers (Fig. 8-43). Electrostatic sprayers apply 10 to 50 gallons per acre of pesticide in the form of small, electrically charged droplets. Droplets average about 50 microns

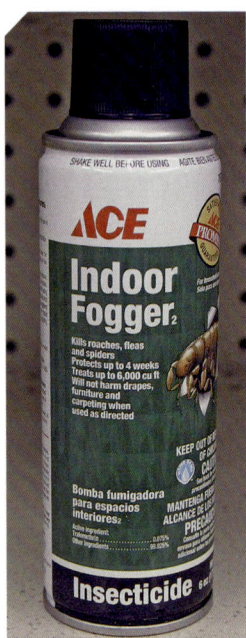

FIGURE 8-44

Aerosol generators and foggers produce a fine insecticide mist that remains suspended in the air for a long period of time, penetrating cracks and inaccessible areas and killing insects on contact.

in diameter and receive an electrostatic charge as they leave the sprayer volute. Because plant material is grounded to the earth, the spray droplets are attracted to the plant surfaces. The negatively charged spray droplets repel each other, so they typically do not clump together to form larger-sized droplets. Electrostatic sprayers are usually powered by a tractor PTO. A transformer connected to the tractor's electrical system creates an electrical charge of about 15,000 to 20,000 volts. Volutes of different configurations direct the spray droplets toward surfaces being treated. These sprayers appear to be more effective if spray droplets only travel a short distance from the sprayer to the target. As the distance increases, the effect of the electrostatic charge diminishes.

Aerosol Generators and Foggers (Fig. 8-44). Aerosol generators and foggers produce small airborne particles of pesticide. These units work for insect control in confined spaces such as residences, greenhouses, and warehouses.

The insecticide-laden fog produced by aerosol generators remains suspended in the air for long periods. It penetrates small cracks and inaccessible areas, killing insects on contact. Sometimes outdoor fogging controls mosquitoes and other biting or irritating insects in locations such as recreational areas. Effective insect control in outdoor areas depends mainly on proper weather. The conditions must keep the fog confined and airborne within an area long enough to contact target insects.

Thermal fog applicators use heat to generate pesticide aerosols. Other types use bifluid nozzles with high-velocity air to produce extremely fine droplets.

Chemical Injection Pumps. Chemical injection pumps inject undiluted liquid pesticides directly into the nozzles, where they mix with water being simultaneously pumped from a water tank. Some injection pumps draw liquid pesticides directly from original containers, eliminating the need for mixing chemicals or cleaning tanks. When used with sprayers, chemical injection pumps allow you to apply one or more chemicals during an operation. With this equipment you can vary the concentration of pesticide mixture during application. Some units have electronic devices that regulate the concentration of pesticide applied.

Many future possibilities exist using chemical injection systems. For example, experimental orchard sprayers use sensors and a computer system to apply pesticide amounts proportional to tree volume. They shut off the spray between trees and where trees are missing.

CHEMIGATION

Injection pumps allow you to apply pesticides through irrigation systems, a practice known as chemigation (Fig. 8-45). Applying pesticides using irrigation systems is an effective and efficient way to deliver them, since these systems are already optimized to thoroughly cover a target area. Chemigation is not a perfect solution, however, and chemigation systems must have devices in place to prevent possible contamination of the water supply by backflow of irrigation water. For instance, regulations require automatic shut-off devices on injection pumps that can stop pesticides from being injected into the system when the irrigation water flow stops.

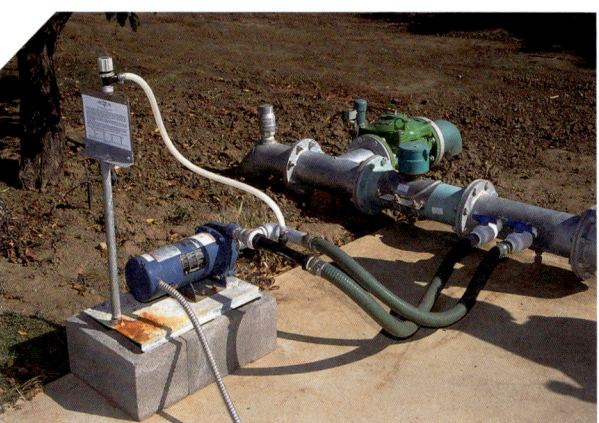

FIGURE 8-45

Small injection pumps are used to meter pesticides into irrigation water, a technique known as chemigation.

Chemigation should be used only when water and pesticides can be distributed uniformly by the irrigation system. At best, uneven delivery of pesticides via irrigation systems may result in unsuccessful control of the target organism; at worst, it can result in environmental contamination, contribute to resistance, and waste money and natural resources.

There are three types of chemigation systems:
- sprinkler systems
- surface systems
- micro-irrigation (drip or trickle) systems

List types of chemigation systems, and describe the situations in which they can be used.

Sprinkler Systems

There are several types of sprinkler systems that can be adapted for chemigation purposes. These include
- center-pivot
- self-propelled linear or lateral move
- solid set
- hand-move lateral
- side roll lateral
- tow-line lateral
- traveling big gun

In many states other than California, center-pivot and self-propelled linear systems are the most popular sprinkler systems used for chemigation. Properly designed, calibrated, and operated, they deposit liquids uniformly during chemical applications. Certain systems are not appropriate for chemigation with pesticides but can be used to apply fertilizers. These include systems that discharge water directly into the wheel track, like water-powered center-pivot systems.

Because center-pivot systems are not used much in California, be sure to check with dealers, your local cooperative extension, or other experts to ensure that your center-pivot system is correctly installed and properly adjusted to field conditions.

Traveling gun systems can be used for chemigating, but only in low wind conditions. Because of the way these systems produce spray, large guns have poor application uniformity and are susceptible to wind drift of major proportions.

Solid set, hand-move, and side roll lines are examples of stationary systems. These systems differ from self-propelled types in that they are stationary and do not move during irrigation. The greatest limitation with stationary systems is distortion of the sprinkler pattern by wind. Consideration must be given to pipe spacing, riser height, and nozzle size to ensure uniformity in application. A manifold must also be used to thoroughly mix the pesticide with the water so that it is delivered uniformly throughout the system (see Kansas Department of Agriculture 1990).

Surface Systems

Furrow and flood (sometimes also called surface or gravity flow) irrigation systems are not recommended for chemigation, since they provide relatively poor uniformity of distribution. Soil-applied chemicals may not reach intended targets, since these systems are often unable to wet the tops of ridges or beds. You must pay strict attention to detail when preparing a field in which you will use a surface chemigation system, since the size and length of the rows influence the amount of water applied and uniformity of deposition. In addition, a slight downhill grade is needed, especially in crops planted on flat ground, to increase the uniformity of water and pesticide movement across the entire field.

Chemigation should be used only when there is uniform water distribution. The first few times you irrigate will likely have the poorest uniformity and the greatest deep-seepage losses. There are several ways to improve uniformity and reduce runoff or deep seepage, including using surge valves or surge irrigation. Water application of 2 to 2.5 inches is a practical minimum for

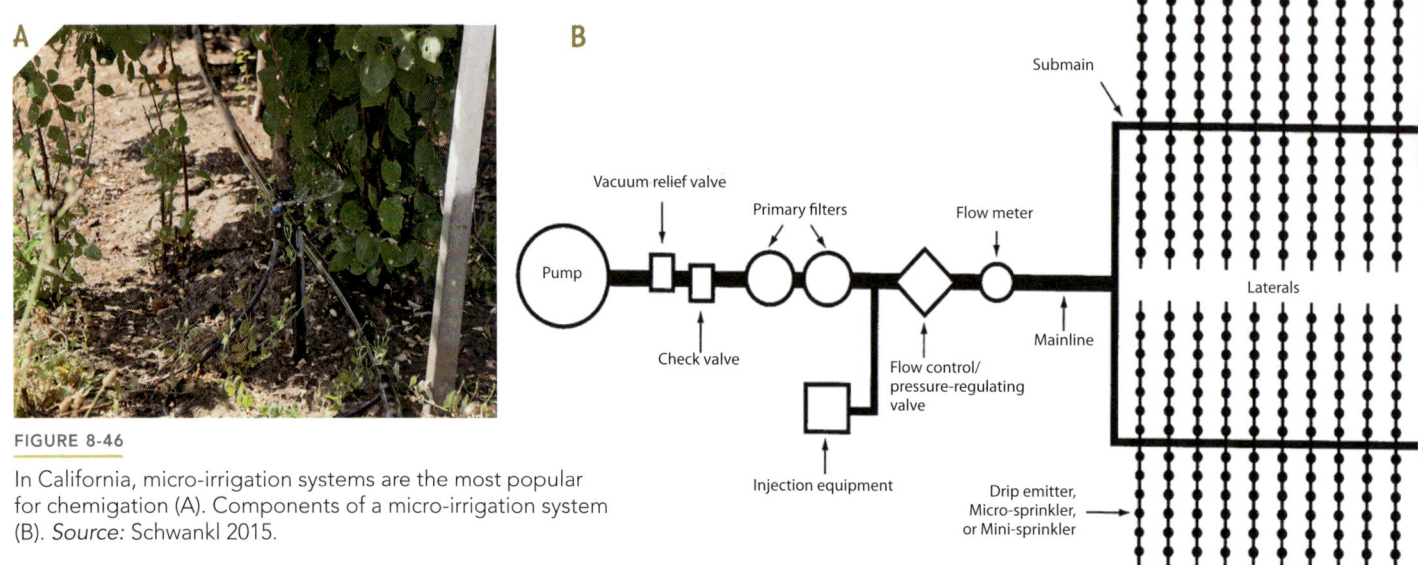

FIGURE 8-46

In California, micro-irrigation systems are the most popular for chemigation (A). Components of a micro-irrigation system (B). *Source:* Schwankl 2015.

most furrow or flood systems. Follow regulations that apply to the collection and use (or reuse) of pesticide-contaminated tailwater. Tailwater collected can be reapplied on the same field or you can use it on other crops for which the chemical is appropriate.

Micro-irrigation Systems

In California, micro-irrigation systems are the most popular for chemigation. There are three types of micro-irrigation systems: surface drip, subsurface drip, and micro-sprinklers. All three types of micro-irrigation systems are made up of the same basic components (Fig. 8-46). Applications are generally made to the root zone or limited areas of surface soil. This practice allows you to carefully control the amount and timing of pesticide and water delivery so they match the exact needs of the crop. These systems limit weed growth, since only a portion of the soil is wetted. A well-maintained micro-irrigation system minimizes runoff because of the low application rates, and deep percolation losses can also be minimized if the correct amount of water is applied. You must pay close attention to micro-irrigation systems, because emitters clogged by dirt or chemical precipitates will deliver less than the desired amount of liquid. Plants near clogged emitters may become water stressed and could die from lack of water if an orifice becomes completely blocked.

Parts of a Chemigation System

In addition to the existing water delivery system, a chemigation setup contains the following components:
- a tank to hold concentrated pesticide
- an agitation assembly to keep concentrate mixed and in suspension throughout the injection cycle for uniform application
- a platform to support the tank, pump, and piping
- a series of specially designed valves (many are packaged as a unit) to prevent water and backflow contamination, control chemical dispersion through the system, and drain the system after use
- an injection system to deliver pesticide from the tank in controlled amounts
- a metering pump (either diaphragm or piston operated) that functions both with required safety equipment and the pesticide formulation

- a low-pressure switch that will stop the water pump motor when water pressure falls below levels effective for proper pesticide distribution
- interlocking electrical or hydraulic controls that will automatically shut down the pesticide injection pump in response to the low-pressure switch
- a calibration setup to help properly calibrate the injection system

Tanks and Agitators

When you select a tank or reservoir for a chemigation system, you are using the same criteria as when selecting a tank for conventional chemical application systems. Tanks for chemigation systems, however, should be large enough to contain all the pesticide needed to treat the entire area without requiring a refill. They should also be self-emptying and should connect to the system with relatively short hoses so that less material is retained in the system after you complete the application. Other selection criteria for pesticide tanks can be found in "Pesticide Tanks" earlier in this chapter. This section will also help you recognize wear in various tank materials.

Agitators are covered in "Agitators" (see Figures 8-10 and 8-11). The type of agitator you select will depend on the pesticide. You must check the pesticide label to find out whether you can use a hydraulic agitator or if mechanical agitation is required.

Valves

Chemigation systems require the use of a series of specially designed valves that prevent flow of pesticides into water drawn from tanks or wells. A valve assembly can consist of a check valve, an air or vacuum relief valve, and a low-pressure drain valve. This assembly will be located immediately adjacent to the discharge head of the pump. In addition to these three valves (often packaged in a single unit), an injection line check valve that prevents the flow of water back toward the pesticide supply tank must be installed between the pesticide injection pump and the irrigation pipeline. Finally, a solenoid-operated valve must be installed at the pesticide tank to prevent water from entering the tank when either the pump or the entire system is shut down. This valve can be eliminated in systems containing a second vacuum relief valve between the positive displacement pesticide injection pump and the injection line check valve.

Chemical Injection Systems

A mechanically durable, reliable, and accurate chemical injection system, specifically designed for chemigating, is essential. Like the chemical supply tank, wettable parts should be made from stainless steel or other nonreactive materials. To help ensure uniform applications, a delivery accuracy of plus or minus 1% is desirable within the minimum to maximum operating range. It also should be easily adjusted while running.

A wide variety of approved chemical injection devices are available; they are classified as either passive (no outside power is needed) or active (an outside power source is required). The primary passive injection device operates on the venturi principle, where, under the proper conditions, a flow constriction in the pipeline creates a vacuum because of the increased velocity of flow. A less-common passive device is the batch tank system. Active injection devices include positive displacement pumps such as diaphragm, piston, roller, and gear pumps. Injection pumps can typically be adjusted over a range of different injection rates to provide a continuous and relatively uniform concentration of chemical in the irrigation water. They should be mechanically rigged with internal and external components made of chemically resistant, noncorrosive materials.

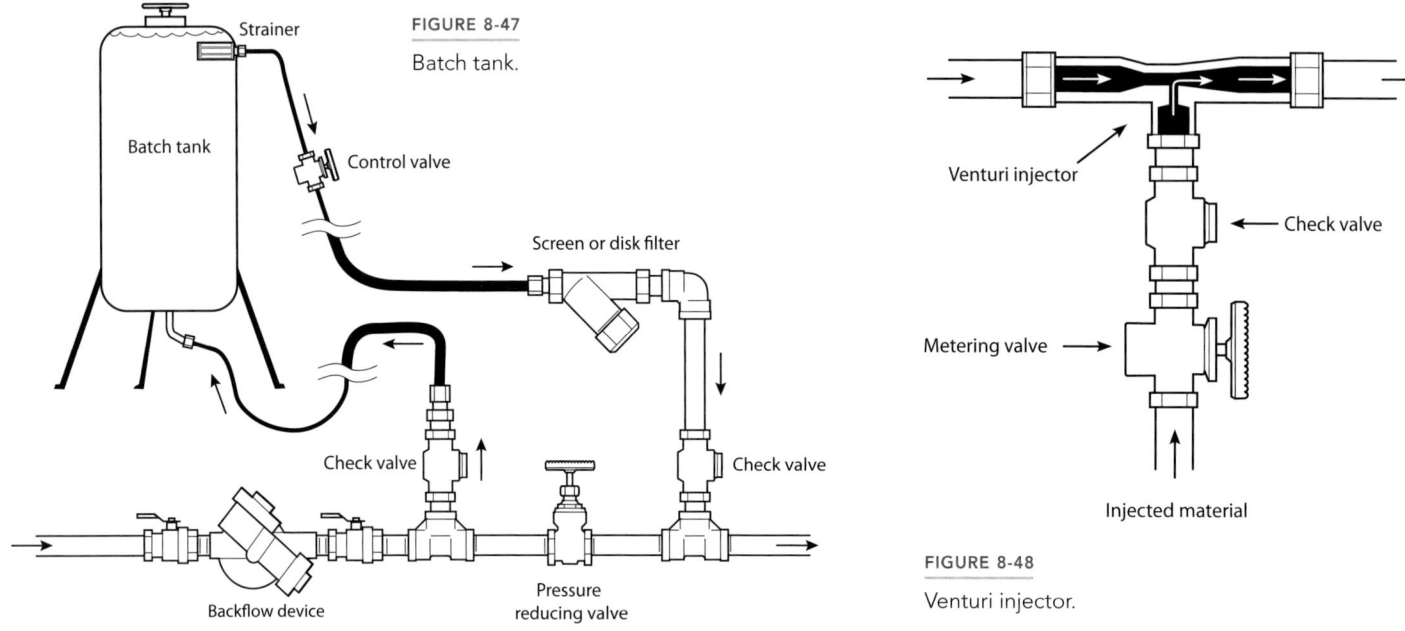

FIGURE 8-47
Batch tank.

FIGURE 8-48
Venturi injector.

PASSIVE SYSTEMS

Batch Tank Injection Systems. Some of the earliest injector systems used batch tanks (Fig. 8-47). These relatively inexpensive and simple systems consist of a tank that is plumbed into the irrigation system so that a portion of the irrigation water flows through it. The tank must be able to withstand the operating pressure of the irrigation system. Since there is often pressure loss as water flows through the batch tank system, the tank must be plumbed across a pressure differential so that the batch tank inlet is at a higher pressure than the tank outlet. Examples of micro-irrigation system components that can cause a pressure differential are a partially closed valve or a pressure-reducing (pressure-regulating) valve. The rate that the material is injected is influenced by the flow rate through the tank and the concentration of injection material in the tank at any given time.

The batch tank is filled with the chemical (most frequently, fertilizer) to be applied. During irrigation, water is allowed to flow into the batch tank, where it displaces some of the tank's contents, forcing them into the irrigation system. Initially, the liquid leaving the batch tank is of high chemical concentration, but with time the concentration in the batch tank becomes more diluted as it mixes with water. The chemical injection starts out at a higher concentration and declines in concentration during the injection period. Batch tanks are appropriate if the objective is to inject a total amount of chemical (e.g., fertilizer) during a long injection period. Batch tanks are not appropriate if a constant injection concentration is required.

Venturi Injection Systems. Injection devices using the venturi principle (Fig. 8-48) have been used for many years in a wide variety of industrial and agricultural applications. A venturi is a specially shaped constriction in a device's water flow path. As the flow passageway at the venturi section becomes smaller, the velocity of the flowing fluid increases such that a vacuum is formed at the venturi's throat section. An opening located in the venturi's throat allows air or a fluid to be "sucked" in and mixed with the water stream. To create this effect, the inlet pressure to the venturi must be at least 15 to 20% greater than the outlet pressure. This is achieved by plumbing the venturi device across a system pressure differential (e.g., a partially closed valve) (Fig. 8-49) or using a small pump that draws water from the micro-irrigation system and forces it through the venturi injector (Fig. 8-50). The injection rate of a venturi-type injector depends on the size of the venturi section (½-inch to 2-inch sizes are available) and on the pressure difference between the inlet and the outlet of the venturi.

PESTICIDE APPLICATION EQUIPMENT 227

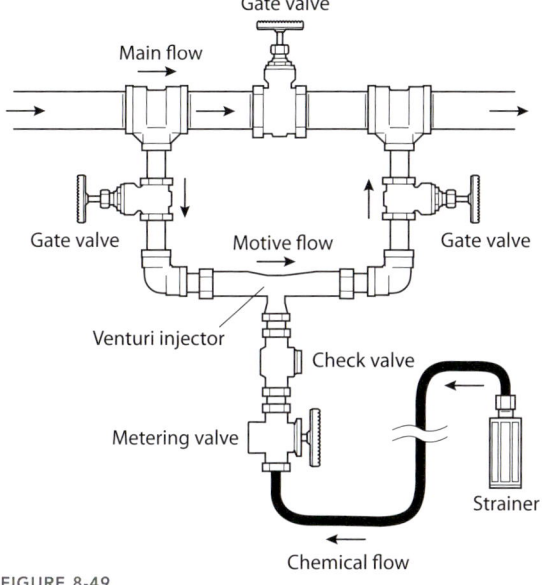

FIGURE 8-49

Venturi across a pressure drop setup.

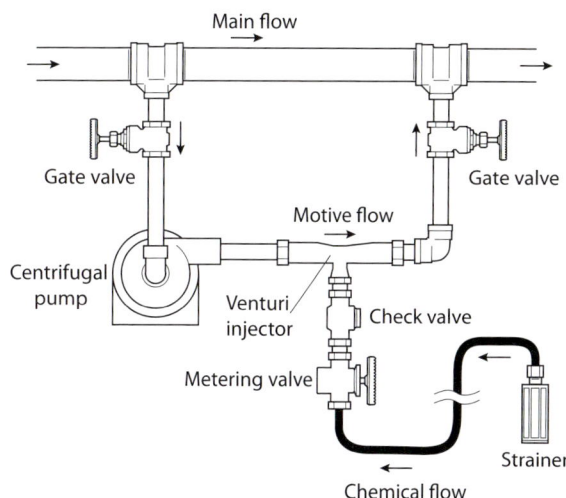

FIGURE 8-50

Venturi with small pump.

The venturi injector delivers a more constant chemical injection rate than does a batch tank. However, the injection rate of a venturi injector can change (or even stop) if the pressure changes upstream or downstream in the micro-irrigation system. This can occur if irrigation sets (applications) with different flow rates are operated from the same water supply pump. A venturi injector installation in which the venturi is plumbed across a pressure differential (see Fig. 8-49) is particularly sensitive to such changes, and it is often inconvenient to readjust the injector. The injector is usually installed parallel with the micro-irrigation system pipeline, with valves that can be closed to isolate the injector from the irrigation system when injection is not occurring. A venturi injector installation using a small pump in conjunction with the venturi eliminates the need to install the venturi across a pressure drop, and it also minimizes the venturi's sensitivity to irrigation system pressure fluctuations. However, this type of installation requires an electrical or gasoline power source.

ACTIVE SYSTEMS

Positive Displacement Pump Injection Systems. Positive displacement pumps have a relatively small capacity and deliver a very constant rate of injection. The pump can use a cylinder-piston configuration or a flexible diaphragm to inject a liquid at a pressure higher than that of the irrigation system. Electrically driven, gasoline engine–driven, and water-driven (Fig. 8-51) pump injectors are available. Positive displacement pumps provide the most accurate and con-

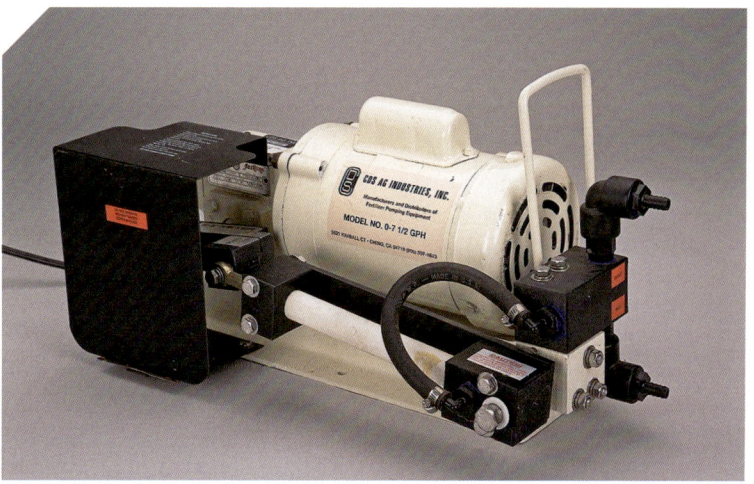

FIGURE 8-51

Cylinder-piston positive displacement injector pump.

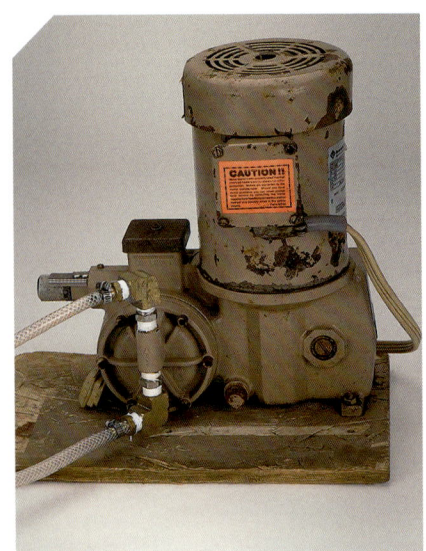

FIGURE 8-52

Diaphragm positive displacement injector pump.

stant injection rate, but they are also the most expensive injection devices. They do not need to be installed across a pressure drop since they are externally powered.

Positive displacement pump injectors are available as constant-rate pumps and as proportional pumps. Constant-rate pumps inject at a set rate (often adjustable) no matter what the flow rate is in the irrigation system. Proportional pumps (frequently water-driven) inject at a rate dependent on the flow rate passing through the injector or through the irrigation system. For the electrical or gasoline-driven pumps, the injector is linked to the irrigation system via a flow meter. For example, a proportional positive displacement injector set at 1:250 would inject 1 gallon of material for every 250 gallons of water passing through it. The proportional rate setting can be adjusted, as can the stock tank mixture concentration, to control the injected material's concentration in the irrigation system (for more information, see Schwankl and Prichard 2001).

PUMPS

Diaphragm pumps. You can calibrate diaphragm pumps so they provide injection rates that are continuous and uniform, as required by irrigation systems that move. The advantages of using a diaphragm pump over other pump types include

- lower maintenance costs on average
- easier adjustments to injection rates during operation

Because of its small number of moving parts and limited number of parts exposed to chemicals during the injection process, a diaphragm pump generally costs less to maintain over its lifetime than other pump types. Another advantage of lower rates of wear, corrosion, and leakage is a reduction in hazards to people and the environment from accidental pesticide releases (see Fig. 8-52).

The main disadvantage of installing a diaphragm pump is its up-front cost, which is generally higher than other pumps.

Piston pumps. Many chemigation systems use piston pumps because they are able to operate at a constant rate, even when pressure in the irrigation system is irregular (Fig. 8-53). This ability to maintain a consistent injection rate is the piston pump's main advantage.

There are two major disadvantages of piston pumps in chemigation: their mechanical complexity and the difficulties people face when calibrating them. First, these pumps have many moving parts that are regularly exposed to chemicals that wear and corrode those parts. Piston pumps, therefore, require more maintenance and have a shorter working life than other pump types. Leaks caused by worn seals are known to leak chemicals onto the system's platform and the soil around the platform, which creates hazards for people and the environment. Second, people often experience problems calibrating piston pumps because of the challenge of adjusting the pump stroke. In order to properly adjust the stroke length, you must stop the pump, make the adjustment, then restart it to measure the new injection rate. This process is time consuming and can be frustrating, because it usually takes several cycles of stopping, adjusting, starting, and measuring output of the pump to accurately calibrate the system.

Other pumps. Several other pump types can be used in chemigation systems. These include roller pumps, gear pumps, and centrifugal pumps. These pump types are used in irrigation systems that do not require the high level of accuracy needed for moving systems, such as wheel-lines, hand-lines, and drip/trickle systems.

AUTOMATED CONTROLS

In California, you are required to install automated controls on irrigation systems used to apply pesticides. An interlocking irrigation pump and chemical injection device will ensure that chemical injection stops when pumping stops. Automated controls help keep chemicals out of the water supply by preventing backflow of pesticides toward the pump and irrigation pipeline when the flow of water stops.

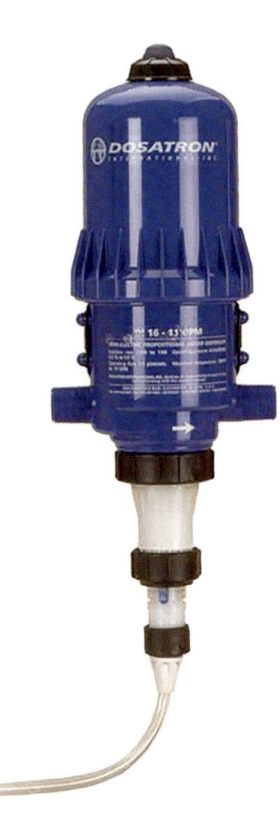

FIGURE 8-53

Water-driven injector (piston) pump.

A Mainline Single Check Valve
B Low Pressure Drain
C Air Vacuum Relief Valve
D Pressure Switch
E Interlocking System Controls
F Solenoid Operated Valve
G Pesticide Injection Pump
H Injection Line Check Valve

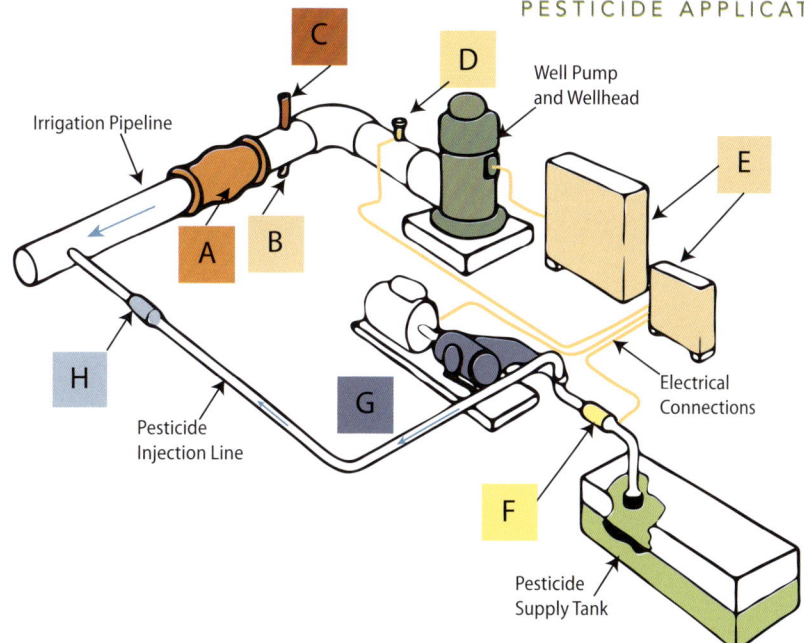

FIGURE 8-54

Schematic of a pesticide injection system with the eight required items, including interlocked system controls (E).

For chemigation setups that power the irrigation pump and the sprinkler system drive with separate electric motors, the electric controls for the two motors must be interlocked (Fig. 8-54). With this setup, as soon as one motor stops working, the other motor shuts down.

For chemigation systems that use internal combustion engines, chemical injection can be powered by belting the pump to the drive shaft or an accessory pulley of the engine (Fig. 8-55). In this setup, when the engine shuts down, both the injection and irrigation pumps will stop, as regulations require.

In addition to the interlocking control system, California requires the use of a pressure switch connected to the irrigation pipeline. The pressure switch stops the water pump motor when water pressure falls below levels effective for proper pesticide distribution. At this point, the interlock activates to shut down the injection system.

CALIBRATION SETUP

A good chemigation setup will include a calibration tube as part of the hose connecting the chemical injection pump and the supply tank. During calibration you can use it to measure the flow rate created by the pump. A typical calibration tube will be clear, resistant to breakage, graduated in units of volume (pints, ounces, milliliters, etc.), and will accommodate the fluid produced by the system over at least 5 minutes. If your system does not include a calibration tube, you can install a pressure relief (or regulating) valve at the end of the injection pump output hose.

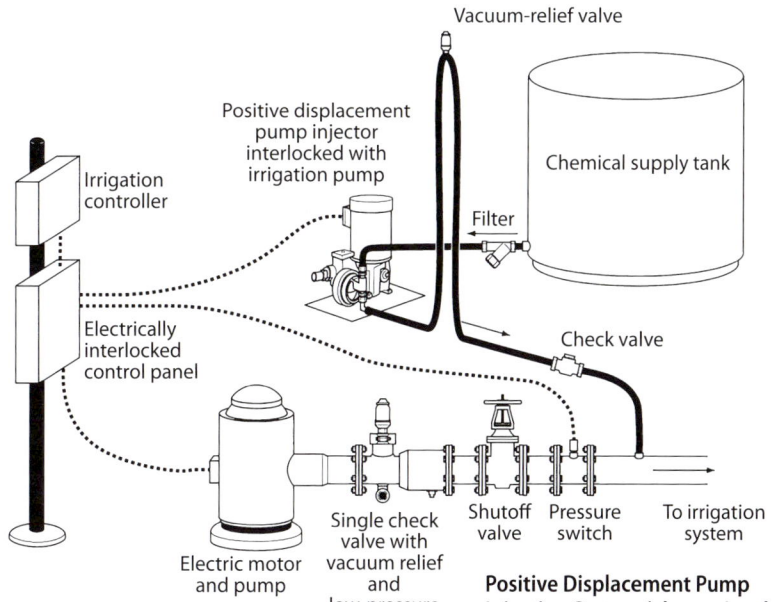

FIGURE 8-55

Minimum requirements for antipollution devices and arrangement of equipment for applying chemicals through the irrigation system (engine drive).

TABLE 8-6

Guide for selecting dust and granule application equipment

	Type	Uses	Suitable formulations	Comments
	bulb applicator	Forcing dusts into small cracks and crevices.	dusts	Simple, easy to use.
	compressed air duster	Applying dusts in confined spaces such as wall voids.	dusts	Avoid breathing dust.
	mechanical duster	Landscape and small agricultural areas.	dusts	Avoid drift. Do not breathe dust. May have bellows to disperse dust.
	power duster	Vine crops and some special applications. Also used in buildings.	dusts	Equipped with blower to disperse dusts. Drift hazard considerable.
	hand-operated granule applicator	Landscape, aquatic, and some agricultural areas.	granules or pellets	Suitable for small areas. Easy to use.
	mechanically driven granule applicator	Turf and other landscape areas. Also commonly used in agricultural areas.	granules or pellets	Requires accurate calibration.
	powered granule applicator	Agricultural areas, usually row crops. Also used in some large landscape applications.	granules or pellets	Frequent servicing and cleaning required. Some units have blowers to disperse granules. Others distribute granules along a boom.

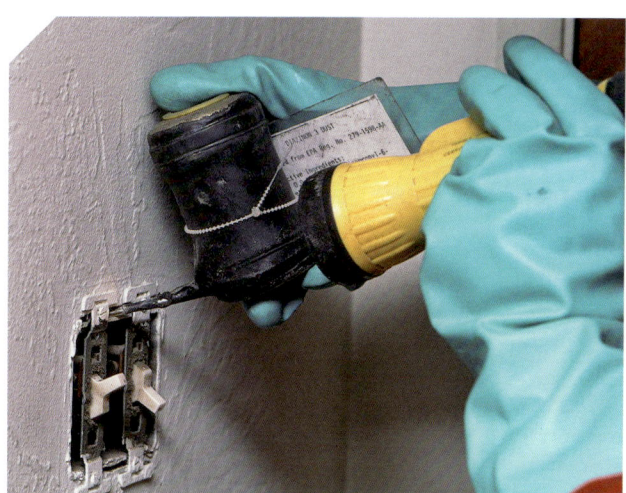

FIGURE 8-56
Bulb applicators can be used to apply dusts to small, confined areas such as electrical outlets and cracks and crevices.

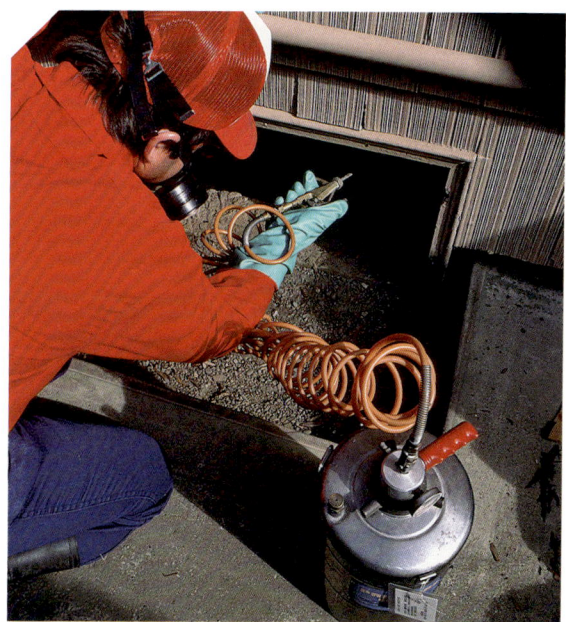

FIGURE 8-57
A compressed air duster may be used to apply pesticide dusts in enclosed areas, wall voids, crawl spaces, and attics.

In this situation, you will set the pressure so it equals the irrigation line pressure at the injection point and direct the flow into a graduated measuring can for at least 5 minutes. For detailed information on monitoring and calibration of chemigation systems, see Chapter 9.

Dust and Granule Application Equipment

Do not mix granules or certain dust formulations with water; apply them dry and undiluted. This requires special equipment, and there are unique problems with this type of application. Because dust formulations are highly susceptible to drift over great distances if applied during windy conditions, outdoor uses of dusts are limited, although sulfur dust is used frequently in grapes. Their greatest use is for pest control in buildings and other confined areas. There are also formulations to control external parasites on livestock, poultry, and pets.

Granules are the dry formulations used most for pest control in landscape, agricultural, and aquatic situations. These are usually incorporated into the soil or applied to bodies of water. Table 8-6 is a guide for selecting dust and granule application equipment.

DUST APPLICATORS

> List the types of application equipment used to apply dusts, and describe the situations in which each should be used.

The function of a dust applicator is to combine the dust with air and spread it evenly over an area. You can choose from several types of dust application equipment. When using any type of dust application equipment, there is a risk of drift and inhalation, so take all necessary precautions when using dust formulations.

Bulb Applicators (Fig. 8-56). Hand-held bulb applicators apply dusts to small, confined areas, cracks, and crevices. Squeezing the bulb, which is made of rubber or a similar flexible material, expels dust-bearing air through a small tube. Some bulb dusters have attachments to extend the reach of the tube and direct the dust. Some applicators have plastic tubes to make them safer for use around electrical outlets, while others have metal tubes made of brass. These attach to a cone or cap that may be made of aluminum or plastic. Depending on the type of bulb applicator, it may have a filler spout or a funnel accessory to help you fill the chamber without spilling the dust.

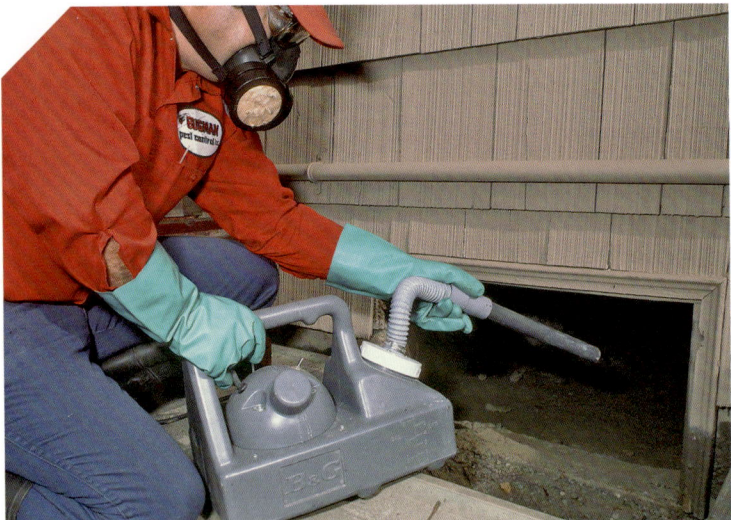

FIGURE 8-58

Power dusters are used to broadcast dust into confined areas. They have a blower to carry dust to treatment surfaces.

Compressed Air Dusters (Fig. 8-57). Compressed air dusters move dusts through a nozzle or hose when a trigger is compressed. Some compressed air dusters have an adjustment knob to control the amount of dust released when the trigger is compressed. High-velocity air picks up some pesticide from an airtight chamber and distributes it as a fine powder. Manufacturers package dust formulations of some pesticides in aerosol cans. You apply these in the same way as liquid aerosols. However, a common problem associated with dusts is their tendency to cake inside the aerosol applicator. Moisture or high humidity enhances caking. Manufacturers overcome this problem by incorporating anti-caking materials into the formulation.

Mechanical Dusters. Mechanical dusters have either a crank-operated fan and agitator or a lever-operated bellows. These devices force dust-laden air out of a hopper. The pesticide dust passes through an orifice in the applicator or through a hose aimed by the operator. Most mechanical dusters have back or chest straps. Smaller units are carried by hand.

Power Dusters. Power dusters use fans powered by electric or gasoline motors (Fig. 8-58). The small, hand-held units work well in structural settings. These units are either battery powered or plug into a standard electrical outlet. Lightweight gasoline engines power larger backpack units. From a hand-held flexible hose, operators direct pesticide dusts at targets up to 15 feet away.

Large power dusters for agricultural crops attach to tractors. Growers use them to apply dusts in date palm gardens and to row or vine crops. There may be several nozzles on a boom. Each nozzle connects by large-diameter flexible tubing to a central blower that mixes the dust with air. Extension tubes or fan-shaped air volutes direct dusts onto target plants. These units may cause environmental problems because of drift hazards associated with dust formulations.

GRANULE APPLICATORS

Granule applicators may be hand-operated, mechanically driven, or engine powered, depending on the needs of the application site. Aquatic weed managers mount granule applicators in boats for some aquatic applications.

Because granules are of varying sizes and shapes, equipment must accommodate size differences. Pellet formulations are granules of identical size and shape. When applied through specially designed applicators, pellets allow for accurate calibration. This provides more uniform application rates than are possible with irregularly shaped granules. Often, granules require incorporation into the soil. Usually, operators attach tillage equipment behind the granule applicators to incorporate granules at the time of application.

Risks associated with the use of granules for pest control include accidental exposure of wildlife and pets, and, when using nonpowered equipment, reliance on keeping a steady pace to ensure even distribution.

List the types of application equipment used to apply granules, and describe the situations in which each should be used.

Hand-Operated Granule Applicators. Hand-operated granule applicators usually strap to the operator's chest. Granules pass through an adjustable opening at the bottom of a cloth, metal, or plastic hopper and drop onto a spinning plate operated by a hand crank. The operator walks at a steady pace while turning the crank to achieve an even distribution of granules.

Drop Spreaders. Several types of drop spreaders (Fig. 8-59), also known as mechanically driven granule applicators, are available. Some have ground wheel–driven metering devices attached to a hopper. Drop spreaders are the most accurate and flexible spreaders available for granules. To control the rate of application, adjust the openings that granules pass through. All the granules fall within the wheelbase, so slight overlapping of the wheels with each pass is necessary for uniform coverage. Read the pesticide label and booklets that come with the spreader so you are familiar with the settings and can determine which setting is best for your specific application.

Common problems associated with drop spreaders include
- skips from granules not dropping evenly or consistently on certain spots during an application
- too little or too much overlap
- uneven spreading when turning corners
- hopper openings in the bottom clogging due to the granules clumping together during moist conditions

Powered Granule Applicators. Small gasoline engines power backpack applicators. These applicators are similar to those used to apply liquids or dusts over a limited area. A blower connected to a flexible hose aids in dispersing the granules. The operator aims the tube at the target area while walking slowly.

Another type of powered granule applicator consists of a long boom attached to a tractor or truck. Granules are augered down the boom and metered out at preset spacings. This provides for accurate calibration and even distribution of granular pesticides.

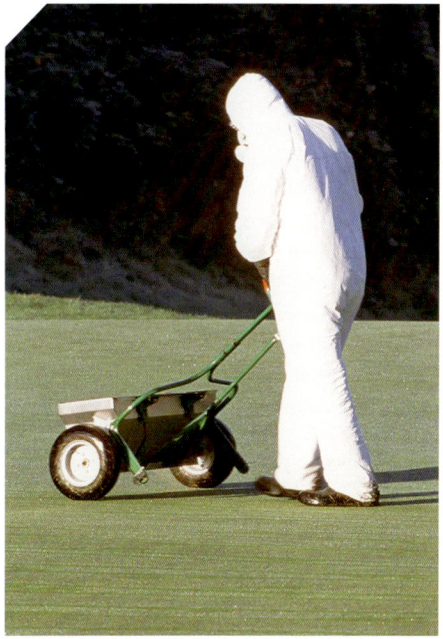

FIGURE 8-59

A mechanically driven granule applicator may be used to apply pesticide granules to agricultural crops. Smaller versions are used for application of granular pesticides to turf.

Livestock and Poultry Application Equipment

Pest managers use several methods to apply pesticides to livestock and poultry. Those described here are used for the external application of liquids or dusts. Several methods are used to apply pesticides to the animal's skin. In addition, veterinarians administer systemic pesticides to protect animals from internal and external parasites. Animals receive systemic pesticides through feed, by subcutaneous injections, and by mouth as pastes, capsules, or tablets.

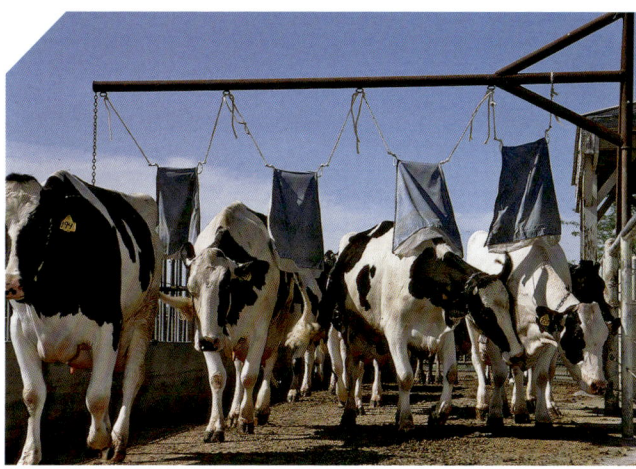

FIGURE 8-60

Certain types of pesticides are applied to livestock by means of dust bags or face and back rubbers. Small amounts of dust or liquid are deposited onto the animal each time it rubs against the device.

Livestock Face and Back Rubbers and Dust Bags

Manufacturers package dry or liquid pesticide formulations into dispensing bags or other dispensing containers. Livestock managers hang or mount these in areas frequented by the animals (Fig. 8-60). As the animals contact these packages, usually to scratch themselves, small amounts of pesticide are released onto their bodies. This effectively controls many different species of external parasites.

Poultry Dust Boxes

Poultry managers put dust formulations of specific pesticides in poultry dust boxes to control insects and mites infesting laying hens. Hens instinctively wallow in the boxes and pick up the dust on their feathers and skin.

Dipping Vats and Spray/Dip Machines

Livestock managers use dipping vats and spray or dip machines to control external parasites on cattle, sheep, and other large animals. They dip or spray animals so that they become totally covered with liquid pesticide. Animals enter and leave these devices through ramps.

Bait Application Equipment

Pesticide bait formulations require special application methods. A major problem associated with baits is exposing nontarget organisms to toxic pesticides. Bait stations or bait applicators can help prevent such exposure.

Bait Stations

> List types of bait application equipment and explain how they work.

Bait stations hold supplies of poisoned food and attract target pests. Use types that prevent children, pets, and nontarget animals from contacting the baits (Fig. 8-61). Bait stations help control flies around poultry and livestock quarters. Other types control squirrels in agricultural and right-of-way locations. Special designs also control rodents in warehouses and residential areas. Manufactures make special bait stations for managing cockroaches, ants, snails, and other invertebrates. Occasionally, bait stations are used for controlling pest birds.

Place bait stations out of the reach of nontarget organisms, pets, and children. Hang fly bait stations above poultry or livestock in poultry houses, loafing sheds, or barns. For pest bird control, managers secure V-shaped troughs high up in trees. They bait these with poisonous seeds or grains. For rodents, locate bait stations in crawl spaces, attics, and other out-of-the-way places.

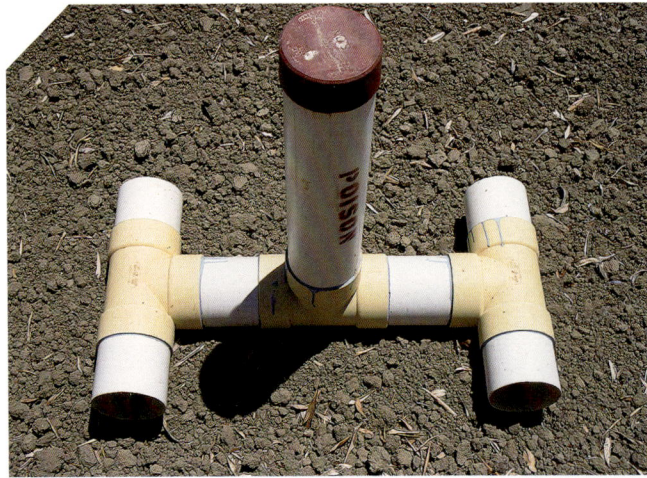

FIGURE 8-61

Bait stations are helpful in preventing nontarget organisms from being exposed to the pesticide.

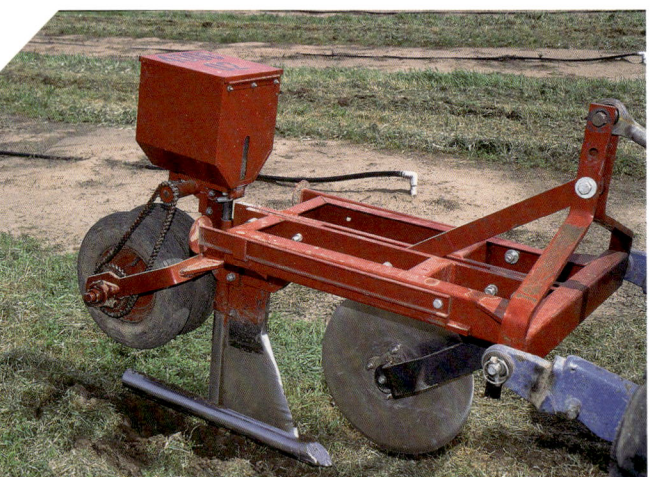

FIGURE 8-62

This burrowing device is used to apply poisoned bait for control of gophers; it forms an artificial burrow that intersects with the natural burrows made by gophers. Poisoned grain is deposited in the artificial burrow.

BAIT APPLICATORS FOR GOPHERS AND MOLES

There are commercially available applicators for applying poisoned baits to control gophers and moles. Use hand-operated models to inject small quantities of poisoned bait directly into an underground burrow made by the gopher or mole. For larger areas infested by gophers, tractor-mounted mechanical bait applicators form baited artificial burrows that intersect natural burrows (Fig. 8-62). Gophers explore the artificial burrows and feed on the bait.

Application Equipment Maintenance

Effective pesticide application depends on properly maintained and adjusted application equipment. Regular inspections and periodic maintenance programs help you avoid accidents or spills caused by ruptured hoses, faulty fittings, damaged tanks, or other problems.

Inspect application equipment for wear, corrosion, or damage before each use. Replace or repair faulty components. Thoroughly clean equipment after every application. Wear PPE, including rubber gloves and eye protection, when cleaning or repairing the equipment. When not in use, store equipment in a way that prevents deterioration or damage.

LIQUID APPLICATION EQUIPMENT

Preventing Problems

Take the following preventive steps to reduce problems of sprayer malfunction or breakdown and to maintain uniform and accurate application.

Use clean water. Water that contains sand or silt causes rapid pump wear and can clog screens and nozzles. Whenever possible, use water pumped directly from a well and make sure all filling hoses and pipes are clean. If you pump water from ponds or irrigation canals, filter it before putting it into the sprayer tank. Also, measure the pH of the water to be sure it is adequate for the intended pesticide use. Chapter 3 describes how to check and adjust pH.

Keep screens in place. Filter screens remove foreign particles from the spray liquid. It is a nuisance to remove collected debris from the screens, but debris accumulation indicates that the screens are doing the job for which they were designed. Removing screens because they keep plugging only increases wear on pumps and nozzles. Make sure screens are the proper size for the type of pesticide being applied. If excessive plugging does occur, try to eliminate the cause, for example, by changing water sources.

Use chemicals that are compatible with the sprayer and pump. Spray chemicals are corrosive to some metals and deteriorate rubber and plastic components. Recognize limitations in existing spray equipment. Avoid problems by modifying the equipment to accommodate the corrosive pesticides. Otherwise, use the equipment only for chemicals that are not corrosive. Sometimes it is possible to replace parts of a sprayer with corrosion-resistant materials.

Properly clean nozzles. Spray nozzles are made to precise specifications. Never use any metal object to clean or remove debris. These may damage the orifice, adversely changing the spray pattern and spray volume. Clean nozzles by flushing with clean water or a detergent solution. Remove stuck particles with a soft brush. Nozzle suppliers sell special brushes for this purpose. Always wear rubber gloves when handling or cleaning spray nozzles. Never blow through them with your mouth, because nozzles usually contain pesticide residues. Use an air compressor if needed, but protect your eyes and skin (Fig. 8-63).

Flush sprayers before use. Use clean water to flush new sprayers and sprayers coming out of storage. Flushing removes foreign particles, dirt, and other debris. The manufacturing process may leave metallic chips, dirt, or other residue in the tank or pump. Storage always subjects spraying equipment to the possibility of being contaminated with dirt, leaves, rodent debris, and rust.

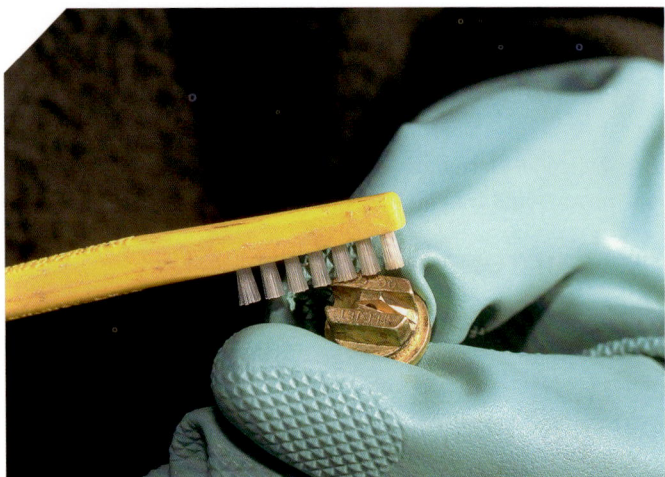

FIGURE 8-63

To clean a clogged nozzle, use compressed air or water for flushing the orifice. Never put your mouth to a nozzle. Use a soft brush to remove stuck objects. Do not use any type of metal device to remove debris, because you may damage the orifice.

Clean sprayer after use. Cleaning spray equipment at the end of each job is important. Clean your sprayer according to the instructions on the label of the last pesticide used. Following the label's directions will ensure that your efforts will remove most residues that can contaminate future tank mixes or damage crops or treated surfaces. Avoid leaving pesticide mixtures in a sprayer overnight or for longer periods of time. Prolonged contact increases chances of corrosion or deterioration of sprayer components. Some pesticides settle out and may be difficult to get back into suspension after being left in an idle sprayer. After mixing them with water, certain pesticides lose their effectiveness quickly. Finally, pesticides left in an unattended sprayer may present a hazard to people, wildlife, or the environment.

If possible, apply leftover spray material to an appropriate (registered) target site. Otherwise, treat unused pesticide mixtures as hazardous wastes. Additionally, some pesticides are difficult to remove entirely from the tank, and you will need to use special cleaners to thoroughly remove their residues. Check the pesticide label, because some of these recommend the use of specific cleaners. You may want to use separate tanks if you apply a difficult-to-clean pesticide, especially when using herbicides.

Clean the sprayer and flush out the tank at the application site whenever possible. If this is not possible, contain the wash water and use it for mixing other pesticides of the same type. Remember that repeated cleaning in a particular location can result in contamination of that area unless you carefully contain wash water. Should you be unable to use the contaminated water in your next tank mix, have it transported to a Class I disposal site as a hazardous waste. Never drain rinse water onto the ground or into sewer or septic lines. See "Sprayer Storage" later in this chapter for more detailed instructions for cleaning equipment before storage.

Inspection and Maintenance

Perform regular inspections and periodic maintenance on spraying equipment. This keeps it in good operating condition and ready for use. Take care of simple maintenance, such as greasing bearings and drive lines, while inspecting the equipment. Always check for the following problems:

- weakened hoses
- leaking fittings
- damage to the tank or tank protective coating
- broken regulators or gauges
- worn nozzles
- worn bearings
- damaged tires (if equipped)
- other mechanical defects or wear

PESTICIDE APPLICATION EQUIPMENT

TABLE 8-7

Troubleshooting problems associated with poor sprayer performance

Problem	Possible cause
uneven spray pattern	clogged nozzles worn nozzles mismatched nozzle sizes nozzle screens not uniform boom not level hoses to nozzles or boom sections not uniform in size pressure not adjusted to operating range of nozzles foam in spray tank
clogged nozzles	rust, sand, or other contaminant in spray tank improper or missing filter screens incompatible spray mixture poorly mixed spray ingredients agitator not working properly failure to use marine grease on mechanical agitator fittings
pressure too low	worn pump nozzles too large nozzles excessively worn air in pressure system pesticide mixture foaming broken or maladjusted pressure regulator needed pressure is beyond the capacity of the pump pump speed too slow drive belts slipping restricted or defective suction hose clogged suction strainer
pressure too high	pump speed too fast pressure regulator not working bypass system blocked, restricted, or undersized nozzles too small filter screens clogged
pump not primed	air trapped in the system suction line not completely full of liquid worn pump drive belts slipping shear pin broken on drive line foam in tank suction line blocked leak in suction hose
pesticide mixture settles out in tank	agitator insufficient or not working properly incompatible mixture tank and hoses not properly cleaned before use pH too high or too low
pulsating pressure	worn piston pump seals highly foaming tank mix
excessive drift	nozzles too small pressure too high application made during windy weather spray boom to high nozzles improperly aligned temperature too high while applying volatile materials treated surfaces not receptive failure to use a drift control agent

Equipment with a self-contained engine requires additional maintenance. Check oil and water levels regularly. Change air filters, oil filters, and motor oil according to the manufacturer's recommendations. Clean and service batteries.

By spending a few minutes each day inspecting and servicing spray equipment, you increase the length of its useful life. Performing regular maintenance tasks also helps to avoid costly breakdowns and possibly dangerous leaks. Develop a checklist for servicing and inspecting equipment so you remember what needs to be done. The checklist can also serve as a service record.

Even when equipment is maintained, leaks can occur in the field. As soon as you notice the problem, stop the application and repair or replace the sprayer before resuming work.

Sprayer Troubleshooting

A sprayer may not exhibit any external sign of trouble, but it still may not be functioning at an optimal level. Problems such as lack of pressure, too much pressure, or inadequate output at the nozzles require troubleshooting to locate and correct the cause. Table 8-7 is a guide to troubleshooting problems associated with poor sprayer performance.

Sprayer Storage

Improperly storing spraying equipment can shorten its useful life. Before storing a sprayer, decontaminate and clean it thoroughly. Wear rubber gloves and other appropriate PPE to avoid contact with pesticide residues. Remove, clean, and reinstall all filters. Partially fill the tank with clean water and add a commercial neutralizing cleaner (or ½ pound of detergent to 30 gallons of water). Circulate this solution through the system for at least 30 minutes and flush it out through the nozzles. Refill the sprayer about half full. Add more commercial cleaner according to directions or add 1 quart of household ammonia to each 25 gallons of water. Circulate this solution for about 5 minutes and flush a small amount through the nozzles. Shut off the sprayer and let the solution remain in the tank for 12 to 24 hours.

> Describe how to properly store application equipment.

While the cleaning solution is soaking in the tank, thoroughly wash all external parts of the sprayer. Use a detergent or ammonia solution or a commercial cleaner. Scrub residue off all surfaces using a bristle brush. Rinse external parts with clean water. You may also want to make note of any nonstandard parts or additions like nozzle turrets and check them carefully, since these components can retain unexpected pesticide residues.

If the sprayer may be in freezing conditions before you use it again, winterize it. Circulate an antifreeze solution in the pump, control, and bypass lines before storage. Remember to remove and properly dispose of the antifreeze solution before using the sprayer again.

To prevent rusting, touch up scratched areas on all painted surfaces of the trailer, boom, tank, and accessories. Lubricate bearings to prevent them from rusting during storage.

Remove and clean nozzles and nozzle strainers. Store these in a clean plastic bag to keep them free of dirt.

After the tank has finished soaking, flush the solution out and rinse with clean water. Seal nozzle outlets with corks or plastic bags to prevent insects or dirt from getting into the lines. Remove and clean all remaining filter screens and store them in a clean plastic bag. Remove O rings from filters and strainers and store them in a plastic bag to prevent them from becoming brittle. Cover the tank loosely to prevent dirt, insects, and rodents from entering during storage. Do not close the tank cover tightly, as this may permanently distort its rubber seal. Store the sprayer inside a building, preferably covered with a tarp for additional protection. Block up equipment that has rubber tires to remove weight from the tires and bearings. You can remove small pumps and store them in a can of new, lightweight motor oil to prevent rusting. However, if pumps have rubber or neoprene parts, do not expose them to oil.

Remove hoses used on hand-held nozzles. Coil these and hang them around a pail, basket, or other large round object. This prevents sharp bends that might cause cracks in the rubber. Never hang hoses over a nail, rack, or board. Store hoses in an area away from direct sunlight.

Release the tension from the pressure regulator and remove the O ring seal. Lubricate the internal cylinder of the regulator and reassemble without the O ring. Place the O ring in a plastic bag and tie it to the regulator.

Before using spray equipment again after it has been in storage, be sure to flush the system thoroughly with clean water.

Dust and Granule Applicators

Thoroughly clean dust and granule applicators after each use. Be sure to remove all pesticides and pesticide residue. Once clean, lubricate chains, auger bearings, and other moving parts according to the manufacturer's instructions. Inspect the equipment for wear and corrosion. Repair rusted or corroded areas to prevent them from getting worse.

Dust Applicators

Before using a dust applicator, inspect it carefully. Check the inside of the bulb or chamber to make sure it is dry and free of residue or potential obstructions. Next, inspect the screw threads where the nozzle or application tip is attached and make sure they are clean. Then make sure that the application tip is securely attached. Finally, inspect the application tips and extensions for cracks and replace any damaged or worn accessories.

After use, clean the equipment with a nylon brush using soap and water. Make sure parts that contact dry pesticide are thoroughly and completely dry before reuse. Carefully inspect the cap, screw threads, and application tubes for cracks and other parts for damage or obvious wear. If you find any flaws (such as cracks in plastic or corrosion in metal parts), remove and replace the worn parts before using the applicator again.

Granule Applicators

Before using granule applicators, inspect them for wear and to make sure there are no pesticide residues left in the hopper or anywhere else on the machine. Remove and replace worn or damaged parts and check to be sure there are no blockages before loading the equipment. Check to make sure the gear cover is in place on applicators that have one; this helps protect moving parts that are easily damaged by dirt or pesticide residue.

Empty and thoroughly wash granule applicators after every use. Normally, cold water is all that you will need to remove pesticide residue from the equipment; however, some pesticides will require scrubbing or the use of hot water to loosen built-up residues. It may be useful to close the spreader so the hopper can be filled completely with water and then drained. If you have to use abrasive cleaners, be careful not to damage the equipment as you work.

Lubricate granule applicators only if the manufacturer recommends it. Be careful of too much lubrication, because grease can increase buildup of pesticide residues and dirt that can damage an applicator's moving parts. Read the manufacturer's recommendations carefully to find out if your equipment requires lubrication before taking this step.

Granule Applicator Storage

Granule applicators should be housed inside, away from sun, heat, and moisture. Store equipment only after it is clean and completely dry, with the rate setting at its highest, and the mechanism open, or "on." Any pesticide remaining in or on the equipment can cause corrosion, as can moisture and heat, especially in combination. Storing equipment wide open helps ensure that it remains dry and free of pesticides. Avoid placing anything on top of stored granule applicators, because extra weight can deform the hopper or wheels.

Maintaining Chemigation Equipment

Periodic monitoring of chemigation systems can help you ensure that they are operating safely and effectively. The following items should be inspected thoroughly before you begin chemigation activities:

- main pipeline check valve
- vacuum relief valve
- low-pressure drain
- chemical injection line check valve
- main control panel for the irrigation system and pumping plant
- chemical injection pump safety interlock
- injection system (inline strainer, manual valve, and chemical storage tank)
- irrigation pump
- injection pump
- power source

Repair or replace any parts you find that are damaged or worn. Be sure to recalibrate the system any time maintenance has been performed and parts have been replaced.

Flushing Irrigation and Injection Systems

Chemigation equipment must be thoroughly flushed after each use in order to ensure safe operation during the next application. After completing an application, run the irrigation system for at least 10 minutes to flush out any chemicals that may remain. You may have to run the system for more than 10 minutes if you are using drip irrigation, as water takes longer to run through low-volume systems. For any irrigation system type that shuts down automatically at the end of an application, be sure to flush it as soon as possible after shutdown is complete. You must also flush systems that have been shut down because of a malfunction or loss of water pressure. Do this as soon as you can after discovering the shutdown. In both of these situations, it is best to flush the system for at least 30 minutes, just to be sure all traces of the pesticide have been run out of the system.

Use clean water to flush your injection system after each use to prevent pesticides from accumulating. It is best to flush the injection system as you are irrigating, so that whatever pesticides you flush out are applied to the same site.

Chapter 8 Review Questions

1. Match the type of application equipment to its major limitation.

1. low-pressure sprayer	a. works only for low-volume applications because of its small tank and inability to produce high pressure
2. controlled droplet applicator	b. requires very accurate calibration to achieve correct application rates at both low and high volumes
3. power duster	c. does not penetrate dense foliage, and droplets cannot travel far unless the unit is equipped with a blower
4. powered backpack sprayer	d. applications limited to low wind conditions because of elevated drift potential; equipment also uses highly concentrated formulations, so hazards to pesticide handlers may be increased
5. ultra-low-volume sprayer	e. can cause environmental problems because of drift hazards

2. Match the application situation to its appropriate liquid applicator.

1. You want to carefully control the amount and timing of both water and pesticide to match the exact needs of the crop.	a. aerosol generator or fogger
2. You need to control insects in a warehouse.	b. air blast sprayer
3. You need to move spray into dense foliage or treetops in a vineyard or orchard.	c. low-pressure sprayer
4. You need to inject liquid pesticides into the soil.	d. chemigation using a micro-irrigation system
5. You need to control tall weeds without damaging the crop underneath them.	e. controlled droplet applicator
6. You need to make very low-volume herbicide applications and want to minimize drift.	f. wick applicator

3. When should you avoid using a metal or coated metal sprayer tank?
   - ☐ a. The pesticide formulations you use can react with metal.
   - ☐ b. The weather is regularly wet or air is excessively humid.
   - ☐ c. The soil is moist and a heavy sprayer will compact soil too much.

4. Which of the following pumps is best to use with abrasive pesticide formulations?
   - ☐ a. piston pump
   - ☐ b. gear pump
   - ☐ c. diaphragm pump

5. If you are using a wettable powder and you think you might have to shut the sprayer's pump down during an application, you should NOT use a _____.
   - ☐ a. closed mixing system
   - ☐ b. thermoplastic tank
   - ☐ c. hydraulic agitator

6. Which part of a sprayer controls its application rate, droplet size, and spray pattern?
   - ☐ a. pumps
   - ☐ b. nozzles
   - ☐ c. pressure regulators

7. You know a pump is worn and may need to be replaced when _____.
   - ☐ a. pressure is too low
   - ☐ b. spray pattern is uneven
   - ☐ c. drift is greater than expected

8. Worn nozzles cause which of the following problems?
   - ☐ a. Pump speed increases unexpectedly.
   - ☐ b. Spray mixtures become contaminated.
   - ☐ c. Spray patterns are obviously uneven.

9. Match the nozzle with its spray pattern and uses.

1. flat-fan nozzles	a. These nozzles produce a high-pressure single stream of pesticide. They are used for spraying distant objects, for crack and crevice treatments in and around buildings, and for banding fluids in row crops.
2. even-spray nozzles	b. These nozzles create more spray droplets in the center and fewer droplets on the side so that the pattern tapers off at each end. They are used with soil-applied herbicides, fungicides, and insecticides.
3. disc-core nozzles	c. These nozzles produce an even distribution of droplets in a fan-shaped pattern. They are used when you don't want the herbicide, fungicide, or insecticide spray to overlap.
4. solid stream nozzles	d. These nozzles produce a hollow cone spray pattern. They are used for high-pressure and high-flow-rate applications of insecticides and fungicides.
5. flooding nozzles	e. These nozzles produce a wide fan angle of up to 160 degrees. They are used to apply fertilizers, and occasionally, herbicides.

10. When using a wettable powder, flowable, or dry flowable formulation, you should avoid using nozzles made out of _____.
    - ☐ a. ceramic
    - ☐ b. stainless steel
    - ☐ c. brass

11. In California, which of the following irrigation systems is used most often for chemigation?
    ☐ a. center-pivot sprinkler systems
    ☐ b. micro-irrigation systems
    ☐ c. self-propelled linear systems

12. Match the application situation to its appropriate dust or granule applicator.

1. You want to disperse granules over a limited area with the aid of a blower.	a. compressed air duster
2. You want to control the amount of dust released when compressing the trigger.	b. bulb applicator
3. You want to strictly control both the application rate and accurate placement of granular pesticides.	c. power duster
4. You need to apply dusts to small confined areas, cracks, and crevices.	d. drop spreader
5. You need to apply dust in a date palm garden.	e. powered granule applicator

13. Use of a bait station designed for specific pests helps to _____.
    ☐ a. reduce populations of beneficial organisms
    ☐ b. prevent children, pets, and other animals from accessing baits
    ☐ c. increase populations of the pest's predators and parasites

14. What single piece of equipment can help you accurately adjust to changing conditions as you make an application?
    ☐ a. check valves
    ☐ b. electronic sprayer controllers
    ☐ c. surge chambers

15. Nonstandard sprayer parts or additions like nozzle turrets have which of the following problems?
    ☐ a. They can retain a surprising amount of pesticide residue if not checked carefully.
    ☐ b. They are challenging to troubleshoot if the operator is unfamiliar with the parts.
    ☐ c. They cannot be switched out easily when changing formulations or application sites.

16. Which of the following can be used to remove stuck particles from a nozzle you are cleaning?
    ☐ a. steel brush
    ☐ b. thin copper wire
    ☐ c. soft brush

17. For which types of equipment will you need to lubricate chains, auger bearings, and other moving parts after use to ensure they remain in good working condition?
    ☐ a. air blast and backpack sprayers
    ☐ b. foggers and aerosol sprayers
    ☐ c. dust and granule applicators

18. **What should you do if you find yourself cleaning application equipment in the exact same location every day?**
    ☐ a. Collect wash water and dump it in a different location after each cleaning.
    ☐ b. Recycle wash water for use wetting roads to keep dust problems at a minimum.
    ☐ c. Contain wash water and use it in your next tank mix of the same pesticide.

19. **Which parts should always be removed from large liquid sprayers that will be stored for extended periods?**
    ☐ a. nozzles, strainers, filter screens, and O rings
    ☐ b. tank covers, spray shields, tires, and valves
    ☐ c. nozzle turrets, pressure gauges, gas caps, and hoses

20. **Why should you store granule applicators with the rate setting at its highest and the mechanism open, or "on"?**
    ☐ a. Leaving equipment this way makes it easier to use after storage.
    ☐ b. Storing equipment this way helps ensure that it remains dry and free of pesticides.
    ☐ c. It keeps the hopper and other mechanisms from warping or becoming deformed.

Chapter 9
Calibrating Pesticide Application Equipment

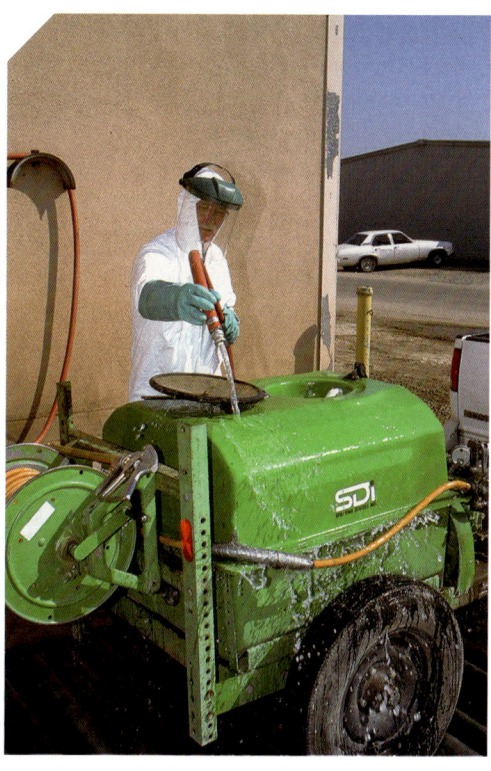

Why Calibration Is Essential... 246
Equipment Calibration Methods....................................... 248
Calculation for Active Ingredient, Percentage Solutions,
and Parts Per Million Dilutions... 269
Using System Monitors and Controllers............................ 276
Chapter 9 Review Questions 276

Knowledge Expectations

- Define calibration and explain why accurate calibration is essential to safe, effective pest control.
- List the tools needed for calibration activities.
- Describe how to calibrate liquid sprayers and be able to calculate speed, gallons per minute (for low- and high-pressure sprayers), and nozzle output using formulas.
- Describe how to determine the correct amount of pesticide needed for a particular application.
- Describe methods used to determine how much pesticide to put into the hopper or tank for a specific application rate over the total area of the application site.
- Describe the best way to change the output of various types of pesticide application equipment and the consequences of each change.
- Describe how to calibrate dry applicators.
- Describe what you need to know before you can dilute a pesticide correctly.
- Be able to calculate the active ingredient concentration of pesticides using formulas.
- Calculate the area of various shapes (circle, square, rectangle, triangle, and irregular shapes).
- Explain how system controllers can impact the calibration of equipment and calculations necessary to apply pesticides effectively.
- Explain the importance of properly calibrating sensors that are part of a system controller.

> Define calibration and explain why accurate calibration is essential to safe, effective pest control.

The term calibration refers to all the adjustments you make to be sure you apply the correct amount of pesticide to the treatment area. Failure to calibrate equipment properly is a cause of ineffective pesticide applications and creates hazards for people during mixing and application. In addition, inaccurate calibration always carries the potential for excessive or illegal residues remaining on treated surfaces.

This chapter discusses the steps you need to take to calibrate any type of pesticide application equipment. It does not discuss common calibration shortcuts and quick calculations. These are applicable only in specific situations or for certain types of application equipment. However, these handy techniques may be available in equipment manuals or trade journals and publications. Learn the principles of proper calibration first. Then, if appropriate, adopt a quick calibration method that applies to your equipment and special needs.

To calibrate your equipment you must first determine the amount of pesticide to apply—the application rate. *Check the pesticide label for this information.* You may need to adjust ground speed and equipment output or modify application patterns to achieve the desired rate. Once you have calibrated your equipment, check and test it periodically to be sure the calibration stays accurate. Many operators fail to understand how rapidly equipment becomes maladjusted or worn. As a result, application equipment is usually not calibrated often enough.

Table 9-1 is a list of helpful conversion factors to use when calibrating pesticide application equipment.

Why Calibration Is Essential

The main reason for calibrating application equipment is to figure out how much pesticide to put into the tank or hopper. Without proper calibration, you cannot ensure that you will apply the correct amount of chemical. Calibration is necessary for

- effective pest control
- protecting human health, the environment, and treated surfaces
- preventing waste of resources
- controlling the volume of water applied to a given area (for liquid applications)
- complying with the law

Effective Pest Control. Manufacturers of pesticides spend millions of dollars researching ways to use their products. Their research includes determining the correct amount of pesticide to apply to effectively control target pests. Using less than the labeled amount of pesticide may result in inadequate control—a waste of time and money. Inadequate amounts of pesticide also lead to problems such as pest resistance and resurgence. Using too much pesticide has adverse effects on natural enemies, target surfaces, and the environment. Applying higher than label rates also wastes materials, but more important, it is illegal.

Human Health Concerns. If you apply pesticides at higher than label rates, you could endanger the health of people in the area from the increased concentration. In addition, illegal residues may result if a pesticide is overapplied. If residues are above allowable tolerances on produce, regulators may confiscate an entire crop to protect consumers. Poorly calibrated equipment may also expose application equipment operators and fieldworkers to concentrations of pesticide for which they are not adequately protected.

TABLE 9-1

Useful conversion factors for calibration

Standard measure	Metric conversions
Length	
1 ft = 12 in	1 in = 25.4 mm = 2.54 cm
1 yd = 3 ft	1 ft = 304.8 mm = 30.48 cm
1 mi = 5,280 ft	1 yd = 914.4 mm = 91.44 cm = 0.914 m
	1 mi = 1,609 m = 1.61 km
	1 mm = 0.03937 in
	1 cm = 0.394 in = 0.0328 ft
	1 m = 39.37 in = 3.281 ft
	1 km = 3,281 ft = 0.6214 mi
Area	
1 sq in = 0.007 sq ft	1 sq in = 6.45 sq cm
1 sq ft = 144 sq in = 0.000023 sq ac	1 sq ft = 929 sq cm
1 sq yd = 1,296 sq in = 9 sq ft	1 sq yd = 8,361 sq cm = 0.8361 sq m
1 ac = 43,560 sq ft = 4,840 sq yd	1 ac = 4,047 sq m = 0.405 h
	1 sq cm = 0.155 sq in
	1 sq m = 1,550 sq in = 10.76 sq ft
	1 h = 107,639 sq ft = 2.47 ac
Volume	
1 tsp = 0.17 fl oz	1 fl oz = 29.6 ml = 0.02961
1 tbs = 3 tsp	1 pt = 473 ml = 0.4731
1 fl oz = 2 tbs = 6 tsp	1 qt = 946 ml = 0.9461
1 cup = 8 fl oz = 16 tbs	1 gal = 3785 ml = 3.7851
1 pt = 2 cups = 16 fl oz	
1 qt = 2 pt = 32 fl oz	1 ml = 0.034 fl oz
1 gal = 4 qt = 8 pt = 128 fl oz = 231 cu in	1 l = 33.8 fl oz = 2.113 pt = 1.057 qt = 0.264 gal
Weight	
1 oz = 0.0625 lb	1 oz = 28.35 g
1 lb = 16 oz	1 lb = 454 g = 0.4533 kg
1 ton = 2,000 lb	1 ton = 907 kg
1 gal of water = 8.34 lb	1 gal of water = 3.783 kg
	1 g = 0.035 oz
	1 kg = 35.27 oz = 2.205 lb

List the tools needed for calibration activities.

Environmental Concerns. Improper pesticide concentrations may cause environmental problems. Calibrating equipment to maintain application rates within label requirements helps protect beneficial insects and wildlife. It also reduces the potential for contaminating surface and groundwater and the air.

Protecting Treated Surfaces. Certain pesticides are phytotoxic and damage treated surfaces when used at higher than label rates. Manufacturers evaluate these potential problems while testing their chemicals to determine safe concentrations. Using too much pesticide also increases chances of building up excessive residues in the soil. These buildups sometimes seriously limit the types of crops that people can grow in an area.

Preventing Waste of Resources. Using the improper amount of pesticide wastes time and adds unnecessary costs to the application. Not only are pesticides expensive, but the fuel, labor, and equipment wear and tear required to make extra applications are costly, too.

Legal Aspects. Applicators who use pesticides improperly are subject to criminal and civil charges, resulting in fines, imprisonment, and lawsuits. Applicators are liable for injuries or damage caused by improper pesticide application.

Equipment Calibration Methods

Sidebar 9-1 lists the few simple tools you need to calibrate pesticide application equipment. Put these items in a small toolbox and use them only for calibration purposes (Fig. 9-1). Keep your tools clean and in good working condition; make equipment calibration a professional operation. Liquid application equipment and dust or granular application equipment require different calibration techniques.

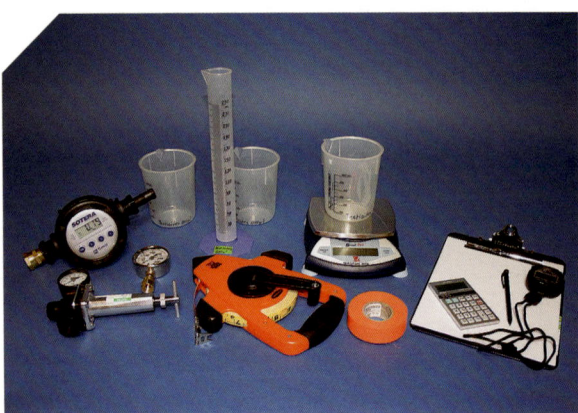

FIGURE 9-1

A few simple tools are required for calibrating a pesticide sprayer. These include a stopwatch, measuring tape, several calibrated containers, a scale, pocket calculator, pressure gauge, flowmeter, and flagging tape.

SIDEBAR 9-1

TOOLS NEEDED FOR CALIBRATION

1. **Stopwatch.** Use a stopwatch for timing travel speed and flow rates. Never rely on a wristwatch unless it has a stopwatch function.
2. **Measuring tape.** Use a 100-foot moisture- and stretch-resistant measuring tape for marking off the distance to be traveled and measuring spray swath width.
3. **Calibrated container.** Use a 1- or 2-quart container, calibrated for liquid ounces, for measuring spray nozzle output.
4. **Scale.** Use a small scale capable of measuring pounds and ounces for weighing granules collected from a granule applicator. The most accurate weight measurements come from scales that have maximum capacities from 5 to 10 pounds.
5. **Pocket calculator.** Use a pocket calculator for making calculations in the field.
6. **Pressure gauge.** Use an accurate, calibrated pressure gauge that has fittings compatible with spray nozzle fittings for checking boom pressure and for calibrating the sprayer pressure gauge.
7. **Flowmeter.** Use a flowmeter attached to a flexible hose or filling pipe for measuring the amount of water put into a tank. You can also use this device for measuring tank capacity and for determining the amount of liquid used during a calibration run. Both mechanical and electronic flowmeters are available. If these are not available, a calibrated 5-gallon pail can be used instead.
8. **Flagging tape.** Use colored plastic flagging tape for marking off measured distances when determining applicator speed.

CALIBRATING PESTICIDE APPLICATION EQUIPMENT

> **SIDEBAR 9-2**
>
> ## SERVICING SPRAY EQUIPMENT
>
> - Flush tank and pumping system with clean water to remove debris and dirt.
> - Inspect hoses for cracks and leaks and replace if necessary.
> - Clean and replace all filter screens.
> - Check nozzles for wear and replace if necessary or if in doubt. All nozzles must be clean.
> - Lubricate all bearings and appropriate moving parts.
> - Make sure pressure gauge is working properly by testing it against another gauge known to be accurate.

List the variables that must be measured to calibrate a sprayer.

Describe how to calibrate liquid sprayers, and be able to calculate speed, gallons per minute (for low- and high-pressure sprayers), and nozzle output using formulas.

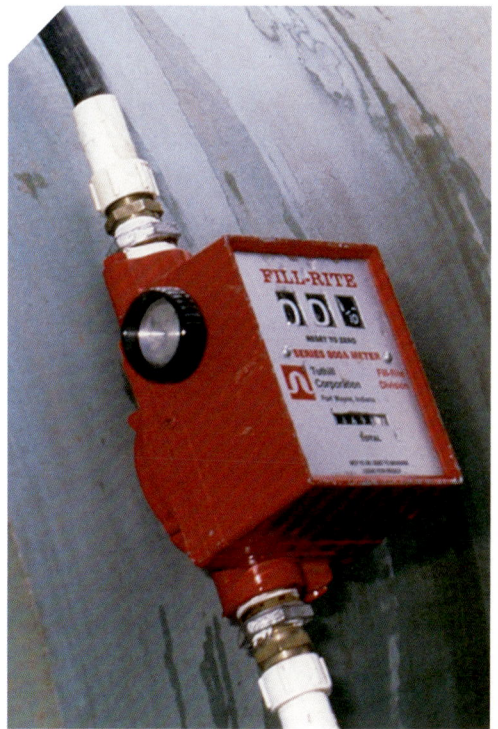

FIGURE 9-2

Flowmeters, similar to the one shown, can be used to measure the volume of spray tanks.

NOTE: Pesticide application equipment and the discharge from application equipment being calibrated may contain pesticide residue. Always wear chemical-resistant gloves and other personal protective equipment (PPE) to prevent pesticide contamination of your eyes, hair, skin, clothing, and shoes. Read Chapter 6 for information on selecting the proper PPE.

CALIBRATING LIQUID SPRAYERS

To monitor pump and nozzle wear, you must frequently calibrate liquid spraying equipment. Abrasive pesticides, such as wettable powders, increase the rate of wear. Pump wear decreases the amount and pressure of fluid output. Nozzle wear increases the volume of output. This usually lowers the output pressure and may produce a poor spray pattern. For more about how to recognize and deal with wear in various components of a sprayer, see Chapter 8; to learn which pesticide formulations are abrasive, see Chapter 3.

The goal is to determine how much area each tank of spray covers when the equipment moves at a known speed and operates at a known pressure. You need to measure these four factors:

- tank capacity
- travel speed
- flow rate
- spray swath width

Before making any calibration measurements, be sure to service the sprayer. Follow the servicing directions outlined in Sidebar 9-2.

Tank Capacity. Physically measure the capacity of the spray tank, or tanks if the equipment has more than one. Never rely on manufacturer's tank size ratings. They may be approximate or may not take into account fittings installed inside the tank. Also, the capacity of spray lines, pump, and filters influences tank volume. To accurately calibrate your equipment, you need to know exactly how much liquid the spray tank holds.

Situate the sprayer on a perfectly level surface. Be sure the tank is completely empty; then close all valves to prevent water leaks. Add measured amounts of clean water until you completely fill the tank. Use a flowmeter attached to a hose (Fig. 9-2), or a bucket or other container of known volume. A 5-gallon bucket works well for smaller sprayers. Be sure to calibrate and mark the bucket before using it to fill the tank. If you are not using a flowmeter, use smaller-volume calibrated containers to top off the tank. Record the total volume of water you put into the tank. Paint or engrave this figure onto the outside of the tank for permanent reference.

While filling the tank, calibrate the tank's sight gauge. Make marks on the tank or gauge as you put in measured volumes of water. If the unit does not have a sight gauge, mark volume increments on a dipstick. Then, always keep this dipstick with the tank. Use 1-gallon marks for tanks with a capacity of 10 gallons or less. Use increments of 5 or 10 gallons for tanks having a total capacity of 50 gallons or less. On larger tanks, use increments of 10 to 20 gallons. Once you calibrate the sight gauge or dipstick, you can measure how much liquid is in the tank when it is not entirely full. Always return tanks to a level surface when reading the sight gauge or dipstick.

Travel Speed. Always measure travel speed under actual working conditions. For instance, if you are calibrating an orchard sprayer, take the water-filled tank to the orchard. Calibrate row crop and field sprayers in the fields you plan to treat. Tractors travel faster on paved or smooth surfaces than on soft dirt or clods. Never rely on tractor speedometers for mile-per-hour measurements. Tractor wheel slippage and variation in tire size due to wear produce as much as a 30% difference in actual versus indicated speed. When calibrating a backpack or hand-held sprayer, walk on terrain similar to the area that you plan to spray.

Using a 100-foot tape, measure off any convenient distance. It can be more or less than 100 feet, but calibration accuracy increases if you use longer distances (from 200 to 300 feet). Sometimes multiples of 88 feet are chosen because 88 feet is the distance covered in 1 minute while traveling 1 mile per hour. In orchards or vineyards, a given number of tree or vine spaces of known length provides a convenient reference. Indicate the beginning and end of the measured distance with colored flagging tape.

Have someone drive (or walk, if calibrating a backpack sprayer) through the measured distance. Maintain the speed desired for an actual application. Choose a speed within a range appropriate for the application equipment. When using a tractor, note the throttle setting, gear, and rpm of the engine. The use of a positive throttle stop is helpful so you can always return the engine to the same speed. Be sure to bring the equipment up to the actual application speed before crossing

---

SIDEBAR 9-3
CALCULATING THE TRAVEL SPEED OF APPLICATION EQUIPMENT

Step 1. Convert minutes and seconds into minutes by dividing the seconds (and any fraction of a second) by 60.

EXAMPLE
Your trip took 1 min and 47.5 sec.

$$47.5 \text{ sec} \div 60 \text{ sec/min} = 0.79 \text{ min}$$

Add these amounts together:

$$1 \text{ min} + 0.79 \text{ min} = 1.79 \text{ min}$$

Step 2. Get the average run time by adding the converted minutes from each run and dividing by the number of runs.

EXAMPLE
Three runs were made.

Run 1 = 1 min, 47.5 sec = 1.79 min
Run 2 = 1 min, 39.8 sec = 1.66 min
Run 3 = 1 min, 52.0 sec = 1.87 min
Total = 5.32 min

5.32 min ÷ 3 runs = 1.77 min/run average time

Step 3. Divide the measured distance by the average time. This will tell you how many feet were traveled per minute.

EXAMPLE
The measured distance is 227 feet.

$$227 \text{ ft} \div 1.77 \text{ min} = 128.25 \text{ ft/min}$$

Step 4. If you wish to determine the speed in miles per hour, divide the feet per minute figure by 88 (the number of feet traveled in 1 minute at 1 mile per hour).

EXAMPLE

$$128.25 \text{ ft/min} \div 88 \text{ ft/min/mi/hr} = 1.46 \text{ mi/hr}$$

the first marker. Use a stopwatch to determine the time, in minutes and seconds, required to traverse the measured distance (Fig. 9-3). For best results, repeat this process two or three times and take an average. Follow the procedure in Sidebar 9-3 (p. 250) to calculate the actual speed of the equipment. You can also use a GPS unit to check the measurements you take using the flagging tape and stopwatch to ensure your accuracy.

Flow Rate. Measure the actual output of the sprayer when nozzles are new, then periodically thereafter to accommodate for nozzle wear. Manufacturers provide charts showing output of given nozzle sizes at specified sprayer pressures. However, you should check output under actual conditions of operation. Manufacturer's charts are most accurate when using new nozzles. Used nozzles may have different output rates because of wear. However, even new nozzles may have slight variations in actual output. Sprayer pressure gauges may not be accurate, which further adds error to the output estimate determined from charts.

Measure liquid sprayer output in gallons per minute (gpm). Select from one of the two methods described below, depending on the type of sprayer you are calibrating. The first method works for low-pressure sprayers, air carrier sprayers, and small hand-held units. It involves collecting a volume of water emitted out of individual nozzles over a measured time. The second method, for air carrier and high-pressure sprayers, measures output of the sprayer over a known period.

Collection method for low-pressure, air carrier, and small hand-held sprayers. Calibrate low-pressure sprayers by measuring the amount of spray emitted from nozzles using clean water only. These include low-pressure boom sprayers, backpack sprayers, and controlled droplet applicators. If the sprayer has more than one nozzle, collect water from each separately, which allows you to compare each nozzle's output and points out any malfunction or wear. You need a stopwatch and calibrated container for making measurements. Wear chemical-resistant gloves to avoid skin contact with water that might be contaminated with pesticide residues. Stand upwind from the nozzles to prevent fine mist or spray from contacting your face and clothing. Wear eye protection to prevent getting spray droplets in your eyes.

For low-pressure power sprayers used in agricultural, right-of-way, and landscape applications, fill the tank at least half full with water. Start the sprayer and bring the system up to normal operating pressure. Operate hydraulic agitators if they will operate during the application. This is important because hydraulic agitators divert some liquid from the nozzles and often lower the pressure in the system. Most power sprayers have a limited operating pressure range depending on the type of pump and type of power unit. Never attempt to operate equipment beyond its normal working range, because this may damage the pump. If you are calibrating a PTO-driven sprayer, be sure that

FIGURE 9-3

Measure a known distance when calculating the speed of travel of the application equipment. Use a stopwatch to time the travel of the sprayer through the measured distance.

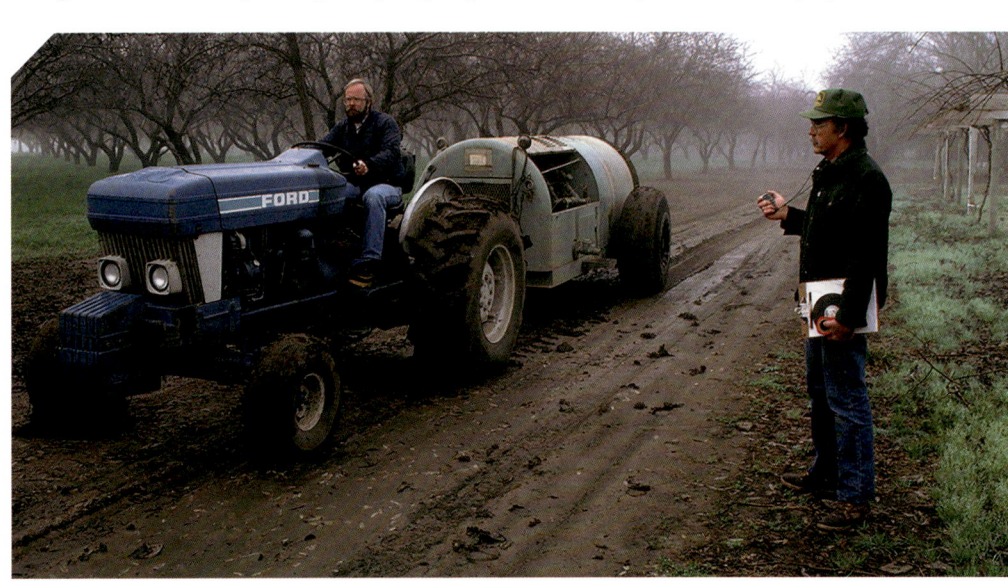

> **SIDEBAR 9-4**
>
> **SAMPLE RECORD OF NOZZLE OUTPUT**
>
> | Nozzle | Volume (fl oz) | Time (sec) |
> |---|---|---|
> | 1 | 12.5 | 23.2 |
> | 2 | 12.0 | 22.5 |
> | 3 | 15.5 | 24.8 |
> | 4 | 14.5 | 26.1 |
> | 5 | 19.0 | 27.2 |
> | 6 | 13.0 | 23.9 |

the tractor engine speed (rpm) is the same as that used in the speed calibration. If this is not the same, the pump output pressure will be different. Adjust the pressure to the requirements of the spray situation and nozzle manufacturer's recommendations. Check the pressure by attaching a calibrated pressure gauge at either end of the boom, replacing one of the nozzles. Open the valves to all nozzles and note the pressure, make adjustments as necessary, then remove the gauge.

While all nozzles are operating at the proper pressure, collect about 15 to 30 fluid ounces of liquid from each nozzle (Fig. 9-4). Use a stopwatch to determine the time in seconds required to collect each volume.

When calibrating backpack sprayers, pump the unit as you would during an actual application. Collect spray in a calibrated container for a measured time. Compressed air sprayers lose pressure during operation, so you must frequently pump them up. To calibrate, fill the tank about half full with water. This provides a sufficient volume of air to keep the pressure more uniform.

For some types of controlled droplet applicators, you can disconnect the hose and orifice from above the spinning disc or cup. After doing this, collect liquid into a calibrated container over a measured time. The liquid must flow through the orifice.

Record the volume of liquid collected from each nozzle or orifice and the time in seconds required to collect each amount. Use a format similar to the form in Sidebar 9-4. Determine the output in fluid ounces per second for each nozzle by dividing the volume by the number of

> **SIDEBAR 9-5**
>
> **CALCULATING GALLONS PER MINUTE OUTPUT FOR LOW-PRESSURE SPRAYERS**
>
> **Step 1.** Determine the gallons per minute (gpm) output of each nozzle (from Sidebar 9-4) by dividing the fluid ounces collected by the time (in seconds) and multiplying the result by 0.4688.
>
> **EXAMPLE**
>
> | Nozzle | Output (fl oz) | ÷ | Time (sec) | = | Output per sec | x | 0.4688 | = | gpm |
> |---|---|---|---|---|---|---|---|---|---|
> | 1 | 12.5 | ÷ | 23.2 | = | 0.539 | × | 0.4688 | = | 0.253 |
> | 2 | 12.0 | ÷ | 22.5 | = | 0.533 | × | 0.4688 | = | 0.250 |
> | 3 | 15.5 | ÷ | 24.8 | = | 0.625 | × | 0.4688 | = | 0.293 |
> | 4 | 14.5 | ÷ | 26.1 | = | 0.556 | × | 0.4688 | = | 0.261 |
> | 5 | 19.0 | ÷ | 27.2 | = | 0.699 | × | 0.4688 | = | 0.328 |
> | 6 | 13.0 | ÷ | 23.9 | = | 0.544 | × | 0.4688 | = | 0.255 |
> | | | | | | | | Total output | = | 1.640 |
>
> **Step 2.** Compute the percentage of variation from the rated nozzle output. Divide the actual gallons per minute output by the rated output. Subtract 1 from this number and multiply by 100.
>
> **EXAMPLE**
>
> | Nozzle | Actual gpm | ÷ | Rated gpm | = | | − | 1.00 | = | | × | 100 | = | Percent variation |
> |---|---|---|---|---|---|---|---|---|---|---|---|---|---|
> | 1 | .253 | ÷ | 0.250 | = | 1.012 | − | 1.00 | = | 0.012 | × | 100 | = | 1.2 |
> | 2 | .250 | ÷ | 0.250 | = | 1.000 | − | 1.00 | = | 0.000 | × | 100 | = | 0.0 |
> | 3 | .293 | ÷ | 0.250 | = | 1.172 | − | 1.00 | = | 0.172 | × | 100 | = | 17.2 |
> | 4 | .261 | ÷ | 0.250 | = | 1.044 | − | 1.00 | = | 0.044 | × | 100 | = | 4.4 |
> | 5 | .328 | ÷ | 0.250 | = | 1.312 | − | 1.00 | = | 0.312 | × | 100 | = | 31.2 |
> | 6 | .255 | ÷ | 0.250 | = | 1.020 | − | 1.00 | = | 0.020 | × | 100 | = | 2.0 |

seconds required to collect it. Convert ounces per second into gallons per minute by multiplying the result by the constant 0.4688. This constant represents 60 seconds per minute divided by 128 fluid ounces per gallon.

Output among nozzles will usually vary. In the example in part 1 in Sidebar 9-5 (p. 252), the output ranges from 0.250 gallon per minute to 0.328 gallons per minute. Assume that the rated capacity (as

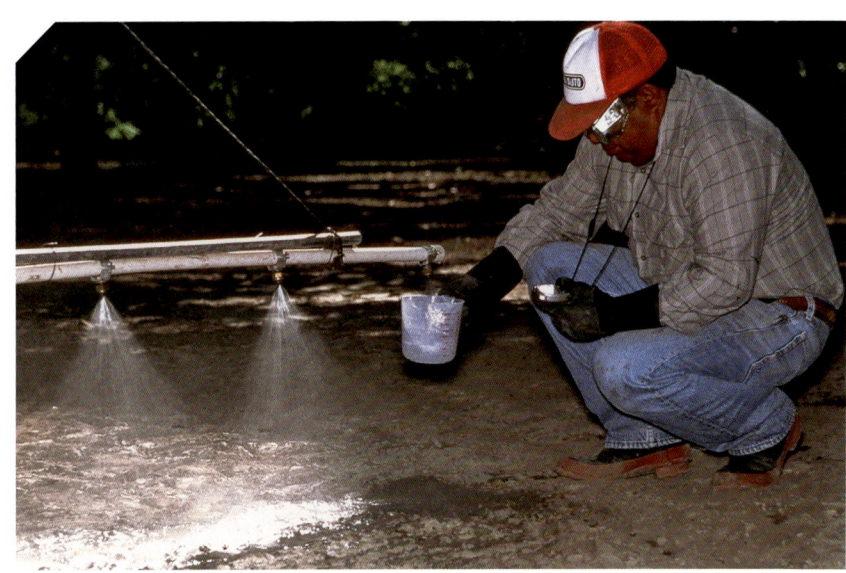

FIGURE 9-4

To determine the output from each nozzle, collect liquid over a measured period of time. Make sure the sprayer is operating at the pressure that would be used under actual field conditions. Wear rubber gloves and eye protection, because the liquid may contain traces of pesticide.

SIDEBAR 9-6

Recalculating Output after Replacing Worn Nozzles

Step 1. Replace worn nozzles (numbers 3 and 5 in this example) and re-measure the output of all nozzles on the boom. Recalculate the gallons per minute for each nozzle. Add these rates together to determine the total output of the sprayer.

EXAMPLE

Nozzle	Output (fl oz)	÷	Time (sec)	=	Output per sec	×	0.4688	=	gpm
1	12.5	÷	23.2	=	0.539	×	0.4688	=	0.253
2	12.0	÷	22.5	=	0.533	×	0.4688	=	0.250
3	13.3	÷	24.5	=	0.543	×	0.4688	=	0.255
4	14.5	÷	26.1	=	0.556	×	0.4688	=	0.261
5	15.2	÷	28.3	=	0.537	×	0.4688	=	0.252
6	13.0	÷	23.9	=	0.544	×	0.4688	=	0.255
							Total output	=	1.525

Step 2. Check to see that all nozzles are within 5% of the rated capacity of these nozzles.

EXAMPLE

Nozzle	Actual gpm	÷	Rated gpm	=		−	1.00	=	Nozzle actual flow rate	×	100	=	Percent variation
1	0.253	÷	0.250	=	1.012	−	1.00	=	0.012	×	100	=	1.2
2	0.250	÷	0.250	=	1.000	−	1.00	=	0.000	×	100	=	0.0
3	0.254	÷	0.250	=	1.016	−	1.00	=	0.016	×	100	=	1.6
4	0.261	÷	0.250	=	1.044	−	1.00	=	0.044	×	100	=	4.4
5	0.252	÷	0.250	=	1.008	−	1.00	=	0.008	×	100	=	0.8
6	0.255	÷	0.250	=	1.020	−	1.00	=	0.020	×	100	=	2.0

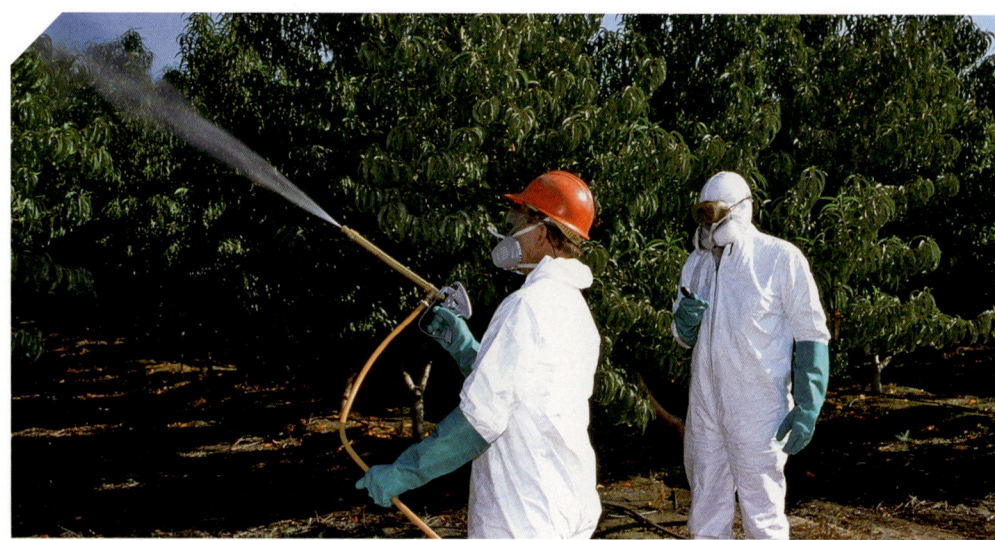

FIGURE 9-5

It is not possible to collect the sprayed liquid from some types of sprayers. To determine the amount of liquid expelled by these sprayers: (1) fill the tank to a known level; (2) run the sprayer under normal conditions for a timed period; and (3) refill the tank to its original level, measuring the amount of water used.

given by the manufacturer) for these nozzles at the recommended operating pressure is 0.250 gallon per minute. The variation among nozzles should not be greater than 5%. The output of any nozzle should not exceed the manufacturer's rated output by more than 10%. Figure the percentage of variation as shown in the example in part 2 in Sidebar 9-5 (p. 252). Divide the actual output by the rated output. Subtract 1.00 from this figure, then multiply by 100 to obtain the percentage of variation. Nozzles 3 and 5 in this example exceed these amounts and therefore must be replaced. However, whenever you replace any nozzles, recheck the flow rate of all the nozzles. Changing one nozzle may affect the pressure in the whole system. After changing nozzles, readjust the pressure regulator to maintain the desired pressure. Part 1 of Sidebar 9-6 (p. 253) shows how to recalculate the output in gallons per minute after replacing worn nozzles.

Spray check devices are calibration aids that provide a visual representation of the spray pattern. Place this portable device under a boom and collect the output from several nozzles. After collection, rotate the device from a horizontal to a vertical position. The liquid drains into a series of evenly spaced glass vials. Floats inside these vials rise to the top of the liquid. You then can see variations in liquid levels, pinpointing nozzle problems and poor nozzle height adjustment.

Measured release method for air carrier or high-pressure sprayers. Due to the air-carrying capacity and high pressures of larger sprayers, it is difficult (and often unnecessary) to collect the spray from the nozzles. Instead, you can find the output of the sprayer over time by measuring how much water the sprayer used.

Start by moving the sprayer to a level surface and fill the tank to its maximum with clean water. Fill the tank to a level that you can duplicate when refilling. A convenient technique is to fill the tank with clean water to the point where it just begins to overflow. In this situation, you must keep the hose out of the water at all times (always maintain an air gap). Use low-volume, low-pressure water, such as from a garden hose, for topping off the tank. Check for leaks around

FIGURE 9-6

A spray swath is the horizontal width being covered with spray material during a single pass. Swath width is measured differently, depending on the type of pesticide application.

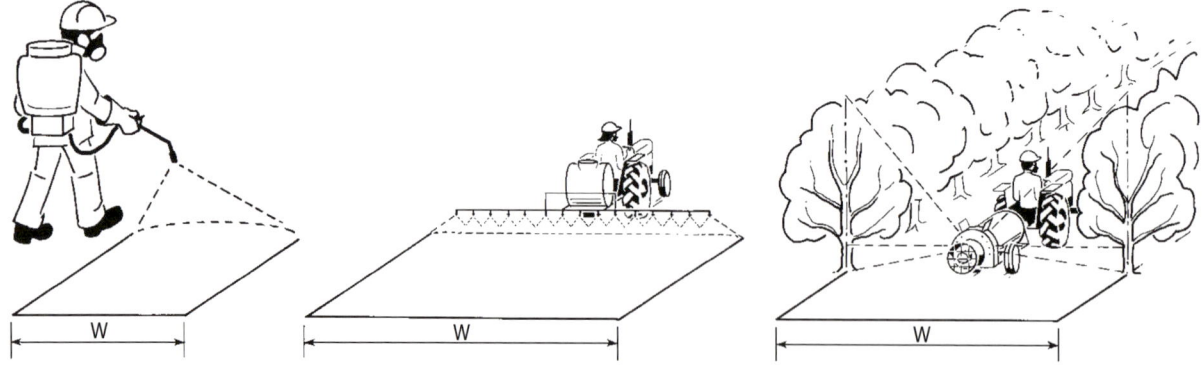

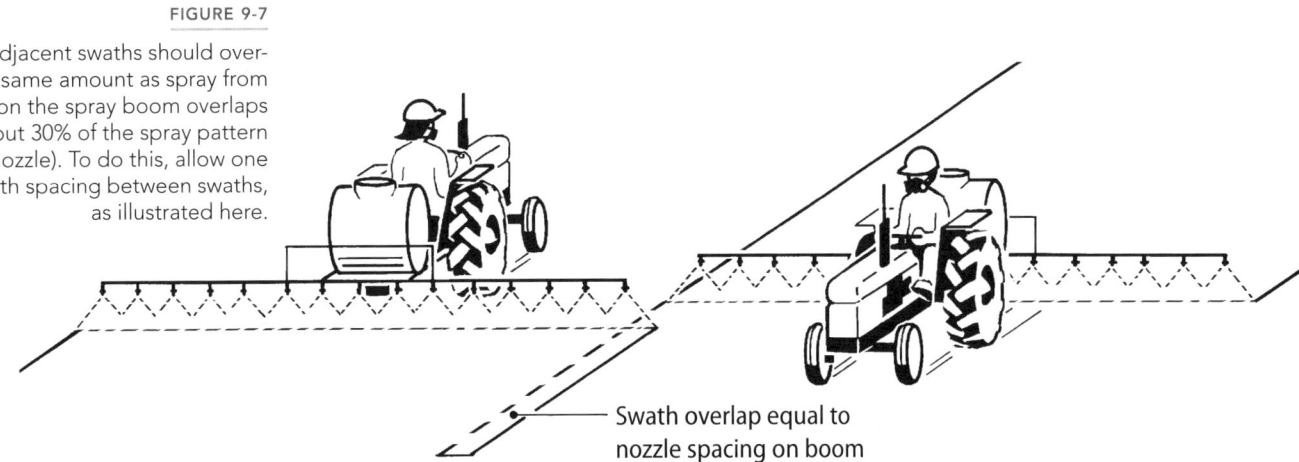

FIGURE 9-7

Spray from adjacent swaths should overlap by the same amount as spray from nozzles on the spray boom overlaps (usually about 30% of the spray pattern of one nozzle). To do this, allow one nozzle-width spacing between swaths, as illustrated here.

tank seals and in hoses. All nozzles must be clean and operating properly or the results will be inaccurate.

Stand upwind and operate the sprayer at its normal operating speed and pressure. Open the valves to all nozzles, starting a stopwatch at the same time. Continue to run the sprayer for several minutes, then close the valves to all nozzles. Record the elapsed time that the nozzles operated (Fig. 9-5).

Use a flowmeter attached to a low-pressure filling hose to refill the sprayer to its original level. (Using a site gauge or dipstick can result in inaccurate measurements.) Record the number of gallons of water used; this volume is the amount of liquid sprayed during the timed run. Repeat this process two more times to get an average of sprayer output. Determine the sprayer output in gallons per minute by using the calculations shown in Sidebar 9-7 (p. 260).

Swath Width. The final measurement needed to complete calibration is the width of the spray swath being applied by the sprayer. Figure 9-6 illustrates spray swath widths for various application situations. For multiple-nozzle boom-type sprayers, the swath is the width of the boom plus the distance between each pair of nozzles. Do not assume that all the nozzles on the boom are spaced the same distance apart. An accurate measurement of swath width must take into account the actual spacing between nozzles on the boom, so measure these distances carefully. You can also calculate swath width by multiplying the number of nozzles by the nozzle spacing, if nozzles are evenly spaced. When making a pesticide application with a boom sprayer, overlap the spray by the same amount as the overlap of the nozzles on the boom (Fig. 9-7). Adjust the boom height so that there is approximately a 30% overlap of spray from adjacent nozzles on the boom (Fig. 9-8).

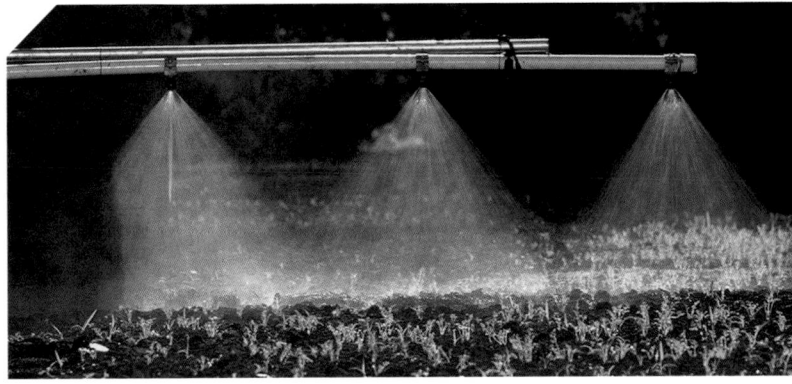

FIGURE 9-8

Under normal conditions, flat-fan nozzles on a spray boom must be spaced so there is a 30% overlap of the spray emitted by adjacent nozzles. This provides a uniform distribution of spray.

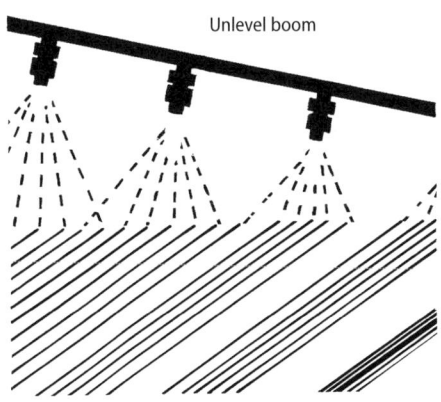

FIGURE 9-9

An unlevel spray boom will cause an uneven pesticide application.

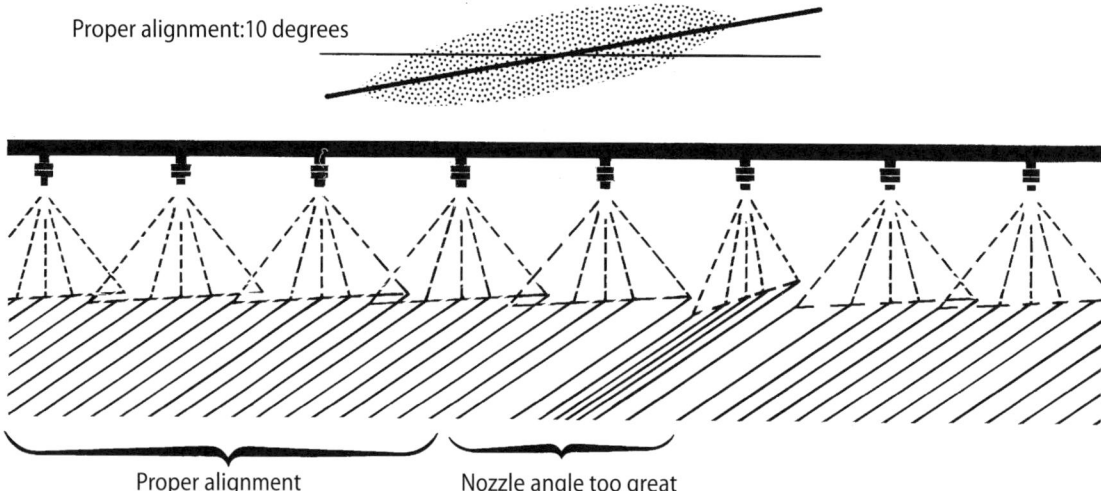

FIGURE 9-10

The spray pattern will be uneven if nozzles are not aligned properly on the spray boom. Rotate nozzles about 10 degrees from the axis of the boom to prevent droplets from adjacent nozzles from touching, but still allow for proper overlap of the spray pattern.

Position nozzles at the exact height they would be during an actual application. Check the spray boom to make sure it is level. An unleveled boom causes uneven spray distribution (Fig. 9-9, p. 255). Align fan nozzles properly to give an even spray distribution (Fig. 9-10).

When applying spray as separate bands or strips, the swath width is equal to the combined width of each band. It does not include the unsprayed spaces between bands (Fig. 9-11).

When spraying crop plants on both sides of an air blast sprayer in an orchard or vineyard, the spray swath is equal to the width of the tree or vine row (Fig. 9-12). If you spray only one side of the row, the swath is one-half the width of the tree or vine spacing (Fig. 9-13). Use a tape measure to determine tree or vine row width. Take several measurements within the orchard or vineyard to check if row spacing is uniform and consistent. Average the results if you find any variation (Fig. 9-14, p. 258).

FIGURE 9-11

Swath width from banded applications is determined by adding the widths of the individual bands.

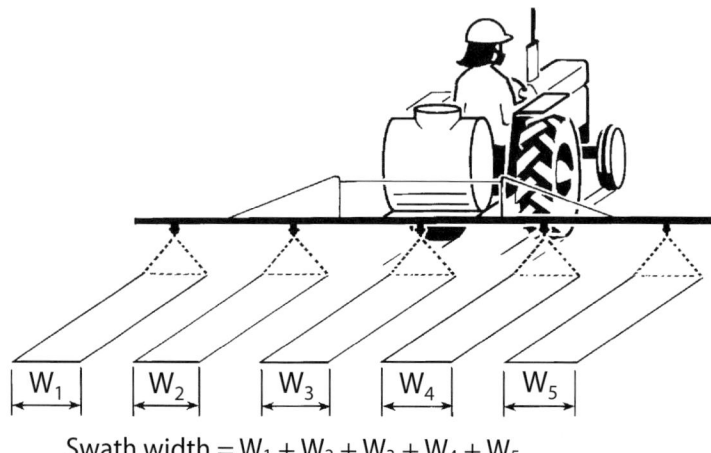

Swath width = $W_1 + W_2 + W_3 + W_4 + W_5$

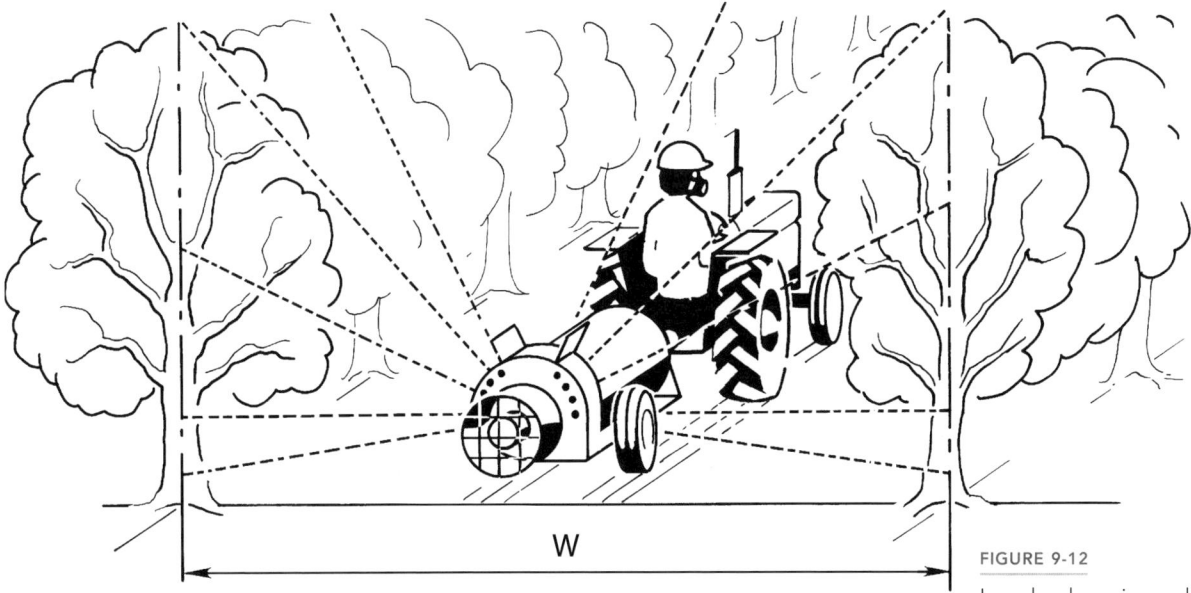

FIGURE 9-12

In orchards or vineyards, if plants on both sides of the sprayer are being sprayed simultaneously with an air blast sprayer or high-pressure boom sprayer, the swath width is the distance between plant rows.

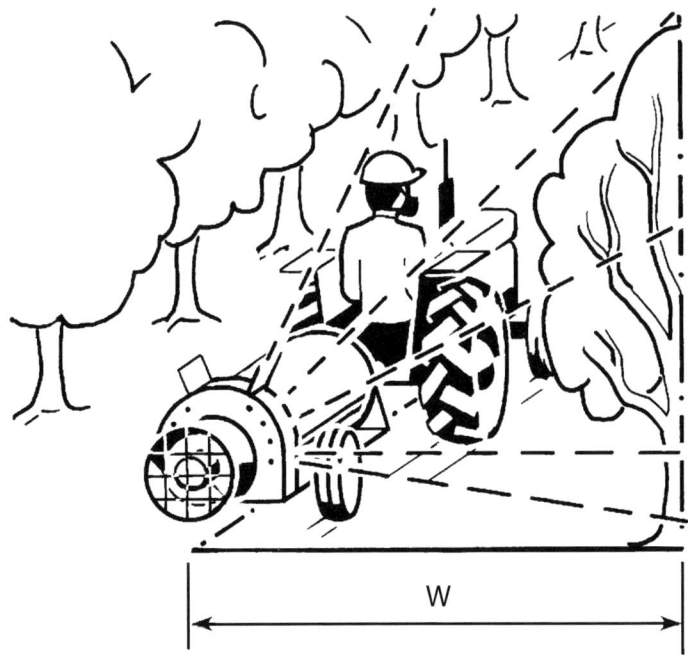

FIGURE 9-13

When spray is emitted from only one side of an orchard or vineyard air blast sprayer, the swath width of each pass is one-half the plant row spacing.

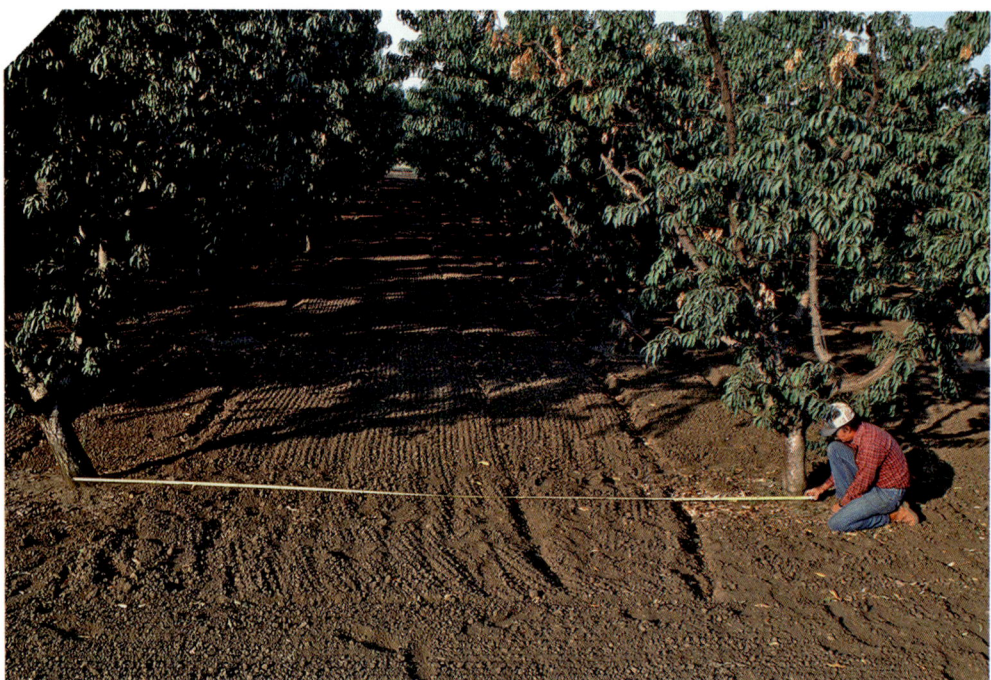

FIGURE 9-14

Swath width for pesticide sprays in orchards and vineyards should be measured from the center of one tree or vine row to the center of the adjacent row. Take several measurements in different locations to check for variation in plant spacing. If variation exists, average the measurements.

It is convenient to know the number of trees or vines per acre. This allows you to adjust an air blast sprayer to apply a given volume of water per acre. After spraying out a tank of known volume, count the number of trees or vines completely sprayed. Then, calculate the area that you sprayed. You can increase or decrease travel speed slightly to apply less or more liquid per acre. You can also change nozzle sizes.

Measure the swath width for herbicide strip sprays in orchards and vineyards to the center of the tree or vine row. Do not include overlap (Fig. 9-15). Unless you apply the herbicide to the entire orchard or vineyard floor, the actual sprayed area is less than the total planted area.

Some applications use an inverted U-shaped boom to apply pesticides to the tops and both sides of vines or plants in a row. Sometimes these booms cover a row on each side of the tractor. The swath width for this type of equipment is equal to the distance between opposing nozzles (Fig. 9-16).

You can inject pesticides into the soil by using special subsoil chisels spaced along a tractor-mounted toolbar. Assume that you are applying pesticides to the entire subsurface area in most soil injection applications. The swath width is equal to the number of chisels multiplied by the space between the chisels on the toolbar (Fig. 9-17, p. 260). When you inject pesticides as bands, the swath width is the sum of all the band widths, similar to surface band applications.

Measure the swath width of a backpack sprayer from the spray pattern produced on the ground in a test run. Keep the nozzle at the height held during an actual application. Maintain this height to prevent variation in swath width. Nozzles on these types of sprayers usually provide a uniform spray pattern. Overlap swaths only enough to ensure a uniform application pattern. Use the same method to measure swath width of controlled droplet applicators.

CALIBRATING PESTICIDE APPLICATION EQUIPMENT 259

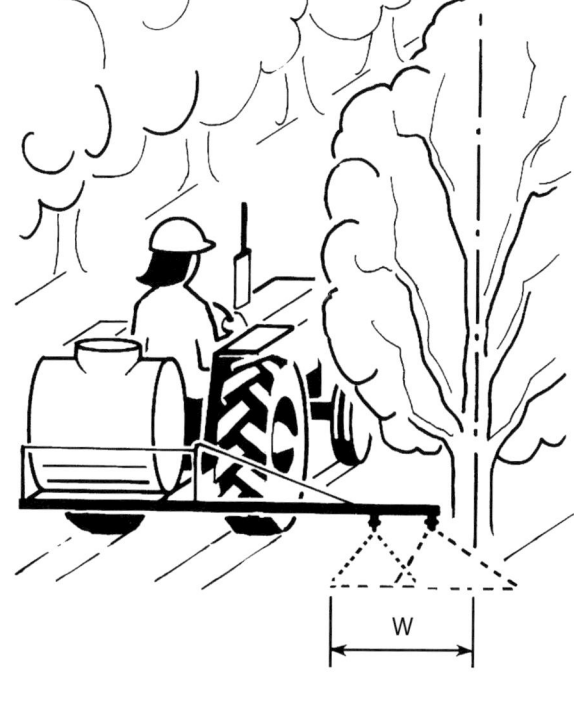

FIGURE 9-15

Swath width for herbicide strip sprays in orchards and vineyards should be measured only to the center of the tree or vine row and should not include overlap.

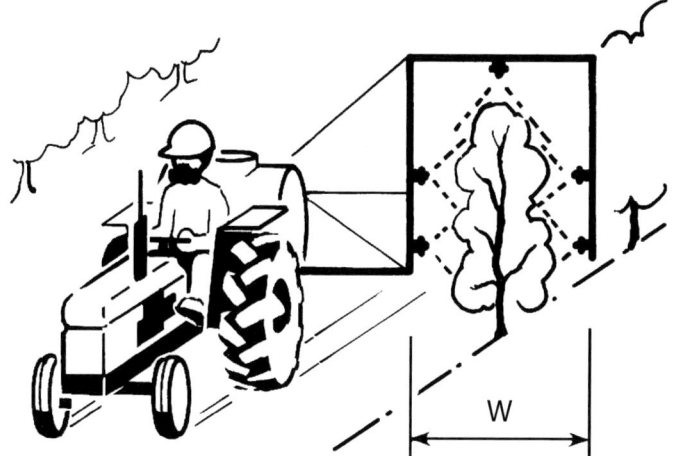

FIGURE 9-16

Spray can be applied to both sides of a plant or vine row through a specially designed, horseshoe-shaped boom arrangement. Several plant rows can be sprayed at the same time with these applicators. Spray swath width is the distance between opposing nozzles. If multiple rows are sprayed, the swath width is the sum of the distances.

Describe how to determine the correct amount of pesticide needed for a particular application.

Describe methods used to determine how much pesticide to put into the hopper or tank for a specific application rate over the total area of the application site.

Determining the Amount of Pesticide to Use. Use tank volume, travel speed, flow rate, and swath width to calculate the total area covered with each tank of material. Knowing this value allows you to determine how much pesticide to put into the tank. Choose from two calculation methods: One for pesticides applied by the acre; the other is for applications made by the square foot, such as landscape treatments or sprays in confined areas. Sidebars 9-8 (p. 261) and 9-9 (p. 263) describe the formula used to make each type of calculation.

Figure 9-18 (p. 262) is an example of how to combine calibration formulas onto a single sheet for field use. This example shows a calibration worksheet designed for orchard sprayers. You can make similar sheets for other types of pesticide sprayers.

To prevent waste of pesticide material, accurately measure the area you plan to treat. Then, mix only the amount of chemical needed.

SIDEBAR 9-7

CALCULATING OUTPUT IN GALLONS PER MINUTE FOR HIGH-PRESSURE SPRAYERS

Step 1. Record the elapsed time during each trial run and the amount of liquid sprayed.

EXAMPLE

Run	Time	Volume
1	1 min 45 sec	37.5 gal
2	1 min 30 sec	33.5 gal
3	1 min 50 sec	38.0 gal

Step 2. Convert the time from minutes and seconds to minutes by dividing the seconds by 60 and adding this decimal to the minutes.

EXAMPLE

Run	Min.	Sec.	Sec. ÷ 60	Min.
1	1	45	0.75	1.75
2	1	30	0.50	1.50
3	1	50	0.83	1.83

Step 3. Divide the collected gallons for each run by the minutes to obtain gallons per minute.

EXAMPLE

Run	Gal.	÷	Min.	=	gpm
1	37.5	÷	1.75	=	21.4
2	33.5	÷	1.50	=	22.3
3	38.0	÷	1.83	=	20.8

Step 4. Add the gallons per minute and divide this total by the number of runs (3 in this example) to get the average output in gallons per minute.

EXAMPLE

Run	Output (gpm)
1	21.4
2	22.3
3	20.8
Total	64.5
Average	21.5

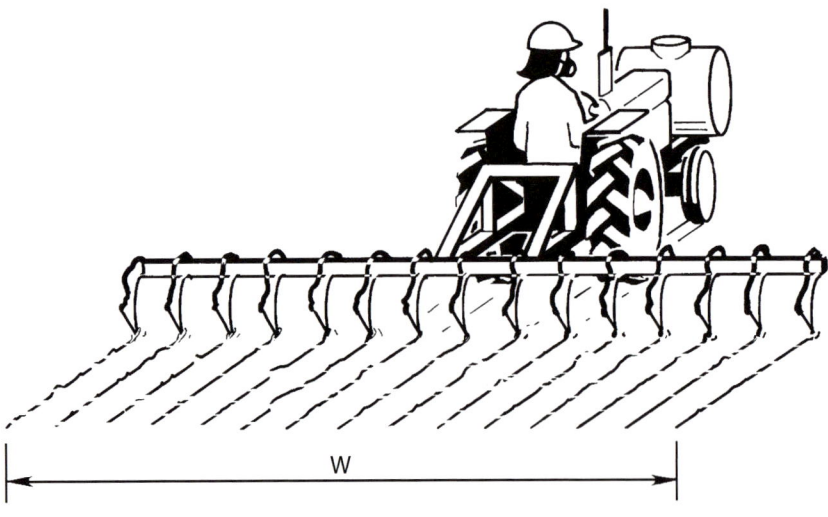

FIGURE 9-17

Subsoil chisels spaced along a tractor's toolbar are used to inject pesticides into the soil. When pesticides are injected into the soil, the swath width is usually considered to be the width of the toolbar.

> **SIDEBAR 9-8**
>
> ## Calculating How Much Pesticide to Put into the Spray Tank: Pesticides Applied on a Per-Acre Basis
>
> **Step 1.** Determine the area that can be treated in 1 minute. Multiply the spray swath width by the travel speed, then divide that number by 43,560 (the number of square feet in 1 acre). The result will be the acres treated per minute. In the example is Sidebar 9-3, the travel speed was calculated to be 128.25 feet per minute.
>
> **EXAMPLE**
>
> Assuming that the swath width is 12 feet, the calculation would be
>
> $$(12 \text{ ft} \times 128.25 \text{ ft/min}) \div 43{,}560 \text{ sq ft/ac} = 0.0353 \text{ ac/min}$$
>
> In this example, when a swath 12 feet wide is being sprayed, 0.0353 acre is covered in 1 minute.
>
> **Step 2.** Determine the gallons of liquid being applied per acre. Divide the gallons per minute figure by the acres per minute.
>
> **EXAMPLE**
>
> $$1.525 \text{ gal/min} \div 0.0353 \text{ ac/min} = 43.2 \text{ gal/ac}$$
>
> **Step 3.** Determine the number of acres that can be treated with a full tank. Divide the actual measured volume of the spray tank (or tanks) by the number of gallons per acre being applied. Assume that the tank holds 252.5 gallons when filled.
>
> **EXAMPLE**
>
> $$252.5 \text{ gal/tank} \div 43.2 \text{ gal/ac} = 5.84 \text{ ac/tank}$$
>
> **Step 4.** Determine how much pesticide to put in the tank. Multiply the number of acres per tank by the recommended rate per acre of pesticide; check the pesticide label for this information. (If the label calls for "active ingredient" see the "Active Ingredient Calculations" section in this chapter.)
>
> **EXAMPLE**
>
> | Recommended rate per acre | x | Acres per tank | = | Amount of pesticide to put in tank |
> |---|---|---|---|---|
> | 1.5 lb/ac | × | 5.84 | = | 8.76 lb |
> | 3 qt/ac | × | 5.84 | = | 17.52 qt |
> | 2 gal/ac | × | 5.84 | = | 11.68 gal |
> | 1 pt/ac | × | 5.84 | = | 5.84 pt |

Changing Sprayer Output

Describe the best way to change the output of various pesticide application equipment and the consequences of each change.

Once you calibrate a sprayer, you have determined its output rate for a specific speed. There may be times when you need to change this output rate. These include

- accommodating variations in foliage
- different plant spacing
- special requirements of the treatment area
- the need to travel at a faster or slower speed
- compensating for nozzle or pump wear

You can make several adjustments, either alone or in combination, to effectively increase or decrease sprayer output within a limited range.

Changing Speed. The simplest way to adjust the volume of spray being applied is to change the travel speed of the sprayer. A slower speed results in more liquid being applied, while a faster speed reduces the application rate. You may need these adjustments when swath width changes slightly. This would be the case in orchards or vineyards where plant spacing differs from block to block (Fig. 9-19, p. 264). Changing the travel speed eliminates the need for altering the concentration of chemical in the spray tank. However, there are limits to the amount of speed change you

ORCHARD SPRAYER CALIBRATION WORKSHEET

Grower: D. BROWN   Date: 1-29-2016   Sprayer Type: AIR BLAST

CHECK:
- ☑ 1. Filter screens and strainers clean?
- ☑ 2. Tank clean and free of scale and sediment?
- ☑ 3. Pressure gauge operating?
- ☑ 4. Nozzles working properly?

Sprayer operating pressure: 100 psi

I-A. GALLONS/HOUR (Method 1—using nozzle chart from manufacturer's catalog)

Nozzle Size	Number (N)		Rated Output (gallons/minute)		Minutes per Hour		Gallons per Hour
D2-25	8	×	0.25	×	60	=	120
D4-25	8	×	0.45	×	60	=	216
		×		×	60	=	
				TOTAL GALLONS PER HOUR		=	336

I-B. GALLONS/HOUR (Method 2—measurement)
1. Fill sprayer to verifiable level.
2. Run sprayer for a measured period of time (T), spraying under the same conditions as in the orchard.   T = 3.53
3. Refill sprayer, measuring the amount of water used (GAL) in gallons.   GAL = 20.4
4. Calculate: gallons/hour = (GAL × 60)/T   TOTAL GALLONS/HOUR = 346.7

II. MILES/HOUR
1. Establish distance (D) in feet.   D = 253
2. Measure elapsed time for sprayer to travel the distance. Make 3 runs and average results.
   a. First run time = 1.05 minutes.
   b. Second run time = 1.15 minutes.
   c. Third run time = 1.13 minutes.
3. Average of three runs (T) = 1.11 minutes.
4. Calculate miles per hour:
   MPH = (D/T)/88   MPH = 2.59

III. ACRES/HOUR
1. Measure width of tree row (W) in feet.   W = 22
2. Calculate miles per acre:
   miles/acre = (43,560/W)/5,280   MILES/ACRE = 0.375
3. Calculate acres per hour:
   acres/hour = MPH/(miles/acre)   ACRES/HOUR = 6.91

IV. GALLONS/ACRE
   (gallons/hour)/(acres/hour) = gallons/acre   GALLONS/ACRE = 50.17

V. ACRES/TANK
   Tank size = 500 gallons/tank
   (gallons/tank)/(gallons/acre) = acres/tank   ACRES/TANK = 9.97

VI. AMOUNT OF PESTICIDE/TANK
   Recommended amount of pesticide/acre = 2.5 lb.
   (pesticide/acre) × (acres/tank) = pesticide/tank   PESTICIDE/TANK = 24.9 lb.

VII. CALIBRATION CHECK
1. Tree spacing (S) = 22 × 22 feet   S = 484
2. Trees per acre (T) = 43,560/S   T = 90
3. Count the actual number of trees sprayed (N) with one tank: N = 918
4. Actual acres sprayed = N/T   ACTUAL ACRES = 10.2
5. Calculated acres per tank (from "V" above)   CALCULATED ACRES/TANK = 9.97
6. Percent accuracy = calculated acres/actual acres × 100   ACCURACY = 97.7%

Active Ingredient: Chlorothalonil
(tetrachloroispthalonitrile)   40.4%
Inert Ingredients: 59.6%
Total   100.0%
Keep Out of Reach of Children
WARNING – AVISO
Si usted no entiende la etiqueta, busque a alguien
(If you do not understand the label, find someone to explain it to you in detail.) See side panel for additional precautionary statements.

FIGURE 9-18

An orchard sprayer calibration worksheet can be helpful in recording and computing the figures necessary for calibration. Similar worksheets can be developed for other types of sprayers. In this example, notice the difference between the rated output of the nozzles and the actual output. Nozzles are worn.

SIDEBAR 9-9

CALCULATING HOW MUCH PESTICIDE TO PUT INTO THE SPRAY TANK: PESTICIDES APPLIED BY THE SQUARE FOOT

Step 1. Determine how many square feet can be treated in 1 minute. Multiply the speed as determined by the procedures in Sidebar 9-3 by the swath width. In this example, assume a single-nozzle hand-operated sprayer is being used to apply a swath width of 2.5 feet at a speed of 128.25 feet per minute.

EXAMPLE

$$128.25 \text{ ft/min} \times 2.5 \text{ ft} = 320.63 \text{ sq ft/min}$$

Step 2. Determine the volume of spray, in gallons, that will be applied to 1 square foot. Divide the gallon per minute output from Sidebar 9-5 of the sprayer by the number of square feet per minute. For this example, assume that the backpack unit sprays 0.05 gallon per minute.

EXAMPLE

$$0.05 \text{ gal/min} \div 320.63 \text{ sq ft/min} = 0.000156 \text{ gal/sq ft}$$

Step 3. Find out how many square feet can be sprayed with one tank. Divide the number of gallons per square foot into the measured tank capacity. For this example, assume that the tank holds 3 gallons.

EXAMPLE

$$3 \text{ gal/tank} \div 0.000156 \text{ gal/sq ft} = 19{,}230 \text{ sq ft/tank}$$

Step 4. Determine how much pesticide to put in the tank. The pesticide label will recommend the amount of pesticide to apply, normally, in the volume per square foot (or per 100 or 1,000 square feet) or per acre. If the label calls for "active ingredient," see "Active Ingredient Calculations" in this chapter.)

EXAMPLE A
If the label recommends the dosage rate per 1, 100, or 1,000 square feet, multiply that rate by the square feet per tank as determined in step 3:

Label recommendation	x	Square feet per tank	=	Amount of pesticide to put in tank
3 fl oz per 1,000 sq ft	×	19,230	=	57.69 fl oz
¾* fl oz per 1,000 sq ft	×	19,230	=	14.42 fl oz
1 oz per 100 sq ft	×	19,230	=	192.3 oz

Note: The fraction ¾ is converted to its decimal equivalent, 0.75, to complete this calculation.

EXAMPLE B
If the pesticide label recommends the dosage rate in units of pesticide per acre, convert square feet per tank (from step 3) to acres per tank by dividing it by 43,560 (the number of square feet in 1 acre):

$$19{,}230 \text{ sq ft/tank} \div 43{,}560 \text{ sq ft/ac} = 0.441 \text{ ac/tank}$$

Then, multiply the label rate per acre by the number of acres per tank:

Label recommendation	x	Acres per tank	=	Amount of pesticide to put in tank
1.5 lb/ac	×	0.441	=	0.662 lb (10.6 oz)
3 qt/ac	×	0.441	=	1.323 qt (42.2 fl oz)
2 gal/ac	×	0.441	=	0.882 gal (7.1 pt)
1 pt/ac	×	0.441	=	0.441 pt (7.1 fl oz)

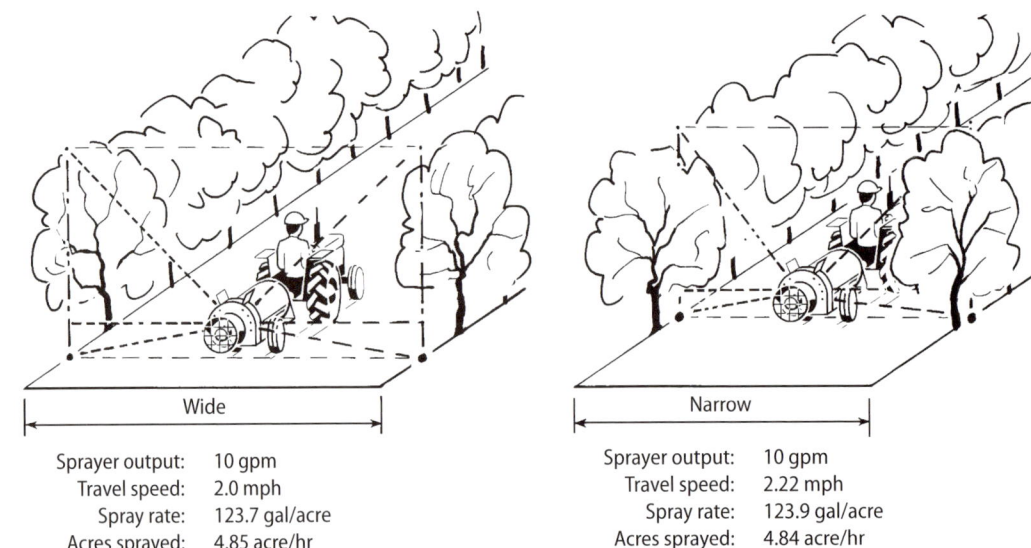

FIGURE 9-19
Changes in row spacing in an orchard or vineyard affect the amount of spray being applied per acre. Increasing or decreasing ground speed can accommodate for the difference in spacing so the correct amount of pesticide per acre will be applied. Variations in the size of trees or vines may also influence the rate of application.

Sprayer must travel faster to keep spray application rate the same.

can make. Operating application equipment too quickly is a common error and results in poor coverage. Operating it too slowly results in runoff, waste, and an increase in application time and cost. To determine how much to increase or decrease your speed, put in the new swath width and rework the calculations shown in Sidebar 9-8 (p. 261) or Sidebar 9-9 (p. 263).

Changing Nozzle Size. The most effective way to change the output volume of a sprayer is to install nozzles of a different size. Larger nozzles increase volume, while smaller ones reduce volume. Changing nozzles usually alters the pressure of the system and requires an adjustment of the pressure regulator. Adjust the output volume of disc-core nozzles by changing either the disc or the core. Sometimes you need to replace both. Be aware that changes in either the core or disc also change the droplet size and spray pattern. Use tables included in nozzle manufacturers' catalogs as a guide for estimating the output of different combinations. Whenever you change any nozzles, recalibrate the sprayer and refigure its new total output.

Changing Output Pressure. As nozzles begin to wear, the spray volume increases. When a pump begins to wear, it becomes less efficient and the nozzle output drops off. Adjusting the pressure regulator to increase or decrease output pressure changes the spray volume slightly: increasing pressure increases the output, while decreasing pressure lowers it. However, to double the output volume you must increase the pressure by a factor of four. This is usually beyond the capabilities of a spraying system, as the working pressure range of the sprayer pump limits this adjustment. Whenever pressure in the system changes, measure the nozzle output again (see Sidebar 9-5, p. 252). Then, rework the calibration calculations. Increasing pressure breaks the spray up into finer droplets, increasing the likelihood of spray drift. Lowering pressure too much reduces the effectiveness of nozzles by reducing their ability to form appropriately sized droplets.

CALIBRATING DRY APPLICATORS

The methods for calibrating dry applicators are similar in many ways to those used for liquids. Granules vary in size and shape from one pesticide to the next, influencing their flow rate from the applicator hopper. You should calibrate granule applicators for each type of granular pesticide you apply. Also, recalibrate this equipment each time weather or field conditions change, especially if humidity increases.

Describe how to calibrate dry applicators.

Before starting to calibrate a dry applicator, be sure that it is clean and all parts are working properly. Most equipment requires periodic lubrication. Calibrating granule applicators involves using actual pesticides, so wear the label-prescribed PPE. Some formulations are dusty and may require respiratory protection. Always wear chemical-resistant gloves to prevent contact with residues on the equipment. You must measure three variables when calibrating a dry applicator:
- travel speed
- output rate
- swath width

Travel Speed. Determine travel speed in feet per minute in the same manner as you would for liquid applicators. Follow the instructions given in Sidebar 9-3. Fill up the applicator hoppers so you can measure speed under actual operating conditions.

Output Rate. To determine the output rate, fill the hopper or hoppers with the granular pesticide. Most granule applicator hoppers have ports with adjustable openings for granules to pass through. Refer to the manufacturer's instructions to determine the approximate opening for the rate and speed you need. Once you set the approximate opening, use one of the following three methods to determine the actual output rate.

1. *Measure the quantity of granules applied to a known area.* The easiest way to calibrate a granule applicator is to collect and weigh the granules applied to a known area. Use this method when working with broadcast applicators. Spread out a plastic tarp of known size on the ground. Then operate the broadcast applicator at a known speed across the tarp (Fig. 9-20). Place the granules collected by the tarp into a container and weigh them. Use the calculations shown in the example in Sidebar 9-10 (p. 266) to figure the amount of granular pesticide applied per acre or other unit of area.

2. *Collect a measured amount of granules over a known period of time.* Collecting and weighing measured quantities of granules is similar to calibrating a liquid boom sprayer with multiple nozzles. Use this method for granule applicators with multiple ports. While operating the applicator at a normal speed, collect granules from one port at a time. Record the time required to collect each sample. Weigh samples separately, then use the calculations shown in Sidebar 9-11 (p. 267) to find the output rate.

3. *Refill the hopper after a measured period of time.* Use this method with hand-operated equipment or when applying small quantities. It also works best when you have several applicators on a boom. Fill the hopper or hoppers to a known level and operate the equipment for a measured time. When finished, weigh the quantity of granules required to refill the hoppers to their original levels. Use the calculations shown in the example in Sidebar 9-12 (p. 268) to compute the output rate. Settling of granules in the hoppers may cause this method to be less accurate than the first two methods listed above.

FIGURE 9-20

To determine the area of granules being applied, measure the swath width across a plastic tarp and multiply this by the length of the tarp.

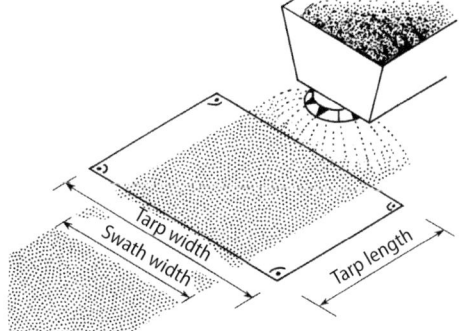

Area measurement: swath width × tarp length

Swath Width. To measure the swath width, operate the equipment under actual field conditions. Whenever possible, place cans, trays, or other containers at even intervals across the application swath. Use these to collect granules. Weigh the granules collected in each container separately to determine the distribution pattern. You can operate some spreaders over a strip of black cloth or plastic. This gives you a rapid visual assessment of granule distribution and swath width. Applicators that apply bands or inject granules into the soil do not have devices to disperse granules from side to side. Determine swath width by adding the widths of individual bands.

Application Rate. Use the example in Sidebar 9-13 (p. 268) to calculate the actual rate of granules being applied per acre or other unit of area. If your calculations do not correspond to the labeled rate, adjust the equipment and repeat the calibration procedure. Motorized and hand-operated applicators apply granules at a fixed output, independent of ground speed. When ground speed increases, you apply fewer granules per unit of area. When ground speed decreases, you apply more material. With this type of equipment you can adjust the application rate by adjusting the size of the port opening and by changing the speed of travel.

The output of ground wheel–driven granule applicators varies according to the ground speed. If ground speed increases, the applicator runs faster and the output rate is greater. When the ground speed slows down, output decreases because the applicator runs slower. The result of

---

SIDEBAR 9-10

CALCULATING GRANULE OUTPUT RATE BY MEASURING THE QUANTITY APPLIED TO A KNOWN AREA

Step 1. Spread a large plastic tarp on the ground. Make sure the tarp is wide enough to contain all the granules that will be distributed by the applicator and is at least 10 feet long. This example uses a tarp 15 feet wide and 10 feet long.

Step 2. Fill the hopper or hoppers of the applicator, adjust the output ports to the correct opening according to the label, and move the applicator across the entire length of the tarp at an even pace while broadcasting granules. Note the travel speed.

Step 3. To determine the swath area, measure the swath width of the granules on the tarp and multiply it by the length of the tarp (the distance traveled). In this example, the swath width is 12 feet.

EXAMPLE

$$\text{Swath area} = 10 \times 12 = 120 \text{ sq ft}$$

Step 4. Transfer the granules on the tarp to a container and weigh them. In this example, the granules on the tarp weighed 4 ounces.

Convert the output in the swath area to a per-acre application rate by converting the weight of the granules to pounds and multiplying by 43,560 (the number of square feet in 1 acre) and dividing by the swath area.

EXAMPLE

$$4 \text{ oz} \div 16 \text{ oz (1 lb)} = 0.25 \text{ lb}$$
$$0.25 \text{ lb} \times 43,560 \text{ sq ft} \div 120 \text{ sq ft} = 90.75 \text{ lb/ac}$$

In this example, the applicator is broadcasting 90.75 pounds of granules per acre. The label of this product calls for an application rate of 80 pounds per acre. To lower the application rate to the listed rate, close the port some or increase the travel speed. Once an adjustment has been made, repeat the calibration procedure to ensure your applicator is calibrated to apply the exact rate required by the label.

SIDEBAR 9-11

CALCULATING GRANULE OUTPUT RATE BY COLLECTING A MEASURED AMOUNT OVER A KNOWN PERIOD OF TIME

Step 1. Adjust the hopper opening according to the manufacturer's instructions suggested for your required application rate. If no information is available, begin with an intermediate setting.

Step 2. Operate the equipment at the speed of an actual application. Collect granules in a clean container, such as a pan or bag, before they drop to the ground. Use a stopwatch to determine the time required to collect each volume. If granules are dispersed through more than one opening, collect and time the output from each. Because some units drop granules onto a spinning disc for dispersal, it may be necessary to disable the disc by disconnecting the drive chain or belt to prevent granule loss during collection. For smaller units, collect the discharge in a bag placed over the outlet. Be sure granules are moved away from the port quickly enough to prevent clogging.

Step 3. Weigh the output from each port separately to detect any variability; if necessary, adjust ports to equalize flow rates. Collections should be weighed in ounces.

Step 4. Determine the output in pounds per hour. Divide each weight by the collection time and multiply by 0.0625 (the number obtained by dividing 1 minute by 16 ounces per pound; this number will convert ounces per minute into pounds per minute).

EXAMPLE

The following is an example of an output collected from a granule applicator with six ports, although the same calculations would apply if only one port were used. Hopper openings were adjusted following the manufacturer's instructions for an application of 200 pounds per acre:

Port	Output (oz)	Time (min)
1	29.5	0.25
2	33.0	0.28
3	31.5	0.26
4	29.0	0.25
5	33.0	0.27
6	30.0	0.26

Port	Output (oz)	÷	Time (min)	=	Output (oz/min)	×	0.0625	=	Output (lb/min)
1	29.5	÷	0.25	=	118.0	×	0.0625	=	7.375
2	33.0	÷	0.28	=	117.9	×	0.0625	=	7.369
3	31.5	÷	0.26	=	121.2	×	0.0625	=	7.575
4	29.0	÷	0.25	=	116.0	×	0.0625	=	7.250
5	33.0	÷	0.27	=	122.2	×	0.0625	=	7.638
6	30.0	÷	0.26	=	115.4	×	0.0625	=	7.213
							Total output per hour		44.420

Step 5. Determine the total output in pounds per minute by adding the individual outputs of each port. In this example the total output is 44.42 pounds per minute.

Step 6. Use the technique shown in Sidebar 9-13 to calculate the rate per acre or other unit of area.

SIDEBAR 9-12

CALCULATING THE RATE OF OUTPUT BY REFILLING THE HOPPER AFTER A MEASURED PERIOD OF TIME

Step 1. Fill the hopper or hoppers to a known level with granules.

Step 2. Operate the equipment for a measured period of time at a known speed.

Step 3. Weigh the amount of granules required to refill the hopper or hoppers to their original level. If multiple hoppers are being used, be sure each is applying approximately the same amount of granules. If a significant variation exists, adjust the ports and repeat steps 1 through 3.

EXAMPLE

In this example, six applicators are used together on a boom. They have been adjusted so that they all apply approximately the same amount of granules.

Hopper	Operating time (min)	Weight of granules (lb)
1	2.5	6.2
2	2.5	6.1
3	2.5	6.1
4	2.5	6.3
5	2.5	6.1
6	2.5	5.9
Total		36.7

Step 4. Convert the output to pounds per minute by dividing the total weight from all hoppers by the time they were operated.

EXAMPLE

36.7 lb ÷ 2.5 min = 14.68 lb/min

Step 5. Use the technique shown in Sidebar 9-13 to calculate the rate per acre or other unit of area.

SIDEBAR 9-13

CALCULATING APPLICATION RATE PER ACRE OR OTHER UNIT OF AREA

Step 1. Determine the acres per minute being treated by dividing the swath width by 43,560 (the number of square feet in an acre) and multiplying the result by the speed of travel. In this example, the swath width is 30 feet and the application speed is 352 feet per minute (4 miles per hour).

EXAMPLE

(30 ft ÷ 43,560 sq ft/ac) × 352 ft/min = 0.242 ac/min

Step 2. Determine the pounds of formulated pesticide being applied per acre by dividing the output rate of the granule applicator (as computed from the calculations in Sidebars 9-10, 9-11, or 9-12) by the acres per minute calculated in step 1. This example uses 44.42 pounds per minute as the output rate.

EXAMPLE

44.42 lb/min ÷ 0.242 ac/min = 183.6 lb/ac

this automatic change in output is that the equipment applies nearly the same amount of material per acre or other unit of area no matter what speed it travels. The equipment has minimum and maximum operating speeds determined by the manufacturer, however. You change the application rate by increasing or decreasing the size of the port openings. In some units, you also change drive gears or sprockets to change the speed of the metering mechanism.

CALIBRATING CHEMIGATION SYSTEMS

Because chemigation systems have many elements, you must check the system thoroughly every time it is used, even before starting your calibration. Check to confirm that the irrigation system contains all of the equipment specified on the pesticide label and/or required by DPR and that the equipment is working properly. One way of testing the functionality of the safety equipment is to start the irrigation system and bring it up to pressure. With the chemical feed tank isolated from the injection system so that no pesticide will be released, start the injection pump and confirm that the injection system interlocked solenoid valve is energized. Manually turn off the irrigation water pump. The following events should occur if the interlock systems and backflow prevention systems are working properly:

- The irrigation water pump will stop.
- The chemical injection pump will stop.
- The chemical injection solenoid valve will close (de-energize).
- The irrigation system check valve(s) will close.
- Air will be drawn into the irrigation system vacuum relief valve.
- A small amount of water will be discharged through the low-pressure drain adjacent to the irrigation system check valve(s).

If any of the irrigation equipment specified on the label is not present or is not functioning properly, it would be a violation of federal and state law to proceed with the chemical application.

Once you have confirmed that the irrigation system is functioning properly, you can proceed with calibration (Sidebar 9-14, p. 270). With the sprinkler system fully pressurized, connect the chemical injection tank to the injection system and start the injection pump. The operator should record a log of the calibration, including the time of day, the system pressure, wind speed and direction, ambient temperature, and any comments regarding observations that may be pertinent, such as odors or passers-by approaching the treated area. The log should be updated frequently during the calibration. If for some reason you must terminate the calibration (or application), continue operating the irrigation system after the chemical injection has stopped to flush the chemical out of the lines.

Calculation for Active Ingredient, Percentage Solutions, and Parts per Million Dilutions

Not all pesticide recommendations call for dry- or liquid-formulated amounts of pesticide per unit of area. Research work sometimes requires a pesticide application rate in pounds of active ingredient (a.i.) per unit of area. Some labels require that pesticides be mixed as a percentage solution or be diluted to parts per million (ppm). Before adding pesticide to the spray tank, read and understand the dilution instructions on the label.

Active Ingredient Calculations

Pesticides are seldom available in their pure state. Manufacturers formulate them into a pest control product by combining them with adjuvants and other ingredients such as carriers and solvents. Therefore, only a portion of any formulated product, whether dry or liquid, is pure pesticide. This portion is the a.i. Some pesticide use guidelines, including those published by the University of California, call for a.i. if there are several formulations available. Because different manufacturers sell different formulations, using a.i. calculations allows you to apply the same amount of actual pesticide to a unit of area no matter what formulation you use.

Active Ingredient: Chlorothalonil
(tetrachloroisophthalonitrile) 40.4%
Other Ingredients: 59.6%
Total: 100.0%

Keep Out of Reach of Children

WARNING—AVISO

Si usted no entiende la etiqueta, busque a alguien para que se la explique a usted en detalle.
(If you do not understand the label, find someone to explain it to you in detail.)
See side panel for additional precautionary statements

FIGURE 9-21

To determine the percentage of active ingredient in a pesticide formulation, check the pesticide label. Liquid formulations list active ingredient as the number of pounds per gallon of formulation. Dry formulations list active ingredient as the total percentage of the weight.

SIDEBAR 9-14

Chemigation Calibration for Low-Volume Sprinklers (Micro-Sprinklers) and Drip (Trickle) Irrigation Systems

Calculation of the amount of pesticide to inject into an irrigation system is based on the wetted area around the emitters, not on the number of acres in the field. To determine the correct amount of pesticide to inject, use the following process.

Step 1. Find the treated area per each emitter (A).

   A = 3.14 × (radius × radius)

EXAMPLE

If the average distance from an emitter to the edge of the wetted area (the radius) measured at the soil surface is 13 inches, then

   A = 3.14 × (13 in × 13 in)
   A = 3.14 × 169 sq in
   A = 530.7 sq in

Step 2. Find the area in square feet that is wetted in each acre (B). 144 is the number of square inches per square foot.

   B = (A × emitters per acre) ÷ 144

EXAMPLE

If there are 300 emitters per acre, then

   B = (530.7 sq in × 300) ÷ 144
   B = 1,105.6 sq ft

Step 3. Find the total area in square feet that is wetted by your system (C).

   C = B × (number of acres covered by system)

EXAMPLE

If the system covers 20 acres, then

   C = 1,105.6 sq ft × 20
   C = 22,112 sq ft

Step 4. Find the amount of pesticide to inject (S). The recommended rate per treated acre of pesticide = R.

   S = (C × R) ÷ 43,560

EXAMPLE

If the desired application rate per treated acre is 1 quart of pesticide, then

   S = (22,112 × 1.0) ÷ 43,560
   S = 0.50 quart of pesticide.

Source: Adapted from Kranz et al. 2008.

SIDEBAR 9-15

CALCULATING LIQUID FORMULATIONS

Assume that a sprayer has been calibrated and found to spray 7.5 acres per tank. You have a recommendation to apply 1.5 pounds of a.i. of chlorothalonil per acre to control rust on snap beans and have been supplied with a liquid formulation containing 4.17 pounds a.i. per gallon. How much chlorothalonil should you put in the tank?

Step 1. Determine the number of gallons of liquid needed per acre by dividing 1 gallon by the pounds of a.i. per gallon and multiplying that by the pounds a.i. per acre.

EXAMPLE

$$(1 \text{ gal} \div 4.17 \text{ lb/gal a.i.}) \times 1.5 \text{ lb a.i./ac} = 0.360 \text{ gal/ac}$$

Step 2. Multiply the known acre capacity of the tank by the gallons per acre.

EXAMPLE

$$7.5 \text{ ac/tank} \times 0.360 \text{ gal/ac} = 2.7 \text{ gal/tank}$$

This is the number of gallons of formulated chlorothalonil that should be put into the tank for spraying 7.5 acres of crop.

SIDEBAR 9-16

CALCULATING POWDER FORMULATIONS

The calibrated sprayer you are using covers 7.5 acres per tank, and you have a recommendation to apply 1.5 pounds a.i. of chlorothalonil per acre for control of rust on snap beans. You are provided with a wettable powder formulation that, according to the label, contains 75% chlorothalonil. How much chlorothalonil should you put into the tank?

Step 1. Convert the percentage of a.i. to a decimal by dividing by 100 (or simply move the decimal point two places to the left).

EXAMPLE

$$75\% = 0.75 \text{ lb a.i./lb formulation}$$

Step 2. Divide the recommended amount of a.i. by the amount of a.i. in the formulation.

EXAMPLE

$$1.5 \text{ lb a.i./ac} \div 0.75 \text{ lb a.i./lb formulation} =$$
$$2 \text{ lb formulation/ac}$$

Step 3. Multiply the pounds of formulation per acre by the number of acres per tank to find out how much material to put into the tank.

EXAMPLE

$$2 \text{ lb formulation/ac} \times 7.5 \text{ ac/tank} = 15 \text{ lb/tank}$$

Describe what you need to know before you can dilute a pesticide correctly.

Be able to calculate the active ingredient concentration of pesticides using formulas.

Labels of pesticides give the percentage by weight of a.i. (Fig. 9-21, p 270). The labels of liquid pesticides also tell how many pounds of a.i. are in 1 gallon of formulation. Use the calculations in Sidebar 9-15 (p 271) to make a.i. calculations with liquid formulations. Use Sidebar 9-16 (p 271) for dry (powder) formulations and Sidebar 9-17 for granular formulations.

Percentage Solutions

Sometimes labels require that the pesticide be mixed as a percentage solution. You mix the product to get a known concentration regardless of the sprayer output rate. Mix percentage

---

SIDEBAR 9-17

Calculating Granular Formulations

You are given a recommendation to apply 0.50 lb a.i. of ethoprop per 1,000 square feet of turf for control of nematodes. You are provided with a granular formulation containing 10% active ingredient (0.1 pound of a.i. per pound of formulation). To what rate should you calibrate the granule applicator?

Step 1. Convert the percent a.i. to a decimal and divide this into the recommended application rate.

EXAMPLE

$$0.5 \text{ lb a.i. per 1,000 sq ft} \div 0.1 \text{ lb a.i. per lb formulation} = 5 \text{ lb formulation}$$

Step 2. Calibrate the granule applicator so that it applies 5 pounds of formulated ethoprop per 1,000 square feet.

SIDEBAR 9-19

Calculating a Percentage Solution: Dry Formulations

The calculations for percentage solutions using dry formulations are similar to the calculations for liquid formulations. First, from the label, determine the percentage of a.i. in the dry formulation. Assume for this example that it is 75% a.i.; 1 pound of dry formulation would contain 0.75 pound of pesticide a.i. You need to mix a 1% spray solution of this formulation in a 264.5-gallon tank.

Step 1. Find the total weight of the liquid in the filled tank by multiplying the volume of the tank by the weight of water per gallon.

EXAMPLE

$$264.5 \text{ gal} \times 8.34 \text{ lb/gal} = 2,205.93 \text{ lb}$$

Step 2. Multiply this weight by 0.01 (1%) to determine the weight of a.i. required to mix a 1% solution.

EXAMPLE

$$2,205.93 \times 0.01 = 22.06 \text{ lb}$$

Step 3. Divide the weight of a.i. by the decimal equivalent of the percentage of a.i. in the formulation. The result is the number of pounds of formulation that should be added to 264.5 gallons of water to achieve a 1% solution.

EXAMPLE

$$22.06 \text{ lb} \div 0.75 = 29.41 \text{ lb formulation}$$

Step 4. Add 29.41 pounds of wettable powder to 264.5 gallons of water to achieve a 1% solution.

SIDEBAR 9-18

CALCULATING A PERCENTAGE SOLUTION: LIQUID FORMULATIONS

To prepare a percentage solution using liquid formulations, you need to know:
- the volume of the spray tank
- the weight of a.i. per gallon of formulation
- the weight of a gallon of water

The weight of water is a constant, approximately 8.34 pounds per gallon. Assume you have measured the volume of the spray tank and find that it holds 264.5 gallons of water. You are given a recommendation to apply a 1% solution of glyphosate for control of aquatic weeds using a high-pressure sprayer with a hand-held spray nozzle. The formulation of glyphosate that you are to use contains 5.4 pounds of a.i. per gallon.

Step 1. Find the total weight of the liquid in the filled tank by multiplying the volume of the tank (264.5 gallons) by the weight of water (8.34 pounds per gallon).

EXAMPLE

$$264.5 \text{ gal} \times 8.34 \text{ lb/gal} = 2{,}205.93 \text{ lb}$$

Step 2. Multiply this weight by 0.01 (1%) to determine the weight of a.i. required to mix a 1% solution.

EXAMPLE

$$2{,}205.93 \times 0.01 = 22.06 \text{ lb}$$

Step 3. Divide the required weight of a.i. by the weight of a.i. in the formulation. The result is the number of gallons of liquid formulation that should be added to 264.5 gallons of water to achieve a 1% solution.

EXAMPLE

$$22.06 \text{ lb a.i.} \div 5.4 \text{ lb a.i./gal} = 4.1 \text{ gal formulation}$$

In this example, one tank of liquid should contain 4.1 gallons of glyphosate formulation. The total volume of water combined with the glyphosate formulation should equal 264.5 gallons, the capacity of the tank. You would therefore use 260.4 gallons of water and 4.1 gallons of formulated glyphosate.

Note: These calculations give a close approximation of the amount of liquid formulation to add to the tank to achieve a known percentage solution. The mathematics for a more exact figure are more complex and unnecessary for this type of work.

SIDEBAR 9-20

CALCULATING A PARTS PER MILLION DILUTION: DRY FORMULATIONS

You are given a recommendation for a 100 ppm concentration of oxytetracycline to be mixed in a 500-gallon tank for control of fire blight on pear trees. The formulation you have is a wettable powder containing 17% a.i.

Step 1. Find the total weight of the liquid in the filled tank by multiplying the volume of the tank by the weight of water per gallon.

EXAMPLE

$$500 \text{ gal} \times 8.34 \text{ lb/gal} = 4{,}170 \text{ lb/tank}$$

Step 2. Determine how many pounds of a.i. are required for 1 pound of spray solution.

EXAMPLE

$$100 \text{ ppm} = 100 \text{ parts a.i.} \div 1{,}000{,}000 \text{ parts solution} = 0.0001$$

Step 3. Determine how many pounds of a.i. are required for a tank of solution, using the weight of the liquid in the tank.

EXAMPLE

$$4{,}170 \text{ lb/tank} \times 0.0001 \text{ lb a.i.} = 0.417 \text{ lb a.i.}$$

Step 4. Divide the weight of a.i. by the decimal equivalent of the percentage of a.i. in the formulation. The result is the number of pounds of formulation that should be added to 500 gallons of water to achieve a 100 ppm solution.

EXAMPLE

$$0.417 \text{ lb a.i.} \div 0.17 \text{ lb a.i./lb formulation} = 2.45 \text{ lb formulation}$$

TABLE 9-2

Parts per million (ppm)

ppm	Decimal solution	Percentage
1 ppm	0.000001	0.0001%
10 ppm	0.00001	0.001%
100 ppm	0.0001	0.01%
1,000 ppm	0.001	0.1%
10,000 ppm	0.01	1.0%
100,000 ppm	0.1	10.0%
1,000,000 ppm	1.0	100.0%

solutions on a weight-to-weight basis (w/w), meaning pounds of a.i. per pound of water. Sidebar 9-18 (p. 273) provides an example of calculating a percentage solution with liquid formulations. Sidebar 9-19 (p. 272) shows the calculations for dry formulations.

PARTS PER MILLION DILUTIONS

You must mix certain pesticides in parts per million (ppm) concentrations. These are the same as percentage solutions. For example, a 100 ppm solution is equal to a 0.01% solution (Table 9-2). The ppm designation represents the parts of a.i. of pesticide per million parts of water. Parts per million dilutions are a common way of measuring very diluted concentrations of pesticides. When calculating parts per million, use the formulas in Sidebar 9-20 (p. 273) if you are mixing dry formulations with water. For liquid formulations, use the formulas in Sidebar 9-21.

DETERMINING THE SIZE OF THE TARGET SITE

If the target site is a rectangle, circle, or triangle, you can use simple measurements and formulas to determine its size. Irregularly shaped sites often can be reduced to a combination of rectangles, circles, and triangles. Calculate the area of each and add them together to obtain the total area (Sidebar 9-22, p. 275).

To apply fumigants, vaporous or mist formulations, or space sprays that must fill the entire inside of a structure or other enclosed space, you need to calculate the volume (cubic feet) of the building, greenhouse, truck, railroad

---

SIDEBAR 9-21

CALCULATING A PARTS PER MILLION DILUTION: LIQUID FORMULATIONS

Assume that a pesticide contains 5.4 pounds of a.i. in 1 gallon of formulation. You are required to prepare a 100 ppm concentration in a 500-gallon tank.

Step 1. Find the total weight of the liquid in the filled tank by multiplying the volume of the tank by the weight of water per gallon.

EXAMPLE

500 gal/tank × 8.34 lb/gal = 4,170 lb/tank

Step 2. Determine how many pounds of a.i. are required for 1 pound of spray solution.

EXAMPLE

100 parts a.i. ÷ 1,000,000 parts solution = 0.0001

Step 3. Determine how many pounds of a.i. are required for a tank of solution using the weight of the liquid in the tank.

EXAMPLE

4,170 lb/tank × 0.0001 lb a.i. = 0.417 lb a.i./tank

Step 4. Divide the required weight of a.i. by the pounds of a.i. per gallon to determine how many gallons of formulation are required. Since this will probably be a small number, convert to ounces by multiplying the result by the number of ounces per gallon (128).

EXAMPLE

0.417 lb a.i./tank ÷ 5.4 lb a.i./gal = 0.0772 gal/tank
0.0772 gal/tank × 128 fl oz/gal = 9.88 fl oz/tank

Adding 9.88 fluid ounces of this formulated pesticide to 500 gallons of water will result in a 100 ppm solution.

> Calculate the area of various shapes (circle, square, rectangle, triangle, and irregular shapes).

SIDEBAR 9-22
CALCULATING THE AREA OF THE TARGET SITE USING VARIOUS SHAPES

Important formulas:
- area of a rectangle = length × width
- area of triangle = ½ × base × height
- area of a circle = 3.14 × radius × radius

Area conversion factors:
- 1 acre = 43,560 sq ft
- 1 mile = 5,280 ft
- 1 mile = 320 rods
- 1 rod = 16.5 ft

To calculate areas for irregularly shaped fields and beds, break the shape into the shapes given above and figure the area for each part. For instance, in the first example, you can divide the field into a rectangle and a triangle; the area of the field is the sum of the area of rectangle A and triangle B.

Example 1. Below, the rectangular area A measures 600 feet by 450 feet and the base of the triangular area B is 300 feet:

area of A = 450 ft × 600 ft = 270,000 ft^2
area of B = 0.5 × 300 ft × 450 ft = 67,500 ft^2
total area = 270,000 ft^2 + 67,500 ft^2 = 337,500 ft^2
total area in acres = 337,500 ft^2 ÷ 43,560 ft^2/acre = 7.75 acres

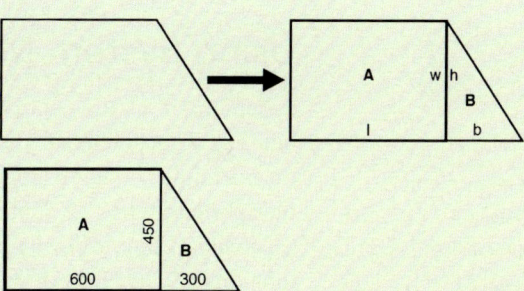

Example 2. This field contains both a rectangular and a half-circle section. To calculate the area, break the shape into a rectangle and a circle. The field area is the sum of the area of rectangle A and one-half the area of circle B. Below, the rectangular area A measures 1,500 feet by 1,200 feet, and the radius of circular area B is 750 feet:

area of A = 1,500 ft^2 × 1,200 ft^2 = 1,800,000 ft^2
area of B = 3.14 x 750 ft^2 [or 3.14 x 750 ft x 750 ft] ÷ 2 = 883,125 ft^2
total area = 1,800,000 ft^2 + 883,125 ft^2 = 2,683,125 ft^2
total area in acres = 2,683,125 ft^2 ÷ 43,560 ft^2/acre = 61.6 acres

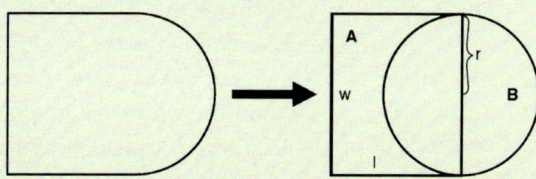

Example 3. The last example is for a field with irregular borders on two of the four sides. To calculate the total area of the field, add the areas of rectangles A, B, and C to the area of triangle D. Below, the rectangular area A measures 600 feet by 450 feet, the squares B and C measure 200 feet by 200 feet, and the base of the triangular area B is 200 feet:

area of A = 450 ft × 600 ft = 270,000 ft^2
area of B = 200 ft × 200 ft = 40,000 ft^2
area of C = 200 ft × 200 ft = 40,000 ft^2
area of D = 0.5 × 200 ft × 225 ft = 22,500 ft^2
total area = 270,000 ft^2 + 40,000 ft^2 + 40,000 ft^2 + 22,500 ft^2 = 372,500 ft^2
total area in acres = 372,500 ft^2 ÷ 43,560 ft^2/acre = 8.55 acres

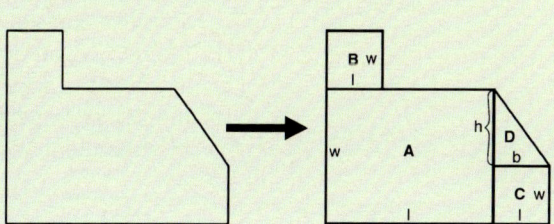

Source: Adapted from Blecker and Thomas 2012.

TABLE 9-3

Pressure changes needed to adjust output because of speed changes with 8015 nozzles at 10 mph at 40 psi applying 30 gpa

Speed (mph)	% Change	Nozzle pressure (psi)	% Change	Spray volume (gpa)
10		40		30
5	−50%	10*	−75%	30
15	+50%	90*	+125%	30

Note: *Outside recommended nozzle pressure.
Source: Bauer 2005.

car, or ship hold. To apply pesticides to bodies of water (not just the surface), you must calculate the volume of the water in the pond or lake. Sometimes the structures or bodies of water are regular in shape. The calculations for these are fairly simple. If the structure or body of water is irregular, you must calculate parts of the structure separately and add them together to find the total volume (see McDonald 1991).

Using System Monitors and Controllers

System monitors and controllers are becoming more popular in achieving accurate application, but they do not eliminate the need for sprayer inspection and calibration. Monitors measure the operating conditions such as travel speed, pressure, and/or flow rate and can alert you to unexpected changes in application rates. Rate (or spray) controllers are monitors with the added capability of automatic rate control. The controller receives the actual application rate from the monitors and compares it with the desired rate. If an error exists, the pressure is regulated to adjust the spray volume. However, nozzles can operate only within a limited range of pressure without either distorting the spray angle or creating off-target drift, so you must be observant during applications to ensure that spray remains even and on target.

Table 9-3 shows a change made in speed and the resulting change required by the pressure regulator. Nozzles that can operate over a wider pressure range are best to use with rate controllers. The controller will adjust the spray volume automatically by adjusting pressure. Since these adjustments are a direct response to various sensors that collect data as part of the system monitor, the sensors must be periodically checked and calibrated. Do not assume that the monitors are foolproof. Consult the manufacturer's operator's manual to properly calibrate and adjust the sensors. Monitors that give travel speed, spray volume, etc. are usually adequate for most sprayer situations. The newer monitors keep track of which booms are being used and the areas they cover so that the calculated area sprayed is very accurate (see Bauer 2005).

> Explain how system controllers can impact the calibration of equipment and calculations necessary to apply pesticides effectively.

> Explain the importance of properly calibrating sensors that are part of a system controller.

Chapter 9 Review Questions

1. **Which of the following defines calibration?**
    - ☐ a. the research you do before an application to be sure you avoid hazards and sensitive areas at the treatment site
    - ☐ b. the review you do of instructions on the label to be sure you apply the pesticide safely at the application site
    - ☐ c. the adjustments you make to be sure you apply the correct amount of pesticide to the treatment area

2. **Why must you regularly calibrate application equipment?**
   - ☐ a. to ensure you are using the correct amount of pesticide for effective pest control
   - ☐ b. to ensure you are using the maximum amount of pesticide allowed by law
   - ☐ c. to ensure that pest problems never reoccur in areas where you apply pesticides

3. **Select the tools that are required for accurate, professional calibration of pesticide sprayers from the list below. Select all that apply.**
   - ☐ a. droplet size chart
   - ☐ b. stopwatch
   - ☐ c. measuring tape
   - ☐ d. wooden toothpick
   - ☐ e. calibrated container
   - ☐ f. magnifying glass
   - ☐ g. flowmeter
   - ☐ h. flagging tape

4. **For sprayer calibration, which four factors need to be measured?**
   - ☐ a. swath width, size of treatment area, travel speed, and sprayer pressure
   - ☐ b. nozzle height, size of treatment area, travel speed, and swath width
   - ☐ c. tank capacity, travel speed, swath width, and flow rate

5. **It takes your equipment 3 minutes to travel 264 feet. How fast, in miles per hour, is the equipment traveling?**
   - ☐ a. 1 mile per hour
   - ☐ b. 2 miles per hour
   - ☐ c. 3 miles per hour

6. **By measuring the output of each nozzle on the spray boom, you discover that the sprayer output is 256 ounces in 30 seconds. What is the output of the sprayer in gallons per minute?**
   - ☐ a. 2
   - ☐ b. 3
   - ☐ c. 4

7. **Which of these will help you the most when determining the amount of pesticide needed for a given application?**
   - ☐ a. calculate nozzle output carefully to account for wear
   - ☐ b. measure the area that you plan to treat accurately
   - ☐ c. ensure the tank holds the correct amount of liquid

8. **Your calibrated sprayer with a 300-gallon tank will cover 4.2 acres. You plan to apply an herbicide at a label rate of 1.5 pounds per acre. How much of this herbicide will you put into the spray tank?**
   - ☐ a. 4.2 pounds
   - ☐ b. 4.5 pounds
   - ☐ c. 6.3 pounds

9. Match the change made to the sprayer with the effect it has on sprayer output.

1. increasing travel speed	a. breaks spray up into finer droplets
2. changing nozzle size	b. alters the pressure of the system and requires an adjustment of the pressure regulator
3. increasing output pressure	c. reduces the application rate

10. What three variables must be measured to properly calibrate dry application equipment?
    - ☐ a. output rate, hopper size, and formulation type
    - ☐ b. swath width, output rate, and travel speed
    - ☐ c. formulation type, travel speed, and output rate

11. Put the following steps for calculating a parts per million dilution of a liquid pesticide in the correct order.
    - ☐ a. Check the label to find out the dilution rate, then calculate how many pounds of a.i. are required for 1 pound of spray solution.
    - ☐ b. Determine how many pounds of a.i. are required for a tank of solution using the weight of the liquid in the tank.
    - ☐ c. Find the total weight of the liquid in the filled tank by multiplying the capacity of the tank, in gallons, by 8.34 pounds per gallon.
    - ☐ d. Divide the required weight of a.i. by the pounds of a.i. per gallon to determine how many gallons of formulation are required.

12. You need to mix a 2% spray solution of a wettable powder formulation containing 50% a.i. in a 20-gallon tank. How much of this formulation would you have to add to the tank in this case?
    - ☐ a. 5.74 pounds
    - ☐ b. 6.67 pounds
    - ☐ c. 7.24 pounds

13. What is the area, in acres, of the irregularly shaped field shown? Given: The base of the field is 2,400 feet, the width of the field is 900 feet, and the field measures 1,500 feet across the top. (1 acre = 43,560 square feet)
    - ☐ a. 34.9 acres
    - ☐ b. 40.3 acres
    - ☐ c. 49.4 acres

14. Rate controllers help increase the accuracy of applications only if nozzles can _____.
    - ☐ a. handle a sufficient range of pressures
    - ☐ b. preserve droplet size if pressure changes
    - ☐ c. prevent leaks when pressure rises

15. Where do rate controllers get the data they need to adjust spray volume accurately?
    - ☐ a. GPS units
    - ☐ b. nozzles
    - ☐ c. sensors

Chapter 10
Using Pesticides Effectively

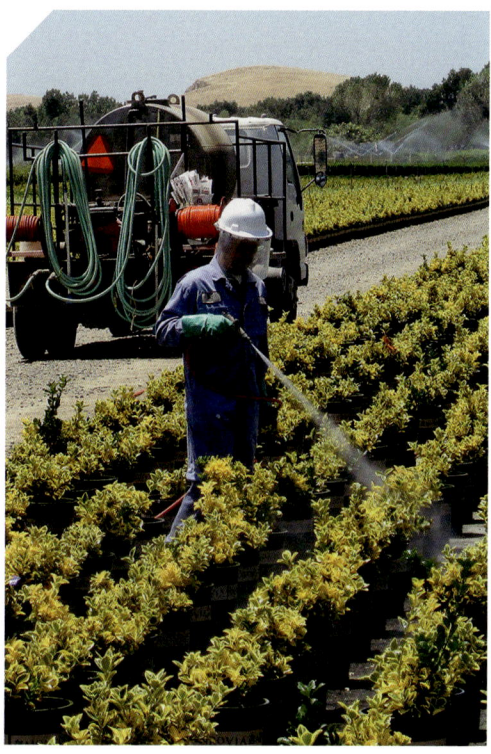

Pest Detection and Monitoring	280
Making Pesticide Use Decisions	287
Choosing the Right Pesticide	289
Making Pesticides More Selective	294
Mixing Pesticides	299
Pesticide Resistance	303
Preventing Offsite Movement of Pesticides	306
Follow-Up Monitoring	316
Chapter 10 Review Questions	317

Knowledge Expectations

- Describe the goals of pesticide applications and how to achieve them.
- Explain how pest identification, scouting, monitoring, and economic threshold data influence pesticide use decisions.
- Provide examples of common pest monitoring methods used before applying pesticides.
- List the factors to consider when selecting and using a pesticide so that the application is maximally effective and hazards associated with its use are reduced.
- Describe how to select the most appropriate pesticide for a particular application.
- Describe the factors that control a pesticide's selectivity.
- Describe procedures, additives, formulation types, and conditions that help keep pesticides on target.
- Explain how a GPS unit can impact the effectiveness of pesticide applications.
- Explain how to determine whether two or more pesticides will be compatible for tank-mixing.
- Describe mixing procedures for
   - a. a single pesticide
   - b. two or more pesticides (tank mix)
- Explain why pesticide resistance is a problem.
- List the factors that contribute to pesticide resistance.
- Describe the different types of drift, including factors that can affect the occurrence of each type of drift.
- Describe ways to prevent other types of offsite movement of pesticides.
- Describe how to implement a follow-up monitoring program to assess the effectiveness of a pesticide application.
- Describe how to evaluate spray coverage and adjust application variables to change coverage as needed.

You must use pesticides effectively as well as safely. The results of a pesticide application should usually be worth any financial or labor investment by
- yielding a profit or quality advantage in crops
- reducing health hazards to people and livestock or poultry
- improving health, appearance, and growth of turf and ornamental plants
- eliminating annoying pests from buildings, workplaces, and homes

This chapter discusses several ways for you to improve pesticide application effectiveness.

Pest Detection and Monitoring

Describe the goals of pesticide applications and how to achieve them.

Pest management decisions must be based on actual site conditions. Therefore, you should understand how to monitor your site to determine whether pests pose a threat. A monitoring program, beginning with regularly performed systematic scouting, records pest types and numbers or damage symptoms so they can be compared over the course of a season. Monitoring often involves counting pest numbers or the number of damage symptoms observed. It also involves counting the number of natural enemies, measuring crop growth, and noting weather and field conditions (Fig. 10-1). For some pests, particularly weeds, surveys are carried out during the season before planting. For all pests, you should monitor before and during the cropping season. A monitoring program includes a good recordkeeping program so that problems can be mapped and analyzed over time (see Flint 2012).

PREDICTING PROBLEMS

Explain how pest identification, scouting, monitoring, and economic threshold data influence pesticide use decisions.

Early detection lets you plan a program for following pest development and activity, which will help you predict if or when treatment is necessary. It also helps if you review the pest history of the farm, landscaped area, building, right-of-way, or other location. Then you will know what pests to expect at different times of the year. If this information is not available, try to get pest history information from a similar location nearby.

Look for conditions that favor pest buildup. For example, some pest insects overwinter in crop residues or field borders. If you see these pests in such areas, there is a strong likelihood they will eventually move into the crop. Weeds that produce seeds provide a seed reservoir for the following year. If this is the case, anticipate large populations of these weeds in following seasons.

USING PESTICIDES EFFECTIVELY

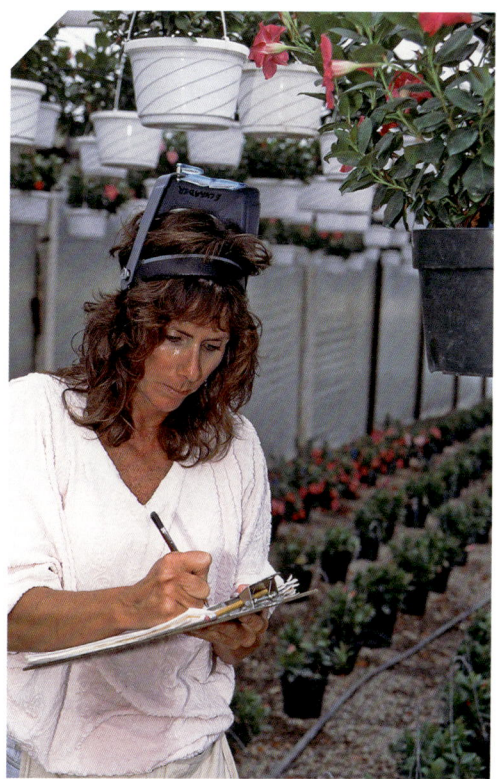

FIGURE 10-1

Keeping monitoring records helps applicators recognize trends in pest numbers or incidence of disease so they can be noted and analyzed over time. A hands-free magnifier makes scouting more efficient.

Vertebrates, such as squirrels, may not be a problem while other food supplies are adequate. However, if conditions change, they may move into cropped or landscaped areas for food. Cockroaches, ants, and rodents need food sources, water, and often shelter before they can seriously infest an area.

Chapter 2 describes how to identify many types of pests. The sidebars in Chapter 2 show you how to use pest identification services. They also describe how to package and ship pests to experts or identification laboratories.

In time, you will learn to recognize the more common pests found in your work situation. When you come across pests you do not recognize, collect samples using traps, nets, or other appropriate methods. If weeds are the problem, dig up samples so roots are included with the rest of the plants. Collect seedlings and/or flowering specimens if they are present. You can also take pictures to send in for identification.

Be careful when handling birds and rodents because they may be diseased. For instance, some flea-infested rodents can vector the plague organism. Birds often carry lice, mites, or biting bugs. Rabies is prevalent in some skunks, bats, and other small mammals. Handle these animals with tongs or heavy gloves to avoid being bitten. Do not contact their urine or feces.

Be sure you recognize natural enemies of pests. Natural enemies may be contributing to the control of the pest problem, eliminating or reducing the need for a pesticide application. Do not mistake natural enemies for pests. To find out more about the natural enemies of the pests in your area, see the UC IPM website, ipm.ucanr.edu/PMG/NE/natenemiespest.html.

Recognizing Key Life History Information. When you monitor pest populations, you learn to recognize their life cycles and stages of development. This information is useful when planning a management program, because success depends on using the right control method at the right time. Some of the things you might learn include the pest's

- preferred habitat
- food or moisture preferences
- time of greatest activity
- seasonal occurrences or life stages

For more information on how life cycles can be used to properly time both pesticide applications and nonchemical control methods, see "Factors Influencing Selection for Resistance" later in this chapter.

Monitoring Weather. Weather greatly influences development of plants and their pests. Wetness from rain, fog, or irrigation is a primary factor that favors most diseases. Temperature is one of several factors that control plant growth, and it determines the rate at which invertebrate organisms develop. For instance, insects complete a generation in less time when temperatures are higher than when weather is cool.

A reliable source of local weather observations is important for determining whether conditions are right for pesticide applications, as well as for making many agricultural decisions, such as planting time, scheduling irrigation, protecting crops from frost, or timing pest management actions.

You can find up-to-date weather information from many sources. The California Department of Water Resources CIMIS program monitors weather variables in many locations throughout the state and reports them online at cimis.water.ca.gov. Also, other organizations, including newspapers, radio stations, and universities, redistribute CIMIS weather data. National Weather Service broadcasts local and regional weather observations and forecasts on NOAA Weather Radio (VHF channels 162.42, 162.50, or 162.55 MHz, depending on location).

ESTABLISHING A MONITORING PROGRAM

Frequent monitoring provides information on the day-to-day populations of pests. The data you gather is what you need to make intelligent decisions. Information you collect may include the density, life stages, and species composition of pest populations. Also include your observations of factors controlling or favoring the pest. You will find that it is difficult to monitor pests while their populations are low and damage is minimal. However, this monitoring is worth the effort. If chemical treatment is necessary, you may learn enough to be able to use less-toxic pesticides. The monitoring information may also help you limit applications to a more restricted area.

Visual inspection is the most common method. It includes any systematic method of searching for pests, pest damage, or evidence of the presence of pests and can be used both before and after pesticide applications to assess pest populations and activity levels. Generally, visual inspection requires thoroughly examining a representative portion of an area in a uniform way. It may include sampling foliage, pulling up a certain number of plants, or walking a prescribed area. Look for patterns of distribution, damage, or activity. Then check for evidence of natural enemies or other mortality factors. Sometimes other organisms may indicate the presence of pests, such as fleas near rodent nests or ants climbing trees or shrubs to collect honeydew from aphids and scale insects.

Provide examples of common pest monitoring methods used before applying pesticides.

The following indicators may provide clues to the presence and identity of some pests:
- seeds
- weed remains from the previous season
- animal burrows
- tracks
- feeding damage
- fecal droppings
- webbing
- insect or mite eggs

Table 10-1 lists some of the useful tools that help you to monitor and observe pests.

Weeds. The most important field information needed for making weed management decisions includes
- what species are present
- the stage of development (seedling, flowering, postflowering)
- whether the relative abundance of different species is changing from previous seasons

Monitor for weeds in the late fall or early winter (after the first rains) to detect emerging winter annuals. Monitor in the late spring to detect emerging summer annuals. Monitor at other times as needed to detect perennial and biennial weeds and weeds not controlled after herbicide applications. Identify all the weed species found growing in an area, preferably while they are in the seedling stage. Watch for any new species.

Use a form similar to Figure 10-2 to keep records of the different weed species and their locations. Map the locations of the weeds you find. Try to estimate the percentage of each weed species relative to the total weed population. Count the numbers and varieties in one or more

TABLE 10-1

Selected invertebrate pest monitoring methods and tools (may also be used for beneficials)

Method or tool	Pest monitored
visual inspection	Most invertebrate species that feed on the outer surfaces of plants and their damage. Evidence of parasitism and predation. Monitoring may require a hand lens or other magnifier.
timed counts	Individuals of exposed beneficial and invertebrate pest species (e.g., lady beetles, caterpillars) or certain types of damage (rolled leaves, twig strikes) that are relatively large and obvious but occur at relatively low density so they are not observed faster than they can be counted.
knockdown techniques: branch beating, shaking plants, or tapping containers over a collecting surface such as drop cloth or clipboard with a white sheet of paper	Adults and larvae or nymphs of easily dislodged invertebrate species, including bugs, lacewings, lady beetles, leaf beetles, leafhoppers, mites, nonwebbing caterpillars, adult parasites, psyllids, thrips, and adult whiteflies.
suction techniques (D-VAC)	Relatively mobile adults and larvae or nymphs of invertebrate species, including bugs, caterpillars, adult whiteflies; beneficial species such as big-eyed bugs, minute pirate bugs, lacewings, and spiders.
sweep nets	Adults and larvae or nymphs of invertebrate species, including weevils, caterpillars, and bugs that are free-living on foliage.
rotary traps	Flying and windborne invertebrates such as winged aphids.
bait traps	Invertebrate pests such as flies, ants, cockroaches, snails and slugs, and certain species of moths.
pheromone traps	Many moths, certain beetles, males of some scales, and other insects; certain parasite adults are attracted to their host's pheromone.
light traps	Night-flying adults of moths, some beetles (e.g., chafers, white grubs, certain scarabs, and some leaf beetles), lacewings, and others.
sticky traps	Adults, including fungus gnats, leafminers, psyllids, shore flies, thrips, whiteflies, winged aphids, and parasites.
pitfall traps	Adult weevils, predaceous ground beetles, ground-dwelling spiders, Collembola, and possibly others such as squash bugs.
carbon dioxide exhalation and shaking	Thrips hidden in buds are stimulated to move by a long, gentle breath into terminals and are dislodged and revealed by shaking plant tips over white or black paper on a clipboard.
indicator or key plants	Most species that feed on the outer surfaces of plants. The same infested plants are inspected before and after treatment to determine whether pest is in the stage that is susceptible to the control action, to compare numbers to previous sampling, and to determine effectiveness of control.
degree-day phenology	Many pests and beneficial species for which temperature development thresholds and rates have been determined.
soil drench or flushes using pyrethrum, soap, or water	Relatively mobile species in soil or hidden places, including centipedes, millipedes, symphylans, and larvae of fungus gnats and shore flies. Thrips and other species in buds may be flushed.
trap boards	Adult weevils, snails.
potato traps	Root-feeding fungus gnat larvae and symphylans, which migrate to feed on underside of potato pieces. Push pieces into soil and pick up and examine the underside of each disc and the soil surface for larvae once or twice a week.
host collection and rearing	Immature stages of species such as parasitoids that feed inside host. Only the adult stage of many insects can be positively identified to species.

Source: Adapted from Flint 2012.

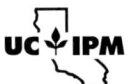

Grape—Early Season Weed Survey
Supplement to UC IPM Pest Management Guidelines: Grape

Grower/Vineyard: _____ Date: _____

Comments: _____

Mechanical Control/Herbicide/Application Date: _____

Record weeds on the form below; use the map to record the location of problematic weeds.

Directions:

1. Survey wine or raisin vineyards in late spring or summer. For table grapes, survey in March (San Joaquin Valley) and January to February (Coachella Valley), after summer annuals have germinated.
2. Pay particular attention to perennials. Check for regrowth of perennials a few weeks after cultivation.
3. Pay attention to wet spots, as these may be problem areas in terms of weed growth.
4. Survey areas around the vineyard as these areas could be a potential source for wind-disseminated seeds, such as marestail and fleabane seeds.
5. Rate infestation either using a numeric scale from 1 to 5 (1 being the lightest), or use "light," "medium," or "heavy."

Summer Annual and Perennial Weeds

Weed	Row middles	Rows
Annual broadleaves		
hairy fleabane (flax-leaf)		
horseweed		
spurge (prostrate/spotted)		
puncturevine		
cudweed, purple		
knotweed, prostrate		
nightshade, black		
pigweed, prostrate		
nettle, burning		
lambsquarters, common		
willowherb, tall annual (panicle willowherb)		
annual morningglories		

Weed	Row middles	Rows
Annual grasses		
junglerice		
barnyardgrass		
crabgrass, large		
foxtail, yellow		
Perennial broadleaves		
bindweed, field		
Perennial grasses		
bermudagrass		
Other perennials		
nutsedge		
Other weeds		

FIGURE 10-2

Keep records of the weed species present in an area to help select appropriate herbicides or other control measures. The form illustrated here was developed for weeds found in vineyards.

randomly selected areas of 1 square yard. Note areas where weeds have produced seeds. Also, keep records of all herbicides used for weed control in the area. This information is useful when plant-back restrictions apply. It also helps you evaluate the effectiveness of previous control efforts. Include in these records the types of cultural methods that were used for weed control.

Look for adjacent weedy areas such as roadsides or ditch banks that may be a reservoir for seeds. Other ways that weeds move into an area include the following:
- Cultivation equipment may move weed seeds or vegetative structures from one site to another.
- Floodwater may carry weed seeds into the flooded area.
- Birds and mammals can move seeds or vegetative structures on their coats, in their feces, and with their nesting materials.

Nematodes. Usually, you must manage nematodes before the crop or other plants are in the ground. Early detection allows enough time to apply a soil treatment before planting. Therefore, take soil samples in autumn for winter- and spring-planted crops or plants. If fumigation is not an option, early detection allows you to select nematode-resistant plant species.

You can use a simple method to determine whether nematodes are present. Check susceptible crops or weeds by digging up plants that look stressed. Inspect the roots for galls, cysts, or swollen root tips. Monitor sandy soils regularly for root-knot nematode infestations when susceptible plants are grown there. If you detect nematodes or know that nematodes have been a problem, arrange for more detailed quantitative sampling. One sample per year should be sufficient.

Take soil samples for nematodes along a long, continuous strip through the area. Keep each sample separate. Sample the soil within the root zone of the plants. Also look for stunted or damaged plants. If you find any, include the infected plants, with roots, in the sampling. Prepare the samples and send them to an identification laboratory as instructed in "Identifying Pests" in Chapter 2. Draw a map of the area that shows locations of healthy and infected plants, soil types, water drainage, and other important features.

Nematodes are usually introduced into new areas via infested soil or plants. Prevent nematodes from entering new sites by using only nematode-free plants purchased from reliable nurseries. To prevent the spread of nematodes, avoid moving plants and soil from infested parts of the cultivated area. Don't allow irrigation water from around infested plants to run off, as this also spreads nematodes. Nematodes can be present in soil attached to tools and equipment used elsewhere, so clean tools thoroughly before storing or moving to a new site (see Perry and Ploeg 2010).

Pathogens. Monitor pathogens by observing plant symptoms or damage or, with certain fungi, by looking for fruiting bodies and other structures. Remember that damaged plant material may serve as an inoculum source for healthy plants. Look for inoculum sources before conditions favor the spread of pathogens. This is important since the most successful control of plant disease pathogens involves suppressing them before infection occurs. Environmental conditions such as temperature, rainfall, or heavy dew are often the controlling factors for pathogen infection or development. Look for a pattern of symptoms:
- Do symptoms occur only on scattered plants?
- Are symptoms concentrated in certain parts of the field?
- Are symptoms generally distributed?

Also, monitor for the presence of insects or nematodes that are capable of transmitting certain pathogens, such as aphids.

Identifying most plant pathogens requires laboratory analysis. Collect damaged plant material according to the instructions in Chapter 2.

Arthropods. You can observe most insects, mites, and other arthropods by visual monitoring. You can also collect plant foliage and examine it with a hand lens or microscope (Fig. 10-3). Use a sweep net to collect certain pest insects found on foliage (Fig. 10-4). However, avoid using sweep nets on tender plants because you can damage them by this technique. Beat foliage onto a white sheet, tray, or pan for a simple way of detecting certain plant-feeding insects. Use these methods to estimate the size of an arthropod pest population or evaluate its rate of increase or decrease. Sometimes the decision to apply a pesticide is based on the number of insects or mites found on a sample of leaves taken from different plants or from sweep net samples. Control decisions are often based on studies that show that until the pest population builds up to a certain size, no economic damage will occur.

Light, especially the ultraviolet spectrum (black light), attracts many night-flying insects. Some pest managers use blacklight traps to attract and kill certain nocturnal insect pests in small areas. These traps also serve as monitoring devices for particular types of insect pests in enclosed areas such as warehouses.

Use sticky traps for catching and monitoring some insect pests. These cardboard or plastic traps have a surface coated with a thick, sticky paste. You can do several things to make sticky traps attractive to target insects. Where you place the traps and the color and shape of the traps attract certain insects. For example, put sticky traps along wall bases or other normal pathways to monitor cockroaches. Use a bright yellow color to attract whiteflies. Hang sticky red or green spheres in trees to catch apple maggot adults or walnut husk flies. You can add attractants to sticky traps or sticky surfaces to attract flies, cockroaches, and other pest insects. Effective attractants include various food, sugar syrups, or chemicals with odors resembling certain food.

Pheromones lure some insects into sticky traps. Pheromones are chemicals produced by insects that attract individuals of the same species. Most pheromone traps use a chemical that mimics the pheromone produced by female insects to attract males for mating. A few mimic pheromones released by males to attract females. As you monitor these traps, you will notice that

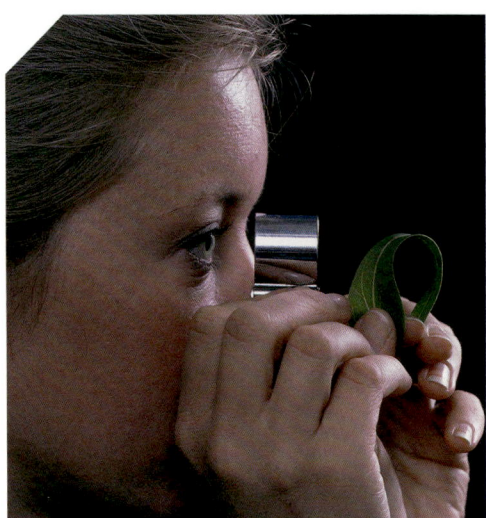

FIGURE 10-3

A hand lens is often needed for detecting, identifying, and monitoring insects, mites, and other arthropods on plant foliage. Hold the lens close to your eye and bring the object being examined up to it until it is in focus.

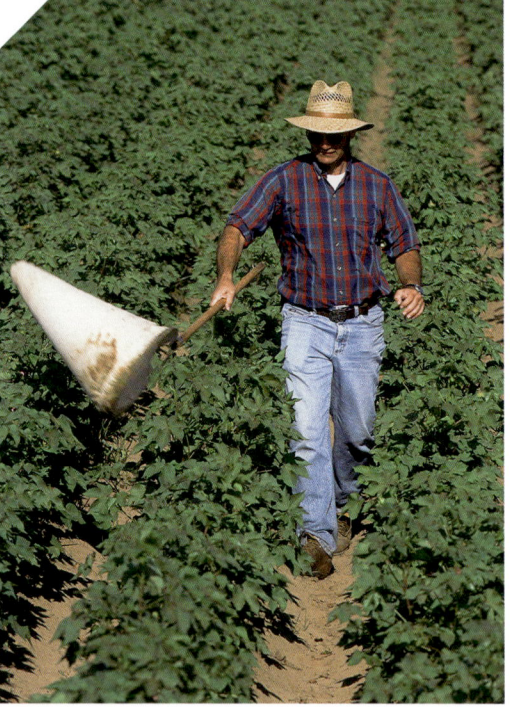

FIGURE 10-4

Use a sweep net to monitor the presence of certain pest insects on plant foliage.

trap catches increase during the time when insects emerge from their pupal stage and begin to mate. Knowing when adults are emerging gives you a good idea of when to apply insecticides for optimal control. For some agricultural pest insects, you can use phenology models to accurately predict egg hatch. This allows you to precisely time insecticide applications. These models use pheromone trap catch information and daily high and low temperatures in the calculations.

The University of California Statewide Integrated Pest Management Program develops phenology models for many insect pests. These are available at the UC IPM website, ipm.ucanr.edu.

Vertebrate Pests. Monitoring for vertebrates requires some understanding of the habits of potential pests. Many species are active only at certain times of the day or night. Other species cease their activities when people are around. Often the best way to monitor for them is to check for evidence of their presence. This includes gopher or ground squirrel burrows, feces of rats or rabbits, or mouse trails. Use animal traps and tracking powders to monitor the activities of vertebrate pests when it is too difficult or time consuming to watch continually for the pests. Some animal traps are spring-loaded devices, such as rat traps, that kill the target animals. Use live traps, which resemble cages, when you must not harm the captured pests (Fig. 10-5).

Use tracking powders to monitor rodent activity in buildings (Fig. 10-6). Spread the powder (cornstarch or flour works well) over an area suspected of being a rodent trail or runway. Tracks left in the dust reveal information about the population size, age of individuals, and areas of activity. This technique is useful in planning the placement and timing of traps or rodenticides. Keep tracking powders on floor surfaces to prevent contaminating counters, furnishings, or other objects in an area. Certain tracking powders contain toxicants that kill rodents. The rodents ingest the poison while cleaning themselves.

> List the factors to consider when selecting and using a pesticide so that the application is maximally effective and hazards associated with its use are reduced.

Making Pesticide Use Decisions

How do you decide when to use a pesticide and what pesticide to use? Health codes require controlling certain pests in restaurants and other public places. In residential and urban situations, take action when the people living and working in these areas can no longer tolerate the pests. Pesticides used in these situations are often selected according to their safety, speed, and effectiveness. In agriculture and other commercial ventures, the economics of pest control must also be considered.

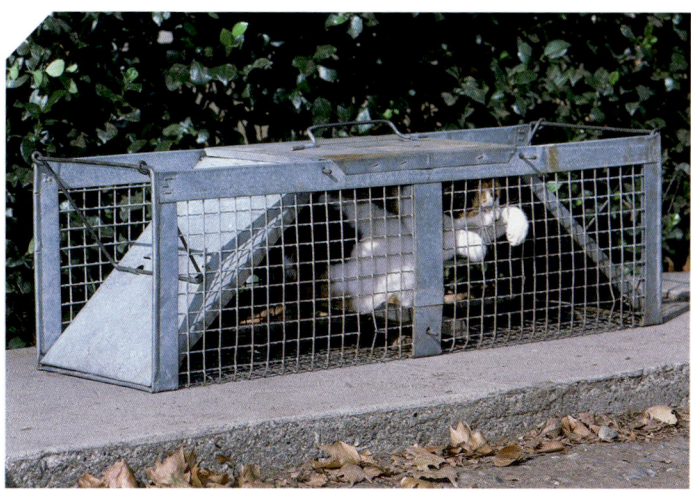

FIGURE 10-5

Live traps can be used to monitor the presence of small animals such as birds or rodents without injuring the animals. Domestic animals, such as this cat, may be accidentally trapped on occasion.

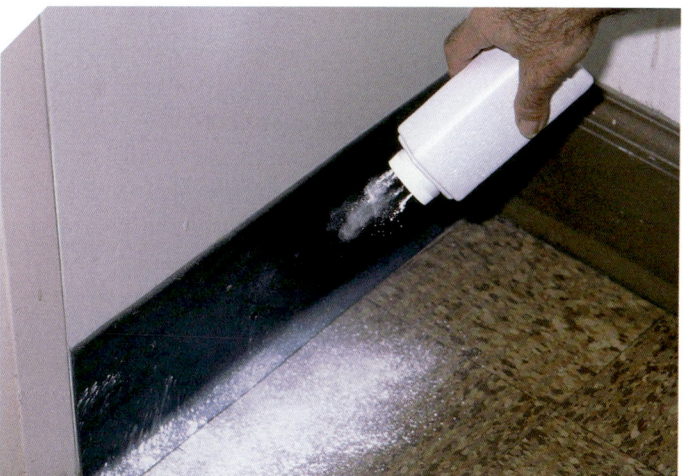

FIGURE 10-6

Tracking powders are used to monitor the activity of small rodents and insects. Toxicants sometimes are added to the powder to kill the animal when it cleans itself.

In most cases, a few individuals of a particular pest probably will not cause economic losses, but as their numbers increase, so does their damage. For some pests, mostly insects, nematodes, and mites, action thresholds (treatment thresholds) have been established. These indicate what population levels can be tolerated without loss and at what level a pesticide application will pay for itself. Such treatment thresholds must be flexible. If the market price for a crop fluctuates, for instance, the threshold of allowable pest damage can be changed to accommodate for this. When the price of pesticides increases or decreases, the tolerable pest injury is adjusted accordingly.

The estimates of pest population densities obtained from sampling are of little value if they cannot be meaningfully related to potential pest damage. The purpose of treatment thresholds is to relate monitoring results to the need for control action. Established decision-making guidelines are available for many pests of agricultural crops, commercial turf, and pests of home and landscape. For California, the UC IPM *Pest Management Guidelines* and the IPM manuals describe pest management actions suggested by University of California experts. Land grant universities in other states provide similar guidelines appropriate to their cropping systems. Use these guidelines to obtain descriptions of pests at a particular site and to assess the risk of damage. Follow the suggested monitoring or sampling procedures. Treatment timing and options using available biological, cultural, physical, or chemical controls are provided.

Treatment thresholds are not static; they are subject to revision based on new pests, new varieties, environmental constraints, new management practices (including new pesticide products), new marketing standards, and variations in commodity prices. Be prepared to be flexible. In new situations, set treatment thresholds low to offset unknown risks and increase monitoring; with experience and experimentation will come the opportunity to revise them.

Calculation and revision of treatment thresholds works well for most situations, except when managing disease. Because prevention is the aim of disease management programs, disease treatment guidelines must predict disease outbreak before it occurs. Therefore, monitoring focuses on quantifying conditions likely to promote pathogen infection, development, or spread.

In comprehensive weed management plans, pest control actions are based on the following measures:

- **Damage thresholds**, which identify the weed population at which a negative impact on the crop is detected.
- **Period thresholds**, which define the period during crop development when crop losses from weed interference are most likely to occur. For instance, certain weeds may seriously reduce the growth of crop seedlings but present much less threat once a crop has developed a substantial canopy.
- **Economic thresholds**, which measure the weed population densities at which control measures must be taken to prevent economic loss.
- **Action thresholds**, which represent the weed population level at which some action is needed to avoid crop loss (see Flint 2012).

For weeds, the most effective time to apply herbicides is before weed seed germination or when weeds are in the seedling stages. Often it is significantly easier and cheaper to apply herbicides before planting or when crop plants are very young. There is no "wait and see" time to allow higher populations to develop, and you should never allow weeds to go to seed. Usually, weeds most seriously affect new, small crop plants. The young plants are more susceptible to competition for light, water, and nutrients. For this reason, the crop stage may be as important as weed numbers in determining treatment needs.

Factors that influence herbicide use decisions include
- favorable weather conditions
- weed species
- growth stage of problem weeds
- growth stage of the crop or desirable vegetation
- amount and type of damage being caused by weeds
- resistance of certain weed species to herbicides

- soil type and condition
- herbicide persistence in the soil
- the economics of chemical control versus mechanical methods such as mowing or tilling

OTHER FACTORS INFLUENCING PESTICIDE USE DECISIONS

Other factors besides cost, effectiveness, and pest susceptibility often have an influence on your decision to use pesticides to control pests. These include

- potential for air pollution and groundwater contamination
- protecting endangered species
- produce packer, handler, or processor restrictions (for agricultural crops)
- cost of training pesticide handlers
- requirements to protect workers in treated areas
- compatibility of restricted-entry and preharvest intervals with necessary cultural practices
- limitations imposed by plant-back restrictions

Choosing the Right Pesticide

Describe how to select the most appropriate pesticide for a particular application.

Choosing the right pesticide or combination of pesticides can be a difficult task. Often you can choose from several pesticides to control a pest in a particular situation. To get information about pesticides for specific uses, consult

- sources of labels such as Internet-based label databases and manufacturers' websites
- University of California farm advisors and county agricultural commissioners
- licensed pest control advisers
- pesticide chemical handbooks
- University of California print and online publications, treatment guides, and *Pest Management Guidelines* (Fig. 10-7)

The University of California Statewide Integrated Pest Management Program's agricultural and urban *Pest Management Guidelines*, including pesticide recommendations, are accessible through the Internet at ipm.ucanr.edu (Fig. 10-8). Up-to-date pesticide use guidelines, pesticide

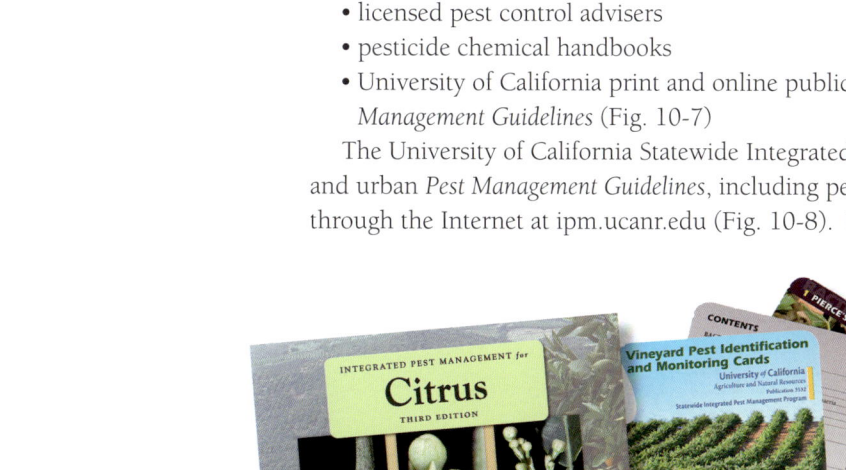

FIGURE 10-7

Pest management manuals are published by the University of California for many different types of crops. These are useful for selecting the proper chemical and other control methods.

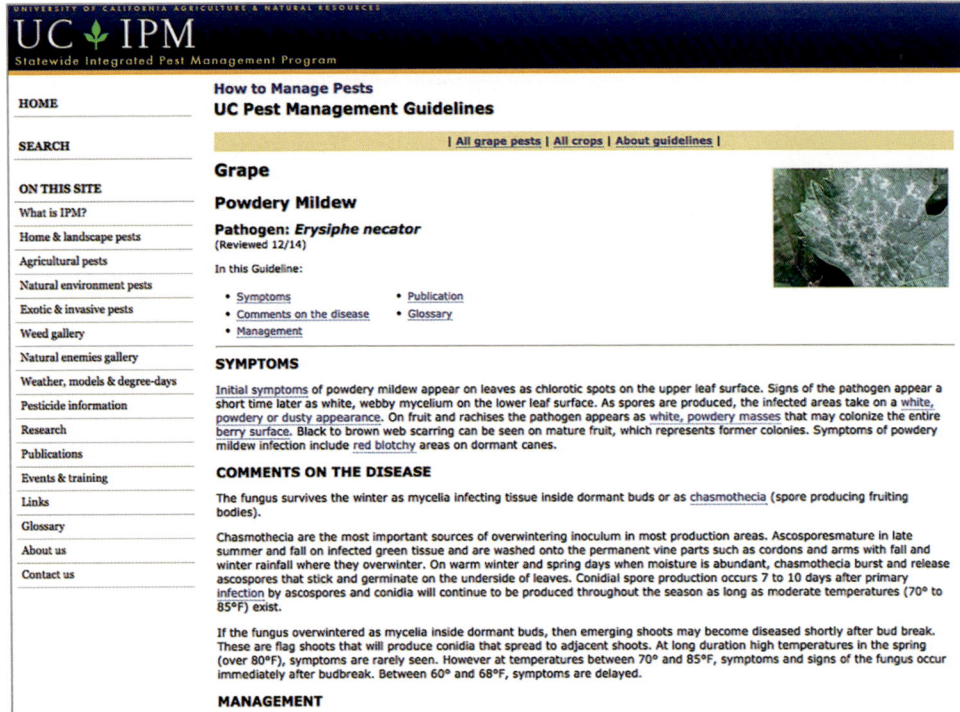

FIGURE 10-8

The University of California Statewide Integrated Pest Management Program maintains an up-to-date listing of pest management guidelines that can be accessed through the Internet.

toxicology information, and other pest management techniques are accessible through this website. You can also buy many UC IPM pest management publications from UC ANR Communication Services, anrcatalog.ucanr.edu. University of California county Cooperative Extension offices can also order these publications for you.

Factors to consider when choosing a pesticide include its
- selectivity
- toxicity
- available formulations
- persistence
- cost and efficacy
- ease of use and compatibility
- effects on beneficial organisms
- movement in and impact on the environment
- restricted-entry intervals and harvest restrictions
- resistance issues

PESTICIDE SELECTIVITY

Describe the factors that control a pesticide's selectivity.

Selectivity refers to the range of organisms affected by a pesticide. A broad-spectrum (or nonselective) pesticide kills a large range of pests as well as nontarget species. A selective pesticide controls a smaller group of more closely related organisms, often leaving beneficials and nontarget organisms unharmed. However, selectivity is not always desirable. There are some definite advantages to controlling multiple pests with a single nonselective pesticide. These include cheaper pesticides (due to a larger market for the manufacturer) and reduced application time and costs.

Pesticide selectivity is controlled by factors such as
- the penetration rate through an organism's outer body covering (or the cuticle of plant tissue)
- the speed at which the toxicant is metabolized by organisms

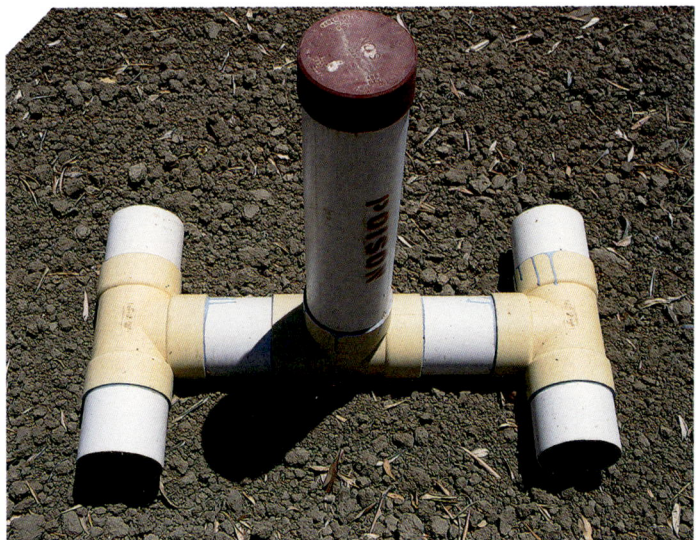

FIGURE 10-9

Use of a bait station, like this one being used for control of ground squirrels, is a method of selectively using pesticides. The bait station excludes most nontarget organisms.

- the way toxicants bind to tissues of different organisms
- the life stage of both target and nontarget organisms
- the pesticide's mode of action

Choose a pesticide or pesticide combination that is suitable for the pest species or range of pest species being controlled. Be sure the materials are capable of controlling the current life stage of these pests. You can determine the suitability of the pesticide by reading its label. If the target site is not on the label, you cannot legally use the material.

Pesticide Formulations. The pesticide formulation influences its selectivity. Granular formulations, for example, do not stick to dry foliage, increasing their selectivity to soil or aquatic pests. Applying a granular systemic formulation to the soil so plant roots take it up is a selective application practice. Pests feeding on plant tissue die, but most natural enemies and beneficial insects do not contact the pesticide. (However, if the pesticide translocates to the nectar or pollen, it may harm pollinators like honey bees and parasitic wasps that feed on nectar and/or pollen.) Liquid sprays and baits containing attractants improve the chances of target pests finding the pesticide. These substances make the pesticide more selective. Putting toxic baits in feeding stations to exclude nontarget animals increases selectivity. You can control squirrels with poisonous bait, for example, if the design of squirrel bait stations excludes dogs and livestock and protects children (Fig. 10-9). For more about pesticide formulations, see Chapter 3.

Adjuvants. You can use some adjuvants to change a pesticide's selectivity as well as to improve the effectiveness of certain pesticides. Use stickers, spreaders, and drift control agents to keep spray mixtures on target. Use surfactants to enhance uptake by target pests, and use attractants to make pesticides attractive specifically to target organisms. For more about adjuvants, see Chapter 3.

TOXICITY OF THE PESTICIDE TO BE USED

Each pesticide has a signal word that indicates the relative hazard of the pesticide. Hazards are modified by such factors as formulation type, persistence in the environment, and amount of pesticide used. For example, microencapsulated formulations are safer for applicators to use than wettable powders.

As a rule, and if you have a choice, select pesticides with the signal word that indicates the lowest level of hazard. DANGER indicates the highest level of hazard, and WARNING, the next-highest level. CAUTION pesticides are preferable and will usually be safer for you to work with. Also, they will often be less harmful to the environment, beneficial insects, natural enemies, and animals. Read all labeling, including the Safety Data Sheet, before making your final decision

TABLE 10-2

Comparison of pesticide formulations

Formulation	Mixing/loading hazards	Phytotoxicity	Effect on application equipment	Agitation required	Visible residues	Compatible with other formulations
wettable powders	dust inhalation	safe	abrasive	yes	yes	high
dry flowables/water-dispersible granules	safe	safe	abrasive	yes	yes	good
soluble powders	dust inhalation	usually safe	nonabrasive	no	some	fair
emulsifiable concentrates	spills and splashes	possible	may affect rubber pump parts	yes	no	fair
flowables	spills and splashes	possible	may affect rubber pump parts; also abrasive	yes	yes	fair
solutions	spills and splashes	safe	nonabrasive	no	no	fair
dusts	severe inhalation hazards	safe	—	yes	yes	–
granules and pellets	safe	safe	—	no	no	–
microencapsulated formulations	spills and splashes	safe	—	yes	–	fair

to ensure that you are working with the least-dangerous and most-effective pesticide for your situation.

PESTICIDE FORMULATIONS

Sometimes you must choose between two or more formulations of the same pesticide to control a target pest. When possible, make your selection based on the type of control desired, safety, cost, and other factors, such as those listed in Table 10-2. For example, emulsifiable formulations of insecticides usually provide quick control but have shorter residual action compared to wettable powders. Whenever you have a choice, consider the safety of pesticide applicators and helpers, as well as known environmental issues. For example, you should select a formulation with a low volatile organic compound (VOC) content whenever possible to reduce air pollution. Select the formulation that is least hazardous to people working or living in the application area. Consider the potential impact on pets, livestock, and poultry.

Evaluate the habits and growth patterns of each pest. Be sure the formulation is suitable for the pest's life stage. Pick a formulation that causes the least impact on the environment. Consider drift, runoff, wind, and rainfall, along with soil type and characteristics of the surrounding area. Cost also influences your selection. Finally, choose a formulation that is compatible with available application equipment.

PESTICIDE PERSISTENCE

Depending on the nature of the pest control problem, consider persistence characteristics when selecting a pesticide. Persistence is desirable in situations where reinfestations are constantly a problem, such as for termite control. Persistent pesticides may be more hazardous in areas where people live and work. Persistence also influences how pesticides move off the target site through leaching and runoff. To protect beneficial insects such as honey bees, low persistence is often as important as low toxicity. Persistence is an important consideration when choosing herbicides, because residues may damage subsequent crops.

Certain types of pesticides, such as some chlorinated hydrocarbons, persist in the environment for a long time. Other pesticides, such as many organophosphates, break down rapidly under normal environmental conditions. We measure the persistence of a pesticide by its half-life—the time it takes for half of what you apply to break down into its component parts. Besides the type of pesticide, other factors influence persistence. For instance, the amount of pesticide applied determines how much of the active ingredient remains after a time.

Pesticide formulation types affect persistence. Microencapsulated and granular formulations tend to release the active ingredient over a longer period. Therefore, only part of the material begins to break down at the moment of application. Pesticides dissolved in oils or petroleum solvents may volatilize more slowly than water-soluble materials and therefore persist longer. Wettable powders used as insecticides have a longer persistence than do emulsifiable concentrate mixtures.

The pH of the water used for mixing pesticides affects the breakdown speed. The pH of the soil or plant or animal tissues may have a similar influence. Tissue or soil that is highly alkaline (higher pH) tends to cause more rapid breakdown of some pesticides than neutral or acidic tissue or soil.

The physical nature of the surface being treated also influences pesticide persistence. Porous surfaces or soils high in organic matter absorb pesticide, reducing the amount of active ingredient available for pest control. Oily surfaces and waxy coatings on leaves and insect body coverings prevent uptake of the pesticide. The oils or waxes may even combine with the active ingredient, reducing toxicity and persistence.

Soil microorganisms break down many pesticides and influence the persistence of pesticides in the soil environment. These organisms include
- bacteria
- fungi
- protozoans
- algae

Water-soluble pesticides that percolate deeper into the soil break down more slowly than those that remain near the surface. This is mainly because fewer microorganisms are present at greater soil depths. Many pesticides break down faster in soils that have diverse populations of microorganisms. High levels of organic matter in the soil often slow degradation because the organic matter binds to the pesticide. This makes the pesticide unavailable to the microorganisms. Repeated use of the same pesticide in the soil can increase the breakdown rate. This increase is apparently the result of either
- a greater soil microorganism population
- an enzyme change in the microorganism population that makes the microorganisms more efficient in decomposing the specific pesticide

Weather affects persistence. For instance, wind and rain remove or dilute pesticides from target surfaces, lessening their effectiveness. High temperatures and humidity cause chemical changes in some compounds, accelerating breakdown. Sunlight produces photochemical reactions that decompose many pesticides. Cooler soil temperatures usually increase pesticide persistence.

COST AND EFFICACY OF PESTICIDE MATERIALS

The cost of a pesticide is an important factor, but be careful not to base selection on cost alone. Check labels to see what rates of active ingredient are required. Convert the cost per pound of active ingredient into cost per unit of area treated. You must balance cost with the degree of effectiveness that can be expected, as well as expected harvest dates. A pesticide that costs 30% more but gives 60% better control is often the better bargain unless it interferes with harvesting or other operations or you need a less-effective pesticide to protect natural enemies.

Unfortunately, the effectiveness of a pesticide is hard to measure, and unbiased opinions are difficult to obtain. Local environmental conditions and methods of application also influence efficacy. Often you must make a value judgment based on personal experience. Keep a notebook and evaluate the results after each application to increase your knowledge of pesticide efficacy.

Weather influences the quality of an application and the efficacy of pesticides. Rainfall shortly after an application can wash off or dilute sprays, while windy conditions produce drift. Some pesticides are more effective in controlling target pests when temperatures are within an optimal range. High temperatures cause some pesticides to be phytotoxic.

Effective pesticide use, therefore, involves
- timing to coincide with optimal weather conditions
- pest susceptibility
- protecting natural enemies, other nontarget organisms (including people and pets), and sensitive areas such as waterways and habitat for endangered species

Ideal conditions are not always possible during pesticide application. Often you must make compromises that may cause your application to be less effective.

EASE OF USE AND COMPATIBILITY WITH OTHER MATERIALS

Pesticides that are simple to use and are compatible with other pesticides have an advantage. Compatibility and ease of use also depend on
- how the pesticide is being used
- what the pesticide is mixed with
- the nature of the treatment area

EFFECTS ON BENEFICIAL INSECTS AND NATURAL ENEMIES

Always try to conserve beneficial insects and natural enemies. If you are using an integrated pest management program, consider how the selected pesticide will work within the goals of the program. This sometimes means compromising for less immediate control of the pest to achieve greater long-term control.

RESTRICTED-ENTRY AND PREHARVEST INTERVALS

The pesticide selected must work within constraints of legally established restricted-entry intervals and the allowable days before harvest. These limitations protect workers, consumers, and the public from excessive residues.

Making Pesticides More Selective

You must ensure that the pesticide you select targets only those organisms that are of concern in the ecosystem, leaving other organisms (like honey bees) unharmed. The way you determine dosage levels, mix and apply the selected pesticide, and time the application has an effect on an application's outcome.

To improve the effectiveness of any pesticide application, you must understand the impact of
- applying pesticides
- applying pesticides using more precise techniques
- applying pesticides using lower dosage rates

PESTICIDE APPLICATION TECHNIQUES AND METHODS

Use specific pesticide application techniques to improve coverage, reduce drift, and achieve better control of pests. Sometimes you can lower the amount of pesticide applied without sacrificing the quality of pest control. Choosing the right application techniques can also reduce human and environmental hazards.

Equipment Operation. Learn how to properly operate pesticide application equipment. For example, the ground speed must always remain constant to ensure even pesticide coverage. Check the nozzles frequently to make sure none have become clogged and that the spray pat-

USING PESTICIDES EFFECTIVELY 295

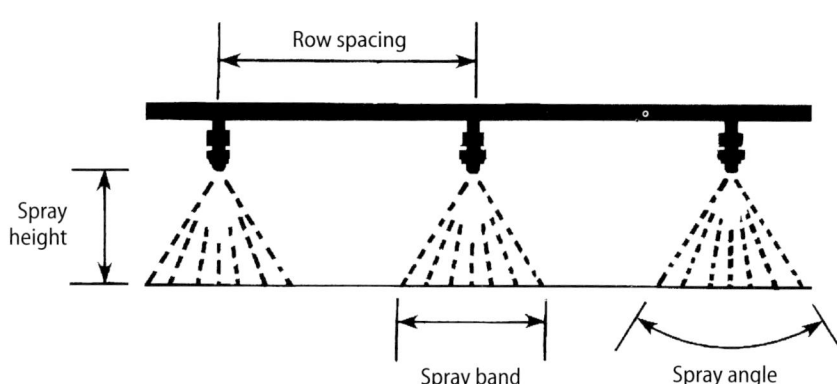

FIGURE 10-10

Boom height must be adjusted to correspond to the type of nozzle being used.

tern remains uniform. Shut off all nozzles during turns to prevent an uneven spray pattern and to prevent contaminating nontreatment areas. When injecting pesticides into the soil, shut off nozzles and raise the boom before making a turn. Leave enough room after the turn to bring equipment up to specified ground speed before restarting the pesticide flow.

Uneven ground causes booms on tractors or other equipment to bounce unless they are well supported and ground speed is slowed. Make sure the boom is always parallel to the ground during application. A tilted boom produces an uneven spray pattern. Adjust boom height to the recommended range specified by the type of nozzles being used (Fig. 10-10).

When using hand spray guns with high-pressure sprayers, keep the application uniform on all parts of the surfaces being treated. Make sure the spray reaches upper foliage or branches of trees or shrubs. Direct the spray to all sides of the plants, but avoid excessive runoff.

Keep the ground speed of air blast sprayers in balance with the volume of air being moved by the fans. This improves even dispersion of pesticide droplets within the plant canopy. Traveling too fast will result in poor coverage because the sprayer blower cannot completely displace the air surrounding the plant as the sprayer passes that plant.

When operating a backpack sprayer, walk at a regular pace and avoid uneven steps. Hold the nozzle steady and keep it a constant distance from the target surface. Maintain constant pump pressure wherever possible.

Preventing Gaps or Overlaps. Pesticide swaths must be uniform, without overlaps or gaps, to make the best economic use of spray materials. In some agricultural settings, the operator can follow furrows or rows to keep the application uniform. In open, unmarked areas, the operator must depend on some other method to prevent overlap or gaps. One method involves using foam markers to mark sprayed areas to prevent overlap or gaps in the application pattern. These markers, attached to the ends of a spray boom, intermittently leave a deposit of long-lasting foam. The operator aligns the application equipment to the foam trail left from a previous pass. In some situations, you can add a colored dye to the spray mixture to show where spraying has taken place.

Remembering the exact point where spraying stopped when leaving the application site to refill spray tanks is a problem. Unless you return to this location, there will be an uneven application. Marking devices help you avoid such problems. In some situations, you can tie colored surveyor's tape to plants to locate where the spraying stopped. In open areas, use marking flags to indicate the location. However, when applying hazardous pesticides, use a marking method that does not require you to contact treated surfaces. Remote-operated foam markers work well.

Electronic positioning devices, such as global positioning systems (GPS), are an accurate way of guiding pesticide application equipment (Fig. 10-11). As the cost of this equipment becomes more reasonable, its usefulness as an application tool increases. You enter swath width and direction of travel into a control unit mounted on the tractor near the operator. The positioning device monitors

Explain how a GPS unit can impact the effectiveness of pesticide applications.

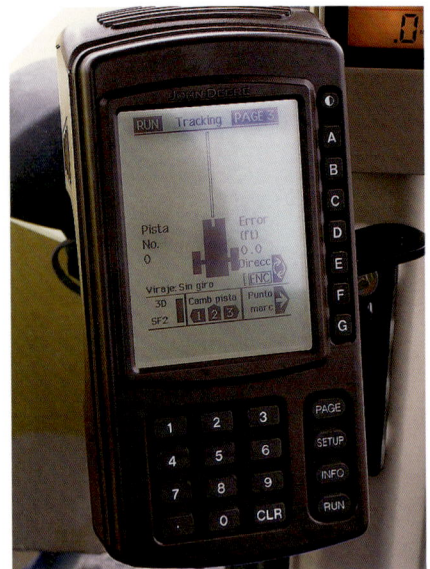

FIGURE 10-11

A GPS unit mounted on your sprayer will guide you back to the exact spot where spraying stopped.

the location of the sprayer and, through readout instruments, guides the operator. When you move the application equipment out of the treatment area for refilling, maintenance, or repairs, the positioning unit electronically records its last location. It can then guide you back to the exact spot where spraying stopped.

Spot Treatments. You can increase selectivity if you apply pesticides as spot treatments rather than to an entire area. In addition, you can reduce the amount of pesticide used by 70 to 90% through spot treatment methods. For example, some weeds may grow in clumps scattered throughout a field after you control all the other weeds by cultivation or with herbicides. Spot treatment involves treating just these clumps or patches rather than the whole field. Periodically, insects and mites congregate in a few areas before dispersing more generally, especially if the infestation is just beginning. Control these pests by treating only the infested plants. In landscaped areas, pests may occur only on certain plant species. Avoid applying pesticides to uninfested plants. Frequently, you need to treat only the edges of fields or landscaped areas for invading pests.

You can use special types of application equipment to improve the effectiveness of spot treatments. Field crop sprayers equipped with chemical injection pumps allow the operator to mix several different pesticides for the same application. The equipment automatically meters concentrated, liquid formulations and dilutes these with appropriate amounts of water.

If you adjust rope wick applicators to wipe herbicides onto target weeds growing above the crop, these become selective, spot treatment devices. Compact, hand-held sprayers allow operators to efficiently apply pesticides as spot treatments to small areas. All-terrain cycles (ATCs) eliminate walking and speed up spot treatment applications.

Band Treatments. In orchards and vineyards, you can apply herbicides as bands within the tree or vine rows. This leaves an area between the rows with a ground cover of weeds or a planted cover crop that you can mow or cultivate. You use only about one-fourth as much herbicide per acre with this method (Fig. 10-12). Mowed weeds between trees or vines reduce soil compaction, prevent erosion, reduce dust, and lower orchard or vineyard floor temperatures. However, weeds in untreated strips may compete with the trees or vines for water and nutrients under certain circumstances.

FIGURE 10-12

Strip spraying is a way of controlling weeds in tree or vine rows while reducing the use of herbicides. Only about one-quarter to one-third of the actual acreage needs to be treated. The area between rows is usually mowed and maintained as a ground cover.

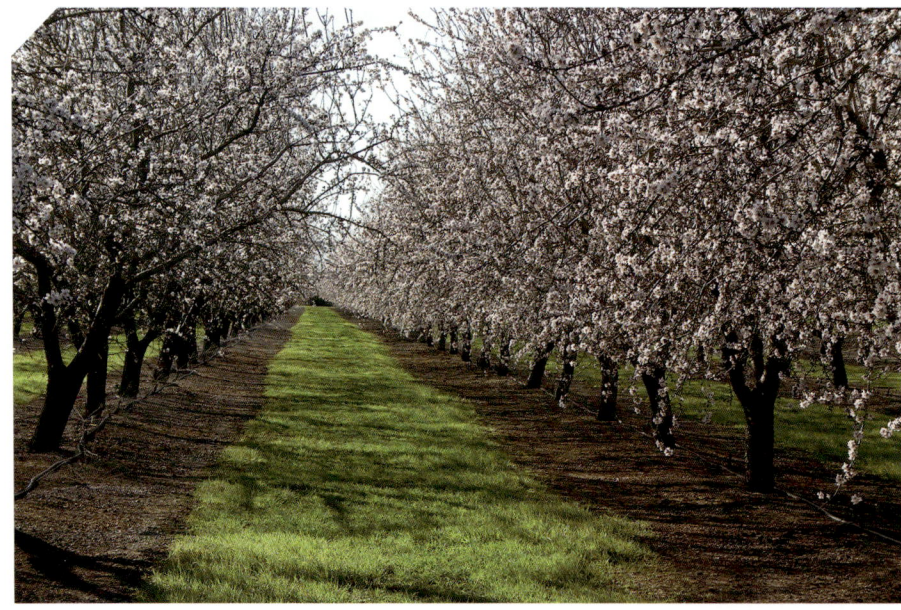

FIGURE 10-13

Applying pesticides to alternate rows or alternate blocks is sometimes done when several sprays are required for control of the same pest. This technique reduces the amount of pesticide used each time by 50%; it also provides locations in the treatment area for the protection of natural enemies.

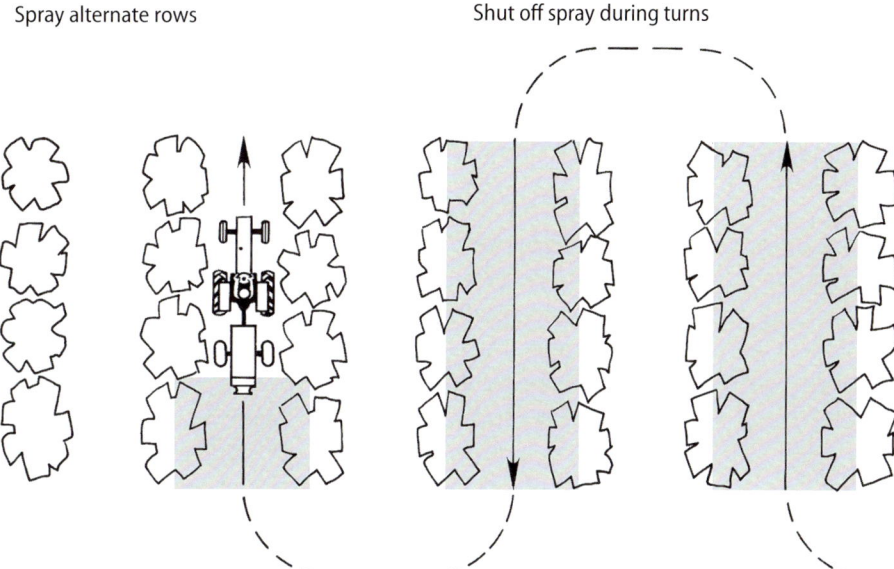

Treating Alternate Rows or Blocks. Spraying alternate rows or blocks in orchards, vineyards, or field crops reduces the amount of pesticide applied. This technique provides some protection to natural enemies in the untreated sections. Use this technique when you need to make frequent treatments for the same pest. Examples include sprays for insects or mites that occur over an extended period. Spray the untreated rows or blocks during the following application (Fig. 10-13). You use only half as much material per application, although the pesticide dilution rate does not change.

Low-Volume Applications. Techniques using low-volume and ultra-low-volume sprays improve the efficiency of pesticide application in certain situations. Because low-volume applications use only about one-fourth as much water carrier, spray mixtures are more concentrated. Ultra-low-volume applications involve highly concentrated mixtures of pesticide combined with a carrier such as vegetable oil. You need special application equipment for ultra-low-volume applications. Sometimes you can lower pesticide amounts by about one-third with low-volume applications and by as much as one-half with ultra-low-volume applications. However, keep the application consistent with label requirements or current University of California recommendations. You can also realize savings of time, fuel, labor, and water. Pesticide applications must be more accurate and calibration more precise when making low-volume applications. Operators using ultra-low-volume equipment work with more concentrated mixtures. This increases the hazards and makes wearing label-prescribed PPE even more important to safeguard your health.

PESTICIDE DOSAGE LEVEL

Sometimes you can lessen the injury to natural enemies and other beneficial organisms by reducing the amount of active ingredient applied to the treatment area for control of certain insects or mites. Use this technique only if the lower dosages are effective against target pests; otherwise it can contribute to an increased population of resistant individuals. Be sure the rate is consistent with pesticide label requirements, current University of California recommendations, or a pest control adviser's written recommendation. Protecting natural enemies helps in long-term management of some insect and mite pest problems, which further reduces the need for additional pesticides. Lowering dosage levels only works when adequate numbers of natural enemies are present before treatment.

APPLICATION TIMING

Proper application timing is important for controlling target pests as well as protecting natural enemies and beneficial insects. Because some pesticides are more effective at different life stages of the pest, time applications with the most susceptible stage. Understanding the biology of the pest will help you determine its susceptible life stages and decide whether a pesticide application will work. You must know a pest's habits, that is, when it is most active and likely to be affected by a pesticide application. Equally, you must know the habits of honey bees and other nontarget organisms so you can avoid the consequences of damaging the ecosystem, such as pest resurgence. See "Protecting Nontarget Organisms" later in this chapter for more about timing applications to avoid bees and other beneficial insects.

Life Stage. The life stage of a target organism influences its response to a pesticide. For instance, young plants are generally more susceptible to herbicides than older ones. Some herbicides are most effective on perennial plants just beginning to flower. These same herbicides are less effective on plants that have not yet begun to flower or have completed their flowering stage. Perennial weeds are more difficult to control once they have developed rhizomes or nutlets. Insects go through several life stages, including eggs, nymphs or larvae, pupae (in some orders), and finally adults. Each insect life stage has different susceptibilities to insecticides. Differences are due to biological and physical characteristics, feeding habits, and the physical location of the organism. Similarly, the success of rodent control with toxic baits depends on the rodent's life stage. For instance, it is always best to initiate control methods prior to the rodent's mating season in order to disrupt or prevent breeding. Be aware that a vertebrate pest's food preferences depend on the time of year, which influences the acceptability of the selected bait. Life stage is also important in disease control efforts. Successful control of pathogens that cause plant disease depends on accurate timing to break the disease cycle. For instance, to control powdery mildew on apricots, you must spray before symptoms are present to disrupt the pathogen's life cycle and prevent infection.

The life stage of nontarget plants in the treatment area is another important consideration. Some herbicides, for example, may be toxic to crop plants as well as weeds once the crop plants have reached a certain growth stage. Check pesticide labels for restrictions on using pesticides during inappropriate life stages of nontarget plants.

Insecticides and miticides applied while perennial plants are dormant may also protect nontarget and beneficial organisms. This technique is often an effective control method for some species of plant-feeding mites, aphids, scales, and other insects that overwinter in dormant plants.

In order to prevent nematode damage in crops and landscapes, your application must be carefully timed to precede or coincide with planting. Nematicides applied before or during planting are much more effective than treatments initiated later in the growth cycle of crops or other desirable plants.

MODE OF ACTION AND PESTICIDE UPTAKE

Pesticides are often grouped by mode of action, which tells you how a pesticide affects the organism it targets and which part of the pest (i.e. stomach, skin, roots) is affected. Knowing how and where a pesticide acts will help you determine the best way to apply that pesticide so that it reaches the intended pest and minimizes damage to other organisms. Consideration of a pesticide's mode of action is also important when you are faced with resistant pests. You can minimize pesticide resistance in target organisms by alternating pesticides with differing modes of action (see "Resistance Management Strategies" later in this chapter for ways to manage pesticide resistance).

Various terms describe methods and routes of pesticide uptake. Pesticides with contact activity pass through the target organism's outer covering (e.g., plant cuticle, arthropod cuticle, or vertebrate skin). Some insecticides and rodenticides are stomach poisons: the target organism must ingest the toxin, which absorbs through linings of the pest's mouth or intestinal tract. Other pesticides have fumigant activity and pass as vapors into the tissues of the target plant or animal. The fumigant enters through respiration or breathing channels or by passing through skin or cuticle. Pesticides can also be taken up systemically, translocating throughout the target plant. Poast (sethoxydim) works this way to kill weeds. Certain pesticides exhibit all these types of uptake. Remember that a pesticide's formulation, as well as weather and soil conditions, can also influence pesticide uptake. For a more thorough treatment of mode of action, see Chapter 3.

Understanding the structural differences, protective coatings, and habits of the pest, as well as how and where a pesticide acts, provides insight into how the pesticide will move into and effect the target organism. You can use this combined knowledge of mode of action and pesticide uptake to increase your application's effectiveness.

Mixing Pesticides

Mixing pesticides requires focus and attention to detail. Forgetting a step in the process or using too much (or too little) of the formulation can cause costly, and sometimes dangerous, problems. Below, you will find an explanation of techniques that can help you mix pesticides safely and effectively. You will also find information about chemical changes that can occur when combining two or more pesticides, as well as resources you can use to determine whether the chemicals you are mixing are compatible.

Effective Methods

Before preparing a tank mix, be sure the spray tank is thoroughly clean and contains no sediments or residues. Evaluate the tank mixture by performing the compatibility test described below.

Testing for Incompatibility

Mixtures of pesticides may be incompatible and may separate or curdle. This clogs spray equipment and wastes the pesticide material. Before preparing a full tank, mix small quantities of the pesticides you will be using to test for incompatibility. Sidebar 10-1 provides instructions for a simple compatibility test that requires only a small investment of time. This simple jar test will not help you determine whether the mixture has changed the chemical effectiveness of any or all the pesticides, however.

When combining chemicals for either the compatibility test or for mixing in the spray tank, add formulations using the following method:

1. Add some of the diluent (usually water) and then add some adjuvants (like surfactants).
2. Add wettable and other powders and water-dispersible granules.
3. Agitate thoroughly and add the remaining diluent.
4. Add liquid products (like flowables and certain adjuvants) and water-soluble concentrates.
5. Add emulsifiable concentrates.

For example, when combining a water-soluble concentrate with a wettable powder, always add the wettable powder first. When mixing an emulsifiable concentrate with a dry flowable, add the dry flowable first (see McDonald 1991).

Field Incompatibility

Sometimes tank mixes seem compatible during testing and after mixing in the spray tank, but problems arise during application. This is known as field incompatibility. The temperature of the water in the tank can cause this problem. It could also be due to water impurities. Sometimes the amount of time the spray mixture has been in the tank causes field incompatibility. Occasionally there are variations among different lots of pesticide chemicals that are great enough to cause an incompatibility. In case of field incompatibility, increased agitation is usually sufficient to recombine the mixture.

Explain how to determine whether two or more pesticides will be compatible for tank mixing.

Describe mixing procedures for
- *a single pesticide.*
- *two or more pesticides (tank mix)*

SIDEBAR 10-1

COMPATIBILITY TEST FOR PESTICIDE MIXTURES

WARNING

Always wear the label-required PPE when pouring or mixing pesticides. Perform this test in a safe area away from food and sources of ignition. Pesticides used in this test should be put into the spray tank once testing is completed. Rinse all utensils and jars and pour rinsate into the spray tank. Do not use utensils or jars for any other purpose after they have contacted pesticides.

TEST PROCEDURE

1. Measure 1 pint of the intended spray water into a clear quart glass jar.
2. Adjust pH if necessary (see Sidebar 3-1).
3. Add ingredients in the following order. Stir well each time an ingredient has been added.

Material to be added	Amount of material to add per 100 gallons of spray mixture
1. Surfactants, compatibility agents, and activators	1 teaspoon for each pint
2. Wettable powders and dry-flowable formulations	1 tablespoon for each pint
3. Water-soluble concentrates or solutions	1 teaspoon for each pint
4. Emulsifiable concentrate and flowable formulations	1 teaspoon for each pint
5. Soluble powder formulations	1 teaspoon for each pint
6. Remaining adjuvants	1 teaspoon for each pint

4. After mixing, let the solution stand for 15 minutes. Stir well and observe the results.

TEST RESULTS

Compatible	Smooth mixture, combines well after stirring. Chemicals can be used together in the spray tank.
Incompatible	Separation, clumps, grainy appearance. Settles out quickly after stirring. Follow instructions below to try to resolve incompatibility; otherwise do not mix this combination in the spray tank.

RESOLVING INCOMPATIBILITY

1. Add 6 drops of compatibility agent and stir well. If mixture appears compatible, allow it to stand for 1 hour, stir well, and check it again. If the mixture appears incompatible, repeat one or two more times, using 6 drops of compatibility agent each time.
2. If incompatibility still persists, dispose of this mixture, clean the jar, and repeat the above steps, but add 6 drops of compatibility agent to the water before anything else is added.
3. If the mixture is still incompatible, do not mix the chemicals in the spray tank. To overcome this problem, you might consider the following alternatives:
   - Use a different water supply.
   - Change brands or formulations of chemicals.
   - Change the order of mixing.
4. Make only one change at a time, and perform a complete test, as described above, before making another change.
   Do not mix the chemicals in the spray tank if incompatibility cannot be resolved.

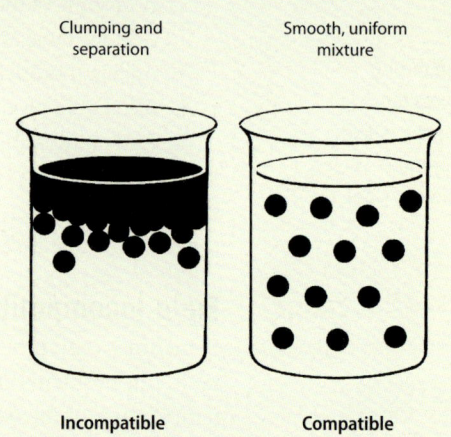

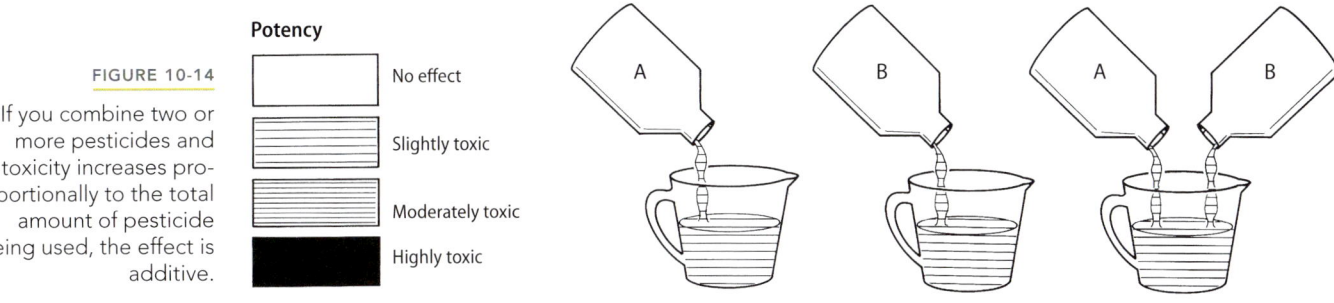

FIGURE 10-14

If you combine two or more pesticides and toxicity increases proportionally to the total amount of pesticide being used, the effect is additive.

Potency:
- No effect
- Slightly toxic
- Moderately toxic
- Highly toxic

Additive effect

Resolving Compatibility Problems in the Spray Tank

You should try several things if pesticide incompatibility develops in the spray tank. First, increase agitation and try to break up the aggregates with a water stream to get the mixture recirculating. If the material still separates, contact your pesticide dealer for an appropriate compatibility agent. Add the agent to the tank and continue agitation.

Changing filter screens to a larger size and cleaning them frequently may help eliminate some of the clumping. If these steps do not resolve the problem, dilute the mixture with additional water and filter off larger particles. If you cannot spray the mixture onto an application site, place it into an appropriate container for disposal. Follow the same procedures you would use to dispose of any other unused pesticide.

CHEMICAL CHANGES WITH PESTICIDES AND PESTICIDE COMBINATIONS

In some tank mixes, pesticides may mix properly in solution but the effectiveness or toxicity of the pesticides in the mixture changes. These changes are due to chemical, rather than physical, reactions between combined pesticides, impurities, or the water used for mixing. Such changes are difficult to recognize because you cannot see them.

Additive Effect

Combining two or more pesticides may result in an additive effect: the toxicity of the combination is no greater than if you used an equal amount of only one of the materials. For example, you apply two insecticides—Compound A and Compound B—at the rate of ½ pound of each per acre. The result on the target insect is no different than if you applied 1 pound of Compound A or 1 pound of Compound B. The results are greater, however, than if you applied just ½ pound of Compound A or ½ pound of Compound B (Fig. 10-14).

Greater Than Additive Effect

Sometimes the toxicity of pesticides being mixed increases above what you expected through an additive effect. You may notice three types of changes: potentiation or synergism, illustrated in Figure 10-15, or a coalescent effect.

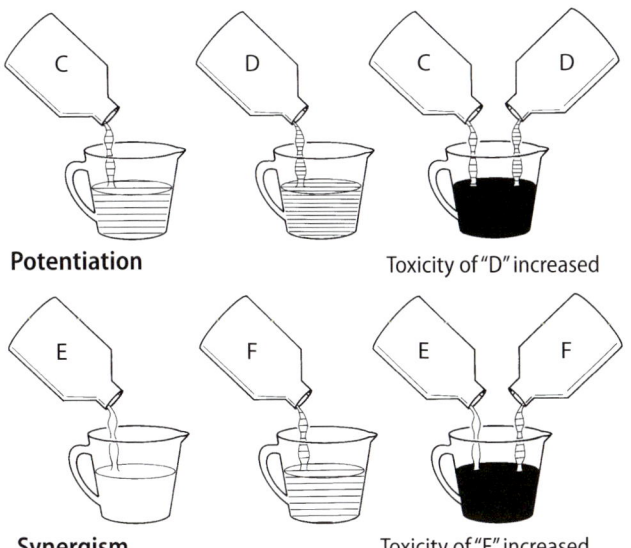

Potentiation — Toxicity of "D" increased

Synergism — Toxicity of "F" increased

FIGURE 10-15

When combined pesticides produce a response greater than what would be expected by the additive effect, the response may be due to potentiation or synergism, as illustrated here.

FIGURE 10-16

Combining pesticides may cancel or reduce the toxic effect of one or both of the components. This is known as an antagonistic effect.

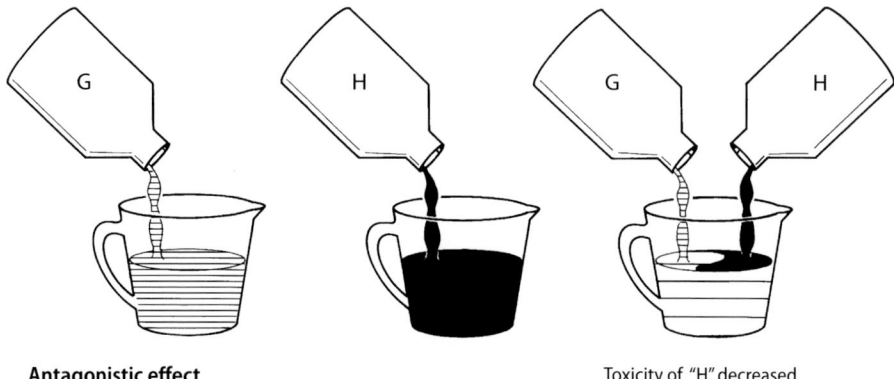

Antagonistic effect　　　　　　　　　　　　　　　Toxicity of "H" decreased

Potentiation. Potentiation increases the toxicity of a pesticide because something mixed with it lowers the pest's tolerance to that chemical. Impurities in malathion, for example, can make malathion more toxic because the impurities inactivate enzymes produced by the pest that normally detoxify malathion. In mixtures of two or more pesticides, one compound may potentiate another in the same way. The result is an effect greater than the expected additive effect.

Synergism. Synergism is another way pesticides increase in toxicity. The chemical you mix with the pesticide may or may not have pesticidal properties but is a synergist that may slow the breakdown of the pesticide or increase its uptake by the pest. For example, piperonyl butoxide has no insecticidal properties, but it is commonly used to increase the toxicity of pyrethrum insecticides. By using this synergist, less of the more-expensive active ingredient is needed.

Coalescent Effect. A coalescent effect occurs when the toxic response from a pesticide mixture is unlike the expected response from either pesticide alone. The combined materials have formed a chemical with a different mode of action.

Antagonistic Effect

Antagonism occurs when a mixture reduces the toxic effect of one or more of the pesticides. For example, if you combine two pesticides, one pesticide may allow the target organism to resist, slow down, or degrade the toxic action of the other (Fig. 10-16).

Deactivation

Deactivation may take place before a spray reaches the intended destination. This usually happens in the spray tank when you mix the pesticides. The quality of the water being used in the spray mixture may cause breakdown, or hydrolysis, of some pesticides. Alkaline water (high pH) commonly shortens pesticide half-life. Sometimes one of the pesticide compounds may change the pH of the spray mixture. Also, one compound may alter or neutralize an electrical charge of the other to reduce its effectiveness. This problem can be especially serious when using herbicides.

Delayed Mixtures

If two pesticides are interactive, problems can occur even when you apply one of them several weeks after the other. An earlier spray may cause deactivation of the second spray. The combination of the two sprays may injure treated plants (become phytotoxic). Check pesticide labels for this type of incompatibility.

Damage to Treated Plants or Surfaces

Pesticide combinations may work well to control target organisms but still create problems. The interaction between the chemicals may cause spotting or staining of sprayed surfaces. They may even damage plant foliage or produce. To avoid this problem, test the mixture on a small area first and observe the results. Chemicals affect some surfaces less than others. Similarly, some species of plants are more sensitive than others. Plant phytotoxicity, however, may not be apparent until several weeks after application.

Sources of Information on Compatibility

Although there are many good reasons to use tank mixes (see "Pesticide Mixtures" in Chapter 3 for a list of the benefits), you must avoid combinations that could damage sprayed surfaces or cause problems with the application equipment. You can get information on pesticide mixtures in the following ways.

Labels

Pesticide labels provide compatibility information for tank-mixing. Many pesticide labels specify other pesticides that can or cannot be mixed with them. These may be specific compounds or general classes of chemicals, such as sulfur-containing compounds or alkaline materials. When making tank mixes, be sure to follow all the instructions on all labels.

Pesticide Manufacturers

You can get specific information on compatibility by visiting the pesticide manufacturer's website or e-mailing the manufacturer or its field representative. Pesticide labels and Safety Data Sheets provide manufacturers' contact information. Chemical dealers usually have the names, e-mail addresses, and telephone numbers of local field representatives. Alternatively, you can find the company using your preferred Internet search engine.

Pesticide Resistance

Explain why pesticide resistance is a problem.

Pesticide resistance is a genetic trait a pest individual inherits that allows it to survive an application of a pesticide that kills most other individuals in the population when applied at label rates. After surviving the pesticide application, the resistant individual then passes the gene(s) for resistance on to the next generation. The more the pesticide is used, the more susceptible individuals are eliminated and the larger the proportion of resistant individuals grows until the pest population is no longer effectively controlled (Fig. 10-17).

FIGURE 10-17

Pest populations develop resistance to pesticides through genetic selection. (A) Certain individuals in a pest population are less susceptible to a pesticide spray than other individuals. (B) These less-susceptible pests are more likely to survive an application and to produce less-susceptible progeny. (C) After repeated applications, the pest population consists primarily of resistant or less-susceptible individuals, and applying the same material or other materials with the same mode of action is no longer effective.

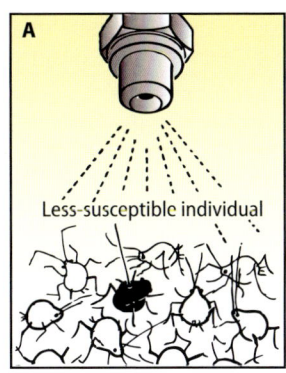
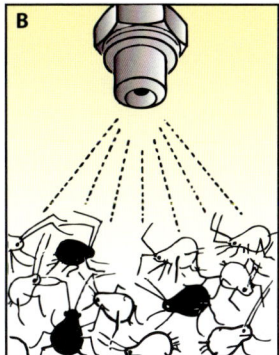
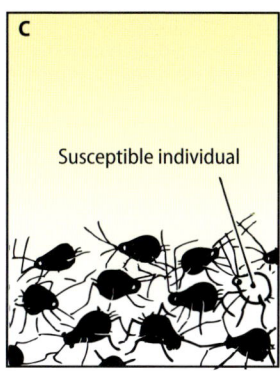

Pesticide resistance is most common in arthropods, with over five hundred species of resistant insects and mites reported worldwide. However, pesticide resistance is increasing with other types of pests as well, with certain populations of bacteria, fungi, vertebrates, and weeds becoming resistant to greater numbers of pesticide products. Frequently, resistance develops in only certain local populations (biotypes) of a species. Elsewhere, populations of that species may still be susceptible to that pesticide.

Several mechanisms may be involved in the development of pesticide resistance. Resistant individuals may naturally possess enzymes that break down the pesticide rapidly or have behaviors that reduce their exposure, or the pesticide may not affect them in the same way as other individuals of their population.

You must also understand the methods used to detect the presence of resistant pests and how to use them. The most important method you can use to fight the development of resistance is monitoring. Monitoring helps you detect tolerance to pesticides in pest populations before resistance becomes widespread. Early detection provides the opportunity to integrate other pest management options to prevent or reduce selection for resistance. For example, combining different weed control practices such as increased cultivation and crop rotation with the use of herbicides can reduce the occurrence of resistant weed biotypes. By alternating pesticide treatments with different modes of action, it may be possible to use some pesticides for a longer period of time because a single pesticide mode of action is no longer the principal source of pest mortality.

Once pesticide resistance has been confirmed, detection and management strategies aid in pesticide selection and in the detection of cross-resistance and multiple resistance.

Factors Influencing Selection for Resistance

Generally, the development of pesticide resistance is similar for insects, mites, fungi, bacteria, weeds, and vertebrates. It involves a combination of genetic, biological, and other operational factors.

> List the factors that contribute to pesticide resistance.

Genetic Factors. Genetic factors that influence the development of resistance are how the organism inherits resistance and how many of the individuals in the population have the genes for resistance. Individuals with the resistance gene are able to tolerate that pesticide and will be able to survive and reproduce. Individuals without the resistance gene cannot tolerate the pesticide and will die. If resistance genes are common, the population inherits them easily. Resistance will spread quickly and may be difficult to manage.

Once a pest exhibits resistance to one pesticide, resistance to others may follow more quickly. This phenomenon, called cross-resistance, occurs when the pest is resistant to two or more pesticides at the same time. Multiple resistance occurs when pests have several distinct mechanisms to withstand pesticide chemicals, allowing them to tolerate several classes of pesticides that are not related to each other chemically. These mechanisms can be focused on the target site (e.g., nerves) of the pest (sometimes called target-site resistance), or cause the organism to detoxify the pesticide after contact or ingestion (nontarget-site resistance). Sidebar 10-2 explains the difference between target-site and nontarget-site resistance.

Populations of resistant individuals within a species are called resistant strains or resistant biotypes. A biotype is any population within a species that has a distinct genetic variation from other populations. Sometimes resistant biotypes may dominate in some areas but not be present in other areas.

Biological Factors. The biology of the pest species influences the rate at which resistance will occur. Biological characteristics include the life span of the pest, its reproductive capabilities, and mobility. Typically, a short-lived, rapidly developing, immobile pest population that produces a large number of offspring will develop resistance rapidly. Resistance evolves more slowly when there are untreated refuges available or when the pest species

---

SIDEBAR 10-2

Types of Herbicide Resistance

There are two types of herbicide resistance to be aware of: target-site and nontarget-site resistance.

TARGET-SITE RESISTANCE

- Most sprayed plants will appear uninjured or only slightly injured.
- Only a few plants will have injury.
- Susceptible plants may still be present, resulting in a few dying or injured plants.

A change in the herbicide rate (i.e., using a full rate or doubling the rate) will not make a difference in the control of weeds exhibiting target-site resistance. To manage these weeds using an herbicide, you must rotate to an herbicide with a different mode of action.

NONTARGET-SITE RESISTANCE

- Most sprayed plants will appear slightly injured to nearly dead.
- Most of the plants will have injury.
- Susceptible plants will be present, especially when resistance is caught early.

Management of weeds with this type of resistance depends on the underlying mechanism of nontarget-site resistance and may involve a change in herbicide rate or management practices.

(insect, pathogen, or vertebrate) is highly mobile. In weeds, resistance is favored by high rates of seed production and germination. High seed production increases the probability of a mutation that may lead to resistance through the process of natural selection.

Operational Factors. Operational factors can be controlled by people. Those that favor resistance include the pesticide's type, persistence, mode of action, and application method (the rate applied, frequency, whether it was mixed with other pesticides, and timing in relation to the dynamics of the pest population).

Management decisions involving these factors can promote or reduce resistance. Repeated use of a single pesticide increases the risk of resistance, especially when other control methods such as biological or cultural controls or pesticides with a different mode of action that would eliminate resistant individuals are not used. Table 10-3 lists the modes of action of different herbicide classes and the number of resistant weed species currently known.

TABLE 10-3

Summary of number of weeds resistant to various herbicide classes in 2016*

Herbicide group**	Site of action	HRAC group	WSSA group	Example herbicide	Total # resistant weeds
ALS inhibitors	inhibition of acetolactate synthase (ALS)	B	2	chlorsulfuron	158
photosystem II inhibitors	inhibition of photosynthesis at photosystem II	C1	5	atrazine	73
ACCase inhibitors	inhibition of acetyl CoA carboxylase (ACCase)	A	1	fluazifop-p-butyl	47
synthetic auxins	synthetic auxins	O	4	2,4-D	32
bipyridyliums	photosytem I electron diversion	D	22	paraquat	31
ureas and amides	inhibition of photosynthesis at photosystem II	C2	7	diuron	28
glycines	inhibition of EPSP synthase	G	9	glyphosate	32
dinitroanilines and others	microtubule assembly inhibition	K1	3	oryzalin	12
thiocarbamates and others	inhibition of lipid synthesis—not ACCase inhibitions	N	8, 16, 26	triallate	10
chloroacetamides and others	inhibition of cell division	K3	15	alachlor	4
PPO inhibitors	inhibition of protoporphyrinogen oxidase	E	14	oxyfluorfen	8
triazoles, ureas, isoxazolidiones	bleaching: inhibition of carotenoid biosynthesis (unknown target)	F3	13	clomazone	5
nitriles and others	inhibition of photosynthesis at photosystem II	C3	6	bromoxynil	4
caratenoid biosynthesis inhibitors	bleaching: inhibition of carotenoid biosynthesis at the phytoene desaturase step (PDS)	F1	12	norflurazon	4
4-HPPD inhibitors	bleaching: inhibition of 4-hydroxyphenyl-pyruvate dioxygenase (4-HPPD)	F2	28	mesotrione	2
glutamine synthase inhibitors	inhibits glutamine synthase	H	28	glufosinate-ammonium	2
mitosis inhibitors	inhibition of mitosis/microtubule polymerization inhibitor	K2	23	chlorpropham	1
cellulose inhibitors	inhibition of cell wall (cellulose) synthesis	L	20, 21, 27	dichlobenil	3
organoarsenicals	unknown	Z	17	MSMA	2
Total number of unique herbicide-resistant weed biotypes					458

Notes: *See weedscience.org for the most recent figures from the international Herbicide Resistance Action Committee (HRAC) and the Weed Science Society of America (WSSA).

Some a.i.'s or products listed may not be currently registered as pesticides or may have had their registration cancelled.

Resistance Management Strategies

To slow the process of natural selection that leads to the development of resistance, implement an IPM program and apply pesticides only when necessary. Use control methods other than pesticides where feasible. Resistant cultivars, biological and cultural controls, and other nonchemical management tactics can be used to reduce the number of pesticide applications and to reduce selection for pesticide-resistant individuals. By using monitoring information and economic thresholds, pesticide applications can be more precisely timed, resulting in fewer applications at more appropriate rates. Monitoring also allows you to select pesticides that specifically target the most bothersome pests, leaving other, less problematic pests alone and reducing the potential for resistance developing across all pests present. Preferred pesticides are selective and short-lived. If repeat applications are required, rotate applications with pesticides that have different modes of action.

Consider the history of pest management practices, especially pesticide use at the site, to reduce selection for resistance. For instance, the risk of resistance is likely to increase in sites where broad-spectrum insecticides have been continually used. Repeat applications of these materials intensify selection pressures and eliminate the natural enemies that may control some insect pests. Using pesticides with different modes of action, on the other hand, may result in lower selection pressure and lower incidences of resistance. This can be very important in managing herbicide and fungicide resistance where mixtures of materials or alternating materials with different modes of action are used to prevent or overcome resistance.

To learn about individual pesticides' mode of action and specific information about managing pesticide resistance, consult the relevant website of the International Resistance Action Committee: the Insecticide Resistance Action Committee (IRAC), irac-online.org; the Herbicide Resistance Action Committee (HRAC), hracglobal.com; or the Fungicide Resistance Action Committee (FRAC), frac.info. For weeds, you may also wish to visit the International Survey of Herbicide Resistant Weeds website, weedscience.org.

Modification of management practices to reduce the development of resistance has been demonstrated by the management of spider mite resistance in San Joaquin Valley cotton in California. Acaricide applications are made one or two times per season using a number of different materials to minimize selection pressure. In addition, broad-spectrum persistent insecticides are avoided to preserve and encourage natural enemy populations. The result is that high levels of acaricide resistance are not common in San Joaquin Valley cotton fields. However, to ensure that these materials remain effective, resistance management practices must be used in conjunction with other IPM strategies.

Preventing Offsite Movement of Pesticides

Preventing Pesticide Drift

Drift can be defined simply as the airborne movement of pesticides to nontarget areas. Offsite movement can be in the form of spray droplet drift, vapor drift, or particle (dust) drift. Studies have shown that a significant percentage of pesticides may never reach the intended target site because of drift, so you must be on the lookout for conditions that favor drift. By avoiding these conditions, it is possible to reduce drift to a tolerable level (see Flint 2012). The most significant factors affecting drift include
- wind speed and direction
- droplet size
- applicator (liquid or dust) proximity to the edges of the treated area
- release height

Assessing Weather Conditions

Significant local variations in weather are common, especially for wind, rain, and temperature, and the most accurate weather observations for a specific location will come from a weather station installed at that site. In-field weather stations placed in key areas may be part of a network of weather stations that use radio telemetry to automatically transmit weather data to a computer that analyzes the data. A computer-assisted weather station generally consists of an electronic data logger, sensing devices, power supply, environmental enclosure, and a support structure, but these can be expensive and hard to maintain.

Stand-alone data loggers are available for monitoring degree-days, chilling hours, frost degree-hours, wind speed, and for tracking the powdery mildew index. These hand-held battery-operated loggers work without having to be attached to a computer; they also measure and accumulate minimum-maximum temperatures.

Electronic devices that continually monitor and record temperatures and other weather variables can store observations on the device or in a computer, and software is available to summarize the data or display graphs or charts. Be sure to set up and maintain the weather instruments according to manufacturers' instructions and calibrate them regularly to ensure accuracy. Dirty, poorly sited, or poorly maintained instruments will give inaccurate measurements that can lead to bad decisions.

Alternatives to expensive computer-aided weather assessment tools and electronic hand-held devices include

- surveyor's tape hung from a tree branch or pole (Fig. 10-18).
- a wind sock
- a visual assessment of wind movement through trees

Using any of these assessment methods will alert you to the wind's relative speed and direction so you can make the best possible application decision (see Flint 2012).

Temperature information can be obtained locally through radio stations or through a number of different sources on the Internet. The National Weather Service broadcasts local and regional weather information on National Oceanic Atmospheric Administration (NOAA) Weather Radio and VHF channels, and it also posts pinpoint local forecasts on the National Weather Service website. Evapotranspiration information is available from the California Department of Water Resources CIMIS program website, cimis.water.ca.gov. Current weather information is also available online by subscription from private weather services that can provide localized forecasts for a fee. The type of information available includes daily agricultural weather forecasts, 7-day temperature and rain forecasts, short-term forecasts, hourly weather observations, and daily weather summaries.

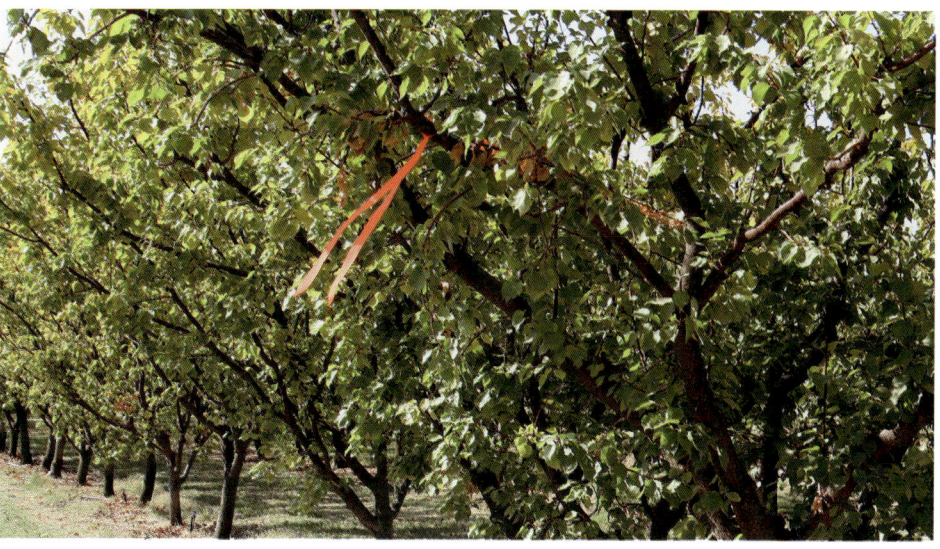

FIGURE 10-18

Surveyor's tape hung from a tree branch is an indicator of relative wind speed and direction, helping you make the best possible application decision.

Describe the different types of drift, including factors that can affect the occurrence of each type of drift.

In California, temperature and other weather information is available through the UC IPM California Weather Database (see the UC IPM website, ipm.ucanr.edu). The weather database provides current and historical daily weather data for approximately 400 weather stations throughout California. Choose a station and obtain daily data over a range of dates and use the data with the degree-day utility or various phenological models to help make management decisions (see Flint 2012).

SPRAY DRIFT

Spray drift occurs more frequently than vapor or dust drift because almost all spray applications result in some offsite movement. You must learn how to reduce the likelihood that sprays move away from the area where you are applying pesticides, whether you perform ground or aerial applications.

Avoid most problems associated with spray drift by paying close attention to spray droplet size, wind direction and speed, and boom or nozzle height. Larger spray droplets are less likely to drift than smaller ones, and droplets released close to the target site are more likely to stay on target (see Table 10-4). Typically, larger nozzle orifices and lower pressures produce larger droplets (see Table 10-5). However, some new nozzles, such as the venturi, or air-induction, nozzles produce larger droplets when used at higher pressures (above 40 psi).

The viscosity (thickness) of the liquid affects droplet size. The viscosity of a liquid is a measure of its resistance to flow: for example, mayonnaise is more viscous than water. As the viscosity of the liquid increases, so does the droplet size, reducing the potential for offsite movement. Formulations such as invert emulsions have a thick consistency that aids in reducing drift. Other formulations produce some spray drift when water droplets begin to evaporate before reaching the intended target. As a result, these droplets become very small and light and may move from the target site. Invert emulsions have less water loss, so more of the pesticide reaches the target. Several drift control additives can help reduce the potential for drift. The number of large droplets can be increased by using certain additives and thickeners. Remember, always follow the label directions when using any spray adjuvant intended for minimizing drift.

Air movement is the most important environmental factor influencing the drift of pesticides from target areas. The movement of air is influenced by the temperature at ground level and the temperature of the air above it, so taking weather readings can help you decide when drift is less likely to occur. Except in the case of temperature inversions, the early morning and evening are

TABLE 10-4

Influence of droplet size on potential distance of drift

Droplet diameter (microns)	Type of droplet	Time required to fall 10 feet	Lateral distance droplets travel when falling 10 feet in a 3 mph wind
5	fog	66 minutes	3 miles
	very fine spray	4.2 minutes	1,100 feet
100	fine spray	10 seconds	44 feet
240	medium spray	6 seconds	28 feet
400	coarse spray	2 seconds	8.5 feet
1,000	fine rain	1 second	4.7 feet

Source: Akesson and Yates 1964.

TABLE 10-5

American Society of Agricultural and Biological Engineers (ASABE) Standard (S-572) characteristics of spray droplets with nozzle catalog code, categories, symbols, and approximate micro sizes and relative comparisons

ASABE Standard				Comparative size*		
Symbol	Category	Code	Approximate VMD§	Relative size	Comparative size	Atomization
VF	very fine	red	<100	○	point of needle (25 microns)	fog
F	fine	orange	100–175	○	human hair (100 microns)	fine mist
M	medium	yellow	175–250	○	sewing thread (150 microns)	fine drizzle
C	coarse	blue	250–375	○	fishing line (250 microns)	light rain
VC	very coarse	green	375–450	○	staple (420 microns)	rain
XC	extremely coarse	white	>450	○	#2 pencil lead (2,000 microns)	thunderstorm

Notes: *Fine droplets are more likely to drift than course droplets; course droplets are more likely to run off. Selecting the correct nozzle will make your application more effective.
§Volume median diameter.

often the best times to apply pesticides. This is because windy conditions are more likely to occur around midday when the temperature near the ground increases. An increase in temperature causes hot air to rise quickly and mix rapidly with the cooler air above it, favoring drift. The best time to spray is when the spray droplets move slowly upward in the absence of windy or inversion conditions. Droplets that travel shorter distances through the air to the target are less likely to drift. Carefully adjusting nozzle height helps reduce the chances that pesticide will move away from the application site through the air.

Low relative humidities, high temperatures, or a combination of both, can also increase the potential for spray drift. Under these conditions, the evaporation rate of water increases, resulting in smaller spray droplets that drift more easily. Avoid spraying during these times.

Reduce outdoor drift problems by spraying when the wind speed is low, by leaving an untreated border or buffer area in the downwind target area, and by spraying downwind from sensitive areas such as residential properties, schools, crops, waterways, or beehives. Be sure to adjust the height of nozzles so that they are spraying pesticide as close to the target as possible while still maintaining proper coverage. For reducing drift indoors, pest control operators must consider the air circulation patterns inside buildings. Turn fans and air conditioners off and close vents where necessary to prevent pesticides from drifting to other areas of the structure. Using low-volatile or nonvolatile pesticides and using only low-pressure treatments can reduce indoor pesticide drift problems (see Randall et al. 2008).

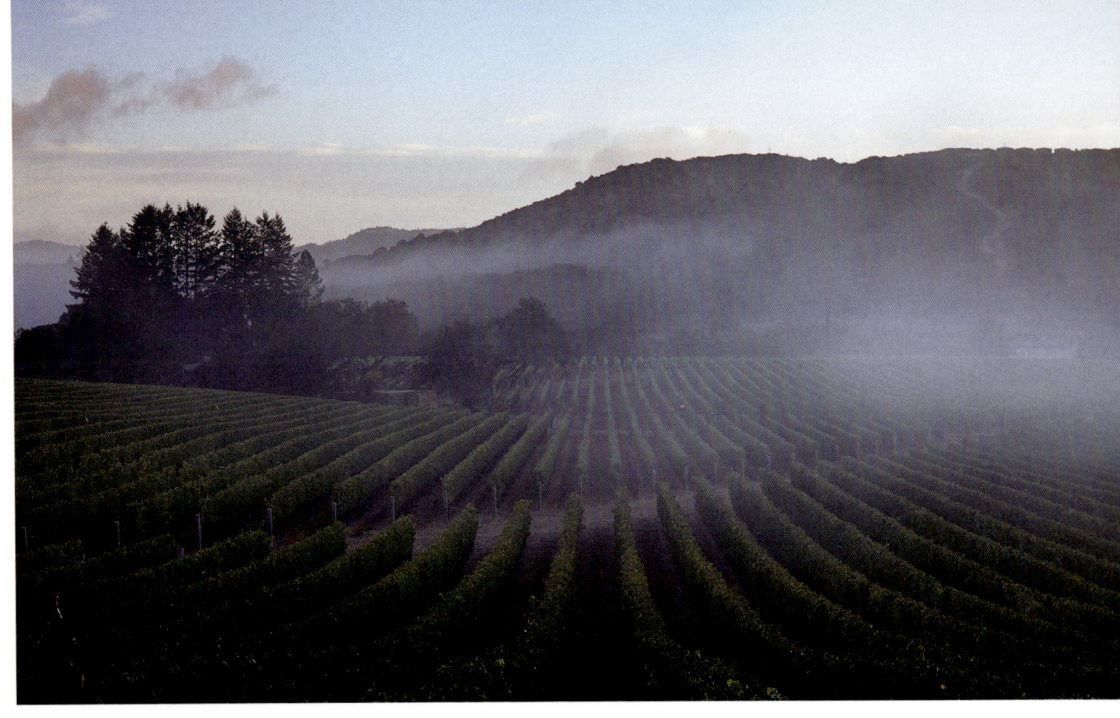

FIGURE 10-19

A temperature inversion is caused by a layer of warm air occurring above cooler air close to the ground. This warm air prevents air near the ground from rising, similar to a lid.

TEMPERATURE INVERSIONS

Temperature inversions can be recognized by noting weather conditions, such as a low fog (as in Figure 10-19), or by observing the movement of dust or smoke. If low fog remains over an area, or if dust or smoke rises little from its source and tends to hang in the air, an inversion is probably present or in the process of developing. Another method of detecting inversions is to place a thermometer at ground level and a second thermometer high above the ground and compare the difference in temperature. If the temperature at ground level is below that found at the elevated thermometer, a temperature inversion exists. Do not apply pesticides under such conditions (see Randall et al. 2008).

VAPOR DRIFT

Vapor drift occurs when a volatile pesticide changes readily from a solid or liquid into a gas, generally when the air temperature is high and the soil is sandy and dry. Pesticides that have volatilized can drift farther and for a longer time than spray droplets, so it is best to choose a pesticide formulated as a low-volatility product to help avoid this hazard. Do not apply volatile pesticides on hot days. Some products can even volatilize several hours after application, so beware if high temperatures are predicted for later in the day (Fig. 10-20). Many products carry

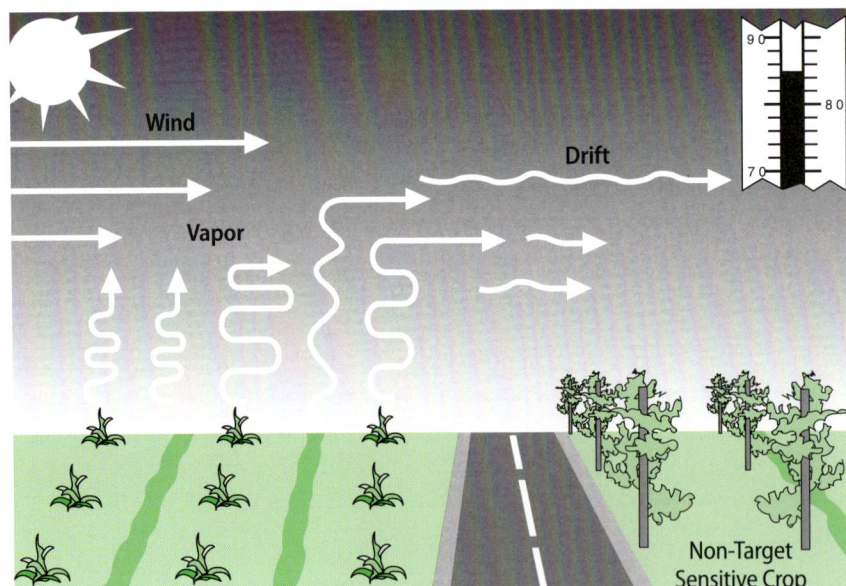

FIGURE 10-20

Vapor drift of pesticides is more likely to occur as heat and wind increase and the relative humidity decreases. *Source*: Randall 2008.

precautions against applying these products when temperatures are above 85°F or expected to reach 85°F. You can also decrease the likelihood of volatilization by injecting the pesticide deep into moist, packed, or tarped soil, or treating the site with water immediately following the application (see Randall et al. 2008).

In addition, the type of application equipment used can increase or decrease emissions. For instance, using a chemigation drip is much more effective than broadcast applications of particular volatile formulations. When dealing with volatile pesticides, carefully check label precautions for product-specific concerns about vapor drift and use DPR's VOC emissions calculator to calculate the volatile organic compound emissions from agricultural applications of nonfumigant pesticides. You can find more information about VOCs from nonfumigant pesticides and instructions for using the calculator on the DPR website, apps.cdpr.ca.gov/voc-calculator.

PARTICLE DRIFT (DUST DRIFT)

Some pesticides can remain active on soil particles for long periods after they are applied. Particle drift occurs when air moves solid particles from the target area during or just after an application. If particles are blown off the target area, contamination or damage to sensitive areas can occur. Take care when using air blast sprayers after certain herbicides have been applied to orchard floors, because they may blow pesticide-contaminated soil into the air.

To prevent particle drift from nearby outdoor pesticide applications from entering a building, be sure to close all windows, vents, and turn off all circulating fans, forced-air heating systems, and air-conditioning units.

For indoor applications of pesticides, reduce particle drift by turning off fans, forced-air heating systems, and other air-circulating equipment. Check pesticide labels for statements related to these concerns (see Randall et al. 2008).

PREVENTING SURFACE WATER AND GROUNDWATER CONTAMINATION

Describe ways to prevent other types of offsite movement of pesticides.

To help prevent surface water and groundwater contamination, the U.S. EPA requires that all pesticide products with directions for outdoor uses must include the environmental hazard statement on the label: "Do not apply directly to water, or to areas where surface water is present, or to intertidal areas below the mean high water mark. Do not contaminate water supplies when cleaning equipment or disposing of equipment wash waters." Pesticides that have the potential to be found in groundwater must bear groundwater warning statements on their labels. Groundwater statements on labels help applicators choose appropriate pesticides where soils are sandy or where extra precautions are needed to reduce contamination risk.

You can reduce the risk of point or nonpoint source contamination greatly by following best management practices (BMPs). BMPs are effective, commonsense practices that emphasize proper mixing, loading, application, and disposal of pesticides. Following these procedures greatly reduces the potential for pesticides to adversely affect the environment.

Use IPM principles. Apply pesticides only when and where necessary and only in amounts adequate to control pests. Following IPM principles, use nonchemical control methods whenever possible. When using pesticides

- Determine the type of pest and the density of the pest population and the proper control method.
- If a pesticide is necessary, select the least-toxic product that will provide adequate control.
- Calibrate pesticide application equipment regularly.
- Use spot treatments or band applications, if possible, to reduce pesticide use.

Identify vulnerable areas. The presence of sandy soil, sinkholes, wells, streams, ponds, and shallow groundwater increases the chance of groundwater contamination. Avoid pesticide application in these locations, if at all possible. Never dispose of empty pesticide containers in sinkholes or dump or rinse sprayers into or near sinkholes (see "Direct Channels" in Chapter 4).

Also avoid contamination of streets, storm sewers, drainage ditches, and other potential sources of runoff to streams and waterways. Do not under any circumstances clean tanks or intentionally discharge water from the tank of any vehicle into a street, along a road, or into a storm drain. For up-to-date lists and maps of groundwater protection areas in California, see the DPR website, cdpr.ca.gov.

Do not mix and load near water. Carry out mixing and loading as far as possible (at least 50 feet) from wells, lakes, streams, rivers, and storm drains. When possible, mix and load pesticides at the site of application. Consider using a sealed permanent or portable mixing and loading pad to prevent seepage into soil.

Keep pesticides away from wells. Do not store or mix pesticides around wells. Poorly constructed or improperly capped or abandoned wells can allow surface water containing pesticides and other contaminants direct entry into groundwater. These wells are sometimes located in or near treated fields and other application sites.

Avoid back-siphoning. Back-siphoning is the reverse flow of liquids into a fill hose. It sucks tank contents back into the water supply. Back-siphoning starts with a reduction in water pressure and can draw very large quantities of pesticide directly into the water source. This happens when the end of the water hose is allowed to extend below the surface of the spray mixture when filling a spray tank. The simplest method of preventing backflow is to maintain an air gap between the discharge end of the water supply line and the pesticide solution in the spray tank. Keep the air gap at least twice the diameter of the discharge pipe. Another method for preventing back-siphoning is to use an anti-backflow device or check valve (see Chapter 8 for additional information about check valves).

Improve land use and application methods. Terraces and conservation tillage can reduce water runoff and soil erosion. Ideally, leave as much plant residue as possible on the soil surface to lessen erosion. Where conservation tillage is not possible, reduce runoff potential by incorporating pesticides into the soil to lower the concentration of product on the soil surface. In ornamental plantings, consider using mulches to reduce water runoff and soil erosion.

Grass buffer strips are very effective in reducing pesticide runoff because they trap sediment containing pesticides and slow runoff water, allowing more runoff water to infiltrate the soil. Leaving untreated grass strips next to streams, ponds, and other sensitive areas can trap much of the pesticide running off treated areas.

Time pesticide applications according to the weather forecast. Pesticides are most susceptible to runoff from heavy rains or irrigation during the first several hours after application. To avoid overspraying an area and causing drift, check the pesticide label for application precautions or restrictions during windy conditions. Wind speed, temperature, and humidity affect the offsite movement of pesticides.

Select products wisely. Whenever possible, use pesticides that are less likely to leach. Read labels for leaching warnings.

Handle pesticides safely. Follow these guidelines to prevent surface or groundwater contamination:
- Immediately contain and control pesticide spills.
- Check application equipment regularly for leaks or damage.
- Mix and load pesticides away from water sources.
- After the pesticide application is complete, follow label directions for proper equipment cleanup and container disposal.
- After applying granular pesticides, sweep or blow any granules from sidewalks, driveways, or patios onto the treatment area.

Clean sprayers at the application site, whenever possible, and at a safe distance from wells, ponds, streams, and storm drains. Spray the rinsate on the treated area or on another site listed on the pesticide label, or use in the next tank mix. Be sure not to exceed label rates (see Randall et al. 2008).

Preventing Pesticide Effects to Sensitive Areas and Nontarget Organisms

To prevent adverse effects on the environment, pesticide users must be aware of sensitive areas, nontarget plants and animals (especially endangered species), and harmful effects on habitat.

Protecting Sensitive Areas

In addition to water sources, sensitive areas include sites where living things could easily be injured by a pesticide. Outdoor sensitive areas include
- schools, playgrounds, recreational areas, hospitals, and similar institutions
- habitats of endangered species
- apiaries (honey bee sites), wildlife refuges, and parks
- areas where domestic animals and livestock are kept
- ornamental plantings, public gardens, and sensitive food or feed crops

Sensitive areas indoors include places where
- people live, work, shop, or are cared for
- food or feed is processed, prepared, stored, or served
- domestic or confined animals live, eat, or are otherwise cared for
- ornamental or other sensitive plants are grown or maintained, such as in malls and buildings

Sometimes pesticides must be deliberately applied to a sensitive area to control a pest. Only applicators who are competent in handling pesticides should perform these applications. At other times, the sensitive area may be part of a larger target site. Whenever possible, take special precautions to avoid application to the sensitive area. Leaving an untreated buffer zone around a sensitive area is a practical way to avoid contaminating it. In still other instances, the sensitive area may be near a site used for mixing and loading, storage, disposal, or equipment washing. The pesticide user must take precautions to avoid accidental contamination of the sensitive area. Check the label for statements that alert you to special restrictions around sensitive areas (see Randall et al. 2008).

Protecting Nontarget Organisms

Pesticides may affect nontarget organisms directly, causing immediate injury, or they may produce long-term consequences through environmental pollution. When pesticides build up in the bodies of animals or in the soil, they accumulate. If you use the same mixing and loading site or equipment cleaning site over a long period, pesticides are likely to accumulate in the soil. When this occurs, plants and animals that come into contact with the soil may be harmed. The following sections discuss some methods you can use to minimize pesticides' effects on nontarget plants; bees and other beneficial insects; and fish, wildlife, and livestock.

Nontarget Plants

Nearly all pesticides can cause plant injury due to chemical exposure (phytotoxicity), particularly if they are applied at too high a rate, at the wrong time, or under unfavorable environmental conditions. Check the pesticide label carefully to ensure you have calculated the application rate correctly and are using the correct application equipment. You must also plan applications ahead of time to ensure that conditions are ideal and that both target and nontarget organisms are at the optimal life stage. For instance, you may want to delay applying herbicides to a crop if it has recently been water stressed, since weakened plants are more likely to experience phytotoxic effects. Use the calibration techniques in Chapter 9 to ensure that application rates and coverage areas remain constant. Most unintended phytotoxic injury is due to herbicides that drift into adjacent areas, though it may sometimes be a consequence of surface runoff. See "Preventing Offsite Movement of Pesticides" earlier in this chapter for methods you can use to avoid drift and surface runoff.

Bees and Other Beneficial Insects

Because bees are such an important part of agricultural ecosystems, applicators must be aware of bee activity when planning pesticide applications. Preventing bee loss is the joint responsibility of the applicator, the grower, and the beekeeper. Check with your local county agricultural commissioner before performing pesticide applications that may harm bees. The commissioner will have contact information for beekeepers who requested notification prior to pesticide applications, as well as the specific bee protection regulations or unique county conditions that can impact your application. You can minimize losses of bees to insecticide poisoning by following a few basic principles:

- Read the label and follow label directions.
- Determine whether bees are foraging in the target area so you can take protective measures.
- Whenever possible, use pesticides and formulations least hazardous to bees. Emulsifiable concentrates are safer than powders and dust formulations. Granules are the safest and least likely to harm bees. Microencapsulated pesticides pose the greatest risk to bees.
- Choose the least hazardous application method. Ground applications are less hazardous to bees than aerial applications.
- Apply chemicals in the evening or during early-morning hours before bees forage. Evening applications are generally safer to bees than morning applications. If unusually warm evening temperatures cause bees to forage later than usual, delay the pesticide application.
- Do not spray crops in bloom except when necessary.
- Do not spray when weeds or other plants around the treatment site are in bloom.
- Do not treat an entire field or area if spot treatments will control the pest.

Table 10-5 lists pesticides according to their impact on honey bees. If a pesticide can harm honey bees, it can also cause problems for other beneficial insects. Often these beneficial insects are valuable allies in keeping pest populations below damaging levels. A pesticide application often harms the beneficial insect population as much as the target pest, so do not spray when beneficial insects are in the target area, except when absolutely necessary.

Fish, Wildlife, and Livestock

Fish kills often result from water pollution by a pesticide and are most likely to be caused by insecticides, especially when small ponds or streams are under conditions of low water flow or volume. Avoid situations where the pesticide you are applying can easily move into water or away from the application site in flowing water. For example, applications to unterraced areas can expose animals below to pesticides moving in water that flows downhill. Read the label to ensure that you leave the required buffer zone between the application site and lakes, streams, or underground water supplies that may feed into bodies of water that support aquatic organisms. To find out more about how to minimize runoff and leaching, see "Preventing Surface Water and Groundwater Contamination" earlier in this chapter.

Bird kills resulting from pesticide exposure can occur in a number of ways. Birds may ingest pesticide granules, baits, or treated seeds; they may be exposed directly to sprays; they may consume treated crops or drink contaminated water; or they may feed on pesticide-contaminated insects and other prey. Granular or pelleted formulations are a particular concern because birds and other animals often mistake them for food. Other formulations (liquid) may be safer when birds and other wildlife are in or near the treated area. Place baits properly so they are inaccessible to pets, birds, and other wildlife and use seed baits that are colored so that nontarget birds will avoid them. For more about methods to keep dry formulations on target, see "Particle Drift (Dust Drift)" earlier in this chapter.

Animals can also be harmed when they feed on plants or animals carrying pesticide residues. Pesticide residues remaining on or in the bodies of dead animals may harm predators. This is called secondary poisoning. Avoid this situation by promptly removing and properly disposing of dead animals from the treatment area. Check the pesticide label for statements about secondary poisoning.

TABLE 10-6

Active ingredients of commonly used pesticides and their effect on bees

Active ingredient	Highly toxic to bees	Toxic to bees	No bee precaution
abamectin	●		
acephate	●		
azadirachtin		●	
azoxystrobin			●
Bacillus thuringiensis ssp. aizawai		●	
Bacillus thuringiensis ssp. kurstaki			●
Beauveria bassiana		●	
bifenthrin	●		
buprofezin		●	
carbaryl	●		
chlorpyrifos	●		
clothianidin	●		
cryolite			●
cyfluthrin	●		
cypermethrin	●		
diatomaceous earth		●	
diazinon	●		
diflubenzuron		●	
dinotefuran	●		
fenpyroximate			●
fipronil	●		
horticultural oil		●	
imidacloprid	●		
kaolin clay			●
malathion	●		
mefenoxam			●
metaldehyde bait			●
novaluron	●		
permethrin	●		
potassium salts of fatty acids (soaps)			●
rotenone		●	
spinosad		●	
sulfur			●
thiamethoxam	●		
zeta-cypermethrin	●		

Key: Highly toxic to bees: Do not apply pesticide or allow it to drift to plants that are flowering.
Toxic to bees: Do not apply pesticide or allow it to drift to plants that are flowering, except when the application is made between sunset and midnight, if allowed by the pesticide label and regulations.
No bee precaution: No bee precaution, except when required by the pesticide label or regulation.

Note: *Some a.i.'s or products listed may not be currently registered as pesticides or may have had their registration cancelled.
Source: Adapted from Hooven et. al. 2013.

Livestock can also be harmed by pesticide applications. The most important source of livestock poisoning by pesticides is through their ingestion of contaminated feed, forage, and drinking water. Contamination often occurs as a result of improper or careless transportation, storage, handling, application, or disposal of pesticides, so be careful when working with pesticides around livestock (see Randall et al. 2008).

Follow-Up Monitoring

Follow up after every pesticide application to determine whether the application was successful. Figure 10-21 is a follow-up checklist. Begin by comparing the amount of pesticide actually used with the anticipated amount. This should vary by no more than 10%. If more or less pesticide was applied, determine the cause. Check sprayer calibration, check tank-mixing procedures, and recalculate the size of the target area. Look for clogged or worn nozzles and wear or blockage in the sprayer pumping system.

Inspect the application site to make sure coverage was adequate and uniform. (Wear PPE if necessary.) Look for

- signs of pesticide runoff
- lack of penetration into dense foliage
- shingling or foliage that is clumping together
- uneven coverage from the top to bottom of large plants

One way to determine whether coverage is uneven includes checking foliage for white residue after a wettable powder application has dried. To find out whether a sprayer has penetrated dense foliage, place water-sensitive paper cards in the treatment area prior to the application. If their color remains unchanged or they show only a few spots, you can adjust your application equipment accordingly to improve your results. Methods for adjusting a sprayer's application rates can be found in Chapter 9.

After an application of insecticides or acaricides, make a second follow-up visit to the treatment area a day or so later. (If the restricted-entry interval has not ended, be sure to wear PPE and avoid unnecessary contact with plant foliage.) At this time, look for signs indicating control of the target pest. Check for damage to natural enemies in the area. In addition, look for other problems, such as phytotoxicity or spotting of painted surfaces. Watch for pest resurgence and secondary pest outbreaks.

Follow up fungicide applications with an inspection to verify that the fungicide suppressed the pathogen.

After applying herbicides, follow up to see which weed species were controlled and which were partially or not controlled. Also look for damage to nontarget plants. Record this information on the treatment record and use it to determine whether you need an additional herbicide treatment.

Record your follow-up observations in the same notebook used to record other aspects of the pesticide application. This information will be useful when you plan future applications for the same pest or in similar target locations.

```
AMOUNT OF PESTICIDE USED
(a) Calculated amount required for job: _____
(b) Actual amount used: _____
(c) Variation—divide (a) by (b) then multiply by 100.
    Subtract answer from 100. (This should be between + 10 and – 10.)

COVERAGE
(a) Uniform _____    or uneven _____
(b) Runoff? _____
(c) Penetration into all areas? _____

EFFECTIVENESS
(a) Target pests controlled or reduced below economic injury level?
    _____
(b) Condition of natural enemies: _____
(c) Secondary pest outbreak? _____

PROBLEMS
(a) Spotting or staining of surfaces? _____
(b) Injury to plants? _____
(c) Other: _____

COMMENTS _____
_____
_____
```

FIGURE 10-21

Pesticide application follow-up checklist.

Margin notes:
- Describe how to implement a follow-up monitoring program to assess the effectiveness of a pesticide application.
- Describe how to evaluate spray coverage and adjust application variables to change coverage as needed.

Chapter 10 Review Questions

1. Match the pesticide application goal with the method(s) used to achieve it.

1. protecting crops from pest damage and/or increasing crop yield	a. placing sticky traps along wall bases or other normal pathways to monitor for certain pests indoors
2. improving the health, appearance, and growth of turf and ornamental plants	b. knowing which pesticide formulations are less likely to leave unsightly residues on plants in public parks
3. eliminating annoying pests from buildings, workplaces, and homes	c. learning to recognize both crop and pest life cycles or stages of development to maximize the effectiveness of your application

2. Understanding the life cycle or stages of pests will help you to _____.
   - ☐ a. schedule pesticide applications without monitoring for pests
   - ☐ b. choose the most effective pesticide to apply
   - ☐ c. create an IPM program that requires no pesticides

3. A common use of a pheromone monitoring trap is to _____.
   - ☐ a. reduce the populations of specific insect pests
   - ☐ b. collect large numbers of different insect species
   - ☐ c. time insecticide sprays for optimal control

4. Which pesticide property would make the material more likely to move with water in surface runoff?
   - ☐ a. high solubility
   - ☐ b. high adsorption
   - ☐ c. high volatility

5. You are spraying for termites in the basement and foundation of a home. In this situation, the pesticide you select should have a long _____.
   - ☐ a. dormancy
   - ☐ b. persistence
   - ☐ c. shelf life

6. What can you do to reduce an insecticide's effect on beneficial insects like honey bees?
   - ☐ a. Use the product when pests are most active, because beneficial insects are less active then.
   - ☐ b. Apply early in the morning or in the evening, because honey bees are less active in the environment.
   - ☐ c. Make an aerial application, because it is much safer for honey bees and other beneficial insects.

7. What can you use to measure a pesticide spray's penetration into the thick foliage of trees?
   - ☐ a. water-sensitive paper
   - ☐ b. wireless chemical sensors
   - ☐ c. pH-sensitive sponges

8. Which of the following problems can be eliminated if your sprayer is equipped with a GPS unit?
   - ☐ a. delivering pesticides too far from the target to reach pests effectively
   - ☐ b. spraying droplets that are too small for field conditions, resulting in drift
   - ☐ c. estimating previous location of equipment incorrectly, causing coverage gaps

9. What is the best source of information on whether two pesticides can be successfully mixed in the same tank?
   - ☐ a. the manufacturer's website
   - ☐ b. the pesticide label
   - ☐ c. the pesticide dealer

10. Put the following list of ingredients in the correct order for adding to a tank mix of two or more pesticides.
    - ☐ a. surfactants
    - ☐ b. emulsifiable concentrates
    - ☐ c. water-soluble concentrates
    - ☐ d. wettable powder
    - ☐ e. diluent

11. Why is it a problem if pests become resistant to the pesticide you normally apply?
    - ☐ a. Pests resistant to that pesticide are often resistant to all products with chemically related active ingredients, so many products will now be ineffective.
    - ☐ b. It causes inconvenience, because you must then seek out other, related pesticide formulations to control pests effectively at this site.
    - ☐ c. Increasing pest populations will attract too many natural enemies (such as parasitic wasps), which often become pests in large numbers.

12. Which of the following situations would increase the likelihood of pesticide resistance?
    - ☐ a. The insect you are trying to control reproduces only once per year.
    - ☐ b. You continually use the same pesticides or pesticides from the same chemical class.
    - ☐ c. You apply a pesticide that has little or no residual effect.

13. Which of the following are types of drift? Select all that apply.
    - ☐ a. pesticides washed off of plant surfaces into a lake during irrigation
    - ☐ b. volatilization of pesticides on a hot, sunny day
    - ☐ c. spray particles trapped in a temperature inversion
    - ☐ d. leaching of pesticides into groundwater after a rainstorm
    - ☐ e. dust particles blown from an application site on a windy day

14. Match the type of offsite movement with the method used to combat it.

1. spray drift	a. Avoid applying on a hot day, especially if soil is sandy.
2. vapor drift	b. Keep nozzles close to the target site while spraying.
3. particle drift	c. Check groundwater protection area maps and limit applications in these areas whenever possible.
4. runoff	d. Turn off fans, forced-air heating systems, and other air-circulating equipment before making an application indoors.
5. leaching	e. Review the weather forecast to make sure it will not rain during the first several hours after your planned pesticide application.

15. Which of the following adjuvants might you add to your tank mix to help reduce spray drift?
    - ☐ a. surfactants
    - ☐ b. attractants
    - ☐ c. thickeners

16. What is the first thing you should look for when returning to perform follow-up monitoring at an application site?
    - ☐ a. indications that pesticide coverage was adequate and uniform
    - ☐ b. evidence of pest damage and presence of natural enemies
    - ☐ c. symptoms of phytotoxicity appearing in nontarget plants

Chapter 11
Reading the Label

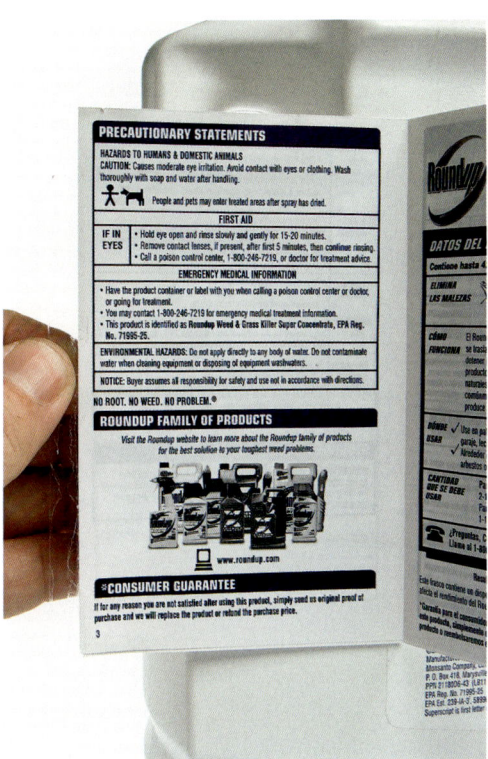

Pesticide Registration and Labeling 321
    Emergency Exemptions and Special Local Need 322
    Pesticide Labels 323
    Safety Data Sheets 328
Chapter 11 Review Questions 331

Knowledge Expectations

- Identify the information found in the different parts of the label and associated labeling information.
- Explain the legal requirement to read, understand, and follow directions on a pesticide label.
- Describe how an employer can ensure that labels and Safety Data Sheets are readily available.
- Describe the type of safety information provided by pesticide labeling and Safety Data Sheets for the pesticide used.

State and federal laws regulate the manufacture, sale, transportation, and use of pesticides. At the national level, the U.S. Environmental Protection Agency (U.S. EPA) is the pesticide regulatory agency. In California, the Department of Pesticide Regulation (DPR) assumes this role. U.S. EPA's authority is a mandate from the Federal Insecticide, Fungicide, and Rodenticide Act (FIFRA).

Originally passed in 1947, this law has undergone several amendments and updates, including the 1992 Worker Protection Standard and the 1996 Food Quality Protection Act. Based on this federal law, U.S. EPA establishes regulations for pesticide registration and labeling and pesticide residue tolerance levels on or in food. These regulations also set standards for using restricted-use pesticides and certifying pesticide applicators. Other federal agencies, including the Department of Agriculture (USDA), the National Institute of Occupational Safety and Health (NIOSH), and the Fish and Wildlife Service (FWS), monitor and regulate some types of pesticide uses.

Pesticide applicators in all states must comply with federal laws. California has enacted additional laws that strive to make pesticide use safer under the special conditions existing here (see Sidebar 11-1). California laws are sometimes more restrictive than federal laws but cannot permit uses or activities prohibited by the federal laws. California laws require reporting the uses of all pesticides in many application locations, such as production agriculture. Each year, managers of agricultural operations and certain other nonagricultural operations must obtain site and operation identification numbers before buying or using pesticides. This chapter describes the requirements for obtaining identification numbers and reporting pesticide uses.

California's pesticide laws are part of the California Food and Agricultural Code. The California legislature passes these laws in response to needs arising within the state or from federal mandates. Regulations are the working rules needed to interpret and carry out these laws. Regulations pertaining to pest control and pesticide use are part of the California Code of Regulations (CCR). DPR develops and proposes pesticide regulations. After receiving comments by mail and from public hearings concerning a proposed regulation, DPR writes a final "Statement of Reasons" and forwards it to the Office of Administrative Law for approval. If approved, it is forwarded to the secretary of state's office to be filed. At this point the new regulation is implemented by DPR.

SIDEBAR 11-1

REASONS FOR PESTICIDE LAWS AND REGULATIONS

1. To provide for the proper, safe, and efficient use of pesticides essential for the production of food and fiber, to protect public health and safety, and to protect the environment.
2. To protect the environment from unnecessary exposure to pesticides by prohibiting, regulating, or controlling uses of these products.
3. To assure agricultural and pest control workers of safe working conditions where pesticides are present.
4. To permit agricultural pest control by competent and responsible licensees and permittees under strict control of the director of the California Department of Pesticide Regulation (DPR) and local agricultural commissioners.
5. To assure consumers, handlers, and fieldworkers that pesticides are properly labeled and are appropriate for the use indicated on the label.
6. To encourage the use of integrated pest management systems favoring biological and cultural pest control techniques augmented by selective pesticides used only when needed to control pests while minimizing harm to nontarget organisms and the environment.

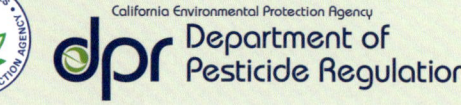

> **SIDEBAR 11-2**
>
> **INFORMATION MANUFACTURERS MUST PROVIDE TO DPR TO REGISTER A PESTICIDE IN CALIFORNIA**
>
> - Exposure information: data on risks of exposure and how people can be protected:
>   - safety related to exposure
>   - mixer, loader, applicator exposure
>   - management of poisoning
>   - toxicology of adjuvants and other components of the formulation
>   - indoor exposure information
>   - if material is a rodenticide, metabolic pathway and mode of action
>   - foliar residue and field restricted-entry data
> - Residue test method
> - Residue data
> - Efficacy
> - Hazard to bees
> - Closed-system compatibility
> - Effects on pest management
> - Inert ingredient hazard
> - Volatile organic compounds: their relationship to air quality
> - Other data as requested by the director of DPR, such as
>   - drift potential
>   - phytotoxicity
>   - contaminants or impurities in the product
>   - analytical and environmental chemistry
>   - effects of tank mixes on the product (compatibility)
>
>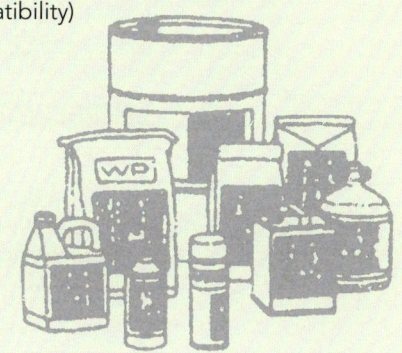

Several other state agencies in California monitor and regulate pesticide use. These include the Department of Public Health, Air Resources Board, Department of Fish and Wildlife, Department of Forestry and Fire Protection (CalFire), Occupational Safety and Health Administration, Waste Management Board, Department of Water Resources, Water Resources Control Board and regional water control boards, and the Structural Pest Control Board. In addition, agricultural commissioners in each county develop pesticide use policies or conditions. These are specific to the needs of their counties. The DPR director must approve county agricultural commissioner policies before they become operative, however. Counties and local governments also may create ordinances governing the use and storage of pesticides within their jurisdictions.

For current pesticide laws and regulations information, obtain a copy of the publication *Laws and Regulations Study Guide* from the California Department of Pesticide Regulation, ATTN: Cashier, P.O. Box 4015, Sacramento, California 95812-4105, or at the DPR website, cdpr.ca.gov/docs/license/pubs/laws_regs_study_guide.pdf.

Pesticide Registration and Labeling

Manufacturers must register pesticides with the U.S. EPA and DPR before they can be used, possessed, or offered for sale in California. These agencies register individual pesticide products. The registration procedure protects people and the environment from ineffective or harmful chemicals. Sidebar 11-2 lists the information that a manufacturer provides to register a pesticide.

The registration procedure includes an evaluation of each chemical. This evaluation establishes how U.S. EPA classifies the material at the federal level. Pesticides are either general-use or restricted-use. A general-use pesticide is one that can be purchased without applicator or handler certification and restricted material permit. California also designates certain pesticides as California Restricted Materials due to state-specific hazards or specific health concerns. With few exceptions, you must obtain a permit from the county agricultural commissioner before buying, possessing, or using any California Restricted Material. Only certified or licensed pesticide applicators can buy, use, or supervise the use of a federal restricted-use pesticide or California Restricted Material.

As part of California's pesticide registration procedure, several state agencies review registration information. These include the California Departments of Food and Agriculture, Fish and Wildlife, Public Health, and Industrial Relations. The Air Resources Board and Water Resources Control Board also review this information. In addition, there is a 30-day public review and comment period. This takes place before DPR makes a decision to register, renew, or reevaluate a pesticide. The public review provides opportunities for interested or concerned people to contribute to registration decisions.

To complete registration, manufacturers supply labels meeting all federal and state requirements. These labels become legal documents and contain important information for users. Some labels refer to other documents, such as endangered species range maps. Agricultural-use pesticide labels also refer to the Worker Protection Standard provisions of Title 40 of the Code of Federal Regulations, part 170 (40 CFR 170). These and other documents referred to on pesticide labels become part of the pesticide labeling.

Emergency Exemptions and Special Local Need

Occasionally, pest problems arise that you cannot control with currently registered pesticides. For example, the commodity, target pest, or site might not be on the registered pesticide label. In some situations, you can request an emergency exemption or a special local need (SLN) registration.

Emergency Exemptions from Registration. Emergency exemptions from registration address urgent, non-routine pest problems for which there are no pesticides registered and no feasible alternatives. Section 18 of FIFRA authorizes U.S. EPA to allow an unregistered use of a pesticide for a limited time if it determines that an emergency condition exists. The regulations governing FIFRA Section 18 (40 CFR 166) define "emergency condition" as an urgent, nonroutine situation that requires the use of a pesticide. DPR forwards Section 18 requests to U.S. EPA only after a full evaluation and only for situations the department determines meet criteria for an emergency condition. If DPR confirms the emergency need and if its scientific review of the residue chemistry, toxicology, and efficacy data demonstrates no unacceptable risks, the request is forwarded. If approved, U.S. EPA will establish a time-limited tolerance (maximum allowable residue levels) to cover any pesticide residues in food that may result. In California, all uses under a Section 18 emergency exemption require a restricted materials permit from the county agricultural commissioner before purchase and use.

Regulations impose strict controls and require recordkeeping for all emergency exemption uses. You must understand the special requirements and responsibilities involved whenever you use pesticides provided with emergency exemptions. DPR prescribes application rates, safety precautions, and other vital application information.

Special Local Need Registrations. Special local need (SLN) registrations are categorized as 24(c) registrations. Section 24(c) of FIFRA allows states to register a new pesticide product not previously registered for any use, or an added use of a federally registered product, as long as there is a demonstrated special local need for such a product. *Special local need* means an existing or imminent pest problem within a state for which the state lead agency (in California, the state lead agency is DPR), based on satisfactory supporting information, has determined that an appropriate federally registered pesticide product is not sufficiently available. States can expand or limit the uses of certain registered pesticides within their jurisdictions. For instance, some SLNs allow uses of pesticides for crops or sites not listed on the label. Others add limitations to the uses of a federally registered pesticide to accommodate area-specific conditions. If the SLN is for use on a food or feed commodity, a tolerance or exemption from tolerance must be established.

You must have the SLN labeling in your possession to use the pesticide for that purpose. The registration numbers for SLN labeling include the acronym "SLN" and the code for the state issuing the registration (CA). These registrations are legal only in the region, state, or local area specified in the labeling. Applying a pesticide having an SLN from another state or region subjects you to civil and criminal penalties.

To find out which SLN registrations pertain to your area, contact any of the following:
- the local county agricultural commissioner's office
- a UC Cooperative Extension farm advisor
- a pest control dealer

PESTICIDE LABELS

The Code of Federal Regulations sets the format for pesticide labels and prescribes the information they must contain. Some packages are too small, however, to have all this information printed on them. In these cases, U.S. EPA requires manufacturers to include the directions for use of the product on accompanying labeling in the form of a booklet, accordion-style foldout, or enclosed leaflet (Fig. 11-1). These booklets, together with the base label, are the complete pesticide label. On metal and plastic containers, manufacturers put these labels in plastic pouches glued to the side of the containers. Paper packages usually have booklets inserted under the bottom flaps. In these cases, the base label attached to the packaging must include a referral statement to the directions for use in the booklet. People who employ pesticide handlers and fieldworkers in California are required by law to provide unrestricted access to complete labels, including the information on an accompanying booklet, and Safety Data Sheets (see "Sections of a Safety Data Sheet" later in this chapter for more about information provided by an SDS).

When to Read the Pesticide Label

Read the pesticide label (Fig. 11-2)
- before buying the pesticide. Make sure the pesticide is registered for your intended use. Confirm that there are no restrictions or other conditions that prohibit using this pesticide at the application site. Be certain its use is suitable under current weather conditions. Also, be sure it controls the life stage of your pest. Find out what PPE and special application equipment you need.
- before mixing and applying the pesticide. Learn how to mix and safely apply the material. Find out what precautions to take to prevent exposure to people and nontarget organisms. Learn what first aid and medical treatments are necessary should an accident occur.
- when storing pesticides. Find out how to properly store the pesticide. Understand the special precautions to prevent fire hazards.
- before disposing of unused pesticide and empty containers. Learn how to prevent environmental contamination and hazards to people. (Before disposal, check with the agricultural commissioner in your area for local restrictions and requirements.)

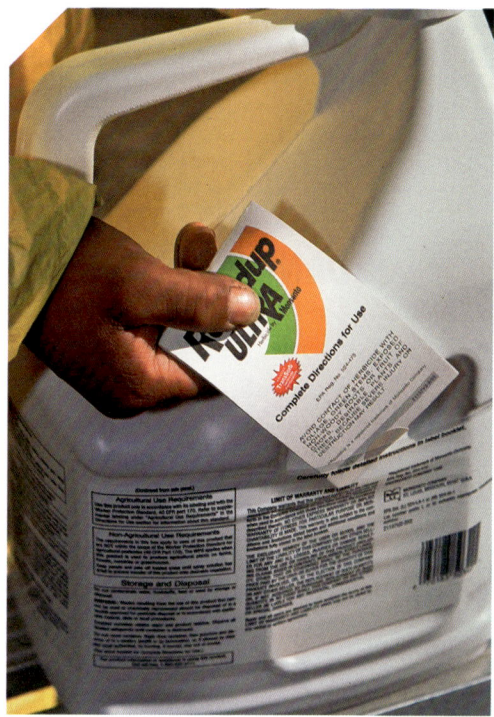

FIGURE 11-1

Supplemental labels are often attached to pesticide packages. Before purchasing a pesticide, make sure you have a complete set of labels.

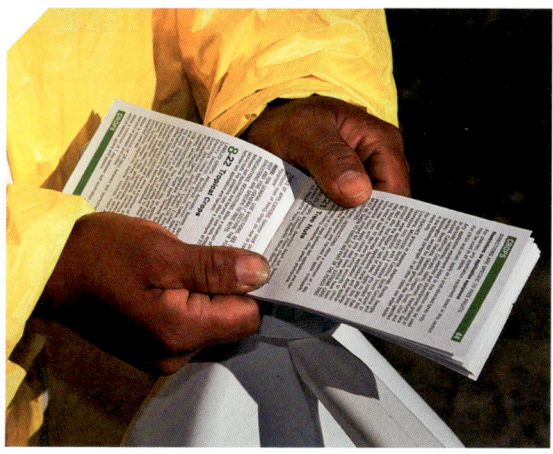

FIGURE 11-2

The pesticide label is a complex legal document that you must read and understand before making a pesticide application. Make pesticide applications in strict accordance with the label instructions.

RESTRICTED USE PESTICIDE
DUE TO ACUTE TOXICITY
FOR RETAIL SALE TO AND USE ONLY BY CERTIFIED APPLICATORS OR PERSONS UNDER THEIR DIRECT SUPERVISION AND ONLY FOR THOSE USES COVERED BY THE CERTIFIED APPLICATOR'S CERTIFICATION.

Knock 'em down 3SL
Herbicide By ToxiK™
A weed, grass, and harvest aid desiccant/defoliant herbicide.

Active Ingredients:

Paraquat dichloride

(tetrachloroisophthalonitrile) 43.2%

Other Ingredients: 56.8%

Total: 100.00%

| Group | 22 | Herbicide |

Water Soluble Liquid

Contains: 3.0 pounds paraquat cation per gallon as 4.14 pounds of dichloride salt per gallon. Contains emetic and stench (odor), and dye

EPA Reg. No. 000-000 EPA Est. 000-XX-000

SCP 1364A-L1 0411 343162

Net Contents 2.5 gallons

KEEP OUT OF REACH OF CHILDREN.
DANGER/PELIGRO
POISON/VENENO

Si usted no entiende la etiqueta, busque a alguien para que se la explique a usted en detalle. (If you do not understand the label, find someone to explain to you in detail.)

©2016 ToxiK, LLC, YourTown, YourState, 01234

FIRST AID
Contains Paraquat, a Bipyridylium Herbicide

If swallowed:
- Call a poison control center or doctor IMMEDIATELY for treatment advice.
- SPEED IS ESSENTIAL. Immediate medical attention is required. If available, give an absorbent such as activated charcoal, bentonite, or Fuller's Earth.
- Have person sip a glass of water if able to swallow.
- Do not induce vomiting unless told to do so by a poison control center or doctor.
- Do not give anything by mouth to an unconscious person.

If inhaled:
- Move person to fresh air.
- The odor of this product is from the stanching agent, which has been added, not from the paraquat.
- If person is not breathing, call 911 or an ambulance.
- Call a poison control center or doctor for further treatment advice.

If in eyes:
- Hold eye open and rinse slowly and gently with water for 15-20 minutes. Remove contact lenses, if present, after the first 5 minutes, then continue rinsing eye.
- Call a poison control center or doctor for treatment advice.

If on skin or clothing:
- Take off contaminated clothing.
- IMMEDIATELY wash with soap and water and rinse for 15-20 minutes. Prolonged contact will cause severe irritation. Contact with irritated skin or a cut or repeated contact with intact skin may result in poisoning.
- GET MEDICAL ATTENTION. Call a poison control center or doctor for treatment advice.

NOTE TO PHYSICIAN:
Administer either activated charcoal (100g for adults or 2g/kg body weight in children) or Fuller's Earth (15% solution; 1 liter for adults or 15ml/kg body weight in children). NOTE: The use of gastric lavage without administration of an adsorbent has not shown any clinical benefit. Do not use supplemental oxygen. Eye splashes from concentrated material should be treated by an eye specialist after initial treatment. With the possibility of late onset corneal ulceration, it is advised that patients with paraquat eye injuries be examined by an eye specialist the day after first presentation. Use treatment that is appropriate for chemical burns. Intact skin is an effective barrier to paraquat however contact with irritated or cut skin or repeated contact with intact skin may result in poisoning.

Have the product container or label with you when calling a poison control center or doctor, or going for treatment.

HOT LINE NUMBER: For 24-Hour Medical Emergency Assistance (Human or Animal) or Chemical Emergency Assistance (Spill, Leak, Fire, or Accident), Call 1-800-000-0000

PRECAUTIONARY STATEMENTS
Hazards to Humans and Domestic Animals

DANGER/PELIGRO
POISON/VENENO

May be fatal if swallowed. Fatal if inhaled. Corrosive. Causes irreversible eye damage. Wear protective eyewear. Do not breathe spray mist. Wear a dust/mist respirator. Do not get in eyes or on clothing. Harmful if absorbed through skin. Avoid contact with skin. Prolonged or frequently repeated skin contact may cause allergic reactions in some individuals. Wash thoroughly with soap and water after handling and before eating, drinking, chewing gum, using tobacco, or using the toilet. Remove and wash contaminated clothing before reuse.

IMPORTANT: Inhalation is an unlikely route of exposure due to low vapor pressure and large spray droplet size, but mucosal irritation or nose bleeds may occur. Prolonged contact with this concentrated product can irritate your skin.

Personal Protective Equipment (PPE) Applicators and other handlers (other than Mixers and Loaders) must wear:

- Long-sleeve shirt and long pants
- Shoes plus socks
- Protective eyewear
- Chemical-resistant gloves - Category A (e.g. barrier laminate, butyl rubber, nitrile rubber, neoprene rubber, natural rubber, polyethylene, polyvinyl chloride (PVC), or Viton®)
- A dust/mist NIOSH-approved respirator with any N, R, P, or HE filter. The respirator should have a NIOSH approval number prefix TC-84A.

Mixers and Loaders must wear:

- Long-sleeve shirt and long pants
- Shoes plus socks
- A dust/mist NIOSH-approved respirator with any N, R, P, or HE filter. The respirator should have a NIOSH approval number prefix TC-84A.
- Chemical-resistant gloves - Category A (e.g. barrier laminate, butyl rubber, nitrile rubber, neoprene rubber, natural rubber, polyethylene, polyvinyl chloride (PVC), or Viton)
- Chemical-resistant apron
- Face shield

② PRECAUTIONARY STATEMENTS (CONT.)

Discard clothing and other absorbent materials that have been drenched or heavily contaminated with this product's concentrate. Do not reuse them. Follow manufacturer's instructions for cleaning/maintaining PPE. If no such instructions for washables exist, use detergent and hot water. Keep and wash PPE separately from other laundry.

Engineering Controls: When handlers use closed systems, enclosed cabs, or aircraft in a manner that meets the requirements listed in the Worker Protection Standard (WPS) for agricultural pesticides [40 CFR 170.240(d)(4-6)], the handler PPE requirements may be reduced or modified as specified in the WPS.

Environmental Hazards: This product is toxic to wildlife. DO NOT apply directly to water, to areas where surface water is present, or to intertidal areas below the mean high water mark. DO NOT contaminate water when disposing of equipment washwater or rinsate.

Paraquat dichloride is toxic to nontarget crops and plants if off-target movement occurs because it desiccates all green plant tissue. Extreme care must be taken to ensure that off-target drift is minimized to the greatest extent possible. Refer to the local state laws, regulations, guidelines, and spray drift information contained in the Directions for Use section for proper application to avoid off-target movement. Do not apply under conditions involving possible drift to food, forage, or other plantings that might be damaged or crops that would be rendered unfit for sale, use, or consumption. Do not apply when weather conditions favor drift from treated areas. To avoid drift, do not make aerial application during periods of thermal inversion.

Physical or Chemical Hazards: This product is mildly corrosive to aluminum and produces hydrogen gas which may form a highly combustible gas mixture. Do not mix or store in containers, spray tanks, nurse tanks, or such systems made of aluminum or having aluminum fittings. This product is compatible with high density polyethylene and rubber lined steel containers.

③ DIRECTIONS FOR USE

It is a violation of Federal law to use this product in a manner inconsistent with its labeling. Knock 'em down 3SL must be used only in accordance with recommendations on this label or in separately published TOXIK supplemental labeling recommendations for this product.

④ **DO NOT** apply this product in a way that will contact workers or other persons or pets either directly or through drift. Only protected handlers may be in the area during application. For any requirements specific to your State or Tribe, consult the agency responsible for pesticide regulation.

DO NOT USE AROUND HOME GARDENS, SCHOOLS, RECREATIONAL PARKS, GOLF COURSES, OR PLAYGROUNDS. (Directions for Use continued on supplemental labeling)

⑤ AGRICULTURAL USE REQUIREMENTS

Use this product only in accordance with its labeling and with the Worker Protection Standard (WPS), 40 CFR part 170. This Standard contains requirements for the protection of agricultural workers on farms, forests, nurseries, and greenhouses and handlers of agricultural pesticides. It contains requirements for training, decontamination, notification, and emergency assistance. It also contains specific instructions and exceptions pertaining to the statements on this label about personal protective equipment (PPE) and restricted-entry interval (REI). The requirements in this box only apply to uses of this product that are covered by the Worker Protection Standard.

For Chemical Fallow, Early Postemergence Broadcast in Peanuts, and Dormant Season Applications, and "Between Cutting" Applications in Alfalfa:
DO NOT enter or allow workers to enter treated areas during the restricted entry interval (RFI) of 12 hours.

For Harvest Aid and Desiccation Applications, Preplant or Preemergence (Broadcast or Banded), and Postemergence Directed Spray: DO NOT enter or allow workers to enter treated areas during the restricted entry interval (REI) of 24 hours

PPE required for early entry to treated areas that is permitted under the Worker Protection Standard and that involves contact with anything that has been treated, such as plants, soil, or water, is:

- Coveralls
- Shoes plus socks
- Protective eyewear (goggles, face shield, or safety glasses)
- Chemical-resistant gloves - Category A (e.g. barrier laminate, butyl rubber, nitrile rubber, neoprene rubber, natural rubber, polyethylene, polyvinyl chloride (PVC) or Viton)

⑰ STORAGE AND DISPOSAL

Do not contaminate water, food, or feed by storage or disposal. Pesticide Storage: Store at temperatures above 32°F.

Pesticide Disposal: Pesticide wastes are toxic. Improper disposal of unused pesticide, spray mixture, or rinse water is a violation of Federal law. If these wastes cannot be used according to label instructions, contact your State Pesticide or Environmental Control Agency, or the Hazardous Waste representative at the nearest EPA Regional Office for guidance in proper disposal methods.

Container Handling [less than 5 gallons]: Non-refillable container. Do not reuse or refill this container. Offer for recycling if available. Triple rinse container (or equivalent) promptly after emptying. Triple rinse as follows: Empty the remaining contents into application equipment or a mix tank and drain for 10 seconds after the flow begins to drip. Fill the container ¼ full with water and recap. Shake for 10 seconds. Pour rinsate into application equipment or a mix tank or store rinsate for later use and disposal. Drain for 10 seconds after the flow begins to drip. Repeat this procedure two more times. Then offer for recycling if available or puncture and dispose of in a sanitary landfill, or by incineration, or if allowed by state and local authorities, by burning.

For minor spills, leaks, etc., follow all precautions indicated on this label and clean up immediately. Take special care to avoid contamination of equipment and facilities during cleanup procedures and disposal of wastes. In the event of a major spill, fire, or other emergency, call 1-800-000-0000, day or night.

CONTAINER IS NOT SAFE FOR FOOD, FEED, OR DRINKING WATER.

⑱ CONDITIONS OF SALE AND LIMITATION OF WARRANTY AND LIABILITY

NOTICE: Read the entire Directions for Use and Conditions of Sale and Limitation of Warranty and Liability before buying or using this product. If the terms are not acceptable, return the product at once, unopened and the purchase price will be refunded.

The Directions for Use of this product must be followed carefully. It is impossible to eliminate all risks inherently associated with the use of this product. Crop injury, ineffectiveness, or other unintended consequences may result because of such factors as manner of use or application, weather or crop conditions, presence of other materials, or other influencing factors in the use of the product, which are beyond the control of TOXIK, LLC or Seller. To the extent permitted by applicable law, Buyer and User agree to hold TOXIK and Seller harmless for any claims relating to such factors.

(Warranty information continued on supplemental labeling)

FIGURE 11-3

This example of a pesticide label illustrates the important sections; these sections are described in the text.

What Pesticide Labels Contain

Refer to the corresponding numbers on the sample pesticide label (Fig. 11-3) for examples of the following pesticide label sections.

1. **Statement of Use Classification.** The U.S. EPA classifies pesticides as either general-use or restricted-use. Federal restricted-use pesticides have a special statement printed on the label in a prominent place (such as the one shown in Figure 11-5). Pesticides that do not contain this statement are general-use pesticides, except where special state restrictions apply. For information, check the DPR list, "California Restricted Materials," which is available from county agricultural commissioners. Some labels have restrictive statements indicating that they are for agricultural or commercial use only. A restrictive statement is different from a statement of use classification.
2. **Brand Name.** A brand name is the name the manufacturer gives to the product. This is the name used for all advertising and promoting. It is also commonly referred to as the product's trade name.
3. **Ingredients.** Pesticide labels list the percentage of active and other ingredients by weight. Other ingredients are all components of the formulation that do not have pesticidal action. Even if they are not considered active, these ingredients may still be toxic, flammable, or pose other safety or environmental hazards. Some, however, are relatively harmless, such as clay. If a pesticide contains more than one active ingredient, the label will state the percentage of each. Manufacturers do not usually individually identify the names or percentages of other ingredients in the pesticide.
4. **Common Chemical Name.** Chemical names of pesticide active ingredients are often complicated. Therefore, manufacturers give most pesticides common, or generic, names. For example, 0,0-diethyl 0(2-isopropyl-6-methyl-4pyrimidinyl) has the common name diazinon. Common names and brand names are not the same, and not all labels list common names for the pesticide.
5. **Chemical Name.** Labels must list all chemicals having pesticidal action (active ingredients) in the product. Chemical names describe the active ingredients' chemical structure and are based on international naming rules.
6. **Formulation.** Labels usually list the formulation type, such as emulsifiable concentrate, wettable powder, or soluble powder. Manufacturers may include this information as a suffix in the brand name of the pesticide. For example, in the name Princep 80W, the "W" indicates a wettable powder formulation. Table 3-6 in Chapter 3 lists definitions for many suffixes used with brand names.
7. **Registration and Establishment Numbers.** The U.S. EPA assigns registration numbers to each pesticide. You need this U.S. EPA number if you are reporting the use of the pesticide. In addition, an establishment number identifies the site of manufacture or repackaging. If the product requires registration in California (but not with U.S. EPA), the Department of Pesticide Regulation will assign a California registration number.
8. **Contents.** Labels list the net contents, by weight or liquid volume, contained in the package.
9. **Signal Word.** An important part of every label is the signal word (Fig. 11-3). The words DANGER and POISON (with a skull and crossbones) indicate that the pesticide is highly toxic. The word DANGER used alone indicates that the pesticide poses a dangerous health hazard. WARNING indicates moderate toxicity, and CAUTION means low toxicity (see "Pesticide Toxicity Categories" in Chapter 3). During the registration process each pesticide is assigned a toxicity category (Category I, DANGER, to Category IV, no signal word required). The level of hazard determines the signal word manufacturers must use on their labels.
10. **Manufacturer.** Pesticide labels always contain the name and address of the manufacturer of the product. Use this address if you need to contact the manufacturer for any reason.
11. **First Aid.** The first aid statement provides emergency information. It tells what to do to decontaminate someone who becomes exposed to the pesticide. It describes the emergency first aid procedures for swallowing, skin and eye exposure, and inhalation of dust or vapors. This section tells you when to seek medical attention.
12. **Precautionary Statements.** Precautionary statements describe the pesticide hazards (Fig. 11-3). Read and follow the instructions given in a precautionary statement. The statement includes as many as three areas of hazard. The most important hazards are those to people and domestic animals.

    The first part of a precautionary statement explains why the pesticide is hazardous, lists adverse effects that may occur if people become exposed, and describes the type of PPE to wear while handling containers and while mixing and applying the product.

The second part of a precautionary statement describes environmental hazards. It tells you whether the pesticide is toxic to nontarget organisms such as honey bees, fish, birds, and other wildlife. Here is where you learn how to avoid environmental contamination.

The third part of the precautionary statement explains special physical and chemical hazards. These include risks of fire or explosion and hazards from fumes.

13. **Directions for Use.** The directions for use are an important part of the pesticide label. It is a violation of the law if you do not follow these instructions. The only exceptions are cases where federal or state laws specify acceptable deviations from label instructions. The directions for use list all the target pests that manufacturers claim their pesticides control. It also includes the crops, plant species, animals, or other sites to which you can apply the pesticides (Fig. 11-3). Here is where you find special restrictions that you must observe. These include crops that you may or may not plant in the treated area (plant-back restrictions, also called rotational crop restrictions). They also include restrictions on feeding crop residues to livestock or grazing livestock on treated plants. These instructions also tell you how to apply the pesticide (including allowable application methods) and provide methods to help you prevent drift. They specify how much pesticide to use, where to use the material, and when to apply it (Fig. 11-4). The directions include the harvest intervals (or preharvest intervals) for all crops whenever appropriate. A harvest interval is the time, in days, required after application before you may harvest an agricultural crop.

14. **Misuse Statement.** The misuse statement reminds users to apply pesticides according to label directions.

15. **Agricultural Use Requirements.** This special statement appears in the Directions for Use section on labels of pesticides approved for use in production agriculture, commercial greenhouses and nurseries, and forests. It refers to the Worker Protection Standard (40 CFR 170). You must use the pesticide according to this standard as well as the requirements on the pesticide label. It provides information on the personal protective equipment (PPE) required for early-entry workers. It also gives the restricted-entry interval for workers (see no. 17, below).

16. **Restricted-Entry Statement.** Usually a period of time must elapse before anyone can enter a treated area unless they are wearing PPE. This period is the restricted-entry interval. Restricted-entry intervals may vary according to the toxicity and special hazards associated with the pesticide. The crop or site being treated and its geographic location also influence the length of this interval. Some pesticide uses in California require longer restricted-entry intervals than those listed on the pesticide label. Check with the local agricultural commissioner for this information.

17. **Storage and Disposal Directions.** This section contains directions for properly storing and disposing of the pesticide and empty pesticide containers. Proper disposal of unused pesticides and pesticide containers reduces human and environmental hazards. Some pesticides have special storage requirements because improper storage causes them to lose their effectiveness. Improper storage may even cause explosions or fires.

18. **Warranty.** Manufacturers usually include a warranty and disclaimer on their pesticide labels. This information informs you of your rights as a purchaser and limits the liability of the manufacturer.

FIGURE 11-4

Many pesticide labels have tables like this one, which shows application rates and directions to control listed pests on specified crop(s). These tables are found in the "Directions for Use" section of the pesticide label.

BRASSICA LEAFY VEGETABLES CROPS AND TURNIP GREENS

All members of the Brassica Leafy Vegetable Group 5, plus Turnip greens, including: Broccoli, Broccoli raab (rapini), Brussels sprouts, Cabbage, Cauliflower, Cavalo broccolo, Chinese broccoli (gai lon), Chinese cabbage (bok choy), Chinese cabbage (napa), Chinese mustard cabbage (gai choy), Collards, Kale, Kohlrabi, Mizuna, Mustard greens, Mustard spinach, Rape greens, Turnip greens

PEST		QUARTS OF THIS PRODUCT PER ACRE	SPECIFIC DIRECTIONS
Flea beetles Harlequin bug Leafhoppers		1/2 to 1	Repeat applications as needed up to a total of 4 times per year but not more often than once every 7 days.
Armyworm Aster leafhopper Corn earworm Diamondback moth Fall armyworm Imported cabbageworm	Lygus bugs Spittle bugs Stink bugs Tarnished plant bug	1 to 2	

FIGURE 11-5

An example of a restricted-use statement found on the top of the first page of a restricted-use pesticide.

RESTRICTED USE PESTICIDE
Due to Toxicity to Fish and Aquatic Organisms
For retail sale to and use only by Certified Applicators, or persons under their direct supervision, and only for those uses covered by the Certified Applicator's certification.

SAFETY DATA SHEETS

In addition to the label, you will also want to review a pesticide's Safety Data Sheet (SDS), formerly known as a Material Safety Data Sheet, or MSDS. The SDS provides detailed information about pesticide hazards (Fig. 11-6). You will find the following information on an SDS:

- the chemical characteristics of active and other hazardous ingredients
- fire and explosion hazards
- health hazards
- reactivity and incompatibility characteristics

FIGURE 11-6

This exerpt of a pesticide's Safety Data Sheet illustrates several sections that can sometimes have different information than is on the product's label e.g., the signal word on an SDS may be different from the label's signal word). The sections pictured include product identification, hazards identification, and regulatory information. Always use the pesticide in accordance with the information provided on the pesticide label.

Safety Data Sheet — syngenta

DACONIL ACTION

Date: 2/5/2014
Replaces: 1/16/2014

1. PRODUCT IDENTIFICATION

Product identifier on label: **DACONIL ACTION**
Product No.: A16422A
Use: Fungicide/Plant Activator
Manufacturer: Syngenta Crop Protection, LLC
Post Office Box 18300
Greensboro NC 27419
Manufacturer Phone: 1-800-334-9481
Emergency Phone: **1-800-888-8372**

2. HAZARDS IDENTIFICATION

Classifications:
Skin Corrosion/Irritation: Category 2
Oral: Category 4
Dermal: Category 4
Inhalation: Category 3
Skin Sensitizer: Category 1B
Carcinogenicity: Category 2
Specific Target Organ Toxicity: Repeated Category 2
Specific Target Organ Toxicity: Drowsiness Category 3
Eye Damage/Irritation: Category 2A

Signal Word (OSHA): Danger

Hazard Statements:
Harmful if swallowed
Harmful in contact with skin
Causes skin irritation
May cause an allergic skin reaction
Causes serious eye irritation
Toxic if inhaled
May cause respiratory irritation
May cause drowsiness or dizziness
Suspected of causing cancer
May cause damage to blood, liver, lung, kidney, spleen through prolonged or repeated exposure.

Hazard Symbols:

15. REGULATORY INFORMATION

Pesticide Registration:
This chemical is a pesticide product registered by the Environmental Protection Agency and is subject to certain labeling requirements under federal pesticide law. These requirements differ from the classification criteria and hazard information required for safety data sheets, and for workplace labels of non-pesticide chemicals. Following is the hazard information as required on the pesticide label:

Warning: Causes substantial but temporary eye injury. Harmful if swallowed May be fatal if inhaled. Prolonged or frequently repeated skin contact may cause allergic reactions in some individuals.

EPA Registration Number(s):

- storage information
- emergency spill or leak cleanup procedures
- LD_{50} and LC_{50} ratings for various test animals
- emergency telephone numbers of the manufacturer

Manufacturers prepare these sheets and make them available to every person selling, storing, or handling pesticides. Ask your employer for them, or, if self-employed, obtain them from the chemical manufacturer or pesticide supplier. You can obtain SDSs for every labeled pesticide, and employers are required to keep them in a clearly labeled, accessible area.

Sections of a Safety Data Sheet

Changes to Occupational Safety and Health Administration (OSHA) regulations have standardized the topics and format of SDSs. These standards mandate that all SDSs contain the following 16 sections.

1. **Identification.** Identification of the product includes the brand name of the product as it appears on the label, as well as any alternate ways to identify the product, such as other trade names or synonyms, chemical name(s), or the U.S. EPA registration number. This section also outlines the product's recommended uses and restrictions on use and provides you with the name, address, and telephone number of the manufacturer. You will also find emergency phone numbers here.

2. **Hazards identification.** This section must state the signal words, along with all relevant symbols or symbol descriptions (Fig. 11-7) and precautionary statements. This section

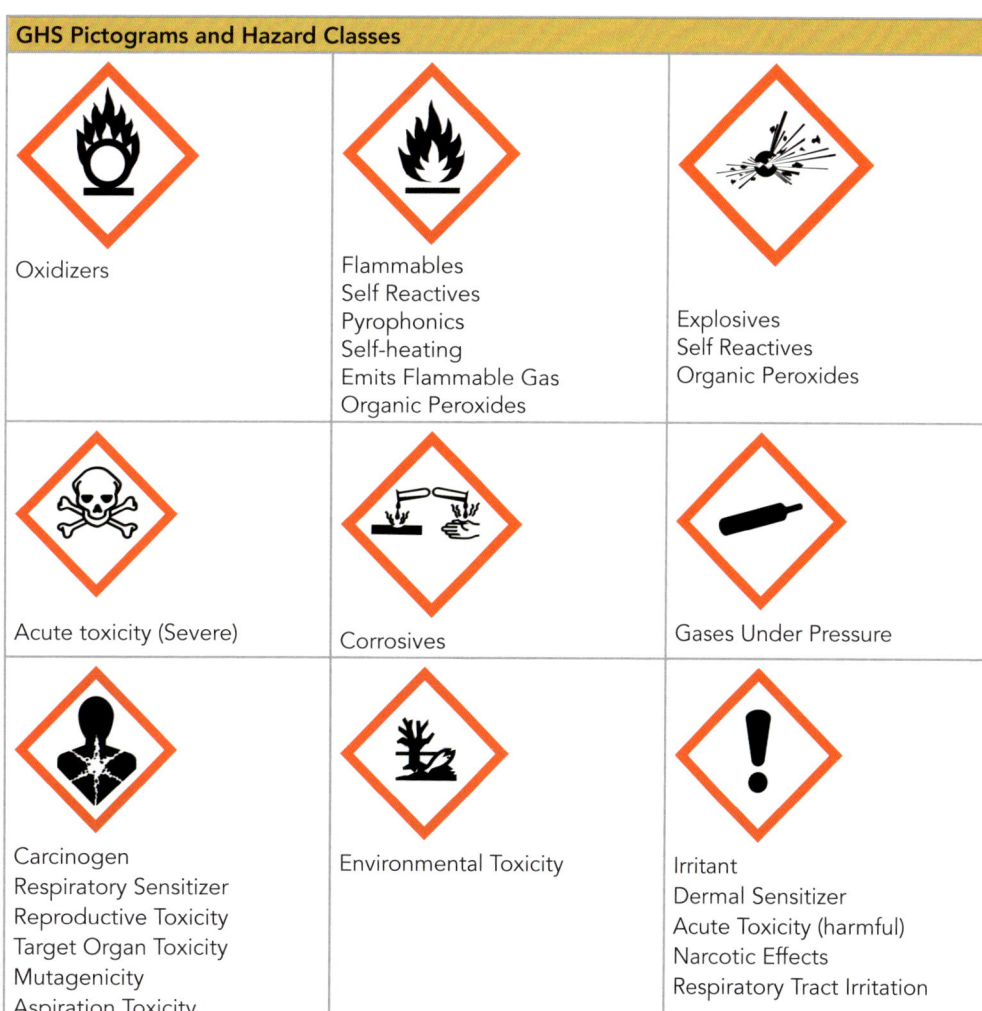

FIGURE 11-7

Hazard classes and pictograms that may be used in section 2 of a Safety Data Sheet, Hazards Identification. Pictograms communicate specific hazards associated with the pesticide.

must also include additional descriptions of hazards that have been identified during the classification process but do not inform the actual class of the pesticide. Information about ingredients that have not been tested for acute toxicity may also be included here in certain circumstances.

3. **Composition/ information on ingredients.** Information about the composition of the pesticide is included in this section. Each classified ingredient, additive, and impurity is listed, along with common names and synonyms, CAS (Chemical Abstracts Service) numbers, or other unique identifiers, and the percentage of each ingredient in the undiluted formulation. You may also see a note about any ingredients that are not revealed because of a trade secret claim.

4. **First aid measures.** Statements in this section provide information needed to assess and respond to exposure incidents, including the various ways people get exposed, major symptoms (both acute and delayed), and the immediate steps you can take to treat the exposed person. Special indications for medical treatment are also found in this section.

5. **Firefighting measures.** This section describes the pesticide's potential to create fire hazards, including hazardous chemicals that may be released during a fire. It includes a list of suitable extinguishing media (e.g., water, foam, dry powder) and, where necessary, unsuitable extinguishing media. In addition, you will find information specifically for firefighters, such as a list of special protective equipment and instructions for avoiding environmental contamination.

6. **Accidental release measures.** During a pesticide spill (accidental release), check this section to find out what PPE, precautions, and procedures you should use to keep the spill contained and begin cleanup. This section lists recommended materials for cleaning up the pesticide and details disposal options.

7. **Handling and storage.** An explanation of the precautions you must take to handle the pesticide safely can be found here. In addition, you can find a description of safe storage conditions for the pesticide.

8. **Exposure controls/personal protection.** This section provides the OSHA permissible exposure limit (PEL) and any other exposure limit used by the manufacturer to describe the maximum allowable exposure. It also lists appropriate engineering controls, personal protection measures, and PPE required to keep you from exposure to the active ingredient or other ingredients that pose health risks.

9. **Physical and chemical properties.** Where they are known, seventeen physical and chemical properties of the pesticide are listed in this section. Properties described include the appearance of the formulation, its odor, flammability or explosive limits, solubility, and viscosity, among others.

10. **Stability and reactivity.** The pesticide's stability and reactivity information is listed in this section. Here you will find a list of chemicals or conditions that create instability, reactivity, or incompatibility during mixing and storage. You can find out how likely it is that you will experience hazardous reactions, as well as the conditions to avoid (like static discharge, exposure to extreme heat, shock, or vibrations) to reduce bad reactions. It also lists hazardous decomposition products to help you avoid unintended exposure to harmful substances.

11. **Toxicological information.** This section details the chronic and acute effects of pesticides through the four likely routes of exposure (inhalation, ingestion, skin, and eye contact) for both long- and short-term exposures. Here you will find numerical measures of toxicity (such as LD_{50} estimates based on animal studies), as well as symptoms related to the pesticide's physical, chemical, and toxicological characteristics. If the pesticide has been found to be a potential carcinogen, that information will be listed here as well.

12. **Ecological information (non-mandatory).** In this section, you may see the pesticide's toxicity to sensitive areas and organisms. For instance, the LD_{50} for honey bees may be listed, as well as information about the pesticide's half-life in soil or in water at certain temperatures. You may also find information about the pesticide's mobility in soil, its potential to bioaccumulate, and other adverse effects it can have on the environment.
13. **Disposal considerations (non-mandatory).** Detailed instructions can be found in this section for safe handling and proper disposal of waste residues, pesticide containers, and contaminated packaging.
14. **Transport information (non-mandatory).** This section may include any information that relates to the local or long-distance transport of the pesticide. For instance, you may see Department of Transportation or other organization's transport hazard class(es) named here, as well as a listing of the pesticide's major environmental hazards. You may also find special precautions for users who will be transporting the pesticide from one place to another, whether moving it from one location to another on the same property or from one town to another.
15. **Regulatory information (non-mandatory).** In this section, you will see safety, health, and environmental regulations that pertain to the pesticide. For pesticides registered for use in California, you may see a Proposition 65 warning message.
16. **Other information.** This section contains information the manufacturer deems important but which does not fit into any of the other sections. It can include revision history or the date of SDS preparation and can also include a brief discussion of the manufacturer's liability or other information about the product (See OSHA 2012).

Chapter 11 Review Questions

1. Match the label part with the information that can be found there.

1. signal word	a. list of the components of the pesticide
2. first aid	b. the word that indicates the toxicity or hazard level of a pesticide
3. precautionary statements	c. the place to look for pests that the manufacturer claims are controlled when exposed to the pesticide, as well as specific sites, plant species, or animals to which the product may legally be applied
4. ingredients	d. information about how to decontaminate someone who has been exposed to the pesticide
5. restricted-entry statement	e. list of specific hazards to people, animals, and the environment for the pesticide
6. directions for use	f. information about how much time must elapse before people can walk through or work in a treated area without wearing personal protective equipment

2. **Which of the following illegal uses can be prevented if you abide by the requirement to read, understand, and follow the instructions on pesticide labels and related materials? Select all that apply.**
   - ☐ a. applying a pesticide that is not registered for the crop you need to treat
   - ☐ b. applying a pesticide during weather conditions listed as restricted for that product
   - ☐ c. applying the product at too low a rate in a given area
   - ☐ d. applying the pesticide too many times in a season in a particular area

3. **Where must an employer store pesticide Safety Data Sheets?**
   - ☐ a. with the pesticide product in the storage area
   - ☐ b. in the sprayer used for applying that pesticide
   - ☐ c. in a clearly labeled, accessible area

4. **Match the document type with the safety information it contains.**

1. SDS	a. how to avoid contaminating the environment while using the product
	b. the personal protective equipment required to safely handle a pesticide
2. label	c. the procedures used for fighting a pesticide fire
	d. information about how to handle pesticide spills

Chapter 12
Pesticide Emergencies and Emergency Response

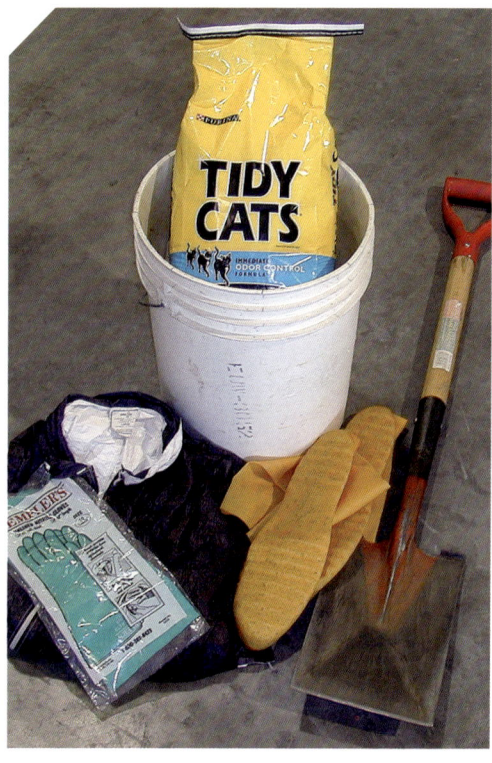

First Aid	335
Pesticide Leaks and Spills	341
Pesticide Fires	344
Stolen Pesticides	344
Misapplication of Pesticides	345
Reviewing Emergency Response to Accidents	346
Chapter 12 Review Questions	346

Knowledge Expectations

- Define first aid.
- Explain the procedures to follow in getting emergency medical treatment for exposure episodes.
- Describe how to set up and execute an emergency response plan.
- Describe pesticide poisoning and overexposure symptoms and signs.
- Distinguish between symptoms of pesticide overexposure and symptoms of common illnesses and heat stress.
- Describe how to identify heat stress and give first aid.
- Describe where to find information about first aid for a person involved in a pesticide incident and explain what to do if
    - a. you get pesticides on your clothing
    - b. you get pesticides in your eyes
    - c. you inhale pesticides
    - d. you swallow pesticides
- List the contents of a well-equipped decontamination facility, including components specific to different formulations.
- List the contents of a pesticide spill kit, including components specific to different formulations.
- Describe what to do when faced with a pesticide leak or spill.
- Describe what to do when faced with a pesticide fire.
- Describe what to do when a pesticide product has been stolen.
- Describe how to respond to the misapplication of pesticides.
- Explain why any incident should be reviewed.

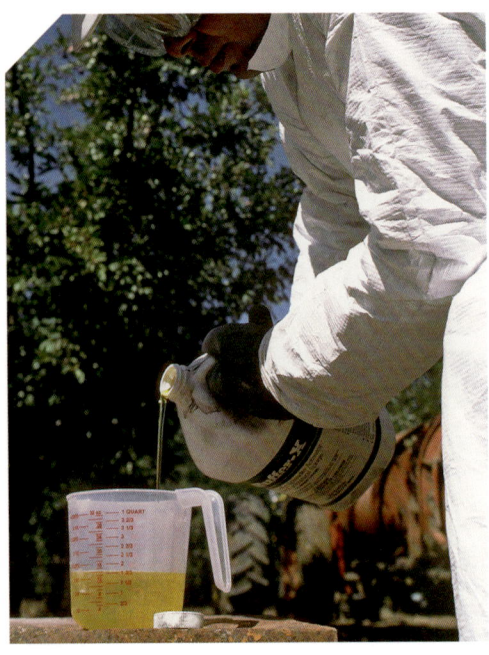

FIGURE 12-1

Any time you work around pesticides, you should be prepared to handle an emergency. Pesticide emergencies may be the result of leaks, spills, fires, thefts, misapplication, or improper storage or handling.

Accidents may occur while you are handling or applying pesticides, even if you are working under the most careful conditions. Pesticides diluted with water are hazardous, but undiluted pesticides are much more dangerous (Fig. 12-1). Pesticide emergencies may be the result of

- leaks
- spills
- fires
- thefts
- misapplication
- lack of care in storage or handling

Whenever you use pesticides, carry with you the names and locations of nearby medical facilities capable of treating pesticide-related injuries. If an accident happens and you have been exposed, seek medical care.

Be prepared to offer first aid to accident victims who get exposed to pesticides. Then, insist they receive prompt medical attention. To help employees locate medical facilities, post the notice shown in Figure 12-2 in a conspicuous place at the work site or in the work vehicle.

FIGURE 12-2

Post a notice like this one in a conspicuous place at the work site. Be sure all employees are shown where this notice is posted.

Emergency Medical Facility

Name of facility:

Location:

Telephone number:

Medical Monitoring for Employees

Name of physician or facility:

Location:

Telephone number:

First Aid

Define first aid.

First aid is the help you give a person exposed to pesticides before they receive emergency help from a medical professional. However, first aid is not a substitute for professional medical care. The precautionary statements section of each pesticide label provides specific first aid information.

Poisoning or exposure can occur if pesticides get onto your skin or into your eyes, if you accidentally swallow them, or if you inhale vapors, dusts, or fumes. The type of exposure determines what first aid and medical treatments are required. Serious pesticide poisoning may stop breathing or cause convulsions, paralysis, skin burns, or blindness. Applying the proper first aid treatment for pesticide exposure may reduce the extent of injury and even save lives. To prepare yourself for such emergencies, enroll in an American Red Cross first aid course that includes cardiopulmonary resuscitation (CPR) training.

Protect yourself when administering first aid to a person suffering from pesticide exposure. Avoid getting pesticides onto your skin. Do not inhale vapors. Do not enter a confined area to rescue a person overcome by toxic pesticide fumes unless you have the proper PPE, including respiratory equipment. Remember, the pesticide that affected the injured person can also injure you.

Explain the procedures to follow in getting emergency medical treatment for exposure episodes.

Get professional medical care at once for anyone who was exposed to a highly toxic pesticide or who shows signs of pesticide poisoning. Call an ambulance or transport the injured person to a medical facility for treatment. In addition to the first aid measures listed below, speed in obtaining medical care often controls the extent of injury. Provide medical personnel with complete information about the pesticide suspected of causing the injury.

EMERGENCY RESPONSE PLANNING

Describe how to set up and execute an emergency response plan.

A carefully thought-out emergency response or contingency plan is one of the most important tools you can have to prevent an emergency situation from becoming a catastrophic event. An emergency response plan can help protect the health and welfare of employees and the community, minimize environmental damage, and potentially reduce liability in the event of an accident. The importance of planning for emergencies cannot be overemphasized. Undertake this planning with painstaking attention.

A pesticide emergency may be caused by a severe weather event such as a tornado or flood or, more likely, an accident or fire. Serious public health and environmental consequences can occur when a tank truck overturns or a hose ruptures, spilling pesticides. An explosion and subsequent fire in a pesticide storage facility could result in serious injuries and environmental contamination, requiring the evacuation of persons downwind from the site of the fire. How you respond to a pesticide emergency may determine whether the incident becomes nothing more than a minor mishap or results in a major chemical release.

Consider the following guidelines when developing an emergency response plan:

- Designate an emergency coordinator. This person must have the knowledge and authority to direct and manage employee responses to a pesticide emergency and to coordinate the efforts of local emergency response agencies such as firefighters, police, and paramedics.
- Maintain a list of emergency response agencies (see Sidebar 12-1). Include names and telephone numbers of all response agencies you may have to call to assist in an emergency. Organize the list in the order to be called.
- Include an outline with your calling list of the information to be passed along during an emergency notification call that contains the following:
  - ◊ name and callback number of the person reporting the incident
  - ◊ precise location of the incident
  - ◊ general description of what has occurred

> **SIDEBAR 12-1**
>
> ## EMERGENCY NUMBERS FOR PESTICIDE ACCIDENTS AND SPILLS
>
> **WHEN PEOPLE HAVE BEEN EXPOSED TO PESTICIDES**
>
> - Dial 9-1-1 for emergency medical assistance. Notify the operator that the problem is a pesticide exposure. Provide an accurate location and information on the type of pesticide involved.
> - After obtaining medical treatment for exposed persons, determine whether a spill has taken place. Follow the instructions below for a spill.
> - Contact the nearest agricultural commissioner's office to report the incident at the website cdfa.ca.gov/exec/county/countymap/.
>
> **FOR PESTICIDE SPILLS ON STATE OR FEDERAL HIGHWAYS**
>
> - Notify the local office of the California Highway Patrol and your local fire department (dial 9-1-1). Inform the emergency operator that a pesticide spill has occurred; provide accurate location and type of pesticide.
> - Contact CHEMTREC at 800-424-9300 for assistance in cleaning up a pesticide spill.
> - Contact the California Office of Emergency Services. Usually a written report will need to be filed. See caloes.ca.gov/home or contact the main office in Sacramento:
>
>   Governor's Office of Emergency Services
>   3650 Schriever Ave
>   Mather, CA 95655, (916) 845-8510
>
> - Contact your local agricultural commissioner's office. Find the commissioner's telephone number for the county where the accident occurred at cdfa.ca.gov/exec/county/countymap/.
>
> **FOR PESTICIDE SPILLS ON LOCAL CITY OR RURAL ROADS OR ON PRIVATE LAND**
>
> - Contact the local police or sheriff and local fire department (dial 9-1-1). Inform the emergency operator that a pesticide spill has occurred. Provide accurate location and type of pesticide.
> - Contact CHEMTEC at 800-424-9300 for assistance in cleaning up a pesticide spill.
> - Report the spill to the California Office of Emergency Services (see caloes.ca.gov/home). Contact your local agricultural commissioner's office. Find the commissioner's telephone number for the county where the accident occurred at cdfa.ca.gov/exec/county/countymap/.

- ◊ the exact name, quantity, and classification of each chemical involved
- ◊ the extent of any injuries
- ◊ potential danger to the environment and persons living in the area

- Prepare a map of your facility to include with your emergency response plan. Show a layout of all chemical storage buildings and bulk storage tanks; access roads; main shut-offs for electricity, water, and gas; perimeter fencing that could hinder access to the pesticide storage facility; the location of fire alarms, firefighting equipment, and personal protective equipment (PPE); and drainage easements on the site. Provide emergency response agencies (in California, these are your county agricultural commissioner and your city or county fire department) with an updated copy of this map whenever changes are made at the facility (Fig. 12-3).
- Provide your emergency response agencies with an area map that shows your facility in relation to the surrounding area. Firefighters, police, and paramedics cannot waste time trying to determine where your facility is located.
- Keep a product inventory of the types and quantities of chemicals stored at your facility. Let your emergency response plan reflect peak season storage. The primary information in the product inventory includes the product names, container volumes, and locations of containers in the storage facility. Also, you must always keep copies of pesticide labels, Safety Data Sheet, and a description of required PPE for the chemicals in storage.
- Maintain an updated list of suppliers who can provide additional equipment and materials that may be needed in the event of an emergency.

The backbone of any emergency response plan is an outline of the exact sequence of actions to take in a crisis. Determine which situations you can handle on your own and which require outside help. Plan step-by-step procedures to respond to various emergencies, such as fires, spills, leaks, and transport accidents. Determine who is responsible for each specific task in the event of an activity, from sounding the alarm to directing the response agencies. Once internal emergency procedures have been established, be sure to share this information with local response agencies. Always keep a current plan on file with local response authorities.

Emergency response or contingency planning is the key to protecting every pesticide mixing, loading, storage, and application site and the surrounding community from a potentially catastrophic situation (see Randall et al. 2008).

RECOGNIZING PESTICIDE POISONING OR OVEREXPOSURE IN PEOPLE

In order to provide the right first aid and communicate with medical personnel responding to the emergency, you must be able to recognize the signs and symptoms of acute pesticide

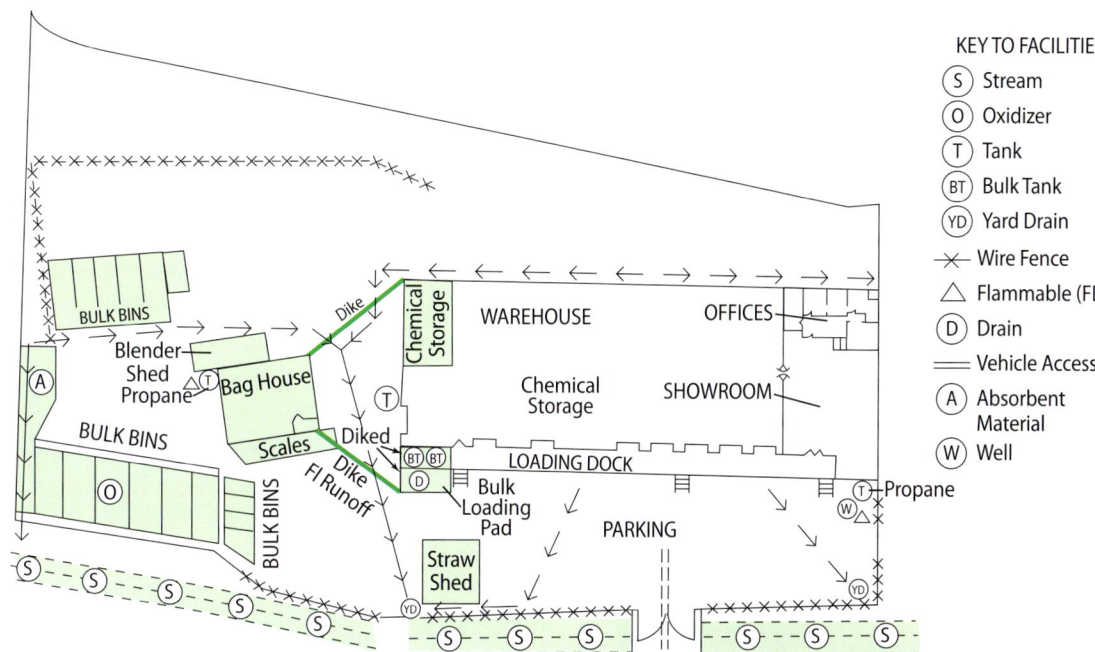

FIGURE 12-3
Include a facility map as part of the emergency response plan. *Source:* Randall 2008.

Describe pesticide poisoning and overexposure symptoms and signs.

poisoning or overexposure. Often symptoms of pesticide poisoning mimic symptoms of heat stress or common illnesses like the flu, so you must note what immediately preceded the onset of symptoms. For instance, has the temperature been unusually high, or has there been a recent pesticide application in or near the site of the incident? The answers to these questions provide the clues needed to properly diagnose illness and respond appropriately.

Poisoning signs are what you can observe in a victim of pesticide poisoning. These can include vomiting, sweating, skin irritation, eye irritation, swelling, or pin-point pupils.

Poisoning symptoms can only be described by the victim, and may include nausea, headache, weakness, burning of the eyes, nose, mouth, or throat, chest pain, body aches, muscle cramps, and dizziness, among others.

Distinguish between symptoms of pesticide overexposure and symptoms of common illnesses and heat stress.

RECOGNIZING AND RESPONDING TO HEAT STRESS

Heat-related illness may mimic certain types of pesticide poisoning. Symptoms of heat illness include tiredness, weakness, headache, sweating, nausea, dizziness, and fainting. Severe heat illness can cause a person to act confused, get angry easily, or behave strangely.

Depending on the severity of the symptoms, first aid for heat-induced illness could encompass any or all of the following actions:

Describe how to identify heat stress and give first aid.

- Call 9-1-1 and notify a supervisor.
- Move workers to an air-conditioned or cool, shaded area where they can rest.
- Cool workers by
  ◊ soaking their clothes with water
  ◊ spraying, sponging, or showering them with water
  ◊ fanning their bodies
- Provide workers with plenty of water, clear juice, or sports beverages to drink.

Describe where to find information about first aid for a person involved in a pesticide incident and explain what to do if
  • you get pesticides on your clothing.
  • you get pesticides in your eyes.
  • you inhale pesticides.
  • you swallow pesticides

IF PESTICIDES GET ON YOUR SKIN OR CLOTHING

Pesticides that get on your skin or clothing can cause serious injury (Fig. 12-4). Some pesticides may cause skin burns or rashes or, through skin absorption, produce internal poisoning. Immediately remove contaminated clothing and wash the affected areas with clean water and soap. Follow the first aid steps listed in the next section.

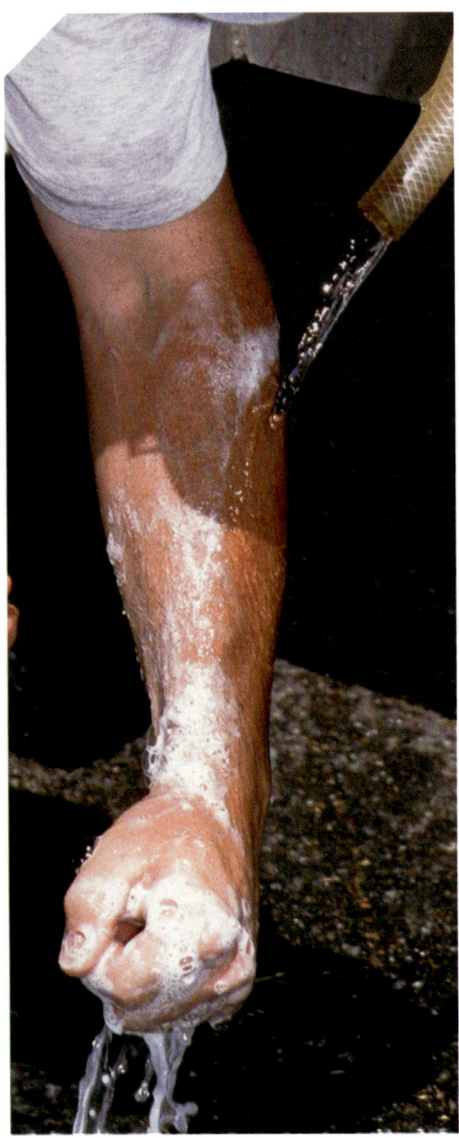

FIGURE 12-4

If pesticides spill on you, the first step is to remove contaminated clothing and wash the affected parts of your body with soap and plenty of water. Do this quickly to avoid serious injury.

First Aid for Skin Exposure

Take the following actions if you or someone else receives skin exposure to pesticides.

- **Leave the contaminated area.** Get away (or remove the victim) from the fumes, spilled pesticide, and further contamination. Do this quickly!
- **Restore breathing.** If the victim has stopped breathing, begin artificial respiration (rescue breathing) at once and continue until breathing resumes or until professional help arrives. If the person has stopped breathing and has no pulse, begin cardiopulmonary resuscitation (CPR) and continue until professional help arrives.
- **Prevent further exposure.** Remove the contaminated clothing and thoroughly wash the affected skin and hair areas. Use soap or detergent and large amounts of water.
- **Get medical attention.** Call an ambulance or have someone transport the injured person to the nearest medical facility as quickly as possible. Let medical providers know the name of the pesticide that caused the injury.

IF PESTICIDES GET IN YOUR EYES

Many pesticides are caustic and cause serious damage if they get into your eyes. Prompt first aid, followed by medical care, helps reduce damage.

First Aid for Eye Exposure

Take the following actions to treat eye exposure:

- **Flush the eyes.** Immediately flush the affected eye or eyes with a gentle stream of clean, temperate, running water (Fig. 12-5). Direct the stream of water away from your eyeball, letting the water run off the bridge of your nose or from the side of your face and into your eye. Hold eyelids open to ensure thorough flushing. Continue flushing for at least 15 minutes (if you wear contacts, flush eyes for 5 minutes, then remove the contacts and continue flushing for 10 minutes). If only one eye is affected, keep the injured eye closer to the ground, so that the water used for flushing will not contaminate your other eye. When flushing your eyes, do not use any chemicals or drugs in the water, since this may increase the extent of injury. If running water is not available, slowly pour clean water from a glass, water cooler, or other container onto the bridge of your nose, rather than directly into your eyes.
- **Obtain medical care.** Always get medical attention if irritation persists after the flushing. Let medical providers know the name of the pesticide that caused the injury.

IF PESTICIDES ARE INHALED

Inhaled chemicals, such as fumigants, pesticide dusts, vapors from spilled pesticides, and fumes from burning pesticides, can cause serious lung injury and may be absorbed into other parts of the body through the lungs. Take first aid measures immediately to reduce injury or prevent death.

Wear a supplied air respirator when entering an enclosed area to rescue a person who has been overcome by pesticide fumes. Cartridge respirators are not suitable for high concentrations of pesticide vapors or deficient oxygen conditions. If you do not have a supplied air respirator, call for emergency help. You will be of more assistance to the injured person by seeking proper emergency help than if you are overcome by the pesticide fumes yourself.

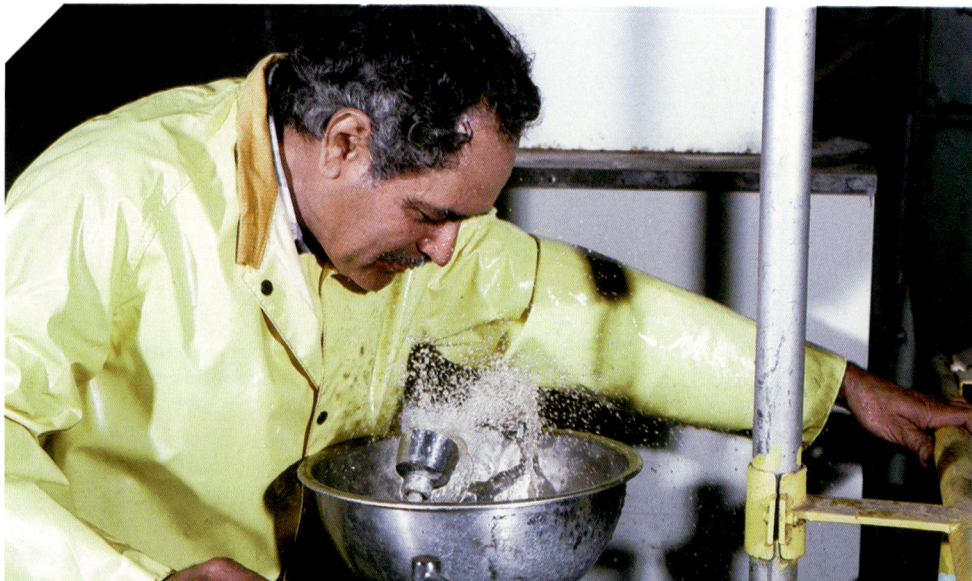

FIGURE 12-5
If you get a pesticide into your eyes, wash them with clean, running water for 15 minutes. Then, if irritation persists, seek medical care.

First Aid for Pesticide Inhalation

Take the following actions if you need to provide first aid to someone overcome by pesticide fumes:

- **Leave the contaminated area or remove an exposed person from the contaminated area.** Anyone overcome by pesticide vapors must get to fresh air immediately. Avoid physical exertion because this places an extra strain on the heart and lungs.
- **Loosen clothing.** Loosening clothing makes breathing easier and also releases pesticide vapors trapped between clothing and the skin.
- **Restore breathing.** If breathing has stopped or is irregular or labored, begin artificial respiration (rescue breathing). Continue assisting until breathing has improved or until medical help arrives. If the person has stopped breathing and has no pulse, begin cardiopulmonary resuscitation (CPR) and continue until help arrives.
- **Treat for shock.** Inhalation injury often causes a person to go into shock. Keep the injured person calm and lying down. Prevent chilling by wrapping the person in a blanket after removing contaminated clothing. Do not administer alcoholic beverages.
- **Watch for convulsions.** If convulsions occur protect the victim from falls or injury and keep air passages clear by making sure the head is tilted back.
- **Get immediate medical care.** Call an ambulance or transport the person to the nearest medical facility. Provide medical personnel with as much information as possible about the pesticide.

IF PESTICIDES ARE SWALLOWED

Two immediate dangers are associated with swallowed pesticides. The first is related to the toxicity of the pesticide and the poisoning effect it will have on a person's nervous system or other internal organs. The second involves physical injury that the swallowed pesticide causes to the linings of the mouth and throat and to the lungs. Corrosive materials, those that are strongly acidic or alkaline, can seriously burn these sensitive tissues. Petroleum-based pesticides can cause lung and respiratory system damage, especially during vomiting. Never induce vomiting if you suspect that the swallowed pesticide is corrosive or petroleum-based. Always read the pesticide label to find out exactly what course of action is recommended.

You can reach regional poison information centers in Sacramento, San Francisco, Fresno, and San Diego by telephone 24 hours a day, 7 days a week. In a poisoning emergency, call the California Poison Control System (CPCS) by using the toll-free number 1-800-222-1222. These centers provide quick, lifesaving information on poisoning treatment. Having the label handy will help the operator react quickly and perhaps save lives.

> **SIDEBAR 12-2**
>
> ## RECOMMENDED DECONTAMINATION EQUIPMENT AND PPE FOR PERSONNEL
>
> - Drop cloths of plastic or other suitable materials on which heavily contaminated equipment and outer protective clothing may be deposited
> - Collection containers, such as drums or suitably lined trash cans, for storing disposable clothing and heavily contaminated PPE that must be discarded
> - Lined box with absorbents for wiping or rinsing off gross contaminants and liquid contaminants
> - Large galvanized tubs, stock tanks, or wading pools to hold wash and rinse solutions; these should be at least large enough for a worker to place a booted foot in and should have either no drain or a drain connected to a collection tank or appropriate treatment system
> - Wash solutions selected to wash off and reduce the hazards associated with the contaminants
> - Rinse solutions selected to remove contaminants and contaminated wash solutions
> - Long-handled, soft-bristled brushes to help wash and rinse contaminated objects
> - Paper or cloth towels for drying PPE
> - Lockers and cabinets for storage of decontaminated clothing and equipment
> - Metal or plastic cans or drums for contaminated wash and rinse solutions
> - Plastic sheeting, sealed pads with drains, or other appropriate methods for containing and collecting contaminated wash and rinse solutions spilled during decontamination
> - Shower facilities for full body wash or, at a minimum, personal wash sinks (with drains connected to a collection tank or appropriate treatment system)
> - Soap or wash solution, single-use washcloths, and single-use towels for personnel
> - Lockers or closets for clean clothing and personal item storage
>
> *Source:* Adapted from NIOSH 1998.

First Aid for Swallowed Pesticides

Act quickly when a pesticide has been swallowed. Follow the pesticide label or poison information center instructions. If you cannot access the pesticide label or CPCS, follow these guidelines:

- **Dilute the swallowed pesticide.** If the person is conscious and alert, give large amounts (1 quart for an adult or a large glass for a child under seven) of water or milk. Do not give any liquids to an unconscious or convulsing person.
- **Induce vomiting.** If the pesticide label indicates, induce vomiting. Make sure the person is kneeling or lying face down or on their right side. If in doubt, do not induce vomiting.
- **Obtain medical care.** Call an ambulance or transport the poisoning victim to the nearest medical facility. Provide medical personnel with as much information as possible about the swallowed pesticide.

SETTING UP EMERGENCY DECONTAMINATION FACILITIES

The decontamination process should consist of a series of procedures performed in a specific sequence. For example, outer, more heavily contaminated items (e.g., outer boots and gloves) should be decontaminated and removed first, followed by decontamination and removal of inner, less contaminated items (e.g., jackets and pants). Each procedure should be performed at a separate station in order to prevent cross-contamination, if possible. The sequence of stations is called the decontamination line.

Stations should be separated physically to prevent cross-contamination and should be arranged in order of decreasing contamination, preferably in a straight line if possible. Separate flow patterns and stations should be provided to isolate workers from different contamination zones containing incompatible wastes. Entry and exit points should be conspicuously marked, and the entry to the contamination reduction zone (CRZ) from the exclusion zone should be separate from the entry to the exclusion zone from the CRZ. Dressing stations for entry to the CRZ should be separate from redressing areas for exit from the CRZ. Personnel who wish to enter clean areas of the decontamination facility such as locker rooms should be completely decontaminated. Information in the following sections are meant to provide examples of best practices and are not required by California regulations (see NIOSH 1998).

> *List the contents of a well-equipped decontamination facility, including components specific to different formulations.*

> **SIDEBAR 12-3**
>
> ### RECOMMENDED EQUIPMENT FOR HEAVY EQUIPMENT AND VEHICLE DECONTAMINATION
>
> - Storage tanks appropriate treatment systems for temporary storage and/or treatment of contaminated wash and rinse solutions
> - Drains or pumps for collection of contaminated wash and rinse solutions
> - Long-handled brushes for general exterior cleaning
> - Wash solutions selected to remove and reduce the hazards associated with the contamination
> - Rinse solutions selected to remove contaminants and contaminated wash solutions
> - Pressurized sprayers for washing and rinsing, particularly hard-to-reach areas
> - Curtains, enclosures, or spray booths to contain splashes from pressurized sprays
> - Long-handled brushes, rods, and shovels for dislodging contaminants and contaminated soil caught in tires and the undersides of vehicles and equipment
> - Containers to hold contaminants and contaminated soil removed from tires and the undersides of vehicles and equipment
> - Wash and rinse buckets for use in the decontamination of operator areas inside vehicles and equipment
> - Brooms and brushes for cleaning operator areas inside vehicles and equipment
> - Containers for storage and disposal of contaminated wash and rinse solutions, damaged or heavily contaminated parts, and equipment to be discarded
>
> *Source:* Adapted from NIOSH 1998.

Decontamination Equipment Selection

Sidebar 12-2 lists recommended equipment for decontamination of personnel and PPE. In selecting decontamination equipment, consider whether the equipment itself can be decontaminated for reuse or can be easily disposed of. Sidebar 12-3 lists recommended equipment for decontamination of large equipment and vehicles. Note that other types of equipment not listed in Sidebars 12-2 and 12-3 may be appropriate in certain situations.

Pesticide Leaks and Spills

List the contents of a pesticide spill kit, including components specific to different formulations.

Treat all pesticide leaks or spills as emergencies. Concentrated pesticide spills are much more dangerous than pesticides diluted with water, but both types should be dealt with immediately. Leaks or spills can occur during transporting, storing, or while using pesticides. Pesticides may be spilled indoors, in enclosed areas, or outside.

Below you will find information that applies to all significant releases of hazardous materials. You should also refer to the Safe Drinking Water and Toxic Enforcement Act of 1986 (Proposition 65) and Section 9030 of the California Labor Code for additional reporting requirements. Before engaging in pesticide application, all pest control businesses must determine

- the definition of *significant spill*
- which agencies must be notified after you call 9-1-1 and the California Emergency Management Agency (CalEMA)

Business owners and managers should contact their local fire department or CalEMA for guidance. For additional information on reporting requirements, visit the California Office of Emergency Services website, caloes.ca.gov/.

SPILL KITS

Keep a spill cleanup kit readily available whenever you handle pesticides or their containers. Also maintain a spill kit at the business location where pesticides are mixed, loaded, and stored, and on each vehicle that transports pesticides. If a spill occurs, you will not have the time or the opportunity to find all of the items needed to respond to the situation.

Include the following in a kit (Randall et al. 2008):
- telephone numbers for emergency assistance

- gloves, footwear, and aprons that are chemically resistant to most pesticides and that comply with the label and SDS PPE requirements
- protective eyewear, as required by the label and SDS
- an appropriate respirator, if either the pesticide label or SDS require the use of one
- containment tubes or pads to confine the leak or spill
- absorbent materials, such as spill pillows, absorbent clay, sawdust, cat litter, activated charcoal, vermiculite, or paper for liquid spills
- sweeping compound for dry spills
- a shovel, broom, and dustpan
- heavy-duty detergent
- a fire extinguisher rated for all types of fires
- any other spill cleanup items specified on all labeling of any products you use regularly
- a sturdy plastic container that holds the quantity of pesticide from the largest pesticide container being handled and that can be tightly closed

Store spill kit items in a plastic container, replace items that have been used or discarded, and keep the contents clean and in working order until needed.

> Describe what to do when faced with a pesticide leak or spill.

What to Do When Leaks and Spills Occur

Immediate Actions
- If the spill occurs on a public roadway, call 9-1-1 and the California Emergency Management Agency, 1-800-852-7550 (see "Reporting," below).
- If anyone has been injured or contaminated, administer first aid. Send for medical help if necessary.
- Rope off the area or set up barricades to keep everyone away from the contaminated site.
- If the spill is indoors, get out of the building. If you have access to the proper PPE, reenter the building to open doors and windows and set up a portable fan.

Contaminated Materials
- Put materials that were contaminated by the spill or have been cleaned up into a sealable drum. Label the drum to indicate that it contains hazardous waste. Include the name of the pesticide and the signal word (DANGER, WARNING, or CAUTION). Because local regulations vary, contact the county agricultural commissioner or the Department of Toxic Substances Control regional office for instructions on how to dispose of the sealed drum and its contents. Under most circumstances, you must send the residue from a pesticide spill to a Class I disposal facility.
- Spills on cleanable surfaces such as concrete require thorough decontamination. Commercial decontamination preparations are available for this purpose, or you can prepare a solution that contains 4 tablespoons of detergent and 1 pound of soda ash dissolved in each gallon of water. Soda ash cannot be used for detoxification of certain pesticides, so check the label or SDS before using this solution. Contact the pesticide manufacturer if you have any questions. For more information, see the section "Cleaning up Pesticide Leaks or Spills," below.

Reporting
When spills occur on public roadways, you must
- call 9-1-1 (or the local emergency response agency)
- call 1-800-852-7550 (or 916-845-8911) and report the spill to the California Emergency Management Agency, California State Warning Center

If the spill causes injury or exposure, you must notify the California Occupational Safety and Health Administration (Cal/OSHA). If the spill occurs in or near a waterway, you must notify the United States Coast Guard; the Department of Fish and Wildlife, Office of Spill Prevention and Response; and the local Regional Water Quality Control Board. Report all leaks or spills of pesticides, no matter where they occur, to the local county agricultural commissioner as soon as

possible. When you call the required agencies, you must provide:
- your identity
- the location, date, and time of the spill, release, or threatened release
- the location of threatened or involved waterways or storm drains
- the substance, quantity involved, and isotope if necessary
- the chemical name (if its toxicity level makes the substance extremely hazardous, report that information, as well)
- a description of what happened

If the spill exceeds federal reporting requirements, you will also need to report
- medium or media impacted by the release
- time and duration of the release
- proper precautions to take
- known or anticipated health risks
- name and phone number where officials can reach you if they need more information

In addition, a written report may be required. Check California and federal statutes and California regulations to find out if a written report is required in your situation and how soon it must be delivered to avoid state and federal emergency notification penalties.

CLEANING UP PESTICIDE LEAKS OR SPILLS

Cleaning up major pesticide spills requires the help of professionals. It is extremely difficult and costly to remove contaminated soil or to prevent or clean up groundwater contamination. The types of pesticide leaks and spills you will most likely encounter will be controllable quantities, such as when a container is damaged or slips to the ground or when diluted pesticide leaks from application equipment. Proper and immediate response to even these small leaks and spills is necessary to minimize damage to human and environmental health. Follow these basic steps when cleaning up a pesticide leak or spill:

- **Clear the area.** Keep people and animals away from the contaminated area. Provide first aid if anyone has been injured or contaminated. Send for medical help if necessary.
- **Prevent fires.** Some liquid pesticides are flammable or are formulated in flammable carriers. Pesticide powders are potentially explosive, especially if a dust cloud forms in an enclosed area. Do not allow any smoking near a spill. If the spill occurs in an enclosed area, shut off all electrical appliances and motors that could produce sparks and ignite a fire or explosion. See "Pesticide Fires," below.
- **Wear PPE.** Before beginning any cleanup, put on the PPE listed on the label for handling the concentrated material. Check the pesticide label for additional precautions. If you are uncertain what has been spilled, wear the maximum protection. This includes chemical-resistant boots and gloves, waterproof protective clothing, goggles, and a respirator.
- **Contain the leak.** Stop leaks by transferring the pesticide to another container or by patching the leaking container (repair paper bags and cardboard boxes with strong tape). Use soil, sand, sawdust, or absorbent clay to form a containment dam around liquid leaks. Common cat litter is a good absorbent material for pesticide cleanup. If the wind is blowing pesticide dusts or powders, cover the spill with a plastic tarp or, if a covering is not available, lightly spray the area with water to prevent offsite movement.
- **Clean up the pesticide.** Proceed to clean up the spill or leak (Fig. 12-6). Brush the containment dam of absorbent material toward the center of a liquid spill. Add additional absorbent material if necessary. Sweep up granule formulations. If the

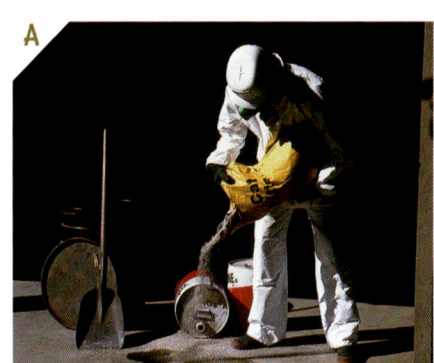
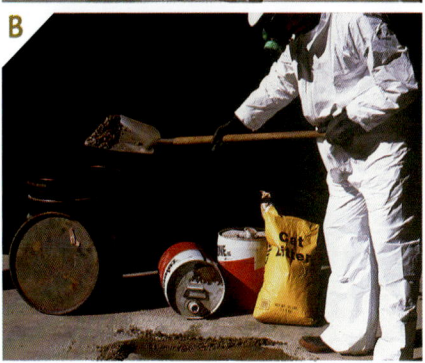

FIGURE 12-6

Cover pesticide spills with an absorbent material (A) and shovel it into a sealable container (B). When the cleanup is completed, seal and label the container and send it to a Class I disposal site. Wear personal protective equipment (required by the pesticide label) during the cleanup.

spill is on soil, shovel out the top 2 to 3 inches of soil for disposal. Place the absorbent or spilled dry product and any contaminated soil in a sealable container. Containers for holding contaminated materials must be suitable for transporting. Label the container with the pesticide name and signal word.
- **Clean nonporous surfaces and safety equipment.** If the spill occurred on a cleanable surface such as concrete or asphalt, use a broom to scrub the contaminated surface with a strong detergent solution. Clean this up again with absorbent material and place it in the container. Equipment such as brooms, shovels, and dustpans must be cleaned or disposed of after use. For instance, brooms cannot be cleaned and so must be discarded, whereas a shovel can be appropriately decontaminated after use and can be kept. When you finish, clean your PPE.
- **Dispose of the material.** Local regulations on disposal of hazardous materials may vary. Check with the local county agricultural commissioner or the California Department of Toxic Substances Control regional office for instructions on how to dispose of the container and its contents.

Pesticide Fires

Fighting pesticide fires requires special care because smoke and fumes generated by burning pesticides cannot be contained; areas endangered by these fumes must be evacuated. Toxic fumes hamper firefighting efforts and require the use of supplied air respirators and protective clothing. Water must be used with caution when fighting pesticide fires. Use it primarily to cool containers and prevent overheated chemicals from exploding. Do not splash or spread toxic chemicals with high-pressure water. It is best to contain small fires with fog, foam, or dry powder rather than water.

Once the fire has been brought under control, all hoses and equipment, including PPE, must be decontaminated. Water and other liquids must be contained, collected, and disposed of as hazardous waste. Residue remaining at the fire site must be removed and disposed of as well.

How to Deal with a Pesticide Fire

Describe what to do when faced with a pesticide fire.

If a pesticide fire breaks out:
- **Call the fire department.** Contact the nearest fire department as quickly as possible (call 9-1-1). Inform them that there is a fire involving pesticides. Provide them with the names of the chemicals contained in the structure or vehicle. If possible, provide Safety Data Sheets to the arriving fire units.
- **Clear the area.** Get people out of the immediate area of the fire; there may be considerable risk of toxic fumes and explosion.
- **Evacuate and isolate the area around and downwind of the fire.** Protect animals and move equipment and vehicles that could be damaged by the fire or fumes or that would impair firefighting efforts. Keep spectators from being exposed to smoke from the fire and runoff from firefighting. Contact the police or sheriff and have downwind residences, schools, and buildings evacuated until the danger has passed.

Stolen Pesticides

Describe what to do when a pesticide product has been stolen.

The first line of defense in any security program is properly trained employees and contractors. They notice much of what occurs in and around a pesticide storage facility or pesticide application business and can provide an early warning when something does not seem quite right or someone is acting suspiciously. Security training and awareness can ensure that these individuals can act effectively as an alert surveillance system. At a minimum, instruct all employees on pesticide inventory control, security of storage facilities and application equipment, and emergency preparedness and response. Individuals must be alert to unusual purchases, threats, or suspicious behavior by other employees or customers (Randall et al. 2008).

Notification Plan

If a breach of security or suspicious activity does occur, contact the appropriate authorities immediately. In addition to alerting the local police department and agricultural commissioner, you must immediately report any threats or suspicious behavior to the local FBI field office. These agencies also must be informed of incidents involving pesticide exposures that occur under circumstances inconsistent with a product's normal use pattern. Information on the location of the appropriate FBI office is available at fbi.gov.

Misapplication of Pesticides

> Describe how to respond to the misapplication of pesticides.

Another form of emergency may exist when pesticides have been misapplied either intentionally, accidentally, or through negligence:
- Intentional misapplication involves intentional use of a pesticide on an unregistered site or knowingly applying pesticides in a manner inconsistent with label directions.
- Accidental misapplication involves unknowingly applying a pesticide to a site not on the label.
- Negligent application involves improper calibration of application equipment as well as improper use and disposal of the pesticide; it also involves applying pesticides at the wrong time or in any other way inconsistent with label requirements.

Making an application mistake is a serious problem; do not compound the damage by failing to take responsible corrective action once the mistake is discovered. You may be financially responsible for damages, both physical and legal, caused by your misapplication of a pesticide. You may be able to reduce the amount of damage and liability by taking prompt action once you discover the error. Of primary importance is the protection of people, animals, and the environment.

Incorrect Amount of Pesticide Applied

Although using insufficient quantities of pesticides usually does not give adequate control of the target pest and is a waste time and money, it generally presents no immediate problems to people or the environment. Using excessive amounts of pesticide, however, can be an environmental threat as well as a danger to human health. This type of problem occurs as a result of
- poor calibration of your application equipment
- faulty mixing of chemicals in your spray tank
- not understanding the label statement regarding application rates

Residues from the pesticide may last longer than expected, or a concentrated application may cause damage to the treated area.

Correcting the Problem. Once an improper application has been discovered, take immediate action. Notify the county agricultural commissioner of the problem and seek information and advice on what remedies to take. Contact the pesticide manufacturer to find out what corrective measures they suggest. Remember, speed is of the utmost importance when trying to reduce damage.

Wrong Pesticide Applied

Lack of attention to your mixing operation or giving the wrong instructions to an employee may result in the wrong pesticide being applied. Besides possible damage to plants or surfaces in the treatment area, using the wrong pesticide exposes you and your workers to unanticipated hazards. For instance, mixing and application might take place without the required PPE, resulting in possible injury to the applicator.

Correcting the Problem. When you discover that you have mixed or applied the wrong pesticide, contact the county agricultural commissioner for help, then call the pesticide manufacturer. Notify people in the application area and keep them away until it can be made safe again.

PESTICIDES APPLIED TO THE WRONG SITE OR CROP

Another form of accident involves pesticides being applied to the wrong site. This can be a serious problem if the site (or crop) is not listed on the pesticide label or if there are workers at the site who are performing cultural operations.

Correcting the Problem. Contact the county agricultural commissioner and the pesticide manufacturer for assistance. Keep people and animals out of the sprayed area until it has been determined that it is safe to return.

Reviewing Emergency Response to Accidents

Accidents happen. The best way to be prepared for accidents is to review emergency responses to past incidents. Good recordkeeping, video or photographic evidence, and first-hand reporting from those involved in the incident can help you and your co-workers understand what went wrong and learn how to respond more effectively to future incidents. Questions to ask include

- What caused the accident?
- What pesticide(s) were involved in the accident?
- How did people respond as the situation unfolded?
- How could people improve their response to the situation?

Emergency response drills are another way to help you understand how to respond in case of an actual emergency. These drills can mimic pesticide fires or spills and will test your knowledge of your company's emergency response plan. Records of these drills can then be reviewed in order to find the strengths and weaknesses of your response plan. Aspects of the plan that were implemented well should be complimented, and areas of weakness can be addressed through additional, focused training.

Explain why any incident should be reviewed.

Chapter 12 Review Questions

1. The help you give people exposed to pesticides before they receive emergency help from a medical professional is called _____.
   - ☐ a. practical treatment
   - ☐ b. first aid
   - ☐ c. emergency care

2. Match the emergency type with the procedures to follow when providing first aid.

1. pesticides on skin or clothing	a. Prevent chilling (from shock) by wrapping the person in a blanket after removing him or her from the accident site and disposing of contaminated clothing.
2. inhaled pesticides	b. After removing contaminated clothing, thoroughly wash the affected areas with soap or detergent and large amounts of water.
3. swallowed pesticides	c. Move the affected person to an air-conditioned or cool, shaded area.
4. heat stress	d. Give the person large amounts (1 quart for an adult or a large glass for a child under seven) of water or milk.

3. Which statements are *true* about first aid response for pesticide exposure to the eye? Select all that apply.
   - ☐ a. Hold eyelids open to ensure thorough flushing.
   - ☐ b. The water should be dripped directly into the eye; don't use an eyewash dispenser.
   - ☐ c. Continuously rinse the eye for 15 minutes.
   - ☐ d. Pour clean water from a glass, water cooler, or other container onto the bridge of the nose, rather than directly into the eye(s).

4. What is considered the backbone of any emergency response plan?
   - ☐ a. an area map that shows your facility in relation to the surrounding area
   - ☐ b. a product inventory of the types and quantities of chemicals stored at your facility
   - ☐ c. an outline of the exact sequence of actions to take in a crisis

5. How can you tell if someone is suffering from acute pesticide poisoning?
   - ☐ a. Find out what immediately preceded the onset of symptoms.
   - ☐ b. Look to see if there are any obvious signs of a pesticide spill nearby.
   - ☐ c. It is impossible to tell unless you are a trained medical professional.

6. Signs that a person is experiencing heat stress can include _____.
   - ☐ a. tiredness and confusion
   - ☐ b. sweating and vomiting
   - ☐ c. body aches and weakness

7. Where should you look for first aid procedures to implement in case of a pesticide exposure incident?
   - ☐ a. publications from your pesticide dealer
   - ☐ b. the pesticide label and Safety Data Sheet
   - ☐ c. documents provided by your local poison control center

8. Put the following decontamination processes in the correct order.
   - ☐ a. removing and cleaning work clothes
   - ☐ b. washing the hands and body
   - ☐ c. removing and cleaning boots and gloves

9. Which of the following items should be part of a well-equipped decontamination facility? Select all that apply.
   - ☐ a. plastic drop cloths
   - ☐ b. containers for holding contaminated PPE
   - ☐ c. brooms
   - ☐ d. long-handled, soft-bristled brushes
   - ☐ e. cat litter
   - ☐ f. single-use washcloths and towels

10. A spill kit should contain which of the following items? Select all that apply.
    - ☐ a. shovel, broom, and dustpan
    - ☐ b. wash and rinse buckets
    - ☐ c. absorbent clay, sawdust, or cat litter
    - ☐ d. PPE as required by the pesticide label
    - ☐ e. large galvanized tubs

11. Which statement is true about proper cleanup procedures for pesticide spills?
    - ☐ a. Remove the top 1 inch of soil to decontaminate soil saturated with a pesticide.
    - ☐ b. Use soil, sand, sawdust, or absorbent clay to form a containment dam around liquids.
    - ☐ c. Use charcoal briquettes to reduce soil contamination and subsequent plant damage.

12. Which of the following actions are recommended in the event of a fire involving pesticides? Select all that apply.
    - ☐ a. Use water jets to put out the pesticide fire.
    - ☐ b. Construct dikes to contain contaminated runoff water.
    - ☐ c. Notify the fire department and inform the firefighters of the nature of the pesticides involved.
    - ☐ d. Contain small fires with fog, foam, or dry powder.

13. In addition to calling 9-1-1 to alert local law enforcement, who else should you notify if pesticides have been stolen?
    - ☐ a. the Department of Pesticide Regulation
    - ☐ b. your local pesticide dealer
    - ☐ c. your local FBI field office

14. What can you do to reduce the amount of damage and liability that can result from a misapplication of pesticides?
    - ☐ a. Call the landowner to report the problem and the steps taken to correct it.
    - ☐ b. Take prompt action to correct and report the error once you discover it.
    - ☐ c. Notify the pesticide dealer to see how they recommend you correct the problem.

15. Why is it important to review the response to a pesticide accident after it has occurred?
    - ☐ a. Looking back at an incident gives everyone a chance to process what happened and move on in a positive way.
    - ☐ b. Reviewing past incidents reduces liability and insurance rates, since employees will be better prepared to respond to emergencies.
    - ☐ c. Thorough review of the response to an accident can help everyone respond more effectively to future incidents.

Answers to Review Questions

CHAPTER 1
1: 1.c; 2.d; 3.a; 4.b
2: 1.c; 2.a; 3.b
3: 1.b; 2.a; 3.c
4: a
5: c
6: b
7: b, c, d, f, g
8: b
9: a
10: c
11: b
12: a
13: c
14: c
15: a

CHAPTER 2
1: b
2: c
3: 1.a; 2.b; 3.b; 4.a
4: c
5: 1.c, h; 2.a, f; 3.b, e; 4.d, g
6: a
7: b
8: a
9: 1.c, e, f; 2.a, b, d
10: 1.b, g; 2.c, d; 3.f, h; 4.a, e

CHAPTER 3
1: a
2: c
3: 1.d, f; 2.b, e; 3.a, g; 4.c, h
4: 1.b; 2.c; 3.a
5: 1.c; 2.a; 3.f; 4.g; 5.h; 6.b; 7.d; 8.e
6: b
7: a
8: c
9: 1.c; 2.e; 3.a; 4.b; 5.d
10: b
11: 1.b; 2.d; 3.a; 4.e; 5.c
12: b
13: c

CHAPTER 4
1: a.T; b.T; c.T; d.F; e.T; f.T
2: 1.c; 2.d; 3.a; 4.b
3: 1.d; 2.a; 3.e; 4.b; 5.c
4: c
5: b
6: a
7: c
8: b
9: a
10: b

CHAPTER 5
1: b
2: a, b, c, d
3: b, c
4: c
5: a, b
6: b
7: c
8: a

CHAPTER 6
1: a
2: a
3: c
4: b
5: 1.a; 2.d; 3.b; 4.f; 5.g; 6.e; 7.c
6: 1.c; 2.a; 3.b
7: a
8: b
9: c
10: c
11: b
12: b
13: a
14: c

CHAPTER 7
1: a, d, e
2: b
3: a
4: c
5: b
6: a.T; b.F; c.T; d.F; e.T; f.T
7: a
8: 1.b; 2.c; 3.a
9: b
10: c
11: b

CHAPTER 8
1: 1.c; 2.b; 3.e; 4.a; 5.d
2: 1.d; 2.a; 3.b; 4.c; 5.f; 6.e
3: a
4: c
5: c
6: b
7: a
8: c
9: 1.b; 2.c; 3.d; 4.a; 5.e
10: c
11: b
12: 1.e; 2.a; 3.d; 4.b; 5.c
13: b
14: b
15: a
16: c
17: c
18: c
19: a
20: b

CHAPTER 9
1: c
2: a
3: b, c, e, g, h
4: c
5: a
6: c
7: b
8: c
9: 1.c; 2.b; 3.a
10: b
11: c, a, b, d
12: b
13: b
14: a
15: c

CHAPTER 10
1: 1.c; 2.b; 3.a
2: b
3: c
4: a
5: b
6: b
7: a
8: c
9: b
10: e, a, d, c, b
11: a
12: b
13: b, c, e
14: 1.b; 2.a; 3.d; 4.e; 5.c
15: c
16: a

CHAPTER 11
1: 1.b; 2.d; 3.e; 4.a; 5.f; 6.c
2: a, b, d
3: c
4: 1.c, d; 2.a, b

CHAPTER 12
1: b
2: 1.b; 2.a; 3.d; 4.c
3: a, c, d
4: c
5: a
6: a
7: b
8: c, a, b
9: a, b, d, f
10: a, c, b
11: b
12: b, c, d
13: c
14: b
15: c

Glossary

abatement. A type of pest control that focuses on reducing the presence of a pest in an area.

abdomen. The rear part of an insect. In people, the body section containing the stomach.

abiotic. Nonliving factors such as wind, water, temperature, and soil type or texture.

abiotic disorders. Noninfectious diseases introduced by adverse environmental conditions, often as a result of human activity.

absorb. To soak up or take in a liquid or powder.

acaricide. A pesticide used to control mites.

accidental misapplication. An unintentional, incorrect application of a pesticide.

accumulate. To increase in quantity within an area, such as in the soil or tissues of a plant or animal.

acetylcholine. A short-acting neurotransmitter, widely distributed in the body, that transmits nerve signals between nerves and muscles, nerves and sensory organs, or nerves and other nerves.

acidic. A solution or substance that has a pH lower than 7.0.

acidifier. An adjuvant used to lower the pH (or acidify) the water being mixed with a pesticide.

action threshold. In pest management, the level of pest damage or pest infestation that warrants a control action.

activator. An adjuvant that increases the activity of a pesticide by reducing surface tension or speeding up penetration through insect or plant cuticles.

active ingredient (a.i.). The material in the pesticide formulation that actually destroys the target pest or performs the desired function.

acute effect. An illness that becomes apparent soon after an exposure to a pesticide occurs.

adaptation. The development of physical and behavioral characteristics that allow organisms to survive and reproduce in their habitats.

additive effect. An increase in toxicity brought about by combining one pesticide with another.

adjuvant. A material added to a pesticide mixture to improve or alter the deposition, toxic effects, mixing ability, persistence, or other qualities of the active ingredient.

adsorb. To gather and hold on a surface, such as pesticides that become attached to soil particles.

aerosol. Very fine liquid droplets or dust particles often emitted from a pressurized can or aerosol-generating device.

aestivation. Dormancy during summer or periods of high temperature or a dry season.

agitator. A mechanical or hydraulic device that stirs the liquid in a spray tank to prevent the mixture from separating or settling.

agricultural commissioner. The official in each county in California who has the responsibility for enforcing the state and federal pesticide regulations and issuing permits for restricted-use pesticides.

agricultural use. A classification of certain pesticides that limits their use to production agriculture settings.

a.i. See *active ingredient*.

air assist sprayer. A sprayer that uses air to move spray droplets to the target surface. See also air blast sprayer.

air blast sprayer. A sprayer that uses a high-powered fan to carry spray droplets to target surfaces. Air blast sprayers are usually used on tall plants such as trees or vines.

air gap. A space between the filling hose and the liquid in a pesticide tank that prevents backflow of pesticide liquids into the water source.

algae (sing., alga). Aquatic, nonvascular plants.

alkaline. A solution or substance that has a pH greater than 7.0.

allowable tolerance. The maximum amount of pesticide residues that may remain on treated produce or other food items once these items become available to consumers.

all-terrain cycle. A three- or four-wheeled motorcycle-like vehicle used for applying low volumes of pesticides in agricultural areas and open lands.

alternate hosts. Plants that support the survival of a pest when its main host is not available.

amphibian. Cold-blooded organism such as a frog, toad, or salamander.

animal kingdom. One of two groups of living organisms, the other being the plant kingdom.

anionic. Materials that contain negatively charged ions; a characteristic of some types of surfactants that helps prevent pesticides from being washed off treated surfaces.

annual. A plant that passes through its entire life cycle in one year or less. Plants can be further divided into summer or winter annuals.

antagonistic effect. Reduced toxicity or effectiveness as a result of combining one pesticide with another.

anther. Male flower part containing pollen.

antibiosis. Production of metabolic substances by an organism (such as a plant) that are toxic or repellent to predators or parasites.

antibiotic. A substance produced by a living organism, such as a fungus, that is toxic to other types of living organisms; sometimes used as a pesticide.

anticoagulant. Chemical that causes death by preventing normal blood clotting.

apiary. A place where bees are kept, such as a beehive.

application pattern. The course the applicator follows through the area being treated with a pesticide.

application rate. The amount of pesticide that is applied to a known area, such as an acre.

application swath. See *swath* and *swath width*.

aquatic. Pertaining to water, such as aquatic weeds or aquatic pest control.

aquifer. An underground formation of sand, gravel, or porous rock that contains water; the place where groundwater is found.

arsenical pesticide. A pesticide that contains some form of arsenic.

arthropod. An animal with jointed appendages and an external skeleton, such as an insect, spider, mite, crab, or centipede.

artificial respiration. See *rescue breathing*.

atmosphere. The air or climate in a given place.

atmosphere-monitoring device. A piece of equipment used to detect and measure vapor levels in an enclosed area. Typically used after fumigation to ensure an area is safe to enter.

attractant. A substance that attracts a specific species of animal to it. When manufactured to attract pests to traps or poisoned bait, attractants are considered to be pesticides.

attractive nuisance. A legal principle referring to an area (such as public or private land) or object that is or could be hazardous to people but that exerts some compelling attraction (especially to children).

auger. A spiral-shaped shaft used for moving pesticide dusts or granules from a hopper to a moving belt or disc for application.

augmentation. The process of building up a population of natural enemies in an area by bringing in additional eggs, larvae, or adults of that species.

avicide. A pesticide used to control pest birds.

axonic. Affecting the axons, or long fibers of nerve cells; impairing normal nerve function by interfering with the conduction of a nerve impulse along a nerve.

backflow. See *back-siphoning*.

backpack sprayer. Also known as a knapsack sprayer, a small, portable sprayer carried on the back of the person making the pesticide application; some are hand-operated, and others are powered by small gasoline engines.

back-siphoning. The process that permits pesticide-contaminated water to be sucked from a spray tank back into a well or other water source.

bacteria (sing., **bacterium**). Unicellular microscopic plantlike organisms that live in soil, water, organic matter, or the bodies of plants and animals. Some bacteria cause plant or animal diseases.

bait. Food or foodlike substance that is used to attract and often poison pest animals.

bait station. A box or similar device designed to hold poisoned bait for controlling rodents, insects, or other pests; usually with baffles or small openings to prevent access to the bait except by the target pest.

band treatment. The application of liquid or dry pesticides in bands or strips, usually to the soil, rather than over the entire area.

beneficial. Being helpful in some way to people, such as a beneficial plant or insect.

beneficial organisms. Living things that prey upon, attack, or parasitize pests or serve as pollinators.

biennial. A plant that completes part of its life cycle in one year and the remainder of its life cycle the following year.

bifluid nozzle. A special nozzle used for producing extremely fine droplets in which fluid is broken up into small droplets by passing through a high-velocity airstream.

binding. A chemical reaction in which molecules of one substance attach to molecules of another substance, forming a bond that can only be broken through another chemical reaction.

bioaccumulation. The gradual buildup of certain pesticides in the tissues of living organisms after feeding on lower organisms containing smaller amounts of these pesticides.

biochemical. A chemical reaction that takes place within the cells or tissues of living organisms.

biological activity. Activity involving the biological processes of living organisms, as opposed to physical or mechanical activity.

biological control. The action of parasites, predators, pathogens, or competitors in maintaining another organism's numerical density at a lower average than would occur in their absence; may occur naturally in the field or be the result of manipulation or introduction of biological control agents by people.

biological factors. Life cycles, life stages, physical attributes, and other factors that protect certain organisms from the toxic effects of pesticides.

biology. The body structure, behavior, and other qualities of a particular organism or class of organisms.

biotic. Of, relating to, or resulting from living things.

biotype. Any population within a species that has a distinct genetic variation from other populations.

blacklight trap. A device that uses ultraviolet light to attract insects.

blocking (photosynthesis). Preventing plants from carrying out photosynthesis by interfering with one or more essential chemical processes.

boom. A structure mounted on a truck, tractor, or other vehicle, or held by hand, to which spray nozzles are attached.

boom applicator. A pesticide application device with multiple nozzles spaced along a boom, making it possible to spray a wide swath; usually used for applying herbicides or other pesticides in large outdoor areas.

botanical. Derived from plants or plant parts.

brand name. A registered or trade name given to a pesticide by its manufacturer or formulator.

breakdown. The process by which chemicals, such as pesticides, decompose into other chemicals.

broadcast application. A method of applying pesticides by dispersing them over a wide area.

broadleaves. One of the major plant groups, known as dicots, with net-veined leaves usually broader than grasses, and whose seedlings have two seed leaves (cotyledons).

broad-spectrum pesticide. A pesticide that is capable of controlling many different species or types of pests. Also known as nonselective pesticide.

brood. A group of young or newly hatched individuals, such as termites.

buffer. An adjuvant that lowers the pH of a spray solution and, depending on its concentration, can maintain the pH within a narrow range even if acidic or alkaline materials are added to the solution.

buffer areas. Parts of a pest-infested site that are not treated with a pesticide to protect adjoining areas from pesticide hazards. Also known as buffer zones or strips.

buffer strips. Areas of a field, usually a minimum of one swath width, left unsprayed to protect nearby structures or sensitive areas from drift. Also known as buffer areas or zones.

buffer zone. See *buffer areas*, *buffer strips*.

caking. The process by which pesticide dusts pack and clump together, preventing proper application.

calibration. The process used to measure the output of pesticide application equipment so that the proper amount of pesticide can be applied to a given area.

California Department of Food and Agriculture (CDFA). The state agency responsible for protecting and promoting agriculture in California.

California Department of Pesticide Regulation (DPR). The state agency responsible for regulating the use of pesticides in California.

carbamate. A class of pesticides commonly used for control of insects, mites, fungi, and weeds. N-methyl carbamate insecticides, miticides, and nematicides are cholinesterase inhibitors; subgroups include dithiocarbamates and thiocarbamates.

carcinogen. A cancer-causing substance or agent.

cardiopulmonary resuscitation (CPR). A procedure designed to maintain circulatory action after breathing and heartbeat have stopped.

carnivore. An animal that eats other living animals.

carrier. The liquid or powdered substance that is combined with the active ingredient in a pesticide formulation; may also apply to the water or oil that a pesticide is mixed with prior to application.

caste. A subgroup with specialized duties within a population of insects, such as worker, soldier, and reproductive termite castes.

cationic. Materials that contain positively charged ions, including cationic materials to improve mixing and absorption by the target pest.

catkin. An inflorescence that hangs down by its own weight; its flowers are usually of one sex.

caustic. Quality of a chemical describing its ability to burn or injure the skin, eyes, or mouth and intestinal lining.

CAUTION. Signal word used on labels of the least-toxic pesticides; pesticides with an oral LD_{50} greater than 500 and a dermal LD_{50} greater than 2,000.

CDA. See *controlled droplet applicator*.

CDFA. See *California Department of Food and Agriculture*.

cephalothorax. The fused head and thorax typical of spiders and other arachnids and many crustaceans.

certified pesticide applicator. A person who has demonstrated through an examination process the ability to safely handle and apply highly hazardous restricted-use pesticides.

certified private applicator. A property owner or manager, or a responsible person employed by the property owner or manager, who has demonstrated through an examination process the ability to safely handle and apply restricted-use pesticides on the property under their control.

chemical control. The use of naturally occurring or synthetic pesticides to manage pest populations in an area.

chemical family. A group of chemicals that have common characteristics, such as chemical structure or environmental persistence.

chemical injection system. The part of a chemigation system that controls the amount of pesticide injected into irrigation water.

chemical name. The official name given to a chemical compound to distinguish it from other chemical compounds.

chemigation. The application of pesticides to target areas through an irrigation system.

CHEMTREC. A chemical-industry-supported organization that provides assistance and advice on pesticide emergencies; telephone 1-800-424-9300.

chlorinated hydrocarbon. A class of pesticide, also known as organochlorine, containing a chlorine atom incorporated into an organic molecule, frequently used for insect and mite control; most early forms such as DDT, chlordane, toxaphene, dieldrin, and dicofol have been banned.

chlorosis. A yellowing or bleaching of normally green leaves due to a nutrient deficiency, disease, pest damage, or other disorder.

cholinesterase. An essential enzyme found in many living organisms, including human beings, that deactivates the chemical acetylcholine that is responsible for transmitting nerve impulses between nerves and between nerves and muscles.

chronic. Of long duration or frequent recurrence.

chronic effect. The harmful effects that occur from small, repeated doses of pesticides over time. Also see *long-term effect*.

chronic illness. An illness that will last for long periods of time, such as cancer, respiratory disorders, and neurological disorders.

Class I disposal site. A disposal site for toxic and hazardous materials such as pesticides and pesticide-contaminated wastes.

Class II disposal site. A disposal site for nontoxic and nonhazardous materials such as household and commercial waste.

classical biological control. A pest control method that uses natural enemies and is directed toward pests that are not native to a geographical area; it involves locating the native home of an introduced pest and finding suitable natural enemies that can be imported, reared, and released into the area where the pest has become established.

climate. Meteorological conditions such as temperature, humidity, precipitation, and other atmospheric conditions over a long period of time. Can refer to local, regional, or global conditions.

closed mixing system. A device used for measuring and transferring liquid pesticides from the original container to the spray tank to reduce the chances of exposure to concentrated pesticides. Special packaging, such as water-soluble bags, is also considered a simple closed mixing system.

coalescent effect. A pesticide mixture that has reacted to form a new chemical with a different mode of action.

common name. The recognized, nonscientific name given to living organisms; also, names of pesticides separate from their brand (trade) names and chemical names.

compatibility agent. An adjuvant that improves the ability of two or more pesticides to combine.

compatible. The condition in which two or more pesticides mix without unsatisfactory chemical or physical changes.

competition. The struggle between different organisms for the same resources, such as water, light, nutrients, and space.

confined area. Places such as buildings or greenhouses, attics, crawl spaces, or holds of ships that may have restricted air circulation and therefore promote buildup of toxic fumes or vapors from a pesticide application.

contact action. When pesticides pass through the target organism's outer covering on contact. Also known as contact activity.

contact poison. A pesticide that provides control when target pests come in physical contact with it.

control agent. Organisms or chemicals that reduce populations of pests, such as natural enemies and pesticides; also, certain types of adjuvants that help reduce spray drift (drift control agents).

continuing education (CE). Approved classes, seminars, or trainings that certified or licensed applicators must take to keep their credentials valid. Topics include pesticide use and safety, California laws and regulations, and pest management.

controlled droplet applicator (CDA). An application device that produces liquid droplets of more uniform size by passing liquid over a notched, spinning disc.

convulsions. Contortions of the body caused by violent, involuntary muscular contractions; a possible symptom of pesticide poisoning.

corrosive materials. Certain chemicals that react with metals or other materials.

cotyledon. The first leaf or pair of leaves of a sprouted seed; grasses (monocots) have one cotyledon, while broadleaved plants (dicots) have two.

coverage. The degree to which a pesticide is distributed over a target surface.

coverall. A one- or two-piece garment of closely woven fabric that covers the entire body except the head, hands, and feet, and must be provided by the employer as personal protective equipment. Coveralls differ from, and should not be confused with, work clothing that can be required to be provided by the employee.

cover crop. A noncrop plant species either grown with the host crop or planted in rotation with annual crops.

CPR. See *cardiopulmonary resuscitation*.

crop rotation. The intentional planting of specific crops in a predetermined order to improve crop health.

crop stage. The stage of development of agricultural crops, such as seedling, flowering, fruit set, etc.

cross-resistance. A condition in which an organism that has developed resistance to one type or group of pesticides is also resistant to other similar or dissimilar pesticides, even though the organism has never been exposed to those pesticides.

cultivar. A cultivated plant variety or strain produced by breeding.

cultural controls. The modification of normal crop or landscape management practices to decrease pest establishment, reproduction, dispersal, survival, or damage.

cumulative effect. Poisoning symptoms that appear only after several repeated doses over a period of time, indicating that the toxic effect is building up in the system of the poisoned individual.

cuticle. The outer protective covering of plants and arthropods that aids in preventing moisture loss.

DANGER. The signal word used on labels of highly hazardous pesticides, which have an oral LD_{50} less than 50 or a dermal LD_{50} less than 200.

DANGER-POISON. The signal word used in combination with the skull and crossbones on labels of pesticides considered to be the most hazardous, having an oral LD_{50} less than 50 or a dermal LD_{50} less than 200. This signal word is also used to identify pesticides that can cause specific, serious health or environmental hazards.

data logger. The storage unit of a computerized weather station.

deactivation. The process by which the toxic action of a pesticide is reduced or eliminated by impurities in the spray tank, by water being used for mixing, or by biotic or abiotic factors in the environment.

decontamination. The process of removing or neutralizing contaminants that have accumulated on people, clothes, and equipment, for instance, thoroughly washing skin exposed to pesticides with soap and water.

deficient oxygen condition. Condition in which the oxygen concentration in air falls below 19%, making an area highly hazardous.

defoaming agent. An adjuvant that eliminates foaming of a pesticide mixture in a spray tank.

defoliant. A pesticide used to remove leaves from target plants, often as an aid in harvesting the plant.

degradation. The breakdown of a pesticide into an inactive or less-active form. Environmental conditions, impurities, or microorganisms can contribute to the degradation of pesticides.

degree-day. The amount of heat that accumulates over a 24-hour period when the average temperature is 1 degree above the lower developmental threshold of an organism.

dehydration. The process of a plant or animal losing water or drying up.

delayed effects. Illnesses or injuries that appear more than 24 hours after exposure to a pesticide.

delayed mixture. An incompatibility or adverse effect between two pesticides that were applied to the same target but at different times.

deposition. The placement of pesticides on target surfaces.

deposition aid. An adjuvant that improves the ability of a pesticide spray to reach the target.

dermal. Pertaining to the skin; one of the major ways pesticides can enter the body.

dermatitis. Inflammation, itching, or irritation of the skin, as can be caused by pesticide exposure.

desiccant. A material that removes water from plants or arthropods or destroys the waxy coatings that protect these organisms from water loss.

detoxify. The process that is used to render a chemical nontoxic. Some organisms can detoxify pesticides through internal biological processes.

dichotomous key. A series of sequentially paired statements that help to identify insects or other living organisms; a type of identification key.

dicot. Plants whose seedlings produce two leaves (cotyledons). Commonly called broadleaves.

diluent. The liquid or powdered material that is combined with the active ingredient during manufacture of a pesticide formulation. Also, the water, petroleum oil, or other liquid mixed with the formulated pesticide before application.

Directions for Use. The instructions found on pesticide labels indicating the proper procedures for mixing and application.

disease. A condition caused by biotic or abiotic factors that impairs some or all of the normal functions of a living organism.

disease triangle. The host plant, causal agent, and favorable environment; when all these elements are present at sufficient levels, a disease outbreak is likely to occur.

dispersion (dispersal). The act of spreading pesticide droplets, dusts, or granules widely over a target area. Also, the spread of living organisms throughout the environment, such as fungal spores.

disposable. Designed to be thrown away after use.

disposal site. See *Class I disposal site* and *Class II disposal site*.

dissolve. To pass into solution.

dormant. To become inactive, such as trees that become bare during winter.

dose. The measured quantity of a pesticide.

DPR. See *California Department of Pesticide Regulation*.

drift. The movement of pesticide particles, spray, or vapor through the air away from the application site.

dry flowable. A dry, granular pesticide formulation intended to be mixed with water for application.

dust. Finely ground pesticide particles, sometimes combined with other materials. Dusts are applied without mixing with water or other liquid.

dyne. The unit of force in the metric system equal to the force that would give a free mass of 1 gram an acceleration of 1 centimeter per second.

early-entry worker. An employee who must enter a pesticide application site to perform cultural activities before the expiration of the restricted-entry interval.

ecological. An approach that considers the interrelationship between living organisms and the environment.

economic damage. Damage caused by pests to plants, animals, or other items that results in loss of income or a reduction of value.

economic injury threshold. The point at which the value of the damage caused by a pest exceeds the cost of controlling the pest, therefore making it practical to use a control method.

ecosystem. The community of organisms in an area and their nonliving environment.

ectoparasitic species. Free living parasites that feed on the surfaces of their hosts.

effective life. The period that an applied pesticide remains toxic enough to adequately control pests.

efficacy. The ability of a pesticide to produce a desired effect on a target organism.

electrostatic. An electrical charge that causes a pesticide liquid or dust to be attracted to the target surface.

emergence. The appearance of a plant through the surface of the soil.

emergency exemption from registration. A federal exemption from regular pesticide registration sometimes issued when an emergency pest situation arises for which no pesticide is registered that has a tolerance on the crop in question.

emulsifiable concentrate. A pesticide formulation consisting of a petroleum-based liquid and emulsifiers that enable it to be mixed with water for application.

emulsifier. An adjuvant added to a pesticide formulation to permit petroleum-based pesticides to mix with water.

emulsion. Droplets of petroleum-based liquids (oils) suspended in water.

encapsulation. A process by which tiny liquid droplets or dry particles are contained in polymer plastic capsules to slow their release into the environment and prolong their effectiveness.

enclosed cab. A compartment with an air filtering system that is installed on a tractor to protect the operator from pesticide exposure.

endangered species. Rare or unusual living organisms whose existence is threatened by human activity, including the use of some types of pesticides.

endoparasitic species. Parasites that live and feed inside their hosts.

engineering controls. Devices that have been developed to protect people as they are mixing, loading, and applying pesticides in a variety of situations, such as enclosed cabs and closed mixing systems.

environment. All of the living organisms and nonliving features of a defined area.

environmental contamination. Spread of pesticides away from the application site into the environment, usually with the potential for causing harm to organisms.

enzyme. A complex chemical compound produced and used by a living organism to induce or speed up chemical reactions without being itself permanently altered.

EPA. See ***U.S. Environmental Protection Agency***.

eradicant. A pesticide that is used to destroy a pest organism, such as a fungus.

eradication. The pest management strategy that attempts to eliminate all members of a pest species from a defined area.

establishment number. A number assigned to registered pesticides by U.S. EPA that indicates the location of the manufacturing or formulation facilities of that product.

estivation. See ***aestivation***.

evaporate. The process of a liquid turning into a gas or vapor.

evolve. To develop gradually. In evolutionary theory, to develop from an earlier biological form.

exclusion. A pest management technique that uses physical or chemical barriers to prevent certain pests from getting into a defined area.

exotic. A pest from another country that is not native to the local area.

exposure. The unwanted contact with pesticides or pesticide residues by people, other organisms, or the environment.

extender. An adjuvant that enhances the effectiveness or effective life of a pesticide by some means such as screening ultraviolet light, slowing down volatilization, or improving sticking qualities.

fallow. Cultivated land that is allowed to lie dormant during a growing season.

farm advisors. University of California specialists in most counties of California who serve as resources for residents of the state on pest management, water management, soil management, nutrition, and many other issues.

Federal Insecticide, Fungicide, and Rodenticide Act (FIFRA). The federal law that regulates pesticide registration, labeling, use, and disposal in the United States.

fencerow. The strip of soil under a fence.

fertilizer. An organic or synthetic substance usually added to or spread onto soil to increase its ability to support plant growth; sometimes mixed and applied with pesticides.

fibrous. Thin, long, multibranching roots that form a dense clump.

field incompatibility. An incompatibility between pesticides mixed together in a spray tank that occurs during application; may result from changes in the temperature of the water used in the mix or changes in the length of time the spray mixture has been in the tank.

fieldworker. An employee of a farming operation who performs cultural practices on crops or agricultural soil.

fieldworker training. Specific training mandated by U.S. EPA and the state of California to protect fieldworkers from pesticide hazards when they work in pesticide-treated areas.

FIFRA. See ***Federal Insecticide, Fungicide, and Rodenticide Act***.

filament. The stalk that supports the pollen-bearing anther in the stamen of a flower.

filamentous. Long and threadlike.

first aid. The immediate assistance provided to someone who is injured, ill, or has been overexposed to a pesticide.

first aid statement. The section of a pesticide label that describes appropriate first aid needed by a person exposed to that pesticide.

fit check. The procedure that must be carried out each time a person puts on an organic vapor filtering respirator and that involves: (1) properly adjusting the straps; (2) closing the filters with the hands and inhaling to check for air leaks around the face seal; and (3) closing the exhalation valve and exhaling to check for air leaks through the filters. Also known as seal check.

fit test. A test that must be performed to check the proper fit of an organic vapor-filtering respirator each time a new respirator is issued.

flowable. Formulations that consist of finely ground particles of pesticide active ingredient mixed with a liquid, along with emulsifiers, to form a concentrated emulsion.

flow rate. The amount of pesticide being expelled by a pesticide sprayer or granule applicator per unit of time.

fog. A spray of very small, pesticide-laden droplets that remain suspended in the air.

foliage. The leaves of plants.

food chain. A hierarchy of different living organisms, each of which feeds on the one below it in the chain.

forecast. A prediction of weather conditions for the near future.

formulation. A mixture of active ingredient(s) combined during manufacture with other materials added to improve the mixing and handling qualities of a pesticide.

frass. Solid fecal material produced by insects.

fruiting bodies. Special structures produced by fungi that contain the spores by which the organisms reproduce.

fry. The life stage of a fish that comes between its larval and juvenile phases.

fumes. Smoke, gas, or vapor; the vapor phase of some pesticide active ingredients.

fumigant. Vapor or gas form of a pesticide used to penetrate porous surfaces for control of soil-dwelling pests or pests in enclosed areas.

fumigation. The process of controlling certain pests by exposing them to an atmosphere of toxic gas inside an enclosed area or under tarped soil.

fungicide. A pesticide used for control of fungi.

fungi (sing. **fungus**). Multicellular lower plants lacking chlorophyll, such as a mold, mildew, rust, or smut; fungal bodies normally consists of filamentous strands called mycelium, and they reproduce through dispersal of spores.

gall. An abnormal swelling of plant tissue, which can be caused by insects, nematodes, and pathogens.

gene. The basic unit capable of transmitting characteristics from one generation of living organisms to the next.

general-use pesticide. A pesticide that has been designated for use by the general public as well as by licensed or certified applicators and that usually has minimal hazards. It does not require a permit for purchase or use.

genetically modified organism (GMO). Any organism whose genetic material has been altered using genetic engineering techniques.

genetic engineering. Intentional alteration of genetic material.

genetic factors. Inherited factors that allow an organism to resist the effect of a pesticide; these might include certain behaviors, timing of life stages, physical attributes, or physiological mechanisms.

genus. The first of the two parts of a living organism's scientific name, it indicates how a species is related to other species in the group.

germinate. To start to grow from a seed or spore into a new individual.

global positioning system (GPS). A worldwide navigation system that uses information received from orbiting satellites.

gnathosoma. The head and mouthparts of mites and ticks.

GPS. See *global positioning system*.

granule. A dry formulation of pesticide active ingredient and other materials compressed into small, pebble-like shapes.

greater than additive effect. A pesticide mixture that has become more toxic than expected. Examples include potentiation, synergism, and coalescent effect.

groundwater. Freshwater trapped in aquifers beneath the surface of the soil; one of the primary sources of water for drinking, irrigation, and manufacturing.

ground wheel–driven. A trailer-mounted dry or liquid pesticide applicator that gets the power to drive a pump, auger, or spinning disc from the movement of one of the trailer wheels as the unit is towed.

habitat. The place where plants or animals live.

habitat modification. Intentionally limiting the availability of one or more of a pest's survival requirements, making the environment less suitable for pest population growth.

half-life. The amount of time it takes for a pesticide to be reduced to half its original toxicity or effectiveness.

hand lens. A small magnifying glass used in monitoring for plant pests.

handler. A person who mixes, loads, transfers, applies (including chemigation), or assists with the application (including flagging) of pesticides; who maintains, services, repairs, cleans, or handles equipment used in these activities; who works with unsealed pesticide containers; who adjusts, repairs, or removes treatment site coverings; who incorporates pesticides into the soil; who enters a treated area during any application or before the REI has expired; or who performs crop advisor duties.

harvest interval. A period of time, as indicated by the pesticide label, that must elapse after a pesticide has been applied to an edible crop before the crop can be harvested legally.

hazard. Something that is potentially very dangerous.

Hazard Communication Program. Part of California's pesticide regulations that requires employers to provide information about pesticides and pesticide applications at the workplace.

hazardous materials. Pesticides that have been classified by regulatory agencies as being harmful to the environment or to people, require special handling, and must be stored and transported in accordance with regulatory mandates.

hazardous waste. A hazardous material for which there is no further use and which must be disposed of only through special hazardous material incineration or by transporting to a Class I disposal site.

heat stress. Potentially life-threatening overheating of the body under working conditions that lack proper preventive measures, such as drinking plenty of water, taking frequent breaks in the shade to cool down, and removing or loosening personal protective equipment during breaks.

HEPA. See *high-efficiency particulate air filter*.

herbivore. An animal that feeds on plants.

herbaceous. A plant that is herblike, usually with little or no woody tissue.

herbicide. A pesticide used for the control of weeds.

hibernate. Passing the winter in a resting or nonactive state.

high-efficiency particulate air filter (HEPA). Special filtering medium designed to remove extremely small particles from the air.

honeydew. The sweet, sticky fluid secreted by plant-feeding insects such as aphids and scales.

hormone. A chemical produced in the cells of a plant or animal that produces changes in cells in another part of the organism's structure.

host. A plant or animal species that provides sustenance for another organism.

host-free area. An area where certain plants that serve as hosts to specific pests are forbidden by law to be grown as a way of controlling some pests.

host-free period. A period of time, usually occurring each year, when certain plants are prohibited from being grown as a way of controlling some pests.

host resistance. The ability of a host plant or animal to ward off or resist attack by pests or to be able to tolerate damage caused by pests.

hydrolysis. A chemical process that involves incorporating a water molecule into another molecule.

hyphae (sing., **hypha**). Threadlike fibers that make up fungal mycelium.

identification key. A written and/or illustrated tool that provides a systematic way to identify and distinguish related living organisms.

idiosoma. The combined thorax and abdomen of mites and ticks.

IGR. See *insect growth regulator*.

impermeable. Having the ability to resist penetration by a substance or object.

impregnates. Items, such as flea collars, that have been manufactured with a certain pesticide in it.

incompatibility. A condition in which two or more pesticides are unable to mix properly or one of the materials chemically alters the other to reduce its effectiveness or produce undesirable effects on the target.

incompatible mixture. The result when two or more pesticides are combined and react to make the mixture unusable.

incorporate. To move a pesticide below the surface of the soil by discing, tilling, or irrigation; also, to combine one pesticide with another.

inert. Not having any chemical activity.

inert ingredients. Obsolete term for ingredients other than the active ingredient in a pesticide formulation. See *other ingredients*.

infection. The establishment of a microorganism within the tissues of a host plant or animal.

infestation. A troublesome invasion of pests within an area such as a building, greenhouse, agricultural crop, or landscaped location.

infiltration. The movement of water into the soil.

inflorescence. The reproductive shoot system of a plant that bears flowers.

ingest. To take into the body through the mouth, such as eating or swallowing.

inhale. To take into the body through the nose or mouth via the lungs.

inherit. To receive a characteristic or quality as a result of its being passed on genetically.

inhibit. To prevent a biochemical reaction within the tissues of a plant or animal.

inoculum. The form of a pathogen that initiates infection.

inorganic. Derived from rock or mineral sources rather than biological or biochemical sources; materials whose molecules do not contain carbon and hydrogen atoms.

insectaries. Laboratories with growth chambers where insects are hatched and reared, often for commercial purposes.

insect growth regulator (IGR). An insecticide that controls certain insects by disrupting the normal process of development from immature to reproductive life stages.

insecticide. A pesticide used for the control of insects; some insecticides are also labeled for control of ticks, mites, spiders, and other arthropods.

instar. The period between molts in larvae of insects. Most larvae pass through several instars; these are usually given numbers such as first instar, second instar, etc.

integrated pest management (IPM). A pest management program that uses life history information and extensive monitoring to understand a pest and its potential for causing economic damage. Control is achieved through multiple approaches including prevention, cultural practices, pesticide applications, exclusion, natural enemies, and host resistance. The goal is to achieve long-term suppression of target pests with minimal impact on nontarget organisms and the environment.

intentional misapplication. The deliberate improper use of a pesticide, such as knowingly exceeding the label rate or applying the material to a site not listed on the label.

interval. The legal period of time between when a pesticide is applied and when workers are allowed to enter the treated area or produce can be harvested. See also *preharvest interval* and *restricted-entry interval*.

introduced pest. A pest that is transported from its native area to a location where it previously did not exist; some pests are introduced accidentally, while others have been introduced intentionally.

inversion. Weather phenomenon in which cool air near the ground is trapped by a layer of warmer air above. Also known as a temperature inversion or inversion layer.

inversion layer. See *inversion*.

invertebrate. Any animal not having an internal skeleton or shell, such as insects, spiders, mites, worms, nematodes, snails, and slugs.

invert emulsion. An emulsion in which water droplets are suspended in an oil rather than the oil droplets being suspended in water.

ion. An atom or molecule that carries a positive or negative electrical charge due to losing or gaining electrons through a chemical reaction.

ionize. The process in which a chemical converts into ions when it dissolves in water or other liquid.

IPM. See *integrated pest management*.

irreversible injury. A health condition caused by certain exposures to some pesticides in which there is no medical treatment or recovery.

irrigation. A method of supplying land or crops with water.

key pest. A pest that regularly causes major damage in a crop or landscape unless it is controlled.

knapsack sprayer. See *backpack sprayer*.

knowledge expectations. The breadth of knowledge about an occupation or procedure, such as pesticide handling, that a person performing this job is expected to have as established by regulations and tested by certification examinations.

labeling. The pesticide label and all associated materials, including supplemental labels, special local needs registration information, and manufacturer's information.

larvae (sing., **larva**). The active, immature form of insects that undergo complete metamorphosis to reach adulthood.

LC_{50}. The lethal concentration of a pesticide in the air or in a body of water that will kill half of a test animal population; values are given in micrograms per milliliter of air or water µg/ml).

LD_{50}. The lethal dose of a pesticide that will kill half of a test animal population; values are given in milligrams per kilogram of test animal body weight (mg/kg).

leaching. The process by which some pesticides move down through the soil, usually by being dissolved in water, with the possibility of reaching groundwater.

legible. Clear enough to be read, easily readable.

lesion. A wound on the outer surface of a plant, animal, or person, usually caused by disease organisms.

lethal. Capable of causing death.

lethal concentration. See *LC_{50}*.

lethal dose. See *LD_{50}*.

liability. Legal responsibility for something, especially costs or damages.

liability insurance. An insurance policy that covers the cost of damages from accidents or the improper use of pesticides.

life stages. The development stages living organisms pass through over time.

ligule. A thin outgrowth or fringe of hairs occurring at the collar region in many grass species.

long-term effect. See *chronic effect*.

Material Safety Data Sheet (MSDS). See *Safety Data Sheet*.

mechanical controls. Devices that exclude, trap, or destroy pests, or modify the environment to make an area unsuitable for pests.

medical facility. A clinic, hospital, or physician's office where immediate medical care for pesticide-related illness or injury can be obtained.

mesh. The number of wires per inch in a screen, such as a screen used to filter foreign particles out of spray solutions; also used to describe the size of pesticide granules, pellets, and dusts.

metabolic inhibitor. A chemical that interferes with normal activity within the cells of living organisms.

metabolism. The total chemical process that takes place in a living organism to use food and manage wastes, provide for growth and reproduction, and accomplish all other life functions.

metamorphosis. The changes that take place in certain types of living organisms, such as insects, as they develop from eggs through adults.

microbial pesticides. Pesticides that consist of bacteria, fungi, or viruses used for control of weeds, invertebrates, plant pathogens, or (rarely) vertebrates.

microencapsulated pesticide. A formulation in which particles of the active ingredient are encased in plastic capsules; pesticide is released after application when the capsules break down.

micro-irrigation systems. Surface drip, subsurface drip, or micro-sprinklers that deliver water to the root zone or limited areas of surface soil to match the exact needs of a plant.

micron. One one-millionth of a meter.

microorganism. An organism of microscopic size, such as a bacterium, virus, fungus, viroid, or mycoplasma.

mimic. To copy or appear to be like something else.

minimal exposure pesticides. High-hazard pesticides identified in California law that have special requirements for handling; only certified commercial applicators may apply or supervise the application of minimal exposure pesticides.

mitigation. The process of making a problem such as a pest infestation less severe.

mitosis. The process by which a cell divides into two daughter cells, each of which has the same number of chromosomes as the original cell.

mixing. The process of opening pesticide containers, weighing or measuring specified amounts, and transferring these materials into application equipment, all in accordance with instructions found on pesticide labels.

mobile. Able to move freely or easily.

mode of action. The way a pesticide reacts with a pest organism to destroy it.

molluscicide. A pesticide used to control slugs and snails.

molting. A process of shedding the outer body covering or exoskeleton in invertebrates such as insects and spiders. Molting usually takes place to allow the animal to grow larger.

monitoring. The process of carefully watching the activities, growth, and development of pest organisms over a period of time, often utilizing very specific procedures.

monocot. A member of a group of plants whose seedlings have a single cotyledon.

mortality. Death.

MSDS. See *Safety Data Sheet*.

mulch. A layer of material intentionally allowed to cover the soil surface in an area.

mutagenic. A chemical that is capable of causing inheritable abnormalities in living organisms.

mycelium (pl., mycelia). The vegetative body of a fungus, consisting of a mass of slender filaments called hyphae.

mycoplasma. A microorganism intermediate between viruses and bacteria, capable of causing diseases in plants.

narrow-range oil. Horticultural oils with 10 to 90% distillation ranges of approximately 60° to 80°F (10 mm hg), and 50% distillation points from 412° to 440°F; used for dormant or summer application.

National Institute for Occupational Safety and Health (NIOSH). The federal agency that tests and certifies respiratory equipment for pesticide application.

native. Animals or plants that are indigenous to an area.

natural enemy. An organism that can kill a pest organism, including predators, pathogens, parasites, and competitors.

natural selection. The process by which organisms best suited to their environment achieve greater reproductive success, and so pass their genetic advantages on to future generations.

necrosis. Localized death of living tissue.

negligent application. A pesticide application in which the applicator fails to exercise proper care or follow label instructions, potentially resulting in injury to people or surrounding areas.

nematicide. A pesticide used to control nematodes.

nematode. Elongated, cylindrical, nonsegmented worms, commonly microscopic; some are parasites of plants or animals.

neonicotinoids. A family of insecticides that mimics the effects of nicotine, disrupting an insect's central nervous system, causing paralysis and death.

neoprene. A synthetic rubber material used to make gloves, boots, and clothing for protection against pesticide exposure.

NIOSH. See *National Institute for Occupational Safety and Health*.

nitrile. An organic cyanide used to create synthetic rubber products. It is also used in pesticide products.

nocturnal. Active at night rather than during the day.

NOEL. No observable effect level; the maximum dose or exposure level of a pesticide that produces no noticeable toxic effect on test animals.

nonionic. An adjuvant that dissolves in the spray solution without producing positively or negatively charged particles.

nonpoint pollution. Pollution from pesticides or other materials that arises from their normal or accepted use over a large general area and an extended period.

nonselective pesticide. A pesticide that has action against many species of pests rather than just a few. See also *broad-spectrum pesticide*.

nontarget organism. Animals or plants within a pesticide-treated area that are not intended to be controlled by the pesticide application.

no observable effect level. See *NOEL*.

notification. See *oral notification* and *posting*.

noxious. Harmful to living organisms, such as a noxious weed.

nymph. The larva of some insects such as mayflies, dragonflies, and grasshoppers that resembles the adult and develops into the adult insect directly, without passing through an intermediate pupa stage.

obligate parasites. Parasites that require living host plants to grow and reproduce.

obsolete. No longer in use; outdated.

occasional pest. A pest that does not recur regularly, but causes damage from time to time as a result of changing environmental conditions or other factors.

ocular. Pertaining to the eye; one of the routes of entry of pesticides into the body.

offsite movement. Any movement of a pesticide from the location where it was applied, through drift, volatilization, leaching, runoff, crop harvest, blowing dust, or by being carried away on organisms or equipment.

oral. Through the mouth, one of the routes of entry of pesticides into the body.

oral notification. A method used to notify workers of pesticide applications on property where they are employed.

organic. A pesticide whose molecules contain carbon and hydrogen atoms; also, plants or animals that are grown without the use of synthetic fertilizers or pesticides.

organic agriculture. Growing of agricultural commodities without the use of certain synthetic chemicals and fertilizers using naturally occurring substances as well as cultural, mechanical, and biological methods.

organic matter. Any material that comes from living organisms; in soil, this would include decaying plant, microbial, and animal matter.

organism. Any living thing.

organochlorines. See *chlorinated hydrocarbons*.

organophosphates. Organic molecules containing phosphorous commonly used as pesticides. Some are highly toxic to people; most break down in the environment very rapidly.

ornamental. Cultivated plants that are grown for purposes other than food or fiber.

OSHA. Occupational Safety and Health Administration. The part of the U.S. Department of Labor that sets and enforces rules that keep people safe and healthy at work.

other ingredients. Ingredients other than the active ingredient in a pesticide formulation. Some may be toxic or hazardous to people.

output rate. The amount of pesticide mixture discharged by pesticide application equipment over a measured period of time.

overwinter. The process of passing through the winter season. Many living organisms survive harsh weather conditions as seeds, eggs, or in certain resting stages.

palmate. Shaped like the palm of a hand, with the veins radiating out from a central location.

panicle. A flower head of a plant in which the lateral branches of the raceme are branched.

parasite. A plant or animal that derives all its nutrients from another organism. Parasites often attach themselves to their host or invade the host's tissues. Parasitism may result in injury or death of the host.

parasitoid. An organism that is parasitic during its immature stages and kills its host as it reaches maturity.

pathogen. A microorganism that causes a disease.

pellet. A pesticide formulation consisting of the dry active ingredient and other materials pressed into uniform-sized granules.

penetrate. To pass through a surface such as skin, protective clothing, plant cuticle, or insect cuticle; also, the ability of an applied spray to pass through dense foliage.

percolation. The process by which water flows downward through permeable soil.

perennial. A plant that lives longer than 2 years; some may live indefinitely.

perianth. The outer structure of a flower, made up of the corolla, the calyx, or both.

permeability. The ability of material (such as geological layers) to allow water and dissolved pesticides to move downward to groundwater freely.

persistent pesticide. A pesticide that remains active in the environment for long periods of time because it is not easily broken down by microorganisms or environmental factors.

personal protective equipment (PPE). Devices and garments that protect handlers from exposure to pesticides. These include coveralls, eye protection, gloves and boots, respirators, aprons, and hats.

pesticide. Any substance or mixture of substances intended for preventing, destroying, repelling, or mitigating any insects, rodents, nematodes, fungi, or weeds, or any other forms of life declared to be pests, and any other substance or mixture of substances intended for use as a plant regulator, defoliant, or desiccant.

pesticide deposition. See *deposition*.

pesticide formulation. The pesticide as it comes from its original container, consisting of the active ingredient blended with other ingredients.

pesticide handler. See *handler*.

pesticide residue. See *residue*.

pesticide resistance. Genetic qualities of a pest population that enable individuals to resist the effects of certain types of pesticides that are toxic to other members of that species.

Pesticide Safety Information Series (PSIS). A series of informational sheets developed and distributed by the California Department of Pesticide Regulation pertaining to handling pesticides, personal protective equipment, emergency first aid, medical supervision, etc.

pesticide use record. A record of pesticide applications made to a specific location.

pest resurgence. See *resurgence*.

petal. One of the showy colored parts of a flower in bloom. The ring of petals forms the corolla of a plant.

PGR. See *plant growth regulator*.

pH. A value used to express relative acidity or alkalinity. Lower numbers indicate increasing acidity; higher numbers indicate increasing alkalinity.

phenology model. A mathematical model that can predict when key events in an organism's development will occur, usually based on biological information about the organisms and temperature data.

pheromone. A chemical produced by an animal to attract other animals of the same species.

photosynthesis. Process by which plants convert sunlight into energy.

physical controls. Activities designed to kill a pest or make the environment unsuitable for survival. Physical controls include mowing, steam sterilization of soil, and installing screens or other barriers.

physiological. Pertaining to the functions and activities of living tissues.

phytotoxic. Injurious to plants.

pistil. The female reproductive part of a flower, which includes the ovary, style, and stigma.

plant-back restriction. A restriction that limits the commodity that can be grown in an area for a designated period of time after a certain pesticide has been used.

plant growth regulator (PGR). A pesticide used to regulate or alter the normal growth of plants or the development of plant parts.

plant kingdom. One of two groups of living organisms, the other being the animal kingdom.

point source pollution. Pollution from pesticides or other materials that arises from spilling or dumping them in one location.

pollinators. Organisms that transfer pollen and fertilize plants; usually refers to bees.

population. A group of individuals of the same species occupying a distinct space and possessing characteristics (such as special adaptations for the habitat) that are unique to the group.

postapplication cleanup. See *decontamination*.

postemergent. An herbicide applied after emergence of a specified weed or crop.

posting. Placing signs around an area to inform workers and the public that the area has been treated with a pesticide.

potency. The toxicity of a pesticide.

potentiation. An increase in the toxicity of a pesticide brought about by mixing it with another pesticide or chemical.

pour-on. A ready-to-use formulation or diluted mixture of pesticide for control of external parasites on livestock. The liquid is usually poured along the back of the animal.

powder. A finely ground dust containing active ingredient and other ingredients. This powder is mixed with water before application as a liquid spray.

power take-off (PTO). A special shaft connected to the rear, front, or side of a tractor and certain other types of equipment that uses the engine of the tractor or other equipment to power external devices such as sprayers, mowers, hydraulic pumps, etc.

PPE. See *personal protective equipment*.

ppm. Parts per million.

precautionary statements. A section on pesticide labels listing human and environmental hazards and personal protective equipment requirements, as well as the product's specific effects on people and animals.

precipitation. Process by which solid particles settle out of a solution, such as a formulated pesticide in a spray tank. Also can refer to rain.

predaceous. Living by hunting and eating other animals.

predacide. Pesticide used for control of predaceous mammals such as coyotes.

predator. An animal that attacks, kills, and eats other animals (prey), consuming several to many prey individuals in its lifetime.

preventive methods. Pest management methods that discourage damaging populations from developing, such as planting weed- and disease-free seed, or growing pest-resistant plant varieties.

prey. An organism that is attacked, killed, and eaten by a predator.

preemergent. The action of an herbicide that controls specified weeds as they sprout from seeds before they push through the soil surface.

preharvest interval. A period of time set by law that must elapse after a pesticide has been applied to an edible crop before the crop can be harvested legally.

preplant. An herbicide that has been incorporated into the soil to control weeds prior to planting crop seeds.

pressure. The amount of force applied by the application equipment pump on the liquid pesticide mixture to force it through the nozzles.

pressure gauge. An instrument on liquid pesticide application equipment that measures the pressure of the liquid being expelled.

private applicator. Individuals who apply pesticides on agricultural property under their control and for their own benefit or needs.

private applicator certification. See *certified private applicator*.

propellant. A material, such as compressed air or gas, used to propel spray liquids or dusts to target surfaces.

protectant. A pesticide that provides a chemical barrier against pest attack.

protective clothing. Garments of personal protective equipment that cover the body, including arms and legs.

protein synthesis. Process by which cells in living organisms build complex chemical chains known as proteins.

protozoan. Minute, single-celled organism belonging to the phylum Protozoa.

psi. Pounds per square inch.

PTO. See *power take-off*.

pupa (pl., **pupae**). In insects having complete metamorphosis, the resting life stage between larval and adult forms.

pyrethroid. A synthetic pesticide that mimics pyrethrin, a botanical pesticide derived from certain species of chrysanthemum flowers.

qualified trainer. A person who is a certified private or commercial applicator, agricultural pest control adviser, registered forester, agricultural biologist, or UC farm advisor, or who has completed a DPR-approved train-the-trainer course.

quarantine. A legally imposed period during which the movement of certain items (such as produce) within a designated area is restricted to prevent the spread of pests.

raceme. A flower stalk with one central stem, with or without a terminal flower, and bearing lateral flowers or small bunches of flowers.

rate. The quantity or volume of liquid spray, dust, or granules that is applied to an area over a specified period of time.

rate controller. An electronic device installed on a pesticide sprayer that adjusts the spray volume automatically by adjusting spray pressure. See also *spray controller*, *system controller*.

recombination. An occurrence in which a pesticide breaks down and combines with other chemicals in the environment to produce a different compound than what was originally applied.

recommendation. A written document prepared by a licensed pest control adviser that prescribes the use of a specific pesticide or other pest control method.

red cell and plasma cholinesterase determination. Blood test used to detect exposure to organophosphate and n-methyl carbamate insecticides.

registration and establishment numbers. Identification numbers assigned by U.S. EPA and the California Department of Pesticide Regulation found on pesticide labels.

regularly handle (pesticides). Categorization of an employee who handles pesticides during any part of the day for more than 6 calendar days in any 30-consecutive-day qualifying period beginning on the first day of handling. Any day spent loading pesticides while exclusively using a closed system or mixing only pesticides sealed in water-soluble packets is not included for any employee who has a baseline blood cholinesterase level established pursuant to California Code of Regulations Section 6728(c)(I).

regulations. Guidelines or working rules that a regulatory agency uses to carry out and enforce laws.

regulatory control. Management of pests by the passage of laws and regulations that restrict activities which would promote pest buildup.

REI. See *restricted-entry interval*.

repellent. A pesticide used to keep target pests away from a treated area by saturating the area with an odor that is disagreeable to the pests.

rescue breathing. Also known as artificial respiration; given mouth-to-mouth to assist or restore breathing to a person overcome by pesticides.

reservoir. A population of pests within a local area; also, an organism harboring plant or animal pathogens.

residual action. The activity of a pesticide after it has been applied. Most pesticide compounds remain active several hours to several weeks or even months after being applied. Also known as residual activity.

residue. Traces of pesticide that remain on treated surfaces after a period of time.

resistance. See *pesticide resistance* or *host resistance*.

respiration. Metabolic process in plants and animals in which, among other things, oxygen is exchanged for carbon dioxide or carbon dioxide is exchanged for oxygen.

respiratory equipment. A device that filters pesticide dusts, mists, and vapors to protect the wearer from respiratory exposure during mixing and loading, application, or while entering treated areas before the restricted entry interval expires.

restricted materials permit. See *restricted-use permit*.

restricted-entry interval (REI). Period of time that must elapse between the application of a pesticide and when it is safe to allow people into the treated area without requiring that they wear personal protective equipment and receive early-entry worker training.

restricted-use permit. Permit issued by county agricultural commissioners that enables growers to possess and apply restricted-use pesticides.

restricted-use pesticide. Highly hazardous pesticide that can be possessed or used only by commercial applicators who have a valid Qualified Pesticide Applicator license or certificate or private applicators who have passed a written exam administered by the local agricultural commissioner.

restrictive statement. A statement on a pesticide label that restricts the use of that pesticide to specific areas or by designated individuals.

resurgence. The sudden increase of a pest population after some event, such as a pesticide application.

reversible injury. A pesticide-related injury or illness that can be reversed through medical intervention and/or the body's healing process.

rhizome. An underground stem of certain types of plants.

rinsate. Liquid derived from rinsing pesticide containers or spray equipment.

rodenticide. A pesticide used to control rats, mice, gophers, squirrels, and other rodents.

rootstock. The underground portion of a plant, such as a root or rhizome; also, on fruit trees and vines, the lower portion of a graft that develops into the root system.

rope wick applicator. A device used to apply contact herbicides onto target weed foliage with a saturated rope or cloth pad.

route of entry. See *route of exposure*.

route of exposure. Any one of the four ways a pesticide gets onto or into the body: dermal (on or through the skin), ocular (on or in the eyes), respiratory (into the lungs), and oral (through the mouth). Also known as route of entry.

rpm. Revolutions per minute.

runoff. Liquid spray material that drips from the foliage of treated plants or from other treated surfaces; also, rainwater or irrigation water that leaves an area and may contain trace amounts of pesticide.

Safety Data Sheet (SDS). An information sheet provided by a pesticide manufacturer describing chemical qualities, hazards, safety precautions, and emergency procedures to be followed in case of a spill, fire, or other emergency. Formerly known as Material Safety Data Sheet (MSDS).

sampling. Collecting several examples of an organism from an area to determine pest identity. Techniques can also be used to get a sense of the size of the population in an area.

saprophyte. An organism that lives on dead or decaying organic matter.

SCBA. See *supplied air respirator*.

scientific name. The unique two-word Latin name, consisting of the genus and species, that scientists assign to each organism, according to taxonomy; a formal way of naming living things.

scouting. Collecting monitoring information in the field; used to detect and assess pest populations in an area.

seal check. See *fit check*.

secondary pest. An organism that becomes a serious pest only after a natural enemy, competitor, or primary pest has been eliminated through pest control.

Section 18 exemption. See *emergency exemption from registration*.

selective pesticide. A pesticide that is effective against only a single or a small number of pest species.

self-contained breathing apparatus (SCBA). See *supplied air respirator*.

sensor. A mechanical device that is sensitive to light, radiation, level, movement, heat, or other stimuli in the environment, and that provides a corresponding output.

sepal. The usually green, leaflike part of a flower that encloses its petals.

service container. Any container designed to hold concentrated or diluted pesticide mixtures, including the sprayer tank but not the original pesticide container.

SDS. See *Safety Data Sheet*.

shelf life. Maximum period of time that a pesticide can remain in storage before losing some of its effectiveness.

shingling. Clumping or sticking together of plant foliage caused by the force of a liquid spray; prevents spray droplets from reaching all surfaces of the foliage and may result in poor pest control.

sight gauge. A device on a pesticide sprayer or configuration of the spray tank that permits the operator to view the level of liquid in the tank.

signal word. One of three words (DANGER, WARNING, CAUTION) found on every pesticide label to indicate the relative hazard of the chemical.

signs. The physical evidence of a pest's presence that can be seen on a host. For example, in plant disease, signs can include visible spores or fruiting bodies.

site. The area where pesticides are applied for control of a pest.

site of action. The location within the tissues of the target organism where a pesticide acts.

skin absorption. The passage of pesticides through the skin into the bloodstream or other organs of the body.

skull and crossbones. The symbol on pesticide labels that indicates that the material is highly poisonous or poses specific, serious health or environmental hazards. Always accompanied by the signal word DANGER and the word POISON. See also *DANGER-POISON*.

SLN. See *special local need registration*.

slurry. A watery mixture containing pesticide powder that leaves a thick coating of pesticide residue on treated surfaces.

soil mobility. A variable characteristic of a pesticide, based on its chemical nature. Highly mobile pesticides leach rapidly through the soil and may contaminate groundwater. Immobile pesticides, or those with low soil mobility, remain tightly attached to soil particles and are resistant to leaching.

soil profile. The characteristics and differences of soil at different depths.

solarization. The practice of using sunlight to heat soil to levels lethal to pests by laying clear plastic on soil surfaces for 4-6 weeks during sunny, warm weather.

soluble. Able to dissolve completely in a liquid.

soluble powder. A pesticide formulation in which the active ingredient and all other ingredients completely dissolve in water to form a true solution.

solution. A liquid that contains a dissolved substance, such as a soluble pesticide.

solvent. A liquid capable of dissolving certain chemicals.

sorptive dust. A fine powder used to destroy arthropods by removing the protective wax coating that prevents water loss.

source reduction. Sanitation practices.

spawn. To reproduce.

special local need registration (SLN). Also known as 24(c) registration; the registration of a pesticide for treatment of a local or specific pest problem where no registered pesticide is available.

species. A subdivision of a genus considered as a basic biological classification and containing individuals that resemble one another and may interbreed.

speed of travel. The speed that the operator moves the pesticide application equipment through the area being treated.

spike. A long cluster of flowers attached directly to a stem, with the newest flowers at the tip.

spore. A reproductive structure produced by some plants and microorganisms that is resistant to environmental influences.

spot treatment. A method of applying pesticides only in small, localized areas where pests congregate, rather than treating a larger, general area.

spray check device. A piece of equipment that measures and visualizes the output from the nozzles on a spray boom, providing rapid visualization of differences in output between nozzles.

spray controller (sprayer controller). A piece of electronic equipment that allows for very accurate metering of pesticide spray. See also *system controller*, *rate controller*.

spreader. An adjuvant that lowers the surface tension of treated surfaces to enable the pesticide to be absorbed.

stamen. The male reproductive organ of a flower.

statement of practical treatment. Obsolete term. See *first aid statement*.

statement of use classification. A special statement found on labels of some highly hazardous pesticides indicating that their use is restricted to people who have been qualified through a certification process.

sterilant. A pesticide used for control of rodents by preventing their reproduction.

sticker. An adjuvant used to prevent pesticides from being washed or rubbed off treated surfaces.

stigma. The part of a flower's female reproductive organ carpel that receives the male pollen grains. It is generally located at the tip of a slender stalk-shaped projection style.

stolon. An aboveground runner stem found in some species of plants.

stomach poison. A pesticide that kills target animals who ingest it.

stunt. To restrict growth; in plants, a common symptom of disease or nematode infestation.

structural pest. An organism (such as a termite or wood rot fungus) that destroys structural wood in buildings.

style. An extension of a flower's ovary, shaped like a stalk, that supports the stigma.

subcutaneous injection. Injecting a substance, such as a drug, under the skin.

sublethal dose. A pesticide dose insufficient to cause death in the exposed organism.

sulfonylureas. A family of herbicides that kills plants when it is taken up by roots and foliage. It is safe for mammals because mammals do not have the enzyme targeted by these chemicals.

summer annuals. Annuals that germinate in the spring, mature and set seed in late summer, and die in the fall.

summer oils. Narrow-range oils applied during the growing season.

superior oils. Term given to more highly refined paraffinic oils in the late 1940s; today, it refers to most oils available (e.g., narrow-range oils) but excludes very heavy dormant emulsions that have low unsulfonated residues. All narrow-range oils are superior oils, but not all superior oils are narrow-range oils.

supplemental label. Additional instructions and information not found on the pesticide label because the label is too small, but are legally considered to be part of the pesticide labeling.

supplied air respirator. A tightly fitting face mask that is connected by hose to an air supply such as a tank worn on the back of the person using the respirator or to an external air supply.

suppression. Pest management strategy that attempts to reduce pest numbers below an economic injury threshold or to a tolerable level.

supreme oils. A specific product (Volek Supreme Oil) but is often used incorrectly to indicate any superior or narrow-range oil. The distillation midpoint of supreme oil is higher and the 10 to 90% distillation range is wider than other narrow-range oil formulations.

surface active agent. See *surfactant*.

surface coverage. The degree to which a spray or dust covers the surface of leaves or other objects being treated.

surface tension. Forces on the surfaces of liquid droplets that keep them from spreading over treated surfaces.

surface water. Water contained in lakes or ponds or flowing in streams, rivers, or canals.

surfactant. Surface-active agent; an adjuvant used to improve the ability of the pesticide to stick to and be absorbed by the target surface.

susceptible life stage. The life stage of a pest organism that is most likely to be affected by a pesticide used to control it; in general, insects are most susceptible during the larval or juvenile stage; weeds are usually most susceptible during the seedling stage.

suspension. Fine particles of solid material distributed evenly throughout a liquid such as water or oil.

sustain. To continue over time without losing effectiveness.

swath. The area covered by one pass of the pesticide application equipment.

swath width. The width of the area covered by spray droplets or granules as the application equipment moves through. The swath width must be measured to calibrate application equipment.

symptoms. Changes in the appearance of an organism due to the activities of a pest. For example, in plant disease, the appearance of lesions, cankers, or discolored leaves. Also, any abnormal condition in people caused by a pesticide exposure that can be felt and described or can be detected by examination or laboratory tests.

synergism. A reaction in which a chemical that has no pesticidal qualities can enhance the toxicity of a pesticide it is mixed with.

synthesized. Materials that are manufactured through chemical processes rather than occurring naturally.

synthetic. A product made artificially by chemical synthesis such as a pesticide or fabric.

system controller. See *spray controller* or *rate controller*.

system monitor. A device that measures a sprayer's operating conditions such as travel speed, pressure, and/or flow rate and can send an alert when unexpected changes in application rates occur. Used in conjunction with GPS units, and spray, rate, or system controllers.

systemic pesticide. A pesticide that is taken up into the tissues of the organism and transported to other locations, where it will affect pests.

tag-along. A liquid or dry pesticide applicator mounted on a wheeled trailer and pulled behind a tractor or other powered vehicle.

tailwater. The water that collects at the lower end of a field during or after irrigation.

tank mix. A mixture of pesticides or fertilizers and pesticides applied at the same time.

target. Either the pest that is being controlled or surfaces within an area that the pest will contact.

temperature inversion. See *inversion*.

thickener. An adjuvant that increases the viscosity of the spray solution so that larger droplets are formed by the nozzles; used to control drift.

thorax. The second of three major divisions in the body of an insect which bears its legs and wings.

threatened species. An organism that is likely to become endangered in the foreseeable future.

threshold. See *economic injury threshold*.

threshold limit value (TLV). The airborne concentration of a pesticide in parts per million (ppm) that produces no adverse effects over a period of time.

TLV. See *threshold limit value*.

tolerance. The ability to endure the impact of a pesticide or pest without exhibiting adverse effects; also, the maximum amount of pesticide residue that is permitted on produce or other edible animal or agricultural crop products.

toxicant. A substance that, at a sufficient dose, will cause harm to a living organism.

toxicity. The potential of a pesticide to poison an exposed organism.

toxicity category. The three classifications of pesticides that indicate the approximate level of hazard, indicated by the signal words DANGER-POISON or DANGER, WARNING, and CAUTION.

toxicity testing. A process in which known doses of a pesticide are given to groups of test animals and the results are observed.

toxicology. The study of toxic substances on living organisms.

tracking powder. A fine powder that is dusted over a surface to detect or control certain pests such as cockroaches or rodents.

trade name. See *brand name*.

training record. Document signed by the trainer, employer, and trainee that records the dates and types of pesticide safety training received.

transgenic plants. Genetically modified organisms.

translocate. The movement of pesticides from one location to another within the tissues of a plant.

transport. To carry somebody or something from one place to another, usually in a vehicle.

treated surface. The surface of plants, soil, or other items that were contacted with pesticide spray, dust, or granules for the purpose of controlling pests.

treatment area. See *site*.

treatment threshold. See *action threshold*.

triazines. A large family of chemicals used to control both broadleaf and grassy weeds, either before or after they emerge, by inhibiting photosynthesis.

triple-rinse. Performing three times the process of partially filling an empty pesticide container, replacing the lid, shaking the container, then emptying its contents into the spray tank.

true leaves. The leaves produced by a plant after the emergence of its cotyledons.

tuber. An enlarged, fleshy, underground stem.

UC ANR. University of California Agriculture and Natural Resources.

UC IPM. University of California Statewide Integrated Pest Management Program.

ultra-low-volume (ULV). A pesticide application technique in which very small amounts of liquid spray are applied over a unit of area; usually ½ gallon or less of spray per acre in row crops to about 5 gallons of spray per acre in orchards and vineyards.

ULV. See *ultra-low-volume*.

umbel. A flower head in which all the flower stalks originate at or near one point. Can be simple or compound.

uniform. Always the same in quality, character, degree, or manner, as in uniform pesticide distribution, uniform size, or uniform mixture.

unloader. A sensitive, valve-like mechanism used on high-pressure applicators that diverts the liquid back into the tank when nozzles are shut off to prevent a rapid buildup of pressure in the system that would possibly damage the pump. When the flow to the nozzles is turned back on, the unloader quickly restores pressure to nozzles.

unregistered crop. Any crop that is not listed on the pesticide label. Pesticides can be applied only to crops that are specifically listed on the label.

unregistered site. Any site, such as a right-of-way or pond, that is not listed on the pesticide label. Pesticides may be applied only to listed or registered crops or sites.

unsulfonated residue (UR). A measure of purity of petroleum oils used as pesticides. Oils used for insecticides and acaricides must have a minimum UR rating based on the grade or type of oil. Oils with higher UR ratings are safer for use on plants.

UR. See *unsulfonated residue*.

U.S. Environmental Protection Agency (U.S. EPA). The federal agency responsible for regulating pesticide use in the United States.

use restrictions. Special restrictions included on the pesticide label or incorporated into state or local regulations that specify how, when, or where a specific pesticide may be used.

vaporize. To transform a spray of droplets to a fog-like vapor or gas.

vapor pressure. The pressure exerted by a material in its gaseous form.

variables. Factors that differ from place to place, or situation to situation. Also, the part of a mathematical equation that does not have a fixed numerical value.

variety. In plants, naturally occurring variants within a subspecies, or strains produced through breeding programs. Also, a collection of varied things, often belonging to the same group.

vector. An organism, such as an insect, that can transmit a pathogen to plants or animals.

vegetative. Relating to or typical of vegetation, plants, or plant growth. Also, asexual reproduction.

vertebrates. The group of animals that have an internal skeleton and segmented spine, such as fish, birds, reptiles, and mammals.

viroid. A microorganism that is much smaller than a virus and is not enclosed in a protein coat; some viroids produce disease symptoms in certain plants.

virus. A very small organism that multiplies in living cells and is capable of producing disease symptoms in some plants and animals.

viscosity. A physical property of a fluid that affects its flowability; more-viscous fluids flow less easily and produce larger spray droplets.

VOC. See *volatile organic compound*.

volatile. Able to pass from liquid or solid into a gaseous stage readily at low temperatures.

volatilization. The process of a liquid or solid passing into a gaseous stage.

volatile organic compound. An organic compound that evaporates at a relatively low temperature and contributes to air pollution.

volute. A metal, duct-like structure used to direct the air flow from a sprayer fan, enabling pesticide-laden air to be directed to treetops or other hard-to-reach areas.

WARNING. The signal word used on labels of pesticides considered to be moderately toxic or hazardous based on their toxicity; they usually have an oral LD50 between 50 and 500 and a dermal LD50 between 200 and 2,000.

watershed. An area of land that drains its surface water into a defined watercourse or body of water.

water-soluble concentrate. A liquid pesticide formulation that dissolves in water to form a true solution.

weather. The state of the atmosphere (temperature, humidity, precipitation, wind conditions) over a short period of time (a day or week) at a specific site.

weather station (electronic). A device that consists of an electronic data logger, sensors, a power supply, an environmental enclosure, and a support structure.

weed. A plant that interferes with human activities, results in economic loss, or is otherwise undesirable.

wettable powder. A pesticide formulation consisting of an active ingredient that will not dissolve in water, combined with mineral clay and other ingredients and ground into a fine powder.

wetting agent. An adjuvant used in pesticide mixtures to lower the surface tension of spray droplets, enabling them to come in close contact and spread out over target surfaces, especially those containing fine hairs or waxy layers.

winter annuals. Annuals that germinate from late fall to early winter, mature and set seed in late winter or early spring, and die in early summer.

work clothing. Garments such as long-sleeved shirts, short-sleeved shirts, long pants, short pants, shoes, and socks; work clothing is not considered personal protective equipment, although pesticide product labeling or regulations may require specific work clothing during some activities.

Worker Protection Standard (WPS). The 1992 amendment to the Federal Insecticide, Fungicide, and Rodenticide Act (F1FRA) that makes significant changes to pesticide labeling and mandates specific training of pesticide handlers and workers in production agriculture, commercial greenhouses and nurseries, and forests. Updated in 2015.

WPS. See *Worker Protection Standard*.

REFERENCES

Akesson, N. B., and W. E. Yates. 1964. Problems related to application of agricultural chemicals and resulting drift residues. *Annual Review of Entomology* 9:285–315, table 1.

Bauer, E., ed. 2005. *Agricultural Pest Control: Plant.* Lincoln: University of Nebraska.

Bird, G. W. 2003. Role of integrated pest management and sustainable development: Historical development of pest management programs. In K. M. Maredia, D. Dakouo, and D. Mota-Sanchez, eds., *Integrated Pest Management in the Global Arena.* Wallingford, UK: CABI Publishing.

Blecker, L. A., and J. M. Thomas. 2012. *National Soil Fumigation Manual.* Fairfax, VA: National Association of State Departments of Agriculture Research Foundation (NASDARF).

California Department of Pesticide Regulation. 2014. *A Community Guide to Recognizing & Reporting Pesticide Problems.* DPR website, cdpr.ca.gov/docs/dept/comguide/commty_guide.pdf.

California Department of Pesticide Regulation. 2015. *Using Pesticides in California.* DPR website, cdpr.ca.gov/docs/dept/comguide/using_excerpt.pdf.

DiTomaso, J. M., and E. A. Healy. 2007. *Weeds of California and Other Western States.* 2 vols. Oakland: University of California Division of Agriculture and Natural Resources Publication 3488.

Dreistadt, S. H. 2016. *Pests of Landscape Trees and Shrubs: An Integrated Pest Management Guide.* 3rd ed. Oakland: University of California Division of Agriculture and Natural Resources Publication 3359.

Dubrovsky, N. M., C. R. Kratzer, L. R. Brown, J. M. Gronberg, and K. R. Burow. 1998. *Water Quality in the San Joaquin-Tulare Basins, California*, 1992-95. U.S. Geological Survey Circular 11595.

U.S. Environmental Protection Agency. 1994. *Pest Smart Update.* Washington, D.C.: Publication EPA-733-N-94-001.

U.S. Environmental Protection Agency. 2014. *Label Review Manual, Chapter 10: Worker Protection Label.* EPA website, epa.gov/sites/production/files/2014-07/documents/chapter10-final-fd-jr.pdf.

U.S. Environmental Protection Agency. 2015. *Protecting Bees and Other Pollinators from Pesticides.* EPA website, epa.gov/pesticides/ecosystem/pollinator/bee-label-info-lrt.pdf.

Feldmann, R. J., and H. I. Maibach. 1967. Regional variation in percutaneous penetration of ^{14}C cortisol in man. Journal of Investigative Dermatology 48(2) (Feb): 181–183.

Flint, M. L. 1998. *Pests of the Garden and Small Farm.* 2nd ed. Oakland: University of California Division of Agriculture and Natural Resources Publication 3332.

Flint, M. L. 2012. *IPM in Practice.* 2nd ed. Oakland: University of California Division of Agriculture and Natural Resources Publication 3418.

FRAC (Fungicide Resistance Action Committee). Website, frac.info.

Hickman, G. W. 2004. *Pest Notes: Lizards.* Oakland: University of California Division of Agriculture and Natural Resources Publication 74120. UC ANR website, ipm.ucanr.edu/PMG/PESTNOTES/pn74120.html.

Hooven, L., R. Sagili, and E. Johansen. 2013. *How to Reduce Bee Poisoning from Pesticides.* Corvallis: Oregon State University PNW 591. OSU Extension website, https://catalog.extension.oregonstate.edu/files/project/pdf/pnw591.pdf.

HRAC (Herbicide Resistance Action Committee). Website, hracglobal.com.

IRAC (Insecticide Resistance Action Committee). Website, irac-online.org.

Kansas Department of Agriculture. 1990. *Chemigation in Kansas*. Topeka: Kansas Department of Agriculture.

Klingman, G. C., and F. M. Ashton. 1975. *Weed Science Principles and Practices.* New York: Wiley.

Kranz, W., C. Burr, J. Hay, J. Schild, and D. Yonts. 2008. *Using Chemigation Safely and Effectively: Training Manual.* Historical Materials from University of Nebraska-Lincoln Extension Paper 915.

Lovatt, C. N. D. Plant growth regulator strategies and avocado phenology and physiology. California Avocado Growers website, californiaavocadogrowers.com/sites/default/files/documents/PRG-Strategies-and-avocado-phenology.pdf.

McDonald, S. A. 1991. *Applying Pesticides Correctly: A Guide for Private and Commercial Applicators*. Washington, DC: US EPA and USDA.

McKenry, M. V., and P. A. Roberts. Phytonematology study guide. Oakland: University of California Division of Agriculture and Natural Resources Publication 4045.

National Institute for Occupational Safety and Health. 1985. *Occupational Safety and Health Guidance Manual for Hazardous Waste Site Activities*. Washington, DC: NIOSH.

National Institute for Occupational Safety and Health. 1998. *Setting Up Emergency Decontamination Facilities*. Washington, DC: NIOSH,

Occupational Safety and Health Administration. 2012. *Hazard Communication Standard: Safety Data Sheets*. OSHA Brief. OSHA website, osha.gov/Publications/OSHA3514.pdf.

Occupational Safety and Health Administration. 2014. *Occupational Heat Exposure*. OSHA website, osha.gov/SLTC/heatstress.

Perry, E. J., and A. T. Ploeg. 2010. *Pest Notes: Nematodes*. Oakland: University of California Division of Agriculture and Natural Resources Publication 7489. ipm.ucanr.edu/PMG/PESTNOTES/pn7489.html.

Pfeiffer, M. 2010. Ground Water Ubiquity Score (GUS). Tucson, AZ: Pesticide Training Resources. PTR website, ptrpest.com/pdf/groundwater_ubiquity.pdf.

Platt, H. D. 1953. Pictorial key to some common adult cockroaches. Atlanta: U.S. Department of Health, Education, and Welfare, Public Health Service Communicable Disease Center.

Randall, C., et al., eds. 2008. *National Pesticide Applicator Certification Core Manual*. Washington D.C.: National Association of State Departments of Agriculture Research Foundation.

Salmon, T. P., and R. A. Baldwin. 2009. *Pest Notes: Pocket Gophers*. Oakland: University of California Division of Agriculture and Natural Resources Publication 7433. UC IPM website, ipm.ucanr.edu/PMG/PESTNOTES/pn7433.html.

Salmon, T. P., and W. P. Gorenzel. 2010a. *Pest Notes: Ground Squirrels*. Oakland: University of California Division of Agriculture and Natural Resources Publication 7438. UC IPM website, ipm.ucanr.edu/PMG/PESTNOTES/pn7438.html.

Salmon, T. P., and W. P. Gorenzel. 2010b. *Pest Notes: Rabbits*. Oakland: University of California Division of Agriculture and Natural Resources Publication 7447. UC IPM website, ipm.ucanr.edu/PMG/PESTNOTES/pn7447.html.

Salmon, T. P., D. A. Whisson, and R. E. Marsh. 2006. *Wildlife Pest Control around Gardens and Homes*. 2nd ed. Oakland: University of California Division of Agriculture and Natural Resources Publication 21385.

Saw, L., J. Shumway, and P. Ruckart. 2011. Surveillance data on pesticide and agricultural chemical releases and associated public health consequences in selected US states, 2003–2007. *Journal of Medical Toxicology* 7:164–171.

Schwankl, L. 2015. Microirrigation systems. UC Davis Fruit and Nut Research and Information website, fruitsandnuts.ucdavis.edu/files/73686.pdf.

Schwankl, L. J., and T. Prichard. 2001. Uniform chemigation in tree and vine microirrigation systems. Oakland: University of California Division of Agriculture and Natural Resources Publication 21599.

Stetson, D. I., and R. A. Baldwin. 2010. *Pest Notes: Birds on Tree Fruits and Vines*. Oakland: University of California Division of Agriculture and Natural Resources Publication 74152. UC IPM website, ipm.ucanr.edu/PMG/PESTNOTES/pn74152.html.

University of California Statewide Integrated Pest Management Program. Website, ipm.ucanr.edu.

Vertebrate Pest Control Handbook Online. Vertebrate Pest Control Research Advisory Committee website, vpcrac.org/about/vertebrate-pest-handbook.

INDEX

An *italic* "f" after a page number, such as 64*f*, refers to a photo or an illustration; an *italic* "t", as in 89*t*, refers to a table or sidebar.

1-naphthaleneacetamide (NAD), 89*t*
1,3-dichloropropene, 143
2,4-D, 74*t*, 89*t*, 94, 183*t*, 305*t*
4-HPPD inhibitors, 305*t*

A

a.i. (active ingredient), 77, 270–272, 326, 330
ABA (abscisic acid), 89*t*
abamectin, 73*t*, 315*t*
abatement laws, 14
abiotic disorders, 56, 57–58
abrasive pesticides
    formulations, 78, 79, 80, 83, 292*t*
    and nozzle selection, 205
    and pump selection, 198, 199*t*, 200, 201
abscisic acid (ABA), 89*t*
absorption, by soil particles, 101
Abutilon theophrasti (velvetleaf), 32
acaricides, 73*t*
ACCase inhibitors, 305*t*
accidents. *See also* environmental hazards; first aid; human exposure to pesticides; spills
    overview, 121, 334
    during applications, 186, 345–346
    clean-up, 342, 343–344
    decontamination process, 340–341, 342
    emergency numbers to call, 165, 329, 336
    fires, 186, 330, 344
    liability for, 105, 190, 248, 345
    planning for, 145, 165–166, 334, 335–336, 346
    reporting, 341, 342–343
    spill kits, 171, 176, 341–342
accumulation of pesticides, 109, 111, 115, 313
acephate, 315*t*
acetylcholine receptor (nAChR) agonists, 74*t*
Achillea millefolium (common yarrow), 35

acidifiers, 90*t*, 93–94
ACRC (Ag Container Recycling Council), 176
Acroptilon repens (Russian knapweed), 35
action thresholds, 16, 288
activators, 90*t*, 92
active ingredient (a.i.), 77, 270–272, 326, 330
active injection devices, 225, 227–228
acute exposure to pesticides, 128–129
additive effect, in mixed pesticides, 301–302
adjuvants, 89–94
adsorption, 101
aerosol cans, 84, 215*t*, 216, 218*t*, 222
Ag Container Recycling Council (ACRC), 176
agitators, 202, 251
agricultural burn permit, 187
Agrobacterium radiobacter, 8, 87
Agrobacterium tumefaciens (crown gall), 8
air assist sprayers, 218*t*, 220, 251–254
air blast sprayers. *See also* sprayers
    calibrating, 251–255, 257
    characteristics, 220–221
    nozzles, 207
    speed of travel, 295
    uses, 218*t*
air pollution, 57*t*
air-purifying respirators, 146, 148–150
air-supplying respirators, 146, 150–151
alachlor, 305*t*
alcohol, and pesticide toxicity, 166
algae, 27, 30, 73*t*, 74*t*
alkali sida (*Malva leprosa*), 32
alkyl dimethylbenzyl, 73*t*
allelopathy, 8
allergies, from pesticides, 127
almond trees, 64*f*
ALS inhibitors, 305*t*
alternate row or block treatments, 297
aluminum and monel nozzles, 205
aluminum fluosilicate, 86
Amaranthus spp. (pigweeds), 33

American Society of Agricultural and Biological Engineers (ASABE), 309*t*
amides, 305*t*
aminopyridine, 73*t*
ammonium caprylic acid, 73*t*
amphibians, 53
animal agriculture pest control, xiv*t*, 85
animal testing, 69–70
anionic surfactants, 91–92
annual bluegrass (*Poa annua*), 31
annual sowthistle (*Sonchus oleraceus*), 35
annual weeds, 28
antagonistic effect, in mixed pesticides, 302
antibiosis, 8
antibiotics, 85
anticoagulants, 85–86
antimicrobials, 73*t*
ants, 36*t*, 48
aphids, 36*t*, 38–39, 44–45
apple scab, 59*f*, 60*f*
application equipment. *See also* nozzles; sprayers
    aerosol dispensers, 84, 215*t*, 216, 218*t*, 222
    agitators, 202, 251
    bait stations, applicators, 234–235
    booms, 295
    chemical injection systems, 218*t*, 225–229, 239, 269–270
    cleaning, 188, 235–239, 238–239
    closed-system mixing units, 157–158, 177–178, 214
    control valves, 212
    controllers, 276
    for dusts, 230*t*, 231–232, 238
    filter screens, strainers, 203–204, 235, 238
    formulation effects on, 292*t* (*See also specific formulations*)
    for granules, 230*t*, 232–233, 264–269
    hand spray guns, 210, 254*f*, 295
    hand-operated equipment, 210, 214–217
    hoses, couplings, fittings, 212–213, 238

learning how to operate, 294–295
for liquids, overview, 195
for livestock, poultry, 233–234
lubricating, 239
maintenance, 122, 196, 235–239, 249
monitors and controllers, 276
powered equipment, 217–222
pressure regulators, gauges, 210–212, 214, 237t, 238, 264, 276
pumps, 197–201, 228, 237t, 238
selection of, 181, 215t, 218t, 230t
spray shields, 214
storing, 237–238, 239
tanks, 196–197, 225, 235–236, 237–238
unloaders, 211
before using, 235, 238, 239
wick applicators, 215t, 217
application rates, 246, 266, 268, 269–274, 276, 327
application records, 188–189
applicators. *See* pesticide applicators
applying pesticides. *See also* application equipment; calibration; handling pesticides
alternate row or block treatments, 297
application patterns, 184–185
band treatments, 296
BMPs (best management practices), 311–312
buffer zones, strips, 111, 183, 184–185, 312
directions for use, 327
equipment problems, 235–237
filling spray tank, 180
liability for accidents, errors, 105, 190, 248, 345
measuring amounts, 178–180
methods, 194–195, 294–297
misapplications, 345–346
notifications to bee keepers, 314
overapplication, 246–248
planning, 163–166, 181–185
preventing gaps and overlaps, 295–296
recordkeeping, 188–189
in sensitive areas, 110–111, 183–184, 313, 331

soil injection, 219, 258, 260f
speed of travel, 182, 184, 261, 264, 265, 276, 295
spot treatments, 296
timing, 298, 308–309, 312, 314
aprons, PPE, 139, 141–142
aquatic pest control, xiiit, 26, 30–31, 82
aquatic wildlife, harm to, 114–115
aquifers, 103f, 104. *See also* groundwater contamination
Argentine ant, 48f. *See also* ants
Armillaria mellea, 60f
Armillaria root rot, 60f
Artemisia douglasiana (California mugwort), 35
arthropod pests, 36–39, 286–287. *See also specific arthropods,* such as spiders
ASABE (American Society of Agricultural and Biological Engineers), 309t
assassin bugs. *See* bugs (true bugs, plant bugs, etc.)
aster family weeds, 35
aster yellows, 65
atmosphere monitoring equipment, 158
atmosphere-supplying respirators, 150–151
atrazine, 74, 75, 183t, 305t
Atriplex semibaccata (Australian saltbush), 33
attractants, 74t, 84, 90t, 94. *See also* pheromones
augmentation of natural enemies, 6
Australian saltbush (*Atriplex semibaccata*), 33
Avena fatua (wild oat), 31
avicides, 73t
azadirachtin, 86t, 315t
azoxystrobin, 76, 183t, 315t

B

Bacillus thuringiensis (Bt), 15t, 87, 113t, 315t
back-siphoning, 312
backpack sprayers, 215t, 217, 218t, 219, 252, 258
backyards, exposure hazards, 123
bacterial diseases, 56t, 62–63, 73t
baits, bait stations, 84, 234–235, 283t. *See also* attractants
band treatments, 296

banned pesticides, 2, 75
barnyardgrass (*Echinochloa crus-galli*), 31
batch tank injection systems, 226
bean plants, 27f
beating, pest monitoring, 283t
Beauveria bassiana, 315t
bed bugs, 44, 87t
bees. *See also* honey bees
characteristics, damage, 48
pesticide impacts, 75, 83, 86t, 111–113, 292, 314–315
as pollinators, beneficials, 38t, 48
beet armyworm, 6f, 24f
beetles, 36t, 38t, 45–46
beneficial organisms, 7, 38t, 75, 111–113. *See also* natural enemies
bentazon, 183t
bermudagrass (*Cynodon dactylon*), 31
biennial weeds, 28
bifenthrin, 76, 183t, 315t
bifluid nozzles, 208, 209t
bioaccumulation of pesticides, 109, 115, 314–316, 331
biological control, 5, 6–9. *See also* natural enemies
biotic and abiotic factors, 56
biotypes, and pesticide resistance, 304
bipyridyliums, 305t
birds
as natural enemies, 8, 38t, 53
pesticide impacts on, 114, 314
as pests, 53, 73t, 281
birdsrape mustard (*Brassica rapa*), 32
black mustard (*Brassica nigra*), 32
black sooty mold, 45
black-tailed hare, 54–55
blacklight traps, 286
blends of chemicals, 90–91
blood test, of cholinesterase levels, 127, 162
blunt spikerush (*Eleocharis obtusa*), 31
BMPs (best management practices), 311–312
bollworm, 21f
booms, 295
boots, PPE, 139, 143, 153, 155
Bordeaux mixture, 15t, 80
border inspection stations, 13
boric acid powder, 15t, 87

botanicals, 86
brass nozzles, 205
Brassica nigra (black mustard), 32
Brassica rapa (birdsrape mustard), 32
breakdown of pesticides, 70, 74, 75, 109
breaking the disease cycle, 59
breeding for pest resistance, 13
Bremia lactucae (downy mildew), 61f
bristletails, 41
bristly oxtongue (*Picris echioides*), 35
broad-spectrum pesticides, 111, 290, 306
broadcast nozzles, 208, 209t
broadleaves, 27
brodifacoum, 73t, 85–86
bromacil, 183t
bromadiolone, 73t, 85–86
bromoxynil, 305t
Bromus rubens (foxtail brome), 31
brown rot of stone fruits, 60f
brush rabbits, 55
bryophytes, 27
Bt (*Bacillus thuringiensis*), 315t
buffer zones, strips, 111, 183, 184–185, 312
buffers (pH), 90t, 93–94
bugs (true bugs, plant bugs, etc.), 36t, 44
bulb applicators, 230t, 231
bull thistle (*Cirsium vulgare*), 35
buprofezin, 74t, 183t, 315t
burn permits, 187
burning pesticide bags, 180, 187
burrowing devices, 234f, 235
butterflies, 38t, 39f, 46

C

cabbage looper, 23f, 24f
cabs, enclosed, 156–157
Cal/OSHA (California Occupational Safety and Health Administration), 342
calculations
    active ingredient (a.i.), 269–272
    amount of pesticide in tank, 259, 261, 263, 271
    application rates, 269–274
    granule applicator output, 265–269
    nozzle output, 252–254
    parts per million solutions, 273, 274

percentage solutions, 272, 273, 274
size of target site, 274–276
sprayer output, 254–255, 260
CalEMA (California Emergency Management Agency), 165, 341, 342
calibration
    checking and testing, 246, 249, 264, 266, 269
    of chemigation systems, 229, 231, 269, 270
    conversion factors, 247t
    defined, 246
    of granule (dry) applicators, 264–269
    of monitors, 276
    sight gauges, dipsticks, 249
    of sprayers
        adjusting output rates, 261, 264, 276
        check devices, 254
        determining pesticide amount, 259, 261, 263
        measuring flow rate, 251–255, 260
        measuring swath width, 254f, 255–258, 259f, 260f
        measuring tank capacity, 249
        measuring travel speed, 250–251
        worksheet, 262
    tools, 248
    why calibrate, 246–248
calibration tubes, 229
California Code of Regulations (CCR), 145, 320
California Department of Fish and Wildlife, 116, 342
California Department of Pesticide Regulation (DPR), ix–xii, 116, 311, 320–322
California Department of Toxic Substances Control, 187, 342, 344
California Department of Transportation (CalTrans), 171
California Emergency Management Agency (CalEMA), 165, 341, 342
California Fish and Game Code, 10
California Food and Agriculture Code, 320
California goldenrod (*Solidago californica*), 35
California Highway Patrol, 165, 169, 171
California Labor Code, 341

California mugwort (*Artemisia douglasiana*), 35
California Occupational Safety and Health Administration (Cal/OSHA), 342
California Office of Emergency Services, 336, 341
California Poison Control System (CPCS), 339
California Public Utilities Commission, 169–170
California Restricted Materials, 321
California Weather Database, 308
CalTrans (California Department of Transportation), 171
Canada thistle (*Cirsium arvense*), 35
cankers, 62–63
Capsella bursapastoris (shepherdspurse), 32
caratenoid biosynthesis inhibitors, 305t
carbamates, 73t, 75, 162, 163f
carbaryl, 75, 89t, 93t, 113t, 315t
Cardaria draba (hoary cress), 32
cardiopulmonary resuscitation (CPR) training, 335
carpet beetle, 45f
carriers (in formulations), 77, 84
cartridge respirators, 148–150
CAS (Chemical Abstracts Service) numbers, 330
cat fleas, 47f. *See also* fleas
Category I-IV pesticides, 70–72, 95, 136, 157
caterpillars, 36t
cationic surfactants, 92
CAUTION pesticides, 70–72, 95. *See also* signal words
CCD (colony collapse disorder), 111, 112
CDAs (controlled droplet applicators), 218t, 219, 252, 258
ceanothus, 11f
cellulose inhibitors, 305t
Centaurea solstitialis (yellow starthistle), 8f, 34f, 35
centipedes, 36t, 37f
centrifugal pumps, 199t, 201
ceramic nozzles, 205
certification and licensing, ix, 190
certified pest-free material, 14
Certified Private Applicator examination, ix

Chemical Abstracts Service (CAS) numbers, 330
chemical cartridge respirators, 149
chemical control of pests, 5, 9. *See also specific pesticides;* pesticide products
chemical groups of pesticides, 73*t*, 74–76
chemical injection pumps, 218*t*, 222
chemical injection systems. *See* chemigation
chemical-resistant clothing, 136–138, 154–155
chemigation
   automated controls, 228–229, 269
   calibration, 229, 231, 269, 270
   equipment maintenance, 239
   system check, 269
   system components, 224–229
   system types, 223–224
CHEMTREC, 165, 336
Chenopodium album (common lambsquarters), 33
Chenopodium murale (nettleleaf goosefoot), 33
chewing lice, 43
children, pesticide exposure, 120, 122, 123, 124, 126, 175, 176
Chinese thornapple (*Datura ferox*), 34
chitin biosynthesis inhibitors, 74*t*
chlorantraniliprole, 113*t*
chlordane, 115
chloride, 73*t*
chlorinated hydrocarbons. *See* organochlorines
chlorine dioxide, 73*t*
chloroacetamides, 305*t*
chlorophacinone, 73*t*, 86
chlorothalonil, 73*t*, 74*t*, 93*t*
chlorpropham, 89*t*, 305*t*
chlorpyrifos, 75, 93*t*, 113*t*, 183*t*, 315*t*
chlorsulfuron, 76, 305*t*
cholinesterase blood test, 127, 162
chronic exposure to pesticides, 128–129
chrysanthemum chlorotic mottle, 65
chrysanthemum stunt, 65
cicadas, 45
CIMIS program, 282, 307
Cirsium spp. (thistle), 35
citrus exocortis, 65

citrus red mite (*Panonychus citri*), 7*f*
citrus stubborn disease, 65
Class I, II disposal sites, 187–188
classical biological control, 6. *See also* biological control
classification
   of pesticides
      by chemical families, 73*t*, 74–76
      by formulation, 77–82
      by modes of action, 74*t*, 76–77, 298–299
      by pest target, 73*t*, 74
   of plants, animals, 20–22
   of weeds, 27
cleaning and maintaining equipment, 188, 235–239, 249
cleaning and maintaining PPE, 139, 144–145, 151, 152–155
cleaning up pesticide spills, 342, 343–344
clomazone, 305*t*
clopyralid, 183*t*
closed mixing systems, 157–158, 177–178, 214
clothianidin, 315*t*
clothing. *See* PPE (personal protective equipment)
clumping of pesticides. *See* incompatibility of pesticides
coalescent effect, in mixed pesticides, 302
cocklebur (*Xanthium strumarium*), 25*f*, 35
cockroaches, 23*t*, 36*t*, 42, 85
Code of Federal Regulations (CFR), 322, 323
cold storage areas, 122
collar region of grasses, 31
colony collapse disorder (CCD), 111, 112
colorants in sprays, 94
common cocklebur (*Xanthium strumarium*), 35
common groundsel (*Senecio vulgaris*), 35
common lambsquarters (*Chenopodium album*), 33
common names, classification, 21–22
common sunflower (*Helianthus annuus*), 35
common yarrow (*Achillea millefolium*), 35

compatibility agents, 90*t*, 92–93
compatibility testing, 299–300
competition, as pest control, 8–9
compressed air dusters, 230*t*, 232
compressed air sprayers, 215*t*, 217, 252
cone nozzles, 207, 209*t*
confused flour beetle, 45*f*
Conibear traps, 10*f*
consperse stink bug, 44*f*
constant-rate pumps, 228
contact pesticides, 74*t*, 76, 298
containers, disposal, 176, 180, 187–188, 327, 331
containers, pesticide. *See* packaging of pesticides
continuing education, 134
control valves, 212
controlled droplet applicators (CDAs), 218*t*, 219, 252, 258
controllers, 276
convergent lady beetle (*Hippodamia convergens*), 7*f*
conversion factors table, 247*t*
Convolvulus arvensis (field bindweed), 34
copper accumulation, 109
copper hydroxide, 15*t*
copper oxychloride sulfate, 15*t*
copper sulfate, 15*t*, 73*t*
corn earworm, 21*f*
corrosive pesticides
   other equipment, 205, 213
   pumps, 198, 228
   tanks, 196, 197
cost of pesticides, 293–294
cottontails, 54–55
county agricultural commissioners
   meetings on laws and regulations, 134
   pesticide policies, 321
   reporting accidents, spills, 336, 341, 342–343, 345, 346
   responsibilities, services, xii, 100
couplings, fittings, hoses, 212–213
coveralls, PPE, 140–141, 155
CPB pheromone, 74*t*
CPCS (California Poison Control System), 339
CPR (cardiopulmonary resuscitation) training, 335
crickets, 36*t*, 41

cross-resistance, 304
crown gall, 62, 63
cryolite, 315t
cucumber beetles, 63
cucumber pale fruit, 65
cucumber wilt, 63
cultural controls, 5, 11–13, 59
curly dock, 25f
cyfluthrin, 113t, 315t
Cynodon dactylon (bermudagrass), 31
cypermethrin, 76, 183t, 315t
Cyperus spp. (nutsedge), 31
cytokinin, 89t

D
D-VAC, 283t
dairies, 12–13
dallisgrass (*Paspalum dilatatum*), 31
damage thresholds, 288
damaged containers, 175
daminozide, 89t
damsel bugs, 44
dandelion (*Taraxacum officinale*), 25f, 35
DANGER pesticides, 70–72, 95, 136, 157. *See also* signal words
data loggers, 307
Datura ferox (Chinese thornapple), 34
Datura stramonium (jimsonweed), 34
DDT, 2, 75, 115
deactivation effect, in mixed pesticides, 302
decontamination processes, 188, 340–341, 342
DED (Dutch elm disease), 62
deergrass (*Muhlenbergia rigens*), 31
defoamers, 90t, 94
degree-day phenology, 283t, 287
demonstration and research pest control, xivt
deposition aids, 90t, 94, 186
depredation permits, 53
dermal exposure to pesticides
    adsorption, 71t, 72, 124–125
    first aid, 337–338
    LD$_{50}$ values, 69f, 71t, 72
    symptoms, 124, 126, 128, 330
desert cottontail, 54–55
desiccants, 77, 86–87
diamethoate, 93t
diaphragm pumps, 198–200, 228

diatomaceous earth, 15t, 87, 315t
diazinon, 73t, 75, 93t, 114–115, 183t, 315t
dicamba, 183t
dichlobenil, 305t
dichotomous keys, 22–23
dicloropropene, 73t
dicots, 27
diflubenzuron, 87t, 315t
Digitaria ischaemum (smooth crabgrass), 31
dimethoate, 113t
dinitroanilines, 305t
dinotefuran, 315t
diphacinone, 73t
dipping vats, 234
dipsticks, for calibration, 249
direct channel pollution, 104, 107
disc-core nozzles, 207
discing, 25
disease cycle, 58–59
disease signs and symptoms, 56–57, 60–61, 285
disease triangle, 58
disposable PPE, 139–140
disposal of pesticides, 102, 176, 180, 187, 327, 331
diuron, 183t, 305t
dormant oil sprays, 88, 114–115
dosage rates of pesticides, 69, 120, 297
DOT (U.S. Department of Transportation), 168, 171, 172
downy mildew (*Bremia lactucae*), 61f
DPR (California Department of Pesticide Regulation)
    certification testing, ix–xii
    endangered species resource, 116
    pesticide regulation, registration, 320–322
    VOC calculator, 311
drainage problems, 57–58
drift hazards
    overview, 104–106, 185–186, 306
    indoors, 309, 311
    liability, 105, 190
    management of
        adjuvants, 90, 94, 186, 308
        droplet size, 106, 182–183, 186, 308–309
        formulation choice, 308

        onsite evaluation, 105, 183–184
        timing applications, 308–309
        troubleshooting, 237t
    particle/dust drift, 81, 107, 311
    spray drift, 105–106, 306, 308–309
    vapor drift, 106, 310–311
    weather effects, 106, 181–182, 185–186, 307–308
drinking and pesticide exposure, 126
drinking water, 102, 103, 110
drop spreaders, 230t, 233
drugs, and pesticide toxicity, 166
dry break couplings, 213
dry flowables, 78, 292t
dumping pesticides, 187
dust and mist masks, 148, 237t
dust applicators, 230t, 231–232, 238
dust bags, boxes, 233f, 234
dust drift, 81, 107, 311. *See also* drift hazards
dust formulations, 81–82, 137, 231–232, 292t. *See also* inert dusts
dust inhalation, 78, 82
Dutch elm disease (DED), 62

E
early-entry workers, 166, 327
earwigs, 36t, 42
eating and pesticide exposure, 126
Echinochloa crus-galli (barnyardgrass), 31
ecological hazards, 331. *See also* environmental hazards; offsite movement of pesticides; wildlife
economic injury thresholds, 16
economic thresholds, 288
ecosystems, 2–3, 26
efficacy of pesticide products, 293–294
electric shock, during application, 186
Electronic Code of Federal Regulations, 14
electronic positioning devices, 295–296
electronic sprayer controllers, 212
electrostatic sprayers, 218t, 221–222
Eleocharis obtusa (blunt spikerush), 31
elm bark beetle (*Scolytus multistriatus*), 62
emergencies. *See also* accidents; first aid; human exposure to pesticides; spills
    decontamination process, 340–341, 342

heat stress, 127, 141, 337
numbers to call, 165, 329, 336
pesticide fires, 186, 330, 344
planning for, 145, 165–166, 334, 335–336, 341–342, 346
reviewing responses, 346
training for, 133
emergency exemptions, 322
emergency response plans, 335–336
emulsifiable concentrates, 79, 292t, 308
emulsifiers, 91, 92
enclosed cabs, 156–157
endangered species, 115–116
Endangered Species Protection Program, 115–116
endothall, 73t
engineering controls, PPE, 156–158
environment
defined, 100
and disease development, 58
pesticide movement in, 100–101 (*See also* offsite movement of pesticides)
environmental hazard statements, 311, 327, 331
environmental hazards
contamination of sensitive areas, 110–111, 183–184, 313, 331
damage to nontarget organisms, 111–116, 298, 313–316
groundwater contamination, 102, 103–104, 107, 110, 311–312
surface water contamination, 102, 107, 110, 114–115, 173, 311–312
enzyme inhibitors, 74t
EPA. *See* U.S. Environmental Protection Agency (EPA)
EPSP synthase inhibitors, 74t
equipment for pesticides. *See* application equipment
eradicants (fungicides), 77
eradication of pests, 4, 14
Erwinia amylovora, 63f
Erwinia rubrifaciens, 62f
establishment numbers, 326
ethephon, 89t
ethoprop, 93t
ethylene, 89t
evaluating pest management, 16
even flat-fan nozzles, 206, 209t

examinations and tests, ix–xii
exclusion of pests, 9–10
exotic weed species, 25
exposure. *See* human exposure to pesticides
extenders, 90t, 92
eye exposure to pesticides, 71t, 79, 125, 128t, 145, 338, 339f
eyewear, PPE, 144–145, 153

F

face masks, PPE, 148. *See also* respirators
face shields, PPE, 145, 153
facial hair, and respirators, 146–147, 150, 151
facility maps, 336, 337f
fall armyworm, 46f
Federal Insecticide, Fungicide, and Rodenticide Act (FIFRA), 68, 320, 322
fenpyroximate, 315t
fertilizers with pesticides, 85, 94–95
fiberglass tanks, 196t, 197
field bindweed (*Convolvulus arvensis*), 34
field incompatibility of tank mixes, 299
fieldworker safety, 166–167
fieldworker training, 132, 133–134, 135
FIFRA (Federal Insecticide, Fungicide, and Rodenticide Act), 68, 320, 322
filter screens, 203–204, 235, 238
fipronil, 183t, 315t
fire blight, 62f, 63
fire hazards, 186, 330, 344
firebrats, 41
first aid
overview, 335
defined, 335
to eyes, 125, 145, 338, 339f
label statement, 326
medical facilities, 334
in mouth, 126, 128t, 339–340
recognizing signs, symptoms, 126–127, 128t, 129, 330, 337
to respiratory system, 125, 128t, 338–339
SDS statement, 330
to skin, 337–338
fish
as beneficials, 38t, 53
control of, 52, 73t, 86t

pesticide impacts on, 114–115, 314
Fish and Game Code, 10
fit testing respirators, 147–148
fitting PPE, 125, 155–156
fittings, couplings, hoses, 212–213
flammable pesticides, 186, 330
flannel bush, 11f
flat-fan nozzles, 205–206, 209t, 255f
fleas, 36t, 47, 84f, 85
flies, 12–13, 36t, 38t, 47
flooding nozzles, 208, 209t
flow rate, measuring, 251–255
flowables, 79, 292t
flowmeters, 249
fluazifop-p-butyl, 305t
flubendiamide, 113t
flushing equipment, 235–236, 237–238, 239
flushing pests, 283t
foam markers, 295
foaming in spray tanks, 94. *See also* defoamers
foggers, 84, 218t, 222
follow-up monitoring, 16, 316
food contamination, 42, 123
food processing plants, 122
Food Quality Protection Act, 320
footwear, PPE, 139, 143, 153, 155
forest pest control, xiiit
formetanate, 93t
formulations of pesticides
and application equipment, 215t, 218t, 230t, 235, 292t
choosing between, 292
defined, 77
and drift hazards, 308
dry flowables, 78, 292t
dusts, 81–82, 137, 292t
emulsifiable concentrates, 79, 292t, 308
flowables, 79, 292t
fumigants, 80–81
granules, 78, 82, 292t, 293, 314
and hazards to bees, birds, 314
invert emulsions, 81
label information, 326
low-concentrate solutions, 80
microencapsulated pesticides, 83, 292t, 293, 314

formulations of pesticides (cont.)
  mixing products, 94–95, 299–303
  and nozzle wear, 204–205
  organic, 68
  pellets, 82, 232, 292t
  persistence of, 293
  and pump selection, 199t
  and selectivity, 291
  slurry, 80
  soluble powders, 78–79, 292t
  suffixes, 77–78
  ultra-low-volume concentrates, 80
  and use of agitators, 202
  volatile pesticides, 101, 106, 310–311
  water-soluble bags or packets, 78, 83, 178
  water-soluble concentrates or solutions, 79, 292t, 293
  wettable powders, 78, 292t
foxtail brome (*Bromus rubens*), 31
FRAC (Fungicide Resistance Action Committee), 306
frost symptoms, 57t, 58
fumigants
  human hazards, 80, 122, 126
  measuring vapors, 158
  packaging, 169
  PPE, 134, 142, 148
  uses, application, 80–81, 299
fungal diseases, 60–61, 285
fungi, 59–62
Fungicide Resistance Action Committee (FRAC), 306
fungicides. *See also specific fungicides*
  chemical families, 73t, 76
  human exposure, 126, 166
  modes of action, 77

G

galls, 62
gas line leaks, 57t
gas masks, 149
gear pumps, 199t, 200–201
geese, 8
general-use pesticides, 321
genetic engineering, 13
genetically modified organisms (GMOs), 13
genus and species names, 21

geology, and leaching risk, 104
gibberellic acid, 89t
global positioning systems (GPS), 295–296
gloves, PPE
  cleaning, 153, 155
  disposable/reusable, 139, 140f, 142
  EPA code letters, 138
  liners, 142
glufosinate-ammonium, 305t
glutamine synthase inhibitors, 305t
glycines, 305t
glyphosate, 74t, 91, 183t, 197, 305t
gnats, 47
goggles, PPE, 144–145, 153
goosefoot weeds, 33
gophers, 54, 235
government agencies. *See regulatory agencies*
GPS (global positioning systems), 295–296
granary weevil, 45f
granular pesticides, 82, 292t, 293, 314
granule applicators, 230t, 232–233, 264–269
granulosis virus, 15t
grape leafhopper, 45f
grapes, 61f
grass buffer strips, 312
grass carp, 53
grass weeds, 31
grasshoppers, 36t, 37f, 38–39, 41
greenhouse whitefly, 45f
greenhouses, nurseries, 122
ground covers, 8
ground squirrels, 54, 55
groundcherry (*Physalis* spp.), 34
groundwater contamination
  overview, 102, 110
  groundwater ubiquity scores, 183t
  leaching, 103–104
  from pesticide storage, 173
  preventing, 311–312
  types of pollution, 107
groundwater protection area (GWPA), 75, 183–184
Groundwater Protection List, 75
groundwater ubiquity score (GUS), 183t
growth inhibitors, 77

growth regulators. *See insect growth regulators (IGRs); plant growth regulators*
GUS (groundwater ubiquity score), 183t
GWPA (groundwater protection area), 75, 183–184

H

habitat modification, 13–14
hail damage, 57t, 58
half-life of pesticides, 70, 101, 331
hand spray guns, 210, 254f, 295
hand-operated equipment, 210, 214–217
handling pesticides
  burning pesticide bags, 180
  cleaning equipment, 188, 235–236, 238–239
  closed systems, 157–158, 177–178, 214
  damaged containers, 175
  disposal of products, 102, 176, 180, 187–188, 327, 331
  and human exposure, 78, 79, 120, 121, 166
  loading, 171–172, 177–178, 292t, 312
  measuring, 178
  opening packaging, 168–169, 178–179, 180
  rinsing containers, 176, 179–180
  SDS statement, 330
  service containers, 169, 174–175
  training, 127, 132–134, 335
hardstem bulrush (*Scirpus acutus*), 31
harlequin bug, 39f
harvest limitations. *See preharvest intervals*
Hazardous Materials Information Center, 172
hazards of pesticides. *See environmental hazards; human exposure to pesticides*
head lice, 43f
headgear, PPE, 139, 142, 155
health. *See human exposure to pesticides; safety*
heat stress, 127, 141, 337
Helianthus annuus (common sunflower), 35
Helianthus tuberosus (Jerusalem artichoke), 35
Helicoverpa zea, 21

hellebore, 86
herbaceous perennial weeds, 28–29
Herbicide Resistance Action Committee (HRAC), 305t, 306
herbicides
   band treatments, 296
   breakdown, and soil properties, 109
   chemical families, 73t, 75, 76
   deactivation in tank, 302
   decision to use, 288–289
   impacts on wildlife, plant diversity, 115, 116
   modes of action, 74t, 77, 289
   and nozzle choice, 205
   and phytotoxicity, 313
   pre- and postemergent, 77
   resistance, 76, 304–306
   and soil erosion, 115
   swath widths, 258, 259f
   transporting, 172
herbivores, as natural enemies, 8
Heterotheca grandiflora (telegraphplant), 35
Hibiscus trionum (Venice mallow), 32
high-pressure hydraulic sprayers, 218t, 220, 254–255
Hippodamia convergens (convergent lady beetle), 7f
history of pest management, 2–3
hoary cress (*Cardaria draba*), 32
honey bees
   characteristics, benefits, 38t, 48
   colony collapse disorder (CCD), 111, 112
   lawsuits, 190
   minimizing losses, 314
   pesticide impacts, 75, 86t, 111–113, 292, 314, 315t
   pesticide label protections, 112
   SDS statement, 331
honeydew, 45
horntails, 48
horseshoe-shaped booms, 258, 259f
horticultural oils, 315t
hose-end sprayers, 215t, 216
hoses, couplings, fittings, 212–213, 238
host plants and disease cycle, 58–59
host resistance, 13
host-free areas and periods, 14
house fly, 47f. See also flies

HRAC (Herbicide Resistance Action Committee), 305t, 306
human exposure to pesticides. *See also specific pesticide formulations;* safety; toxicity of pesticides
   acute *vs.* chronic exposure, 128–129
   emergency numbers to call, 165, 336
   harmful effects, symptoms, 126–127, 128–129, 330, 335, 337
   how pesticides enter the body, 124–126
   lethal dose, lethal concentration, 69–72
   when/where exposure occurs, 120–124, 165–166, 186
humidity, and drift hazard, 106
hydraulic agitators, 202
hydrogen peroxide, 73t
hydroprene, 87t
Hyposoter exiquae parasitic wasp, 6f

I

ice damage, 57t
ice vests, 141
identification keys, 22
identifying pests. *See also specific pests*
   arthropods, 36–38
   bacteria, 62–63
   fungi, 60
   pathogens, 56–57
   resources, 22–24
   vertebrates, 52
   viruses, 64
   weeds, 26–30
IGRs (insect growth regulators), 86t, 87
illness. *See first aid; heat stress*
imazapyr, 73t, 183t
imidacloprid, 73t, 74t, 75, 183t, 315t
impregnates, 85
incompatibility of pesticides, 92–93, 95, 292t, 299–303
Indian tobacco (*Nicotiana quadrivalvis*), 34
indianmeal moth, 46f
indoor hazards
   drift, 104, 105, 309, 311
   pesticide storage, 122–123
   runoff, leaching, 102, 103
   sensitive areas, 111
indoxacarb, 113t
industrial pest control, xiiit, 84
inert dusts, 86–87
inert ingredients, 77, 205, 326, 330

infiltration of water into soil, 102
inflorescence types, 29
inhalation hazards
   dusts, 78, 82
   first aid, 125, 338–339
   fumigants, 80
   label/SDS statements, 326, 330
   symptoms, 128t
injuries. *See first aid; heat stress; spills*
inoculation and disease spread, 58–59, 285
insect growth regulators (IGRs), 86t, 87
Insecticide Resistance Action Committee (IRAC), 306
insecticides
   botanicals, 86
   chemical families, 73t, 74–76
   human exposure, 126
   modes of action, 74t, 77, 298–299
   pests controlled, 86t, 87t, 113t
insects. *See also specific insects*
   body structure, 37f, 38
   generations per year, 39
   monitoring, 286–287
inspection stations, 13
instars, 38
institutional pest control, xiiit, 84
insurance, liability, 190
integrated pest management. *See* IPM (integrated pest management)
International Resistance Action Committee, 306
International Survey of Herbicide Resistant Weeds, 306
invasive plants, 26
inversions, temperature, 106, 181–182, 310
invert emulsions, 81, 308
invertebrate pests, 35–36. *See also specific pests*
inverting agents, 94
IPM (integrated pest management). *See also pest management*
   overview, 4–5
   defined, 2
   and environmental hazards, 311
   Pest Management Guidelines, 23, 288, 289–290
   and pesticide resistance, 306
   program history, 2–3
   program resources, 289–290, 308

Ipomoea spp. (morningglory), 34
iprodione, 74t, 183t
IRAC (Insecticide Resistance Action Committee), 306
iron phosphate, 73t
irrigation practices, 57–58
irrigator boots. *See* footwear, PPE
isoxazolidiones, 305t
ivyleaf morningglory (*Ipomoea hederacea*), 34

J

jackrabbits, 54–55
Jerusalem artichoke (*Helianthus tuberosus*), 35
jimsonweed (*Datura stramonium*), 34
johnsongrass (*Sorghum halepense*), 31

K

K84 strain of *Agrobacterium*, 8
kaolin, 74t, 315t
katydids, 41
key pests, 3
keys, identification, 22
knowledge expectations, for certification and licensing, ix–xi

L

labels, pesticide, 326
   application rate, 246, 327
   chronic toxicity warning, 129
   cleaner information, 236
   compatibility of tank mixes, 303
   damaged labels, 174–175
   environmental hazard statement, 311, 327
   first aid instructions, 125, 126, 326
   formulation, 77–78, 326
   as legal document, 322, 323
   manufacturer's information, 303, 326
   and planning an application, 163–165, 167
   pollinator protection, 112, 327
   PPE description, 134, 136, 137–138, 144, 327
   precautionary statements, 128, 129, 326–327
   preharvest intervals, 123, 327
   respirator requirement, 146, 147t
   sections of, 324–328
   on service containers, 169, 174–175
   when to read, 323
laboratory tests
   pest identification, 26t, 37t, 50t, 56
   of pesticides, 69–70
lacewings, 36t, 38t
lady beetles, 7f
lambda-cyhalothrin, 113t
landscape maintenance pest control, xiiit
larvae, defined, 38
latex stickers, 92
Latuca serriola (prickly lettuce), 35
laws and regulations
   application restrictions, 186
   Category I-IV pesticides, 70
   chemigation, 228–229, 269
   disposal of pesticides, 187–188
   drift liability, 105, 190
   heat stress training, 127
   improper use of pesticides, 248
   injection systems, 222
   label requirements, 323
   pesticide illness training, 127
   pesticide mixing, 177
   pesticide safety training, 132–134
   posting pesticide warnings, 167, 172, 173
   protection of pollinators, 112
   regulatory agencies, 320–321, 322 (*See also* DPR (California Department of Pesticide Regulation); U.S. Environmental Protection Agency (EPA))
   respirators, 145, 146, 147, 148
   SDS statement, 331
   service containers, 175
   tank covers, 196
   transporting pesticides, 169–170, 171
   vertebrate controls, 52, 53
lawsuits, 190
LC_{50} (lethal concentration) of pesticides, 69–70, 71t
LD_{50} (lethal dose) of pesticides, 69–72, 71t
leaching, 101, 103–104, 185t. *See also* groundwater contamination
leaf rust (*Puccinia recondita*), 61f
leaf spots, 56t, 63
leafhoppers, 45
leafminers, 36t
leaks of pesticides, 341–344. *See also* spills
lethal concentration (LC_{50}) of pesticides, 69–70, 71t
lethal dose (LD_{50}) of pesticides, 69–72
lettuce diseases, 61
liability for application accidents, errors, 105, 190, 248, 345
liability insurance, 190
lice, 36t, 43, 43f
licensing requirements, ix, xii, 190
life cycles, development
   and application timing, 298
   arthropods, 38–39
   bacteria, 63
   fish, 52
   fungi, 61
   nematodes, 50
   snails and slugs, 52
   viruses, viroids, phytoplasmas, 65
   weeds, 27–28
light excess/deficiency, 57t, 58
light traps, 283t
lightning damage, 57t
lime, 15t
lime sulfur, 15t
little mallow (*Malva parviflora*), 32
live traps, 287
livestock
   pesticide applications, 85, 233–234
   pesticide impacts on, 115, 314, 316
   weed suppression, 8
lizards, 53
loading pesticides
   best practices, 171–172, 312
   hazards by formulation, 292t
   mechanical systems, 177–178
locusts, 41
London rocket (*Sisymbrium irio*), 32
low-concentrate solutions, 80
low-pressure sprayers, 218t, 219–220, 251–254
low-volume sprays, 297
lubricating equipment, 239
lygus bug, 44f

M

maggots, 47
maintainance of equipment, 122, 196, 235–238, 239, 249

malathion, 75, 93t, 113t, 183t, 302, 315t
Malva spp., 32
mammal pests, 53–55, 73t
management of pests. *See* pest management
mancozeb, 183t
manure-breeding flies, 12–13
marking devices, 295
masks, PPE, 140, 148. *See also* respirators
Material Safety Data Sheet (MSDS). *See* Safety Data Sheet (SDS)
Matricaria matricarioides (pineapple weed), 35
mealybugs, 44–45
measuring pesticides, 178
mechanical agitators, 202
mechanical and physical controls, 5, 9–11
mechanical dusters, 230t, 232
medical care, 334, 335–336. *See also* first aid
medications, and pesticide toxicity, 166
mefenoxam, 315t
mefluidide, 89t
mepiquat chloride, 89t
mesh, defined, 82
mesotrione, 305t
metal tanks, 196t, 197
metaldehyde, 73t, 315t
metam-potassium, 75
metam-sodium, 74t, 75
metamorphosis, 38–39
metconazole, 73t
methomyl, 75, 93t, 113t
methoprene, 87t
methoxyfenozide, 113t
metric conversion table, 247t
mice, 53
microbials, 74t, 87
microencapsulated pesticides, 83, 292t, 293, 314
microorganisms in soil, 293
midges, 47
mini-bulk containers, 177–178
mist masks, 148
mites, 36t, 37f, 38, 39, 40, 73t
miticides, 73t, 74t, 113t
mitochondrial ATP synthase inhibitors, 74t

mitosis inhibitors, 74t, 305t
mixing pesticides
　best practices, 312
　closed systems, 157–158, 177–178
　combining products, 94–95, 301–303
　compatibility testing, 299–300
　hazards by formulation, 292t
　and human exposure, 78, 79, 120, 121
　settling out, 237t
　techniques for, 177
mobility of pesticides in soil, 103–104. *See also* leaching
modes of action of pesticides, 74t, 76–77, 298–299, 304–306
moles, 235
molluscicides, 73t
molting, 38, 39f
Monilinia spores, 60f
monitoring pests, 16
　after applications, 316
　and detecting resistance, 304, 306
　methods and tools table, 283t
　pheromones, 88, 286–287
　and predicting problems, 280–281, 280–282
　programs for
　　arthropods, 286–287
　　disease pathogens, 285
　　nematodes, 285
　　vertebrates, 287
　　weeds, 282, 284f, 285
　signs of presence, 282
　visual inspection, 282, 283t
monitors and controllers, 276
monocots, 27
morningglory weeds, 34
mosquitoes, 14, 36t, 38t, 47
moths, 36t, 38t, 39f, 46
movement of pesticides. *See* offsite movement of pesticides
mowing, 11
MSDS. *See* Safety Data Sheet (SDS)
MSMA, 305t
Muhlenbergia rigens (deergrass), 31
multi-site inhibitors, 74t
mustard weeds, 32

N
N6-benzyl adenine, 89t

NAA (naphthalene acetic acid), 89t
NAD (1-naphthaleneacetamide), 89t
naled, 93t
names of pesticide products, 326, 329
names of plants and animals, 20–22
naphthalene acetic acid (NAA), 89t
narrow-range oils, 88
National Institute for Occupational Safety and Health (NIOSH), 146, 147t, 148
National Organic Program, 14
National Weather Service, 282, 307
natural enemies
　augmented, 6
　imported, 6
　naturally occurring, 6–9, 38t
　pesticide impacts, 75, 111–113, 314
　resources, 281
　and selective pesticide treatments, 297–298
neem, 86t, 113t
nematicides, 73t, 298
nematodes, 48–51, 285
neonicotinoids, 73t, 75
nettleleaf goosefoot (*Chenopodium murale*), 33
Nicotiana spp., 34
nightshade (*Solanum* spp.), 34
NIOSH (National Institute for Occupational Safety and Health), 146, 147t, 148
nitriles, 305t
nitrogen excess, 57t
no observable effect level (NOEL), 70
nonionic surfactants, 91–92
nonpoint source pollution, 107
nonselective pesticides, 111, 290. *See also* broad-spectrum pesticides
nontarget organisms, 69, 111–116, 298, 313–316
nontarget-site resistance, 304
norflurazon, 183t, 305t
notifications of pesticide application, 166
novaluron, 315t
nozzle strainers, 203, 204
nozzles
　calculating output, 251–254
　changing, to change output volume, 264

nozzles (cont.)
   cleaning, 235, 236f, 237–238
   construction and wear, 204–205, 251
   and drift, 106, 182–183, 186, 309
   manufacturers' charts, 251
   spray patterns, 182, 237t, 255–259
   tip codes, 208–209
   types, 205–208
nurse tanks, 214
nutrient deficiencies, 57–58
nutsedges (*Cyperus*), 31
nymphs, 39

O

occasional pests, 3
Occupational Safety and Health Administration (OSHA), 329, 330
ocular exposure. *See* eye exposure to pesticides
Office of Spill Prevention and Response, 342
offsite movement of pesticides
   in air, 104–107 (*See also* drift hazards)
   factors that influence, 100–101, 182–183, 185–186
   groundwater contamination, 102, 103–104, 107, 110, 311–312
   impacts on
      nontarget organisms, 111–116, 298, 313–316
      objects, plants, animals, 105
      sensitive areas, 110–111, 183–184, 313, 331
   leaching, 101, 103–104, 185t
   pollution, 107
   residues, 108–109, 122–123
   runoff, 91, 102, 312
   soil erosion, 102, 115, 312
   surface water contamination, 102, 107, 110, 114–115, 173, 311–312
   in water, 102–104
oil-soluble pesticides, 79, 122, 124, 134
oleander leaf scorch, 63
olive knot, 62
Onopordum acanthium (Scotch thistle), 35
oral exposure to pesticides, 126, 128t, 339–340
oral LD$_{50}$ values, 69f, 71t, 72
organic (OV) cartridges, 146, 147t, 148, 150

Organic Foods Act, 14
Organic Foods Production Act (OFPA), 14
organic matter
   and leaching, 103
   and pesticide breakdown, 109, 293
organic pesticides, 14, 15t
organoarsenicals, 305t
organochlorines, 74–75, 108, 115
organophosphates, 114, 162, 163f
oryzalin, 74t, 183t, 305t
oscillating boom sprayers, 220
OSHA (Occupational Safety and Health Administration), 329, 330
OSHA Title 29 regulations, 147, 148
other ingredients, in pesticides, 77, 205, 326, 330
outdated pesticide products, 176
OV cartridges, 146, 147t, 148, 150
oxyfluorfen, 91, 305t
oxytetracycline, 73t

P

packaging of pesticides, 168–169, 174–175, 177–178
packing shed hazards, 122
paints with impregnates, 85
Panonychus citri (citrus red mite), 7f
paraquat, 74t, 126, 183t, 305t
parasites, parasitoids, 6f, 7, 38t
parasitic wasps, 6f
parathion, 114, 124, 125
particle/dust drift, 81, 107, 311. *See also* drift hazards
particulate respirators, 148–150
parts per million solutions, 273, 274
Paspalum dilatatum (dallisgrass), 31
passive injection devices, 225–227
pathogens, 7, 56–57. *See also specific pathogens,* such as bacteria
peach leaf curl, 60f
pear decline, 65
PEL (permissible exposure limit), 330
pellets, 82, 232, 292t. *See also* granular pesticides
pendimethalin, 183t
penicillin, 85
percentage solutions, 272, 273, 274
percolation. *See* leaching
perennial weeds, 28–29
period thresholds, 288

permethrin, 73t, 76, 113t, 183t, 315t
permissible exposure limit (PEL), 330
permits
   bird control, 53
   DANGER pesticides, 70
   depredation, 53
   vertebrate pest control, 52
persistence of pesticides
   accumulation, 109, 111, 115, 313
   chemical families, 74–75
   defined, 101, 108
   leaching risk, 103
   and pesticide choice, 292–293
   secondary poisoning, 115, 314
personal protective equipment. *See* PPE (personal protective equipment)
PESP (Pesticide Environmental Stewardship Program), 3
Pest Control Aircraft Pilot's Certificate, ix
pest management. *See also* IPM (integrated pest management)
   biological control, 5, 6–9
   BMPs (best management practices), 311–312
   chemical control, 5, 9 (*See also* applying pesticides; pesticide products)
   choosing a pesticide, 289–294
   creating a plan, 3–4
   cultural controls, 5, 11–13, 59
   deciding to use pesticides, 287–289
   goals, 3–4, 280, 287–288
   mechanical and physical controls, 5, 9–11
   other controls, 13–15
   pesticide resistance, 76, 303–306
   predicting problems, 280–281
   treatment thresholds, 16, 288
Pest Management Guidelines, IPM, 23, 288, 289–290
pest resistance. *See* host resistance
pest resurgence, 111
pesticide applicators
   compliance with laws, 320
   liability for accidents, 105, 190, 248, 345
   safety, 162–166, 178, 186, 188
   training, 127, 132–134, 335
   work descriptions, xiii–xivt
Pesticide Environmental Stewardship Program (PESP), 3

pesticide products. *See also* applying pesticides; formulations of pesticides; labels, pesticide; persistence of pesticides
   overview, 68
   active ingredient (a.i.), 77, 330
   characteristics (solubility, adsorption, volatility), 100–101
   chemical families, 73t, 74–76
   choosing a pesticide, 289–294
   cost and efficacy, 293–294
   defined, 9, 68
   disposal, 102, 176, 180, 187–188, 327, 331
   half-life, 70, 331
   inert ingredients, 77, 330
   mixtures, 92–93, 94–95, 292t, 299–303
   modes of action, 74t, 76–77, 298–299
   names, common and brand, 326, 329
   for organic agriculture, 14, 15t
   packaging, 168–169, 174–175, 177–178
   and pest lists, 73t, 74
   registration, 123, 321–323
   regulation, xivt, 70–72, 100, 112
   resistance, 76, 303–306
   shelf life, 175–176
   storing, 173–176, 327, 330, 336
   and temperature, 172, 174
   theft, 344–345
   transporting, 169–172, 173, 331
pesticide resistance, 76, 303–306
pesticide safety training, 132–134
pesticide tanks, 196–197, 225, 235–236, 237–238
pests. *See also* identifying pests
   and application timing, 298, 313–314
   categories
      forest, aquatic, etc., xiii–xivt
      four main groups, 20
      key, occasional, secondary, 3
   defined, 20
   and example pesticides, 73t, 74
   resistant strains, 76, 304–306
   scientific and common names, 20–22
   signs of presence, 24, 52, 57

pests of people, 36t, 42, 48, 281
petroleum oil carriers, 84
petroleum oils, 15t, 73t, 74, 76, 87–88
petroleum solvents, 79, 122, 124
pets, 85, 124
pH of spray solution, 93–94, 293, 302
phenology models, 283t, 287
phenoxy herbicides, 94. *See also* 2,4-D
pheromone traps, 283t, 286–287
pheromones, 15t, 84, 88
phosmet, 93t, 113t
photosynthetic inhibitors, 77
photosystem I, II inhibitors, 74t, 305t
phylloxerans, 45
Physalis spp. (groundcherry), 34
physical control of pests, 5, 9–11
Phytophthora palmivora, 87
phytoplasmas, 59, 65
phytotoxicity, 116, 292t, 303, 313
Picris echioides (bristly oxtongue), 35
pictograms, in SDS, 329f
Pierce's disease, 63
pineapple weed (*Matricaria matricarioides*), 35
piperonyl butoxide, 302
piscicides, 73t
piston pumps, 199t, 201
pitfall traps, 283t
placarding vehicles, 172
Planococcus ficus (vine mealybug), 88f
plant agriculture pest control, xivt
plant-back restrictions, 108, 327
plant breeding, 13
plant bugs. *See* bugs (true bugs, plant bugs, etc.)
plant growth regulators, 88–89
plant hormones, 88–89
plastic nozzles, 205
plastic-coated pesticides, 83
Poa annua (annual bluegrass), 31
pocket gophers, 53
point source pollution, 107
Poison Control System, 339
POISON signal word, 71t, 72
poisoning symptoms, 126–127, 128–129, 330, 335, 336–337
pollinators, 38t, 75, 111–113. *See also* honey bees

pollution
   symptoms, 57t
   types of, 104, 107
polyethylene tanks, 196t, 197
polypropylene tanks, 196t, 197
positive displacement pump injection systems, 227–228
postemergent herbicides, 77
postharvest pesticide use, 123
posting emergency medical notice, 334
posting pesticide warnings, 121, 166–167, 173
potassium salts, 315t
potato family weeds, 34
potato scab, 63
potato spindle tuber, 65
potato traps, 283t
potentiation effect, of mixing pesticides, 301–302
poultry houses, 12–13
poultry pesticide applications, 233–234
powdery mildew (*Uncinula necator*), 61f
power dusters, 230t, 232
PPE (personal protective equipment)
   overview, 134–135
   aprons, 139, 141–142
   cleaning and maintaining, 139, 144–145, 151, 152–155, 340–341
   closed mixing systems, 157–158, 177–178, 214
   coveralls, 140–141, 155
   discomfort of, 156
   disposables, 139–140
   disposal of, 154
   employer responsibilities, 133–134
   engineering controls, 156–158
   EPA code letters, 138
   eyewear, 144–145, 153
   face shields, 145
   fitting, 125, 155–156
      fit checking, 125, 148
      fit testing, 125, 147–148
   footwear, 139, 143, 153, 155
   for fumigants, 134, 142
   gloves, 139, 140f, 142
   headgear, 139, 142
   and heat stress, 127, 141
   limits to protection, 156

PPE (personal protective equipment) (*cont.*)
  pesticide label/SDS information, 326, 327, 330
  residues on, 105, 154–155
  respirators, 146–151
  reusables, 139, 140
  storing, 155
  suits, 139, 141
PPO inhibitors, 305*t*
precautionary statements, 128, 129, 326–327, 329–330
predacides, 73*t*
predators, 7, 38*t*
preemergent herbicides, 77
preharvest intervals, 122, 123
preserved pest specimens, 24
pressure gauges, 211–212
pressure hoses, 213
pressure regulators, 210–211, 214, 237*t*, 238, 264, 276
pressure spray applicators, 84. *See also* aerosol cans
pressure strainers, 203, 204
prevention of pests, 4. *See also* pest management
prickly lettuce (*Latuca serriola*), 35
primary disease infections, 58–59
prometon, 183*t*
prometryn, 75
propanil, 74*t*
propargite, 73*t*, 74*t*
proportional pumps, 228
Proposition 39 warning, 331
Proposition 65, 341
prostrate pigweed (*Amaranthus blitoides*), 33
protectants, repellents, 74*t*, 77, 85
protection of pollinators, 112. *See also* honey bees
psyllids, 45
pubic lice, 43*f*
public health pest control, xiv*t*
public safety, 168
Puccinia recondita (leaf rust), 61*f*
pumps
  choosing, 197–198, 199*t*
  storing, 238
  troubleshooting, 237*t*
  types, 198–201, 228

  used in chemigation, 227–228
puncturevine, 25*f*
purple nutsedge (*Cyperus rotundus*), 31
pyraclostrobin, 76, 183*t*
pyrethrins, 86, 183*t*
pyrethroids, 73*t*, 75–76
pyrethrum, 15*t*, 86, 302
pyriproxyfen, 87*t*

Q
Qualified Applicator Certificate (QAC), ix, xii
Qualified Applicator License (QAL), ix, xii
quarantines, 13–14

R
rabbits, 54–55
rabies, 53
Raphanus raphanistrum (wild radish), 32
raptor mortality, 114
rate controllers, 276
rats, 53, 73*t*, 82, 85–86
recombination of pesticides, 109
recordkeeping, 188–189
recycling containers, 176, 180, 187–188
redroot pigweed (*Amaranthus retroflexus*), 33
refined oils, 88
registration numbers, 322, 326
registration of pesticides, 321–323
registry of certified pest-free material, 14
regulations. *See* laws and regulations
regulatory agencies, 320–321, 322. *See also specific agencies,* such as DPR
regulatory pest control, xiv*t*
repellents, protectants, 74*t*, 85
reporting pesticide accidents, 336, 341, 342–343, 345, 346
reptiles, 53
research pest control, xiv*t*
residential pest control, xiii*t*, 84, 122–123
residue tolerance levels, 70, 123
residues on sprayed surfaces
  on application equipment, 122, 188
  and effective pest control, 108
  in packing sheds, processing plants, 122
  on PPE, 105, 154–155
  reducing hazards of, 109
  at residential sites, 123

  sources of, 78, 81, 87, 292*t*, 303
  spray colorants, 94
  tolerances, 123
resistance to pesticides, 76, 303–306
resources
  compatibility of tank mixes, 303
  in emergencies, 336, 339, 342
  endangered species, 116
  identifying pests, 22–23
  natural enemies, 112, 281
  pest resistance, 306
  pesticide laws and regulations, 321
  pesticides and pest management, xii, 289–290
  phenology models, 287
  transporting pesticides, 171, 172
  weather information, 282, 307–308, 311
respirators
  air-purifying type, 146, 148–150
  air-supplying type, 146, 150–151, 338
  cleaning and maintaining, 151, 152–153
  and enclosed cabs, 156
  and facial hair, 146–147, 150, 151
  filters, 148, 149–150, 156–157
  fit checking, 125, 148
  fit testing, 125, 147–148
  and fumigants, 148, 150
  and medical evaluations, 145, 146
  NIOSH testing and certifying, 146, 147*t*, 148
  OSHA Title 29 regulations, 147, 148
  pesticide label requirements, 146, 147*t*
  restrictions, 138*f*
  reusable/disposable, 139, 140
  when to use, 145, 156
respiratory exposure to pesticides, 125, 128*t*, 338–339. *See also* inhalation hazards
restricted materials permit, 322
restricted-entry intervals, 121, 124, 167, 327
restricted-use pesticides, 100, 321–323, 324–325*f*, 328*f*
retail food stores, 123
reusable PPE, 139
right-of-way pest control, xiii*t*

rimsulfuron, 76
rinsing pesticide containers, 176, 179–180
rinsing pesticide equipment, 235–236, 237–238, 341
river bulrush (*Scirpus fluviatilis*), 31
rodenticides, 73*t*, 82, 85–86
rodents
    handling, 281
    management, 73*t*, 82, 85–86
    types of, 53–55
roller pumps, 199*t*, 200
root knot nematodes, 49*f*, 50*f*. *See also* nematodes
rope wick applicators, 215*t*, 217
rose mosaic virus, 64*f*
rosetting, 64*f*
rosy apple aphid, 45*f*
rotary traps, 283*t*
rotational crop restrictions, 108. *See also* plant-back restrictions
rotenone, 73*t*, 86, 315*t*
routes of pesticide exposure, 69, 70, 124–126
runoff hazards, 91, 102, 312. *See also* pollution; surface water contamination
rushes and sedges, 30–31
Russian knapweed (*Acroptilon repens*), 35
Russian thistle (*Salsola iberica*), 33

S
sabadilla, 15*t*, 86
Safe Drinking Water and Toxic Enforcement Act, 341
safety
    of fieldworkers, 166–167
    of pesticide applicators, 162–166, 178, 186, 188
    of public, 168
    training, 132–134
Safety Data Sheet (SDS), 163, 171, 328–331
safety glasses, 144–145, 153
Salsola iberica (Russian thistle), 33
sampling/sending for identification
    arthropods, 37*t*
    disease pathogens, 56
    nematodes, 50*t*
    weeds, 26*t*
sandbur, 25*f*

sanitation, 11–12
sawflies, 48
scales, 36*t*, 44–45
SCBA (self-contained breathing apparatus), 151
scientific names, 20–21
Scirpus spp. (bulrush), 31
Sclerotinia, 61
Scolytus multistriatus (elm bark beetle), 62
scorpions, 36*t*
Scotch thistle (*Onopordum acanthium*), 35
screens, filters, 203–204, 235, 238
SDS (Safety Data Sheet), 163, 171, 328–331
secondary disease infections, 59
secondary pest outbreaks, 3, 111
secondary poisoning, 115, 314
sedges and rushes, 30–31
seed treatments
    as pest control, xiv*t*
    storing treated seeds, 176
selectivity of pesticides, 290–291, 294–299
self-contained breathing apparatus (SCBA), 151
Senecio vulgaris (common groundsel), 35
sensitive areas for pesticide applications, 110–111, 183–184, 313, 331
service containers, 169, 174–175
servicing sprayers, 236–238, 249
Setaria glauca (yellow foxtail), 31
shelf life of pesticides, 175–176
shepherdspurse (*Capsella bursapastoris*), 32
shipping papers, 171
shrubs, as pests, 73*t*
sight gauges, 196–197, 249
signal transductions, 74*t*
signal words, 70–72, 129, 326, 328*f*, 329
signs *vs.* symptoms of diease, 60–61
silica gel, 87
silverfish, 41
silvicides, 73*t*
simazine, 75, 183*t*
Sisymbrium irio (London rocket), 32
site selection, 11
skin exposure to pesticides

    absorption, 71*t*, 72, 124–125
    first aid, 337–338
    symptoms, 124, 126, 128*t*, 330
skippers, 46
SLN (special local need) registrations, 322–323
slugs, 51–52, 73*t*
slurry, 80
smoking and pesticide exposure, 126
smooth crabgrass (*Digitaria ischaemum*), 31
snails, 51–52, 73*t*
soaps, 15*t*, 89, 315*t*
soda ash, 342
sodium cyanide, 73*t*
sodium hypochlorite, 73*t*
soft rots, 56*t*, 63
soil erosion, and pesticide movement, 102, 115, 312
soil injection applications, 219, 258, 260*f*
soil properties
    and leaching risk, 103–104
    and pesticide breakdown, 109, 293
soil samples, 285
soil tillage, 10–11
Solanum spp. (nightshade), 34
solid stream nozzles, 208, 209*t*
Solidago californica (California goldenrod), 35
solubility of a pesticide, 101
soluble powders, 78–79, 292*t*
Sonchus oleraceus (annual sowthistle), 35
Sorghum halepense (johnsongrass), 31
sorptive dusts, 86–87
sowthistle (*Sonchus oleraceus*), 35
special local need (SLN) registrations, 322–323
species names, 21
speed of travel, during application
    and application rates, 261
    and coverage, 182, 184, 295
    measuring, 250–251
    and pressure changes, 276
Sphaerotheca pannosa, 61*f*
spider mites, 39, 306
spiders, 36*t*, 37*f*, 38, 39
spill kits, 171, 176, 341–342

spills. *See also* accidents
  cleanup, 342, 343–344
  emergency kits, 171, 176, 341–342
  numbers to call, 165, 329, 336
  from packaging, 168–169
  and pollution, 107
  reporting requirements, 336, 341, 342–343
  SDS statement, 330
  during transport, 170–172
spinosad, 315t
spinosyns, 183t
spittlebugs, 45
spores, 60, 61
spot treatments, 296
spray colorants, 94, 293–294
spray drift. *See* drift hazards
spray droplets, 106, 182–183
spray nozzles. *See* nozzles
spray patterns, 182–183, 237t, 255–259
spray shields, 214
sprayers. *See also* application equipment; applying pesticides; calibration
  cleaning, 235–236
  components (*See also* nozzles)
    agitators, 202
    control valves, 212
    electronic controllers, 212
    hoses, couplings, fittings, 212–213, 238
    pressure regulators, gauges, 210–211, 214
    pumps, 197–201
    screens, strainers, 203–204, 235, 238
    spray shields, 214
    tanks, 196–197, 225, 235–236, 237–238
  maintenance, 236–238, 249
  operation of, 294–295
  preventing problems, 235–236
  storing, 237–238
  troubleshooting, 237t
  types of
    air blast hydraulic sprayers, 218t, 220–221, 251–255, 255–259
    backpack sprayers, 215t, 217, 218t, 219, 252, 258
    compressed air sprayers, 215t, 217, 252
    electrostatic sprayers, 218t, 221–222
    hand spray guns, 210, 254f, 295
    high-pressure hydraulic sprayers, 218t, 220, 254–255
    hose-end sprayers, 215t, 216
    low-pressure sprayers, 218t, 219–220, 251–254
    trigger-pump sprayers, 215t, 216
    ultra-low-volume sprayers, 218t, 221
spraying pesticides. *See* applying pesticides; sprayers
spreader-stickers, 90t, 92
spreaders. *See* surfactants
springtails, 40–41
stainless steel nozzles, 205
stainless steel tanks, 196t, 197
standard measure conversion table, 247t
standing water, and pests, 12
statement of use classification, 326
stickers, 90t, 92
sticky traps, 283t, 286
stolen pesticides, 344–345
stomach poisons, 298–299
storing application equipment, 237–238, 239
storing pesticides
  inventory list, 336
  label statement, 327
  safe practices, 173–176
  SDS statement, 330
  security issues, 173, 345
strainers, 203–204
streptomycin, 85
strip spraying, 296
strobilurins, 73t, 76
structure of soils, and leaching, 103
strychnine, 73t, 86
sucking lice, 43
suction hoses, 213
suction strainers, 203
suits, PPE, 139, 141
sulfometuron methyl, 76
sulfonylureas, 73t, 76
sulfosulfuron, 183t
sulfur, 15t, 74t, 315t
summer annuals (weeds), 28
summer oils, 88
sunburn, 57, 58
sunflower (*Helianthus annuus*), 35
sunscald, 57, 58
superior oils, 88
supplemental labels, 323
supplied air respirators, 146, 151, 338
suppression of pests, 4
supreme oils, 88
surface tension, 91
surface water contamination, 102, 107, 110, 114–115, 173, 311–312
surface-active ingredients, 77
surfactants, 90t, 91–92
surge chambers, 214
swallowed pesticides, 126, 128t, 339–340
swath width, measuring, 254f, 255–258, 259f, 260f, 266
sweep net monitoring, 283t, 286
symptoms of pesticide exposure, 126–127, 128t, 129, 330, 337
symptoms *vs.* signs of disease, 60–61
synergism effect, of mixing pesticides, 301–302
synergists, 76
synthetic auxins, 74t, 305t
synthetic pheromones, 88
system controllers, 276
systemic pesticides, 74t, 76, 82, 85, 91

T

tall morningglory (*Ipomoea purpurea*), 34
tank capacity, measuring, 249
tank mixes, 92–93, 94–95, 292t, 299–303
tanks, 196–197, 225, 235–236, 237–238
Taphrina spores, 60f
Taraxacum officinale (dandelion), 25f, 35
target-site resistance, 304
TC numbers, 146, 147t, 148, 149, 150, 151
tebuthiuron, 73t
telegraphplant (*Heterotheca grandiflora*), 35
temperature
  and pesticide transport, storage, 172, 174
  recording, 307–308
temperature inversions, 106, 181–182, 310

termites, 36t, 42–43, 292
tests and examinations, ix–xii
texture of soils
   and herbicide breakdown, 109
   and leaching, 103
thermoplastic tanks, 196t, 197
thiamethoxam, 315t
thickeners, 90t, 94
thiocarbamates, 305t
thiram, 166
thistle, 35
threshold limit value (TLV), 70
thrips, 36t, 43–44, 283t
ticks, 36t, 37f, 38, 40
timed counts, 283t
timing of applications, 298, 308–309, 312, 314
tip codes of nozzles, 208–209
Title 29 regulations, 147, 148
TLV (threshold limit value), 70
tobacco budworm, 24f
tolerance levels, residues, 70, 123
tomato fruitworm, 21f, 24f
tomatoes, 62–63
toxaphene, 115
toxicity of pesticides, 315t. *See also* human exposure to pesticides; persistence of pesticides
   to bees, 75, 86t, 111–113, 292, 314–315
   Categories I to IV, 70–72
   chemical families, 74–75
   combinations of pesticides, 95, 166, 301–303
   in environment, 100–101, 110–116 (*See also* environmental hazards; offsite movement of pesticides)
   LC_{50} (lethal concentration) values, 69–70, 71t
   LD_{50} (lethal dose) values, 69–72
   no observable effect level (NOEL), 70
   phytotoxicity, 116, 292t, 303, 313
   plant and animal testing, 69–70
   plant symptoms, 57t, 58
   residue tolerance levels, 70, 94, 123
   SDS statement, 330
   signal words, 70–72, 129, 326, 328f, 329
   threshold limit value (TLV), 70

toxicity tables, 112
tracking powders, 82, 287
tractor cabs, 156–157
training, 127, 132–134, 335
transgenic plants, 13
transporting pesticides, 169–172, 173, 331
trap boards, 283t
trapping pests, 10
traps, for pest monitoring, 283t
travel speed, during application, 182, 184, 250–251, 261, 276, 295
treated seeds, xivt, 176
treatment thresholds, 16, 288
tree tobacco (*Nicotiana glauca*), 34
treehoppers, 45
trees, as pests, 73t
triallate, 305t
triazines, 73t, 75
triazoles, 305t
triclopyr, 183t
trifloxystrobin, 76, 183t
trigger pump sprayers, 215t, 216
triple-rinsing pesticide containers, 176, 179–180
trucks, and pesticide transport, 170, 171–172, 331
true bugs, 36t, 44
tumble pigweed (*Amaranthus albus*), 33
tungsten carbide nozzles, 205
twig borers, 36t

U
U.S. Coast Guard, 342
U.S. Department of Transportation (DOT), 168, 171, 172
U.S. Environmental Protection Agency (EPA)
   CCD information, 112
   Endangered Species Protection Program, 115–116
   pesticide labels, 323
   pesticide registration numbers, 326
   pesticide registrations, 100, 321–322
   pesticide residue tolerances, 70, 123
   PPE code letters, 138
   respirator requirements, 146–147
   toxicity categories, 129
UC Cooperative Extension, xii, 134
UC IPM California Weather Database, 308

ultra-low-volume concentrates, 80, 297
ultra-low-volume sprayers, 218t, 221
ultraviolet inhibitors, 92
Uncinula necator (powdery mildew), 61f
unloaders, 211
ureas, 305t
USDA National Organic Program, 14, 128t

V
vapor drift, 106, 310–311. *See also* drift hazards
variegated cutworm, 24f
vectors, 51, 55, 59, 64, 65
vegetable oils, 15t
vehicle manifests, 171
velvetleaf (*Abutilon theophrasti*), 32
Venice mallow (*Hibiscus trionum*), 32
venturi injection systems, 226–227
Venturia inaequalis, 60f
vertebrate pests
   amphibians and reptiles, 53
   birds, 53
   fish, 52–53
   habitat modification, 13
   mammals, 53–55
   monitoring, 287
   trapping, 10
vine mealybug (*Planococcus ficus*), 88f
viroids, 59, 65
virucides, 73t
viruses, 59, 64–65
visual inspection of plants, 282, 283t
VOC (volatile organic compound) emissions, 311
volatile pesticides, 101, 106, 310–311

W
walnut bacterial disease, 62f
warfarin, 86
WARNING pesticides, 70–72, 95, 136. *See also* signal words
wash water disposal, 237
wasps, 36t, 38t, 48
waste pesticide products, 176, 179, 187
water damage to pesticides, 174
water deficiency/excess, 57–58
water pH, 93–94, 302
Water Quality Control Boards, 187–188, 342

water supplies, drinking, 102, 103, 110
water tables, 104
water treatment plants, 102
water-dispersible granules, 78, 292t
water-sensitive cards, 316
water-soluble bags or packets, 78, 83, 178
water-soluble concentrates or solutions, 79, 292t, 293
waterproof clothing, as PPE, 137
weather effects
    abiotic disorders, 57t, 58
    and development of pests, 58, 281–282
    drift management, 106, 181–182, 185–186, 307–308
    pesticide breakdown, efficacy, 109, 293, 294
    and safe applications, 181–182
weather stations, 282, 307–308, 311
weed control. *See also* herbicides
    ground covers as, 8
    mowing, 11
    and natural enemies, 8, 38t
Weed Science Society of America (WSSA), 305t
weeds. *See also specific weeds*
    overview, 24–25
    classification, 27, 28–29
    common pest weeds, 30–35
    development, life cycles, 27–28
    how they are pests, 25–26
    identifying, 26–30
    monitoring, 282, 284f, 285
    reproduction, dispersal, 25, 29f, 30
    sampling/sending for identification, 26t
    seeds, 25, 30
weevils, 45–46
wells, contamination, 104, 312
western flower thrips, 43f
western malarial mosquito, 47f
western yellowstriped armyworm, 24f
western-X disease, 65
wettable powders, 78, 292t
wetting agents. *See* surfactants
whiteflies, 44–45
wick applicators, 215t, 217
wild oat (*Avena fatua*), 31
wild radish (*Raphanus raphanistrum*), 32
wildlife, 114–115, 314
wilts, 62
wind injury, 58, 307
wind, and drift hazard, 106, 186, 307

winter annuals (weeds), 28
wood finishes with impregnates, 85
woody shrubs, as pests, 73t
work clothing. *See* PPE (personal protective equipment)
Worker Protection Standard (WPS), 133–134, 135, 320, 322, 327
worker training, 132–134, 335
wounds, and disease spread, 59, 64, 65
WPS. *See* Worker Protection Standard
WSSA (Weed Science Society of America), 305t

X

Xanthium strumarium (common cocklebur), 35
Xanthomonas vesicatoria, 62f
Xylella fastidiosa, 63

Y

yellow bud mosaic, 64f
yellow foxtail (*Setaria glauca*), 31
yellow nutsedge (*Cyperus esculentus*), 31
yellow starthistle (*Centaurea solstitialis*), 8f, 34f, 35
yellowjacket, 48f. *See also* wasps

Z

zeta-cypermethrin, 113t, 315t
zinc phosphide, 73t